Immune Deficiency and Cancer

Epstein-Barr Virus and Lymphoproliferative Malignancies

Immune Deficiency and Cancer

Epstein-Barr Virus and Lymphoproliferative Malignancies

Edited by
David T. Purtilo

University of Nebraska Medical Center
Omaha, Nebraska

Plenum Medical Book Company • New York and London

Library of Congress Cataloging in Publication Data

Main entry under title:

Immune deficiency and cancer.

Includes bibliographical references and index.
1. Lymphoproliferative disorders—Etiology. 2. Epstein–Barr virus. 3. Immunological deficiency syndromes—Complications and sequelae. 4. Viral carcinogenesis. 5. Cancer—Immunological aspects. I. Purtilo, David T., 1939-   . II. Title. (DNLM: 1. Epstein–Barr virus—Pathogenicity—Congresses. 2. Lymphoproliferative disorders—Etiology—Congresses. WH 700 S9895i 1982)
RC646.2.I45   1984   616.99′449   84-4733

ISBN-13: 978-1-4684-4762-0   e-ISBN-13: 978-1-4684-4760-6
DOI: 10.1007/978-1-4684-4760-6

This book is dedicated to the memory of
Colin, Keith, and James,
and to
a healthy life for Billy, Nathan, and Kenny.

PREFACE

The discoveries of Burkitt, Epstein, and Henle have laid the
foundation for continuing generation of information regarding the
mechanisms of induction of diseases by Epstein-Barr virus. The
discovery of the virus two decades ago resulted from clinical and
basic science collaborative studies on Burkitt lymphoma. Subsequently, nasopharyngeal carcinoma and infectious mononucleosis
have been linked etiologically with the virus. During the first
decade of research following the discovery of the virus, the
mechanisms for the induction of BL, NPC, and IM were sought. At
that time one prevailing view was that individual oncogenic
strains of EBV were responsible for the different disorders.
Paralleling the development of immunology in the 1970's was the
accrual of knowledge about immunological events occurring during
IM. These studies suggest that immune defense mechanisms determine the outcome of this viral infection rather than different
viral strains.

During the early 1970's, Starzl and Penn and Gatti and Good
had noted an increased frequency of malignancy in renal allograft
recipients and children with primary immune deficiency disorders,
respectively. These observations provoked investigators to
restudy the role of immune surveillance against malignancy. At
that time immune surveillance was thought to occur against
tumor-specific antigens; thereby neoplasms were eliminated.
Breakdown of immune surveillance was reasoned to be responsible
for the development of a wide variety of malignancies. However,
after arduous research on experimental models and patients, it
appears that the surveillance is relevant chiefly to virally
induced malignancies in immune deficient individuals. Noteworthy,
is the restricted appearance of only a few histologic types of
malignancy in immune deficient patients. In the child with
inherited immune deficiency, the predominant malignancy is
malignant lymphoma of the B cell type. In children with primary
immune deficiency, more than half of the cases of malignancy are
malignant lymphomas. Similarly, malignancies in renal allograft
patients are predominantly virally linked B cell lymphomas.
Cutaneous squamous cell carcinomas, Kaposi's sarcoma, and uterine

cervical carcinoma which are prevalent could be caused by ubiquitous viruses.

In 1975 we described the X-linked recessive progressive combined variable immunodeficiency disorder (Duncan's disease) which
is manifested as fatal infectious mononucleosis, aplastic anemia,
agammaglobulinemia, or malignant lymphoma. X-linked lymphoproliferative syndrome (XLP) has served as a model for studying viral-
induced diseases governed by immune responses. In a group of 100
patients with XLP approximately two-thirds have developed fatal
infectious mononucleosis, 35% malignant B cell lymphoma, 19% a- or
hypo-gammaglobulinemia, and 17% aplastic anemia. EBV genome has
been identified in all of the surgical biopsy and autopsy tissues
studied. Collaborative studies have revealed immune defects in
individuals prior to infection by EBV which become accentuated
following infection by the virus.

The editor had reasoned that immune deficiency in transplant
patients and other individuals with primary immune deficiency may
allow EBV to evoke various clinical disorders. In 1981, he and
George Klein asked colleagues throughout Europe and North America
to contribute to a volume of Cancer Research. In the November
issue the investigators documented that EBV-induced fatal
lymphoproliferative diseases occurred in immune deficient
allograft recipients and children with primary immune deficiency
disorders. They also noted that often the malignant lymphomas
were polyclonal B cell proliferative disorders simulating
malignant lymphoma. In 1979 George Klein had hypothesized that
polyclonal B cell proliferation in African children at risk for
Burkitt lymphoma could convert to monoclonal malignancy vis-a-vis
an 8;14 reciprocal translocation resulting in a 14q+ aberration.
The Manolovs had described in 1971 this specific chromosomal
alteration. This seminal study has provided an opportunity to
investigate the role of immunoglobulin gene (heavy and light
chains) and oncogene (c-myc and B-lym) rearrangements in the
induction of Burkitt lymphomas.

In this volume we update recent studies on EBV and the role
of immune deficiency in the induction of lymphoproliferative
diseases. On September 22-23, 1982 a symposium was held in Omaha,
Nebraska. Many of the chapters contained herein were the outgrowth of the presentations and discussions at the meeting. I
have asked several investigators to prepare manuscripts for
inclusion in this book. The editor takes responsibility for the
errors introduced in editing these manuscripts.

The continuing elaboration of a very wide spectrum of
diseases provoked by Epstein-Barr virus in individuals with
various types of immunological disorders has been surprising to
many. Epstein-Barr virus was becoming the forgotten virus in

cancer research. Many had assumed that the road blocks to proving that EBV was oncogenic in Burkitt's lymphoma and nasopharyngeal carcinoma would not be overcome. Explosive growth knowledge in molecular virology, immunopathology, cytogenetics, and immunopharmacology has opened new vistas to mechanisms whereby this virus induces many diseases in human beings. We can now diagnose EBV infection accurately and quantitate immunological deficiencies. Improved diagnosis and the advent of new drugs to treat the patients and measures to prevent immune deficiency offer bright prospects for obviating EBV-induced diseases.

The contributors are thanked for their creative product. This book goes beyond reportage by development of testable hypotheses. The research reported here from my laboratory was supported by contributions to the Lymphoproliferative Research Fund and PHHS grant number 30196, awarded by the National Cancer Institute, DHHS, the American Cancer Society RD161, and the Nebraska Department of Health LB506. The expert photographic work of Mr. James Smith and Sergio Diaz is appreciated. Karen Spiegel, who typed the manuscript under the guidance of Ms. Leslie Schmidt, is acknowledged with gratitude. My wife, Ruth Purtilo, Ph.D., is thanked for her consultation and support in my investigation of patients with immune deficiency.

David T. Purtilo, M.D.

Professor and Chairman
Department of Pathology and Laboratory Medicine,
Professor of Pediatrics, and Professor in
Eppley Institute for Research in Cancer and Allied Diseases
University of Nebraska Medical Center
Omaha, Nebraska

PREFACE

CONTENTS

MODEL SYSTEMS FOR EPSTEIN-BARR VIRUS-TARGET CELL INTERACTION

ACQUIRED IMMUNE DEFICIENCY AND LYMPHOPROLIFERATIVE DISORDERS

IMMUNE DEFICIENCY, EPSTEIN-BARR VIRUS (EBV) AND LYMPHOPROLIFERATIVE DISORDERS

David T. Purtilo

Pathology & Laboratory Medicine
University of Nebraska Medical Center
Omaha, Nebraska 68105

INTRODUCTION

This book presents data regarding mechanisms of immunity against and the resulting spectrum of Epstein-Barr virus (EBV) diseases which can ensue depending on the type and degree of immune deficiency occurring in an individual patient. Focus is on lymphoproliferative diseases, especially opportunistic malignant B cell lymphomas, occurring in predisposed immune deficient individuals. However, a growing spectrum of diseases have been recently associated with EBV (1). Empirical evidence that immune deficiency is important in lymphomagenesis stems from reports of lymphomas in renal transplant recipients and in children with inherited immunodeficiency (2).

The concept of immune surveillance (3) considers that the immune system recognizes and responds to tumor-specific antigens of a newly emerging clone of transformed malignant cells and thus eliminates the clone of cells. Regrettably, investigators working in the decade of the 1970's failed to critically evaluate the types of cancers occurring in the immune deficient individuals. They generalized the concept of immune surveillance to include all types of cancer. Vigorous efforts to find tumor-specific antigens and to use immunotherapy in a variety of cancers have been unsuccessful.

Careful scrutiny of the types of cancers seen in individuals with acquired immune deficiencies, such as those in the renal transplant recipients (4) or male homosexuals with the acquired immune deficiency syndrome (AIDS) (5) reveals predisposition to squamous cell carcinoma, Kaposi's sarcoma, and malignant B cell

1

lymphomas. Importantly, all of these cancers could be induced
potentially by specific ubiquitous viruses. For example, Kaposi's
sarcoma has been linked to cytomegalovirus (6), malignant B cell
lymphomas to EBV (7), squamous cell carcinoma to papilloma virus
(8), and uterine cervical carcinoma in transplant recipients and
other women to herpes hominus (9).

Immune surveillance probably provides recognition of viral
antigens and provokes cytotoxic cells to eliminate virally
infected cells (7). Thus, acquired or inherited immunodeficiency
may allow certain ubiquitous viruses to induce unrestrained
proliferation and/or the immune response afflicts genetic damage
in the target cell. Our research efforts can be rationally guided
by the data gained from the empirical observations of the types of
cancers in immune deficient patients (2). Viruses as a potential
cause of cancer may be optimally investigated in high risk
patients with immune deficiency.

The development of testable hypotheses to study high risk
immune deficient patient for etiologic factors in lymphomagenesis
provides an opportunity to gather information to identify the
multi-step events leading to specific cancers and related benign
disorders. A spectrum of disorders can be anticipated in immune
deficient patients (1). The clinical expression probably depends
on whether the immune deficiency is primary or secondary with
respect to the timing of the viral infection. For example, EBV
infection in males with the X-linked lymphoproliferative syndrome
(XLP) can lead to a variety of phenotypes or diseases, i.e.,
aproliferative phenotypes consisting of agranulocytosis, aplastic
anemia, red cell aplasia, or acquired agammaglobulinemia or
proliferative phenotypes of chronic or fatal infectious mononucleosis, pseudolymphoma, or various B cell malignant lymphomas
(10). Moreover, young renal transplant recipients tend to rapidly
develop fatal infectious mononucleosis following primary EBV
infection whereas older patients are apt to slowly progress to
malignant lymphoma due to reactivation of virus.

Acquired immune deficiency is occurring at an ever increasing
frequency. The use of immunosuppressive cytotoxic drugs, irradiation, and allo-transplantation of organs including heart, kidney,
bone marrow, thymus, etc. have resulted in the emergence of
malignant lymphoproliferative diseases in many patients (11,12).
In addition, unusual life-styles such as occurring in a subset of
male homosexuals (5), who are profoundly promiscuous, has resulted
in AIDS. As noted earlier, these individuals acquire
immunoregulatory-immunodeficiency defects and develop malignancies
and opportunistic infections comparable to renal transplant
recipients. Urgently, we must identify individuals at high risk
for developing viral-induced malignancies and associated diseases.
Efforts to quantitate and identify the specific immune defects

responsible for vulnerability to viral agents such as EBV are
underway. Some of the progress resulting from these studies is
contained in this book.

Throughout the book, the recurrent theme is that defective
immune responses to the virus can lead to uncontrolled lymphoproliferative diseases. The information is grouped into six
sections: I Classical EBV-Associated Disorders; II Inherited
Immunodeficiency Syndromes and Lymphomagenesis; III Model Systems
for Investigating EBV and Host or Target Cell Interactions; IV
Acquired Immunodeficiency Disorders; V Genetic Predisposition to
Lymphomagenesis; and VI Prevention and Treatment of Immune Deficient Individuals.

Epstein-Barr Virus

Denis Burkitt discovered the tumor bearing his name (13) and
collaboration with Epstein, Achong and Barr resulted in the identification of this herpesvirus (14). Viral particles could not be
observed in portions of tumor examined directly. However, after
six years of painstaking study, viral particles were observed in
the first electron micrograph examined of tumor which had been
grown in tissue cultures. I think that the host immune response

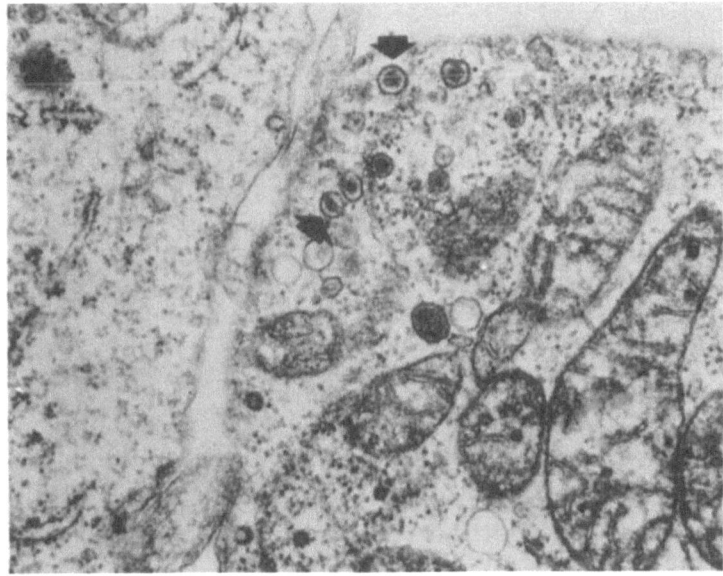

Fig. 1. Electron micrograph depicting Epstein-Barr virus particles X100,000.

had likely prevented the virus from undergoing complete replication in vivo. Establishment of the tumor in culture removed the
immune surveillance effectors and allowed the virus to progress
through its cycle to form particles. This herpesvirus (Figure 1)
is a member of the gamma herpesviruses (15). Other members of the
herpesviruses include varicella-zoster, cytomegalovirus, and
herpes hominus.

    The virus have tropism for B cells bearing viral receptors.
On infecting the cell, EB nuclear-associated antigen (EBNA)
appears. Two pathways can be pursued by the virus: a proliferative (transforming) pathway or a lytic pathway potentially
productive of viral particles may appear. The latter is associated with the appearance of early antigen (EA) and viral capsid
antigen (VCA) (16). Once infected by EBV an individual harbors
the virus in latency life-long. In acquired immune deficiency,
depending on the type and degree, EBV becomes more or less active
and capable of inducing life-threatening disease.

    Section III considers the molecular virology of EBV in
detail. The molecular genetics of EBV genome is being investigated vigorously. Individuals aim to identify transforming
portions of the virus (Figure 2). Latently infected lymphocytes
usually contain multiple copies of the viral genome. Most of the
intracellular viral DNA is in the form of episomal closed circles
(17). Viral DNA is replicated concomitantly with cell DNA by
cellular enzymes. Some EBV DNA may integrate into cell DNA.
Expression of the viral genome is tightly regulated in latently
infected growing transformed cells. Three regions of EBV genome
express RNAs. Two intranuclear and one surface antigen have been
detected. The ability of EBV and cell genomes to exist and function together had led Kieff and colleagues (18) to investigate
whether EBV DNA has regions that are similar to human cellular
DNA. The cellular DNA has specific homology to the third internal
repeat (IR3) in EBV DNA. Binding of IR3 occurs chiefly to

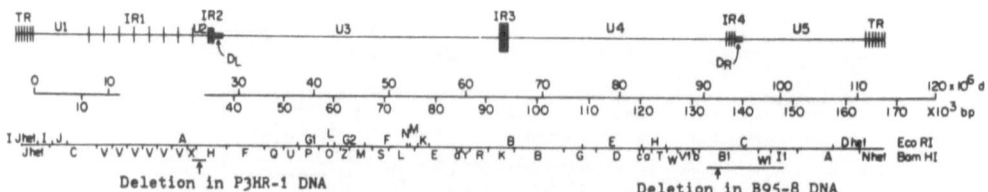

Fig. 2. Physical map of EBV DNA. Abbreviations: TR - terminal
         repeat and IR3 - internal repeat. (With permission of:
         Heller, M., Henderson, A., and Kieff, E. Repeat array in
         Epstein-Barr virus DNA is related to cell DNA sequences
         interspersed on human chromosomes. Proc. Natl. Acad.
         Sci. USA, 79:5916-5920, 1982.)

chromosomes 2, 8, 14, and 22. These chromosomes often undergo cytogenetic rearrangements in Burkitt lymphomas. The cytogenetic alterations in malignant lymphomas and their possible significance is evaluated in Chapter 22. The chromosomes involved in the transposition in Burkitt lymphoma cells contain genetic loci coding for immunoglobulins and oncogenes.

Immune Defense against EBV

EBV and Homo sapiens have harmoniously lived together for eons. The virus is thought to have evolved from a common herpesvirus progenitor approximately 50 million years ago (19). Concurrently, the immune system of human beings has genetically evolved multiple immune effectors to provide failsafe defense against this virus. However, this watertight surveillance mechanism can be broken due to inherited or acquired immune deficiency. Figure 3 summarizes various immune effectors which have been

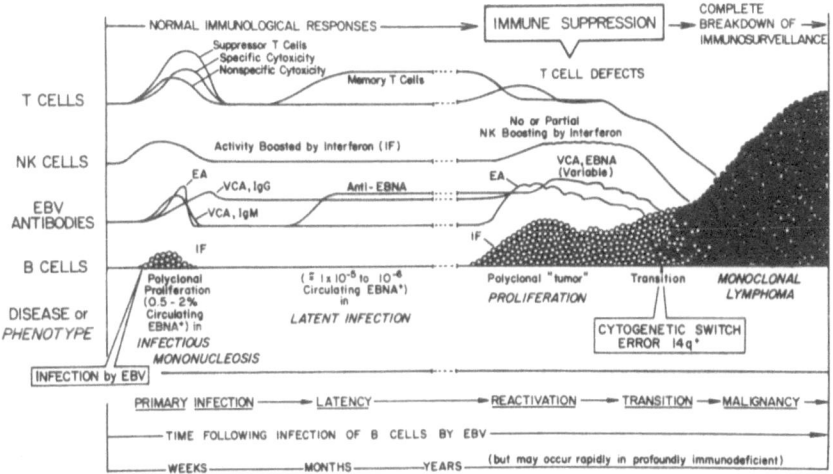

Fig. 3. Hypothesis summarizing cellular and humoral Epstein-Barr virus (EBV) responses. Normal immune responses to primary infection are shown at the left. Reactivation of Epstein-Barr virus and resumption of B-cell proliferation in the immune suppressed renal transplant recipient is shown at right. EA, early antigen; VCA, viral capsid antigen; EBNA, EB nuclear-associated antigen; NK, natural killer cells. (From: Purtilo, D.T. Immune deficiency predisposing to Epstein-Barr virus-induced lymphoproliferative diseases: The X-linked lymphoproliferative syndrome as a model. In: G. Klein and S. Weinhouse (eds.), Advances in Cancer Research. Vol. 34, pp. 279-307, 1981. Published with the permission of Academic Press.)

identified in vitro which may defend against the virus. The right
side of the diagram displays events that may occur following
primary infection in individuals with inherited immune deficiency.
The diagram also illustrates how acquired immune deficiency, as in
a transplant recipient, may lead to defective defense against
primary infection or allow reactivation of EBV. The conversion
from polyclonal B cell proliferation to monoclonal proliferation
is postulated to occur vis-a-vis a specific cytogenetic event.
For example, a reciprocal 8;14 translocation could endow a cell
with capacities to escape regulatory defenses. In Chapter 7
the immunoregulatory defects against EBV in patients with XLP are
discussed. XLP serves as a model for evaluating the role of EBV
in primary immunodeficiency and lymphomagenesis. In Chapter 16
and 17 the consequences of the immune deficiency in cardiac and
renal transplant recipients are considered.

Prospectus on Immunodeficiency and EBV-induced Malignancies

The mechanisms of immune deficiency and the pathogenesis of
diseases associated with EBV form the central theme of this
monograph. In Section I classical EBV-associated disorders
including infectious mononucleosis (IM), nasopharyngeal carcinoma
(NPC), and Burkitt's lymphoma (BL) are evaluated with regards to
immune deficiency. Section II considers the X-linked lymphoproliferative syndrome and Chediak-Higashi disease. Children with
these disorders often die of lymphoproliferative disorders which
are likely evoked by EBV. Model systems for investigating
EBV-target cell interaction comprise Section III Cellular and
molecular biological aspects of the virus are considered. In rac-
addition, the immunobiology of herpesvirus-induced lymphoproliferative diseases in cotton-topped marmosets, which are immune
deficient, are described. A new experimental model which
evaluates the role of immune deficiency to EBV is introduced in a
chapter on murine infection by the virus.

Section IV pertains to acquired immunodeficiency and lymphoproliferative diseases. Data from the Cincinnati Allograft
Transplant Cancer Registry data is summarized through September,
1982. Specific chapters on lymphoproliferative diseases in
cardiac and renal transplant recipients are included. An alarming
prevalence of EBV carrying lymphomas has been documented in renal,
cardiac, and thymic epithelial transplant patients. Two perspectives on AIDS and the role of EBV in lymphomagenesis and lymphadenomegaly in male homosexuals conclude this section.

Genetic factors in lymphomagenesis are summarized in Section
V. Mendelian predisposition to lymphomagenesis and the specific
cytogenetic or chromosomal rearrangements found in malignant
lymphomas are considered. Investigation of oncogenes (20) and

cytogenetic transpositions in oncogenesis, which are at the cutting edge of research, are presented in context of chromosomal damage. Thus the initiating or promoting effects of EBV in lymphomagenesis are considered as part of a multi-step process which might end in a final cytogenetic step (Figure 2). Klein (19) has postulated that in African BL 3 steps occur: 1) EBV initiates B cell proliferation; 2) malaria acts as a mitogenic factor increasing the proliferating pool of B cells; and 3) a specific chromosomal aberration (i.e., 8;14 translocation) is the final step which endows the cell with a capacity to outstrip host defenses. The identification of immunoglobulin loci at the breakpoints on chromosomes 2, 22, and 14 and the localization of human c-oncogene at the breakpoint of chromosome 8 has been provocative. Rowley (21) has proposed that the breakage, transposition, and juxtaposition of the active immunoglobulin genetic loci with oncogene at the breakpoint on 8 activates oncogene and prompts the cell to proliferate.

The final section of this book concerns efforts to prevent and treat individuals with immune deficiency. Our efforts to provide genetic counseling for families with XLP and related disorders are of obvious importance (22). Identification of individuals at risk for inherited immunodeficiency is possible by pedigree analysis and inoculation with ØX174. Males with XLP have a defect in helper or memory T cells which prevents them from switching from IgM to IgG antibodies on secondary challenge with ØX174 (23). Thus high risk males can be monitored for EBV infection and definitively treated with bone marrow transplantation. Moreover, their mothers often show paradoxically high and active EBV antibody titers (24-26). This aids also in the diagnosis of XLP and provides data for genetic counseling.

Immune modulators and anti-viral agents such as interferon are described in treating herpesvirus infections in Chapter 23. In addition, consideration of the antiviral drug, Acyclovir®, is provided in the chapter by Hanto on renal transplant recipients.

Allogeneic bone marrow transplantation has proven successful in immunologically reconstituting individuals with immune deficiency. None of the patients who have received bone marrow transplantation have developed a malignant lymphoma. This treatment thus may prevent lymphomas and cancers in immune deficient children.

The future holds a bright promise for providing definitive genetic correction of inherited immune deficiency. We are presently collaborating with a group in Salt Lake City to identify the XLP locus. Other investigators are pursuing similar projects to isolate genes responsible for other immune deficiencies. Gene transplantation may, in the future, immunologically reconstitute these individuals.

Identification of risk factors and mechanisms responsible for impairing immune surveillance in AIDS patients may provide rationale for developing strategies for intervention (5). Similarly, the development and adaptation of immunosuppressive regimes for retaining immune surveillance against viral infection while providing sufficient immune suppression to prevent rejection of the allograft is being sought.

The comprehensive approach to the investigation of the immune deficient patient described in this text ought to provide both practical and theoretical guides to prevention and rational strategies for curing individuals with life-threatening Epstein-Barr virus infections and related disorders.

REFERENCES

1.   Editorial. New clinical manifestations of Epstein-Barr
           virus infection. Lancet, ii:1253, 1982.
2.   Purtilo, D.T. and Klein, G. Introduction to Epstein-Barr
           virus and lymphoproliferative diseases in immunodeficient
           individuals. Cancer Res., 41:4209, 1981.
3.   Schwartz, R.S. Epstein-Barr virus-oncogen or mitogen? N.
           Engl. J. Med., 2:1307, 1980.
4.   Penn, I. Allograft Transplant Cancer Registry. In: D.T.
           Purtilo (ed.), Immune Deficiency and Cancer: Epstein-
           Barr Virus and Lymphoproliferative Malignancies. New
           York: Plenum Press, 1983.
5.   Sonnabend, J.A., Witkin, S.S., and Purtilo, D.T. The
           syndrome of acquired immunodeficiency. An explanation
           for its occurrence among homosexual men. In: D.T.
           Purtilo (ed.), Immune Deficiency and Cancer: Epstein-
           Barr Virus and Lymphoproliferative Malignancies. New
           York: Plenum Press, 1983.
6.   Drew, M.L., Mintz, L. Miner, R.C., Sands, M., and Ketterer,
           B. Cytomegalovirus and Kaposi's sarcoma in young homo-
           sexual men. Lancet, 1:125, 1982.
7.   Purtilo, D.T. Epstein-Barr virus-induced oncogenesis in
           immune deficient individuals. Lancet, 1:300, 1980.
8.   Howley, P.M. The human papillomaviruses. Arch. Path. Lab.
           Med., 106:429, 1982.
9.   Purtilo, D.T. Viruses, tumors, and immune deficiency.
           Lancet, 1:684, 1982.
10.   Purtilo, D.T., Sakamoto, K., Barnabei, V., Seeley, J.,
           Bechtold, T., Rogers, G., Yetz, J., and Harada, S.
           Epstein-Barr virus-induced diseases in males with the X-
           linked lymphoproliferative syndrome (XLP). Am. J. Med.,
           73:49, 1982.
11.   Hanto, D.W., Frizzera, G., Purtilo, D.T., Sakamoto, K.,

Sullivan, J.L., Saemundsen, A.K., Klein, G., Simmons, R.L., and Najarian, J.S. Clinical spectrum of lymphoproliferative disorders in renal transplant recipients and evidence for the role of Epstein-Barr virus. Cancer Res., 41:4253, 1981.

12.   Bieber, C.P., Heberling, R.L., Jamieson, S.W., Oyer, P.E., Cleary, M., Warnke, R., Saemundsen, A., Klein, G., Henle, W., and Stinson, E.B. Lymphoma in cardiac transplant recipients. Association with the use of cyclosporin A, prednisone and antithymocyte globulin (ATG). In: D.T. Purtilo (ed.), Immune Deficiency and Cancer: Epstein-Barr Virus and Lymphoproliferative Malignancies. New York: Plenum Press, 1983.

13.   Burkitt, D.P. A sarcoma involving the jaws in African children. Br. J. Surg., 46:218, 1958.

14.   Epstein, M.A., Achong, B.G., and Barr, Y.M. Virus particles in cultured lymphoblasts from Burkitt's lymphoma. Lancet, 1:702, 1964.

15.   R.E.F. Matthews (ed.) Classification and Nomenclature of Viruses. New York: Karger, 1982.

16.   Henle, W., Henle, G., and Lennette, E.L. The Epstein-Barr virus. Sci. Am., 241:48, 1979.

17.   Lindahl, T., Adams, A., Bjursell, G., Bornkamm, S.W., Kaschka-Dietrich, E., and Jehn, U. J. Mol. Biol., 102:511, 1976.

18.   Heller, M., Henderson, A., and Kieff, E. Repeat array in Epstein-Barr virus DNA is related to cell DNA sequences interspersed on human chromosomes. Proc. Natl. Acad. Sci. USA, 79:5916, 1982

19.   Klein, G. Immune and non-immune control of neoplastic development: contrasting effects of host and tumor evolution. Cancer, 45:2486, 1980.

20.   Dalla-Favera, R., Bregni, M., Erikson, J., Patterson, D., Gallo, R.C., and Croce, C.M. Human c-myc onc gene is located on the region of chromosome 8 that is translocated in Burkitt lymphoma cells. Proc. Natl. Acad. Sci. USA, 79:7824, 1982.

21.   Rowley, J.D. Identification of the constant chromosome regions involved in human hematologic malignant disease. Science, 216:749, 1982.

22.   Hamilton, J.K., Pacquin, L.A., Sullivan, J.L., Maurer, H.S., Cruzi, P.G., Provisor, A.J., Steuber, C.P., Hawkins, E., Yawn, D., Cornet, J., Clausen, K., Finkelstein, G.Z., Landing, B., Grunnet, M., and Purtilo, D.T. X-linked Lymphoproliferative Syndrome Registry Report. J. Pedi., 96:669, 1980.

23.   Ochs, H.D., Sullivan, J.L., Wedgewood, R.J., Seeley, J.K., Sakamoto, K., and Purtilo, D.T. X-linked lymphoproliferative syndrome: abnormal antibody responses to bacteriophage ØX174. In: R. Wedgwood and F. Rosen

(eds.), Primary Immunodeficiency Diseases.   New York:
Alan R. Liss, 1983.

24.   Sakamoto, K., Seeley, J.K., and Purtilo, D.T.   Persistent
active infection of Epstein-Barr virus in carrier
females of the X-linked lymphoproliferative syndrome.
In: H. Shiota, Y-C. Cheng, and W.H. Prusoff (eds.),
Proceedings of the International Symposium on
Herpesviruses: Clinical, Pharmacological and Basic
Aspects.   pp. 375-379.   Amsterdam-Oxford Princeton:
Exerpta Medica, 1982.

25.   Harada, S., Sakamoto, K., Seeley, J.K., Lindsten, T., Rogers,
G., Pearson, G., and Purtilo, D.T.   Immune deficiency in
the X-linked lymphoproliferative syndrome.   I.   Epstein-
Barr virus-specific defects.   J. Immunol., 129:2532,
1982.

26.   Lindsten, T., Seeley, J.K., Sakamoto, K., Yetz, J., Harada,
S., Bechtold, T., Rogers, G., and Purtilo, D.T.   Immune
deficiency in the X-linked lymphoproliferative syndrome.
II.   Immunoregulatory T cell defects.   J. Immunol.,
129:2536, 1982.

INFECTIOUS MONONUCLEOSIS AND COMPLICATIONS

James Linder and
David T. Purtilo

Department of Pathology and Laboratory Medicine
University of Nebraska Medical Center
Omaha, NE 68105

INTRODUCTION

Infectious mononucleosis (IM) is a febrile illness of older
children and young adults caused by the Epstein-Barr virus (EBV).
The diagnosis is based on the triad of physical, hematologic and
serologic findings. In this chapter we review the discovery of
IM, the typical and atypical cases. We emphasize immunologic
determination of the outcome of the infection by EBV. Several
monographs discuss the historical and clinical aspects of IM (12,
39,54).

History

Investigation of diseases resembling IM date to 1889. Emid
Pfeffer described Druesenfieber (glandular fever), a condition
believed by some to be the first description of IM. This is
unlikely, considering the differences between the two diseases as
clearly articulated by Hoagland (54). Druesenfieber likely
represents infectious lymphocytosis, a non-EBV-viral illness.
Near the turn of the century Turk, and others described illnesses
resembling IM. Not until 1920, however, was the classical
description and term infectious mononucleosis made by Sprunt and
Evans (107). Shortly after the clinical description of IM, Downey
and McKinlay put forth an elegant description of the morphology of
the "atypical" lymphocytes in this illness (21).

In 1932 Paul and Bunnell discovered an antibody in the blood
of IM-patients that agglutinated sheep erythrocytes, so-called
heterophile antibody (87). This prompted heterophile antibody

11

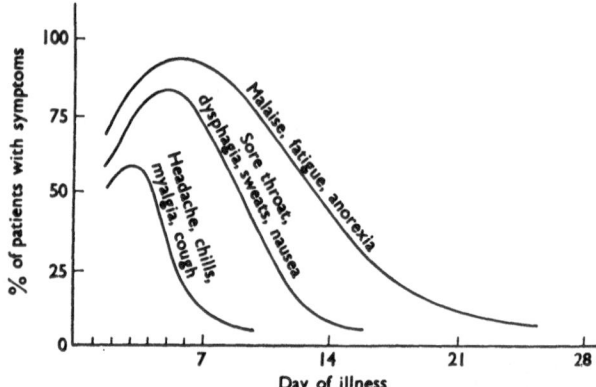

Fig. 1.   Usual symptoms of major clinical symptoms in uncompli-
          cated infectious mononucleosis. (From: Finch, S.C.
          Clinical Symptoms and Signs of Infectious Mononucleosis.
          In: Carter, R.L. and Penman, H.G. (eds.) Infectious
          Mononucleosis. Blackwell, Oxford, 1969. Courtesy of
          Blackwell Scientific Publications Limited.)

determination as a diagnostic test for IM. However, nearly 50
years passed until EBV was identified as the etiologic agent,
after IM occurred in a technician working with the virus (19).
Subsequent studies by the Henles and others confirmed that EBV was
the cause of IM (25,49,51,52).

Clinical Manifestations

        Characteristic symptoms of IM are the insidious onset of
malaise and fatigue, followed by the abrupt onset of sore throat,
sweats, fever, nausea, anorexia, and headache. Less frequent
symptoms include: chills, cough, myalgias, arthralgias, diarrhea,
photophobia, rash, and abdominal pain (Figure 1) (12,13,32).

        Physical examination reveals systemic enlargement of lymphoid
tissues, most pronounced in the pharynx and cervical lymph nodes
(Figure 2). The lymphadenopathy is symmetrical, increasing
rapidly during the first week of illness, then gradually diminishing about three weeks after the onset of symptoms. Lymph
nodes are tender but are not fluctuant or suppurative. Splenomegaly is detected in at least 60% of patients, the exact incidence depending on the diligence and skill of the examiner.

Hematologic Features

        The peripheral blood smear is usually the first objective
laboratory test to suggested IM. The total leukocyte count usually

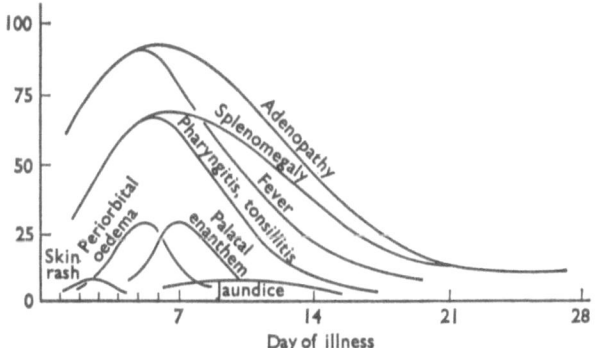

Fig. 2. Usual frequency and duraction of major physical signs in
young adults with uncomplicated infectious mononucleosis.
(From: Finch, S.C. Clinical Symptoms and Signs of
Infectious Mononucleosis. In: Carter, R.L. and Penman,
H.G. (eds.), Infectious Mononucleosis. Blackwell, Oxford
1969. Courtesy of Blackwell Scientific Publications
Limited.)

ranges from 12 x 10^9/1 to 20 x 10^9/1, although it may reach 30 x
10^9/1. Usually, 60-70% of the differential count are lymphocytes,
and in florid cases they may reach 95%. When the leukocyte count
does not exceed 10 x 10^9/1, there usually is still an absolute
lymphocytosis (greater than 4.5 x 10^9/1) (32).

Ten to 20% of lymphocytes are described as "atypical" (Table
1) (Figure 3). The spectrum of morphologic aberrations was elo-
quently stated by Downey and McKinlay (21). The most common atypical cells are medium to large lymphocytes with basophilic cytoplasm, occasionally having azurophilic granules or vacuoles. The
lymphocytes have a scalloped border as they mold around erythrocytes. Nuclei are smudged and may harbor nucleoli. Small
basophilic lymphocytes and lymphoblasts are seen (77,105,118).

Table 1. Morphologic Features of Aytpical Lymphocytes

Increased cell size
Pleomorphism with transition from small to large cells
Smudged or coarse chromatin
Nucleoli
Irregular nuclear shapes
Increased cytoplasm
Scalloping of cytoplasmic boarder around erythrocytes
Cytoplasmic vacuoles or granules
Cytoplasmic basophilia

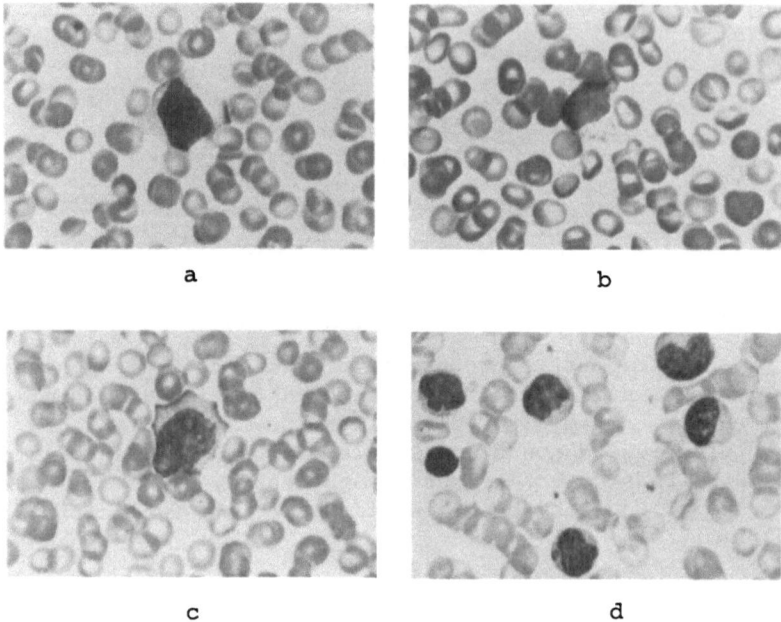

a   b

c   d

Fig. 3.   Atypical lymphocytes of infectious mononucleosis.
          (From: McKenna, R.W. Laboratory Medicine, 10:137,
          1979, with permission of Lipincott/Harper/Row.)

     Other hematologic abnormalities in IM, such as anemia, throm-
bocytopenia, neutropenia, and monocytosis are discussed later
under Complication of Infectious Mononucleosis.

Serologic Features

     Two types of serologic studies aid the diagnosis. The most
common is the demonstration of heterophil antibodies to sheep or
horse erythrocytes (15). Less frequently used is the determination of antibodies to specific components of the EBV.

Heterophile Antibodies

     The concept of heterophile antibodies was introduced by
Forssman in 1911. These antibodies bind to antigens that do not
appear to be related to the antigen that stimulated the antibody
production (66). Antibody in IM patients agglutinates sheep red
blood cells (SRBC). Since antigens on SRBC should have no relation to the agent causing IM, this is a classic example of a
heterophile antibody. Heterophile antibody titer is determined by
the Paul-Bunnell (PB) test, in which SRBC are combined with dilutions of serum to determine agglutination titers (87). Healthy

individuals rarely have titers exceeding 1:56, while the mean titer in IM patients is 1:646 (85). A drawback of the PB test is that heterophile antibodies to SRBC also occur in Hodgkin's disease, leukemia, hepatitis, tuberculosis, and serum sickness (66).

IM- and non-IM-specific heterophile antibodies are distinguished by a simple differential absorption test. The Paul-Bunnell-Davidson (PBD) test measures SRBC agglutination after first absorbing patient serum with suspensions of either guinea pig kidney cells (GPK) or bovine erythrocytes (BE). The IM-specific heterophile antibody is absorbed by BE but not by GPK; while non-IM heterophile antibodies have exactly opposite absorption qualities (15). The differential absorption test is useful in low-titer of heterophile antibody. In such instances, a decrease of SRBC agglutination of at least 16-fold by preabsorbing the serum with BE, with no more than an 8-fold decrease after GPK, is indicative of IM-specific heterophile antibody (85).

The sensitivity of heterophile tests has been improved approximately three-fold by substitution of horse erythrocytes (HRBC) for sheep cells. This is dubbed the horse cell differential absorption tests (HCAT) (72,74).

Rapid slide tests are based on the same principles as the PB and PBD agglutination (16,72). Numerous manufacturers distribute rapid slide tests. In the Monospot® test, patient serum is combined with BE and GPK cell suspension on either half of a microscope slide. A horse cell stroma is then added. Agglutinating activity blocked by BE but not GPK is characteristic of IM heterophile antibody.

Immune adherence hemagglutination (IAHA) is a highly sensitive assay of heterophile antibody (74). Comparison of tests show IAHA and HCAT have similar sensitivity for detecting acute IM. IAHA is the most sensitive method to identify heterophile antibody in symptomatic EBV infection, and is useful when the rapid slide test or HCAT is negative in spite of clinical symptoms suggesting IM.

For over 90% of cases with clinical features of IM, the rapid slide tests are sufficient. When the heterophile titer is at least 1:56 to 1:112 the slide test has a sensitivity of 99% compared to the HCAT (85). Rarely, rapid tests may give false positive results (57,58). Approximately 10% of patients with the mononucleosis syndrome are heterophil negative. Cytomegalovirus, Toxoplasma gondii, and rarely drugs and viruses induce the syndrome. Heterophile negative cases require EBV-specific titers for definitive diagnosis (56).

EBV-specific Serology

Heterophile antibody appears in about 90% of adolescents and adults who have classic signs and symptoms of IM, such as sore throat, fever, lymphadenopathy and lymphocytosis. However, about 10% of adults, 30% of 7-9 year old children, 40% of 3-6 year old children, and nearly all children less than 3 years old will not develop heterophile antibodies after EBV infection (34,109). Since viruses and parasites may cause symptoms identical to IM, without inducing heterophile antibody, specific tests to either confirm or refute EBV as the cause of symptoms are sometimes needed.

EBV-specific serodiagnostic tests detect antibodies against specific components of the EBV, such as the viral capsid antigen (VCA), early antigen (EA), and Epstein-Barr nuclear antigen (EBNA) (51,52). These antibodies may provide evidence for acute EBV infection, or indicate immunity to EBV depending on the antibody, or class of antibody present.

Serodiagnostic tests use lymphoblastoid cell lines transformed by EBV in a principle analogous to the indirect Coombs assay. These cells express EBV antigens, and binding of serum antibody to EBV antigens is demonstrated by immunofluorescence.

Antibody titer to different viral components exhibits a characteristic pattern during the illness (Figure 4). Anti-VCA of both the IgG and IgM class appears in the early phase of infec-tion. In acute IM anti-VCA IgM occurs in high titer early in the illness, and rapidly diminishes during convalescence (22,27,84, 103). By contrast, the titer of IgG anti-VCA during acute symptoms and convalescence may be similar, thus limiting its usefulness for identifying acute IM. However IgG anti-VCA often suggests immunity to EBV, since this antibody persists lifelong after infection. Anti-VCA of the IgA class is also produced in IM. It has been demonstrated in 68% of serum specimens during acute illness and may serve as an adjunct in identifying heterophile-negative EBV infection (29).

An additional marker of acute EBV infection is antibody to EA, which is expressed in lymphoblastoid cell lines in two immu-nofluorescence patterns. In the diffuse form (D), the entire nucleus exhibits antigenic staining while in the restricted (R) form the staining is limited to cytoplasmic aggregates. Anti-EA (D) occurs in 80% of adults with IM during the acute phase of illness. Anti-EA (R) characterizes many EBV pediatric infections (51).

Antibody to EBNA characteristically does not appear until after resolution of symptoms (i.e., one month up to four months).

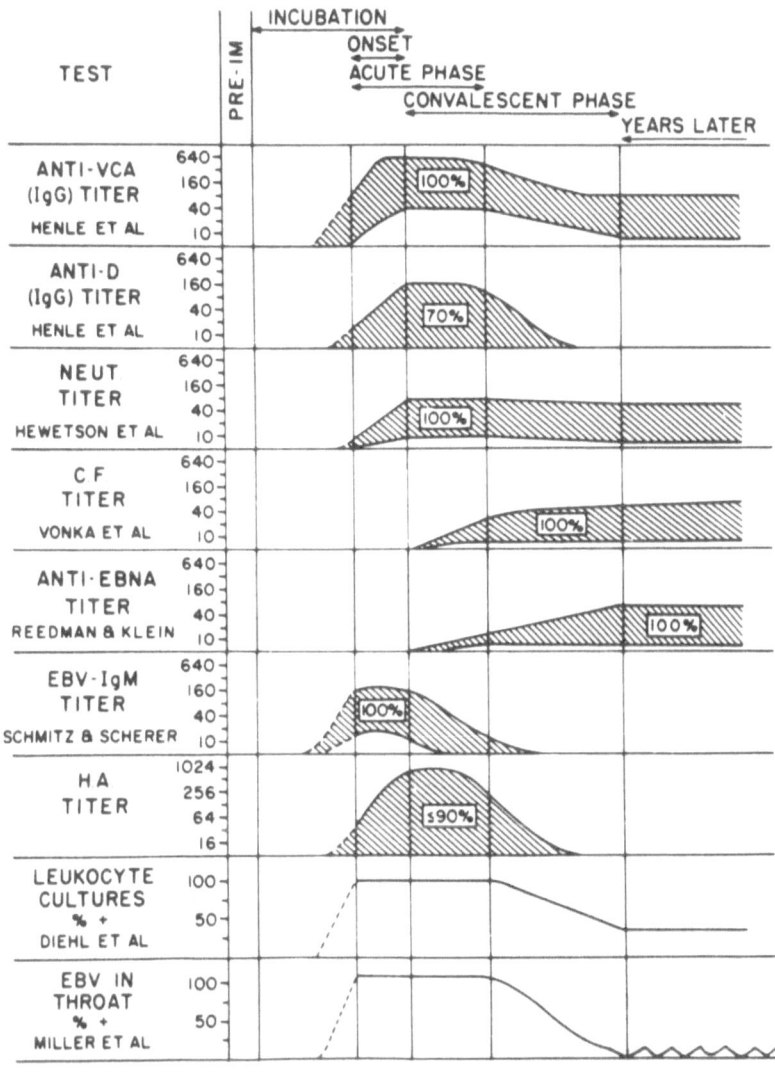

Fig. 4. Schematic presentation of antibody responses, leukocyte cultures and assays for Epstein-Barr virus (EBV) in throat washings during infectious mononucleosis. (VCA = viral capsid antigen; D = diffuse component of early antigen; C.F. = complement fixation; EBNA = Epstein-Barr nuclear antigen; H.A. = heterophile antibody). (From: Henle, W., Henle, G. and Horwitz, C.A.: Epstein-Barr virus-specific diagnostic tests in infectious mononucleosis. Hum. Path., 5:551, 1974 with permission of W.B. Saunders, Co.)

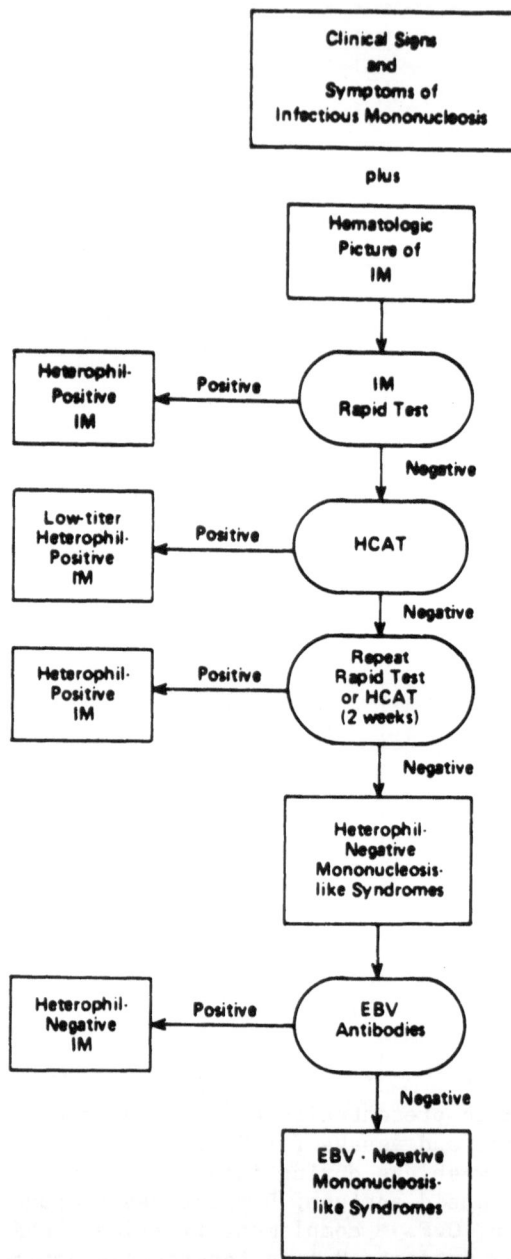

Fig. 5.   Strategy for evaluation of suspected EBV infection.
(From: Ophoven, J.   Infectious mononucleosis: Part 2
Serologic aspects.   Lab. Med., 10:203, 1979.   Courtesy
of Lippincott/Harper & Row.)

Once anti-EBNA appears it persists for life. Since it is present only after resolved illness, it marks immunity to EBV infection, along with anti-VCA of the IgG class.

To summarize succinctly, most patients with IM have pharyngitis, lymphadenopathy and fever; a leukocytosis between $10 \times 10^9/1$ and $20 \times 10^9/1$, with at least 10% atypical lymphocytes; and heterophile antibody. If these features are present, the diagnosis is clear and no further tests are required.

In approximately 5 to 10% of patients, symptoms and blood smears are characteristic of IM, but the rapid slide test is negative. Repeat rapid slide tests may become positive. In other instances, more sensitive methods, such as HCAT and IAHA will detect heterophile antibody and establish the diagnosis. When heterophile antibody is not detectable, EBV-specific serodiagnostic tests are useful. Positive anti-VCA IgM and antibody to the D-component of the early antigen support diagnosis of acute EBV infection, while the absence of these antibodies or the presence of anti-VCA IgG or anti-EBNA indicates remote EBV infection, and suggests the current symptoms are not EBV-related (51). In this event, serologic tests for antibodies to cytomegalovirus, toxoplasma gondii, adenovirus, etc. may explain the mononucleosis-like syndrome (28,56,67). A strategy for the evaluation of suspected EBV infection is presented in Figure 5.

ETIOLOGY AND PATHOGENESIS

It seems appropriate to us that this section on the etiology of IM follows our discussion of diagnosis. Nearly 50 years transpired from the clinical description of IM to identification of EBV as the etiologic agent. The appreciation of the role of EBV in IM is intimately linked to the brilliant investigations of Denis Burkitt of the lymphoma of African children that now bears his name (8). His suggestion that the tumor may have an infectious etiology prompted electron microscopic studies by Epstein, Achong, and Barr, who in 1964 discovered herpesvirus-like particles in cultured Burkitt's lymphoma cells (24). The first indication of that EBV causes IM came in 1967, when a laboratory technician contracted IM while working with EBV. Her serum, which lacked anti-EBV antibody prior to illnes, contained antibody after the onset of symptoms. Furthermore, during her illness it became possible to cultivate lymphocytes from her blood in tissue culture and demonstrate that her lymphocytes expressed Epstein-Barr viral antigens (49). This fortuitous event prompted extensive seroepidemiologic and biochemical studies to define the role of EBV in IM. Evidence for this role is summarized as follows:

1. IM occurs only in individuals who lack circulating anti-
    body to EBV.

2. Individuals possessing anti-EBV are immune to IM.

3. The symptoms of IM are regularly accompanied by develop-
    ment of antibody against the EBV (51).

4. Oropharyngeal secretion of EBV occurs in 70-90% of
    patients for up to 18 months after IM (37,79).

5. B-lymphocytes from patients with IM express EBNA during
    the acute illness (69,99).

6. Patients with IM develop EBV-specific cytotoxic T-cells
    (99,108).

The primary target of EBV infection may be epithelial cells in
the oropharynx, or B-lymphocytes that carry specific EBV-receptors
that are closely associated with the C3d receptor (64,65). In
either case, B-lymphocytes have become infected. Curiously, certain individuals seem to lack the ability to become infected with
EBV. For example, the authors know prominent investigators of the
virus who remain seronegative despite their handling of virally
infected cell lines for decades. Joncas and associates (38) have
proposed that seronegative adults lack EBV receptors.

Infection leads to polyclonal B-lymphocyte activation and
hypergammaglobulinemia (63). The period of acute infection of B-
lymphocytes has been aptly described as an immunologic struggle
(92). Elsewhere in this book Harada and colleagues describe
immune responses to EBV, especially in autoimmune persons. The
combatants are the B-cells infected by EBV and T-cells attempting
to control B-cell proliferation. Immunologic marker studies show
90% of peripheral blood lymphocytes in acute IM are T-cells
(3,18,86). Most of the atypical lymphocytes in IM are actually T-
cells responding to EBV infection B-cells, not viral-infected
lymphocytes. A high percentage of the atypical lymphocytes mark
with monoclonal antibodies as T-suppressor cell subsets (48) and
cytotoxic T-cells (47,99,108). In vivo these T-cells likely
modulate B-cell proliferation. The combination of cellular immune
response to EBV and antibodies against EBV-specific antigens break
the viral production cycle (110). Robinson (98) estimates 5-20%
of circulating B-cells are EBNA positive. He ascertained this by
depleting blood of IM patients of T-cells and then culturing the
B-cells for 18-24 hours and then staining for EBNA.

With resolution of symptoms there is a decrease heterophile
titer, and the establishment of immunity against EBV (Figure 4).
EBV virus genome is probably integrated into DNA of some B-

lymphocytes and epithelial cells of the oropharynx so that latent virus is never completely eliminated. This accounts for persistent titers of antibodies to the VCA and EBNA, which can become elevated when individuals become immunosuppressed and their T-cells are less capable of holding EBV in check. This exaggerated humoral reponse probably is adaptive to compensate for the T-cell defects.

IM is predominantly a disease of young adults who are 15-25 years of age. EBV infection in children is usually asymptomatic, or causes a mild respiratory illness that endows them with immunity to further EBV infection. Numerous epidemiological studies have investigated the relationship between age of EBV-exposure and IM. Not surprisingly, when a large percentage of the children in a population contract EBV-infection at a young age, few adults are susceptible and the incidence of IM is low. Early exposure to EBV occurs most frequently in countries and communities where hygiene and socioeconomic conditions are low (52). This feature is illustrated in Figure 8 in our chapter on Burkitt's Lymphoma (p. 109). In tropical and developing countries most children have EBV antibody by age 6 (50). In affluent societies exposure to EBV is often delayed until adulthood. A study of Yale college freshmen showed only 51% with prior exposure to EBV; of the susceptible 49%, 13% developed during their first year and 74% of those had clinical features of IM (26,102). A similar prospective study of incoming U.S. military academy cadets revealed 36% were susceptible to EBV. During their four years of college, 46% contracted EBV infection and one quarter of these had IM.

The virus is most likely transmitted in the saliva of individuals following EBV infection, making oral contact through kissing or shared drinking glasses a common means of spread (37,79). Transmission of EBV among children is probably made via saliva. This could be airborne or be transmitted on toys and other shared objects. True epidemics of IM have not been substantiated in the period after the clinical and etiologic features of the disease were defined. Outbreaks purported as epidemics in earlier times (80), may reflect non-EBV viral infections, and "epidemics" in military camps may simply reflect aggregation of large numbers of susceptible individuals (113,114).

No differences in susceptibility with regard to sex or race has been found, when socioeconomic and hygienic standards are equal.

COMPLICATIONS OF INFECTIOUS MONONUCLEOSIS

The overwhelming majority of EBV infections in infants, children and young adults pass unnoticed. When IM develops after

EBV infection, the most common complication is the fatigue,
headache and malaise, that impairs performance of college of students. Mononucleosis is the fourth most common cause of absen-
teeism from work among military personnel. Recurrent and chronic
mononucleosis are reported as nonexistent, but have been observed
by us (4). Elsewhere in this volume Tobi describes chronic mononucleosis in detail.

Table 2. Complications of Infectious Mononucleosis

Mechanical	Spleen rupture
	Acute airway obstruction
Nervous system	Fatigue
	Depressions
	Catatonia
	Pseudotumor
	Cranial neuropathies
	Mononeuritis
	Polyneuritis (Guillain-Barre)
	Inappropriate ADH secretion
	Hearing loss
Cardiovascular system	Myocarditis
	Pericarditis
Respiratory system	Interstitial penumonitis
	Pleural effusion
	Mediastinal lymphadenopathy
	Pseudolymphoma
	Opportunistic Staphylococcal or Streptococcal infection
Gastrointestinal system	Transient hepatitis
	Massive liver failure
	Pancreatitis
	Malabsorption
Kidney	Interstitial nephritis
Bone marrow and blood	Anemia, red cell aplasia
	Thrombocytopenia
	Granulocytopenia
	Aplastic anemia
	Cryoglobulinemia
Immune system	Polyclonal B-cell proliferation
	Malignant lymphoma
	Graft-versus-host-like illness
	Acquired agammaglobulinemia
	Chronic mononucleosis
Skin	Rash
Fetus	Rare cardiac and other deformities

Fortunately, serious complications occur in less than 1% of patients. Two uncommon, but well recognized complications are splenic rupture and acute airway obstruction (43,53). Spleen enlargement occurs in about 60% of patients, reaching maximum size during the first three weeks of illness. The enlargement mirror the engorgement of the red pulp with lymphocytes and large pyrinophilic cells. A lymphoid infiltrate of the capsule, trabeculae and walls of blood vessels may weaken the supporting tissue and predispose the spleen to rupture or formation of subcapsular hematoma (100). Trauma or sudden compression of the spleen by contraction of abdominal musculature likely precipitates the actual rupture. In a review of 107 cases reported through 1978, Ruthaw found trauma played some role in 89 cases, the remainder being "spontaneous." In another series by Aung et al., 80% of cases of splenic rupture occurred in males, presumably due to their physical activity (4). The overall incidence of splenic rupture is about 0.2% of cases.

Acute airway obstruction is a rare, dramatic complication of IM (76). It is due to hyperplasia of pharyngeal lymphoid tissue, and edema of pharyngeal soft tissues (43). Often clinicians treat the obstruction of the airway with a high dose of corticosteroid. This usually produces lympholysis and removes the obstruction. The chemosurgery, however, momentarily suppresses immunity. No data is available to allow prediction of long range effects of this treatment.

Given that IM is a systemic disease, diverse organ systems are infiltrated by lymphoid cells. The nervous system, liver, skin, heart, lungs, and blood are among the many organs listed in Table 2 in which manifestations of IM occur.

A wide variety of neurologic diseases are associated with IM and EBV infection (40,42). The severity may range from a mild neuritis, to the Guillain-Barre syndrome causing respiratory failure and death. Other well-documented neurologic manifestations include Bell's palsy, meningoencephalitis, and transverse myelitis (106). Fortunately, these complications affect less than 1% of patients. It is worthwhile to note that the Guillain-Barre syndrome and facial palsy may occur when IM is not clinically apparent, but serologic evidence for EBV infection is present (40). Other complications of IM have been recently reviewed by us (98). The cerebrospinal fluid (CSF) in cases of acute meningoencephalitis contains lymphocytes, especially plasmacytoid forms. Antibodies to EBV may be lacking in the CSF.

Hepatic involvement is present in most patients with IM (68). The most common finding is a mild elevation in liver enzymes, such as alkaline phosphatase, lactate dehydrogenase, serum glutamate exaloacetic transaminase and serum glutamic-pyruvic transaminase (Figure 6) (32).

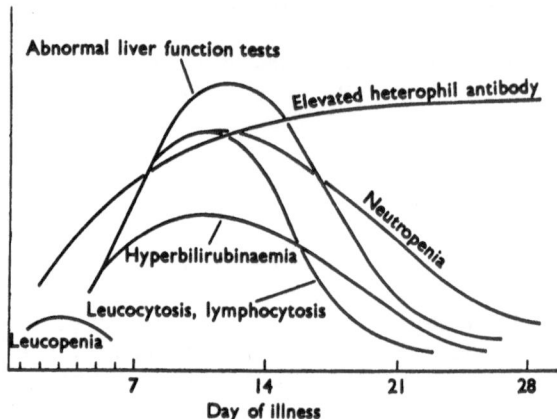

Fig. 6. Major laboratory changes in adults with uncomplicated
         infectious mononucleosis. (From: Finch, S.C.:
         Laboratory Findings in Infectious Mononucleosis.
         In: R.C. Carter and H.G. Penman (eds.), Infectious
         Mononucleosis. Oxford: Blackwell, 1969. Courtesy of
         Blackwell Scientific Publications Limited.)

     Perturbations in liver function tests appear during the second
week of illness and may be accompanied by hyperbilirubinemia.
Abnormal liver function has no strong diagnostic implication in
classic cases of infectious mononucleosis; but in a patient with
hepatitis, IM must be considered as a possible etiology. The
histologic alteration in the liver biopsy are limited to mild
infiltration of the portal tracts of lymphocytes and larger
pleomorphic lymphoid cells, with mild degeneration of hepatocytes.
Many instances of IM with fulminant hepatic necrosis and death
have been recorded (1,2,46), particularly in males with X-linked
lymphoproliferative syndrome and others have been documented
(92,95). See the chapter by Purtilo.

     Cutaneous manifestations are common in IM. Approximately 14%
of patients not on antibiotic therapy develop a mild, transient
morbilliform rash (95). Less common are erythema multiforme,
erythema nodosa, and urticaria (6,89,115). Ampicillin or other
penicillins induce a skin rash in 42-100% of patients 5 to 14 days
after receiving the drug (90). It begins as puritic maculopapular
eruption on the trunk, then spreads to the arms and face. The
mechanism may be related to immune complexes of ampicillin antigens and antibody. Alternatively, this may be a manifestation of
a graft-versus-host reaction, mediated by T-lymphocytes (92).
Whatever the cause, the rash fades about one week after eruption.
These rashes do not indicate an allergy to penicillin or its de-
rivatives.

Cardiovascular effects of IM include abnormal electrocardio-
grams, with nonspecific S-T segment depressions or T-wave changes
that resolve after recovery from IM (54). Cases of fatal myocarditis, acute pericarditis, and heart block with EBV infection have
been reported (35,61,97).

Pulmonary manifestations may include interstitial pneumonitis,
hilar lymphadenopathy, and pleural effusions (81). Opportunistic
infections by pyogenic bacteria - Staphylococci, Streptococci, H.
influenzas and S. pneumonae can occur.

Decreased numbers of platelets, granulocytes, and red cells
are common in IM. In a study by Carter, mild thrombocytopenia
occurred in 50% of IM patients during the first four weeks of
disease (10). The low counts ranged between 100×10^9/L and 140 x
10^9/L, only 5 of 47 patients had platelet counts below 100×10^9.
None of these patients had hemorrhagic complications, and platelet
counts returned to normal levels during convalescence. Severe
thrombocytopenia with purpura and hemorrhage has rarely complicated IM, particularly in children (96). The mechanism of thrombocytopenia may be due to anti-platelet antibody, hypersplenism,
or defective platelet synthesis (23). Disseminated intravascular
coagulation causing thrombocytopenia has been seen in several
patients (D. Purtilo - personal observations.)

Mild granulocytopenia is equally as common as thrombocytopenia
during the first weeks of illness (33,44). Over half of the
patients in Carter's series had counts below 3×10^9/L (11).
Toxic granulation of neutrophils and a predominance of band forms
may persist until approximately the third week of illness. Severe
granulocytopenia or agranulocytosis has been noted (71,119). The
cause of the granulocytopenia may be related to arrest of myeloid
maturation at the promyelocyte or myelocyte stage (104).

Autohemolysis occurred in approximately 25% of 41 IM patients
studied by Kostinas and Cantow, but none of these had clinical
evidence of anemia (71). Hoagland observed hemolytic anemia in
approximately 3% of 500 patients (55). The mechanism of hemolysis
is unclear for most cases. In some instances, the Coombs'
antiglobulin test is positive and the titer of cold antibody to
the i-antigen is increased (9). The role of anti-i is unclear
since up to 70% of IM patients develop this antibody, while only a
fraction have hemolysis (116). Hemolysis has been associated with
anti-i or anti-N antibody, or to a Donath-Landsteiner type antibody (7,111,117).

Hemolysis complicating IM is well-known in patients who have
inherent defect in red blood cells, such as in hereditary spherocytosis, hereditary eliptocytosis, or pyruvate kinase deficiency
(17,59). Red cell aplasia has been found in a male with X-linked

lymphoproliferative syndrome (XLP) (92). Aplastic anemia, with
suppression of megakaryocytes, granulocytes, and erythrocytes is
rare (82), but has been a rather common complication of the IM
phenotype of XLP. Misdiagnosis of medullary histiocytic reticu-
losis has been made in immune deficient individuals who exhibit
atypical response to EBV infections (78).

An iatrogenic complication of IM is the biopsy of either lymph
nodes or the bone marrow. The illness occurs in the age group
most commonly affected by Hodgkin's disease. Lymphadenopathy may
dominate the clinical presentation, other signs and symptoms of IM
may not be present or not appreciated by the patient's physician
(101). Description of pathologic changes in lymph nodes follows.

Hematopathology of Lymph Nodes in IM

Mixed T, B-cell and histiocyte proliferation marks lymph nodes
from patients with acute IM (41). The paracortical zones of the
lymph nodes harbors florid proliferation of lymphocytes in all
stages of differentiation including small lymphocytes, immunoblasts, plasma cells, and large reactive histiocytes. The
numerous mitotic figures could be interpreted as an ominous sign,
but the heterogeneity of the proliferating cells signals the reactive process. The follicles may be large and irregularly shaped,
or inconspicuous depending on the stage of the infection and host-
immune response. The paracortical and follicular expansion may
markedly distort the lymph node architecture, but true nodal effacement is not normally seen. A preserved reticulin pattern and
a prominent fine vascular network is demonstrated with silver
stains. The sinusoids, although somewhat compressed by the
reactive process, remain intact. Commonly, sinus histiocytosis is
prominent, although the cells are small and uniform in contrast to
typical sinus histiocytosis. The sinusoids may also contain
enlarged lymphoid cells, plasma cells, mitotic figures, and
erythro- and nucleo-phagocytosis.

Reactive binucleate immunoblasts in IM can resemble the
Reed-Sternberg cell of Hodgkin's disease. The reactive cell tends
to be smaller than, and has smaller basophilic nucleoli than true
Reed-Sternberg cells. A zone of paranuclear clearing, or hof,
aids in identifying the masquerading Reed-Sternberg cell. In
spite of these differences it may be impossible to discern whether
or not individual cells are true Reed-Sternberg cells. Clearly
the best way to avoid misinterpreting the lymph node of IM as
Hodgkin's disease is by appreciating the patient's clinical
presentation and the overall reactive features of the node
(20,101). Moreover, EBV genome is not present in lymph nodes from
Hodgkin's disease patients.

The quiescent bone marrow in IM is a striking contrast to the immunoblastic proliferation occuring in the lymph nodes. Mild and nonspecific collections of lymphocytes are seen in the bone marrow, and small sarcoid-like granulomas have been noted (60,75). The spleen may show foci of necrosis in the lymphoid sheaths and prominent plasmacytoid cells. Capsular and subendothelial lymphoid infiltrate is common.

Since the principle target of EBV infection is the immune system, it is not surprising that immunologic complications accompany the viral infection. The type and severity of complication depends on the immune competence of the host. For example, the immature immune system of children may be an inhospitable environment for viral proliferation, and yield an asymptomatic course. Nearly half of adolescents develop IM. With normal immune function, antibodies against viral antigens, cytotoxic and memory T-cells appear during the infection. Together antibody-dependent cellular cytotoxicity and the killer functions of T-cells control the acute infection.

With inherited or acquired immunodeficiency a different scenario follows EBV infection. A model of EBV infection in immunodeficiency is the X-linked lymphoproliferative syndrome (XLP) described by Purtilo et al. (91,93). Detailed descriptions of XLP are described in chapters by Harada and Purtilo in this volume. Males with this disorder have immunoregulatory T-cell defect, causing impaired capacity to control EBV-triggered B-cell proliferation and overt cytotoxic activity against body tissue. These patients may develop at least four phenotypes following infection by the virus: (1) chronic or fatal IM, (2) aplastic anemia, (3) a- or hypo-gammaglobulinemia, and (4) malignant lymphoma. Over 100 patients affected with XLP have been studied, and 70% have succumbed to IM or the above complications (94,95).

EBV infection may prove fatal, or possibly trigger lymphoproliferative diseases in numerous other immunodeficiency diseases, such as selective IgA deficiency, ataxia telangiectasia, severe combined immune deficiency, and common variable immunodeficiency (36).

In this book, Penn and Hanto discuss lymphoproliferative diseases in renal transplant recipients, who can develop a fatal IM-like disease, and a spectrum from polyclonal B-cell proliferation to monoclonal lymphoma. These patients all show active EBV infection, similar to males with XLP (45). Such observations underscore the notion that individual variation in immune response, or failure of immune response, determines the clinical outcome of EBV infection.

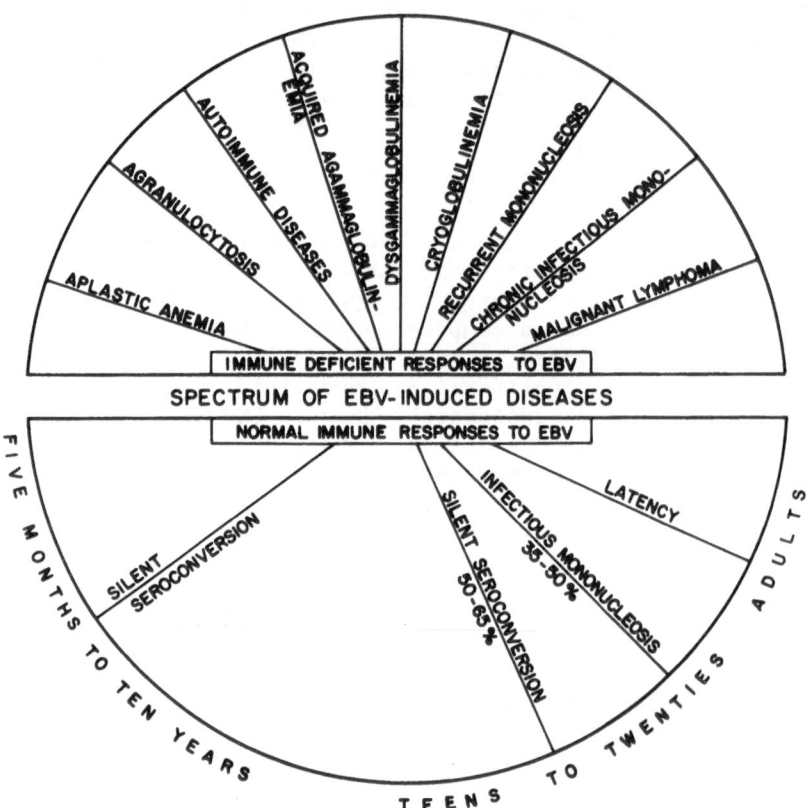

Fig. 7.   Spectrum of diseases and their complications due to
          Epstein-Barr virus infection. (Reprinted by permission
          from: Purtilo, D.T. Epstein-Barr virus-induced diseases
          are determined by immunocompetence. Clinical
          Microbiology Newsletter, 7:47, 1982. Copyright 1983
          by Elsevier Science Publishing Co., Inc.)

     Fatalities are allegedly rare in infectious mononucleosis. In
Penman's 1968 review of the world literature (88) 20 documented
cases of fatal IM were found, nine were due to neurologic complications, three to splenic rupture, three to secondary infection,
two to liver failure and one to myocarditis. He estimated 1 fatality per 3000 cases of IM. The identification of XLP and
related disorders suggests that another class of fatality in IM
can be related to defective immune responses to EBV. No longer
can we rely solely on the classical diagnostic triad of Hoagland
for diagnosis of fatal EBV infections. In many instances the role
of EBV in these deaths is not appreciated. EBV infection in an
immunodeficient host may be misdiagnosed a viral hepatitis,

malignant histiocytosis, aplastic anemia or acute leukemia.
EBV-specific serology may be useful in excluding these illnesses.
The demonstration of EBV genome in tissue is crucial for inves-
tigation of EBV-related diseases.

SUMMARY AND CONCLUSIONS

We have described typical and atypical forms of infectious
mononucleosis. A spectrum of complications can arise according to
the age and immune competence of the individual. The spectrum of
diseases and complications is summarized in Figure 7.

REFERENCES

1. Adkins, B.J. and Steele, R.H.   Death from massive hepatic
        necrosis in infectious mononucleosis. N.Z. Med. J.,
        85:56, 1977.
2. Ainley, N.J. A fatal case of infectious mononucleosis with
        extensive zonal necrosis of the liver. Ulster. Med J.,
        18:219, 1949.
3. Aiuti, F., Rocchi, G., D'Amelio, R., Giunta, S., and
        Fiorilli, M. Lymphoid cells in infectious mononucelosis
        classified according to T and B cell markers. Int. Archs.
        Allergy Apl. Immun., 48:353, 1975.
4. Aung, M.K., Goldberg, M. and Tobin, M.S.   Splenic rupture
        due to infectious mononucleosis. J. Am. Med. Assoc.,
        240:1752, 1978.
5. Ballow, M., Seeley, J., Purtilo, D.T., St. Onge, S.,
        Sakamoto, K., and Rickles, F.R. Familial chronic mono-
        nucleosis. Ann. Int. Med., 97:821, 1982.
6. Bodansky, H.J. Erythema nodosum and infectious mono-
        nucleosis. Brit. Med. J., 2:1263, 1979.
7. Bowman, M.S., Marsh, W.L., Schumacher, M.R., Oyen, R. and
        Reinhart, J. Auto anti-N immunohemolytic anemia in
        infectious mononucleosis. Am. J. Clin. Path., 62:465,
        1974.
8. Burkitt, D.P. A sarcoma involving the jaws in African
        children. Br. J. Surg., 46:218, 1958.
9. Calvo, R., Stein, W., Kochwa, S., and Rosenfield, R.E.
        Acute hemolytic anemia due to anti-i; Frequent cold
        agglutinins in infectious mononucleosis. J. Clin.
        Invest., 44:1033, 1965.
10. Carter, R.L. Platelet levels in infectious mononucleosis.
        Blood, 25:817, 1965.
11. Carter, R.L. Granulocyte changes in infectious mono-
        nucleosis. J. Clin. Path., 19:279, 1966.
12. Carter, R.L. and Penman, H.G. Infectious Mononucleosis,
        Blackwell, Oxford, 1969.

13. Chang, R.S. Infectious mononucleosis. Hall, Boston, 1980.

14. Contratto, A.W. Infectious mononucleosis. A study of one
       hundred and ninety six cases. Arch. Intern. Med.,
       73:449, 1944.

15. Davidsohn, I. and Lee, C.L. The clinical serology of
       infectious mononuclesois. In: R.L. Carter and H.G.
       Penman (eds.) Infectious Mononucleosis. p. 171.
       Blackwell, Oxford, 1969.

16. Davidson, R.J.L. New slide test for infectious mono-
       nucleosis. J. Clin. Pathol., 20:643, 1967.

17. DeNardo, G.L. and Ray, J.P. Hereditary spherocytosis and
       infectious mononucleosis with acquired hemolytic anemia.
       Am. J. Clin. Path., 39:284, 1963.

18. DeWaele, M., Thielemans, C., and VanCamp, B.K.G.
       Characterization of immunoregulatory T cells in
       EBV-induced infectious mononucleosis by monoclonal anti-
       bodies. N. Engl. J. Med., 304:460, 1981.

19. Diehl, V., Henle, G., Henle, W., and Kohn, G. Demonstration
       of a herpes group virus in cultures of peripheral leuko-
       cytes from patients with infectious mononucleosis. J.
       Virol., 2:663, 1968.

20. Dorfman, R.F. and Warnke, R. Lymphadenopathy simulating
       the malignant lymphomas. Hum. Pathol., 5:519, 1974.

21. Downey, H. and McKinlay, C.A. Acute lymphadenosis compared
       with acute lymphatic leukemia. Arch. Int. Med., 32:82,
       1923.

22. Edwards, J.M.B. and McSwiggan, D.A. Studies on the
       diagnostic value of an immunofluorescence test for EB
       virus-specific IgM. J. Clin. Path., 27:647, 1974.

23. Ellman, L., Carvalho, A., Jacobson, B.M., and Colman, R.W.
       Platelet autoantibody in a case of infectious mono-
       nucleosis presenting as thrombocytopenic purpura. Am.
       J. Med., 44:723, 1973.

24. Epstein, M.A., Achong, B.G., and Barr, Y.M. Virus par-
       ticles in cultured lymphoblasts from Burkitt's lymphoma.
       Lancet, 1:702, 1964.

25. Evans, A.S., Niederman, J.C., and McCollum, R.W.
       Seroepidemiologic studies of infectious mononucleosis
       with EB virus. N. Engl. J. Med., 279:1121, 1968.

26. Evans, A.S., Niederman, J.C., and Sawyer, R.N. Prospective
       studies of a group of Yale University freshman. II.
       Occurrence of acute respiratory infections and rubella.
       J. Infect. Dis., 123:271, 1971.

27. Evans, A.S., Niederman, M.C., Cenabre, L.C., West, B., and
       Richards, V.A. A prospective evaluation of heterophile
       and Epstein-Barr virus-specific IgM antibody tests in
       clinical and subclinical infectious mononucleosis:
       specificity and sensitivity of the tests and persistence
       of antibody. J. Inf. Dis., 132:546, 1975.

28. Evans, A.S. Infectious mononucleosis and related syndromes. Am. J. Med. Sci., 276:325, 1978.

29. Evans, A.S. and Niederman, J.C. EBV-IgA and new heterophile antibody tests in diagnosis of infectious mononucleosis. Am. J. Clin. Path., 77:555, 1982.

30. Fiala, M. Heiner, D.C., Turner, J.A., Rosenbloom, B., and Guze, L.B. Infectious mononucleosis and mononucleosis syndromes - clinical, virological and immunological features (Medical Progress). West. J. Med., 126:445, 1977.

31. Finch, S.C. Clinical symptoms and signs of infectious mononucleosis. In: R.L. Carter and H.G. Penman (eds.), Infectious Mononucleosis. p. 19. Oxford: Blackwell, 1969.

32. Finch, S.C. Laboratory findings in infectious mononucleosis. In: R.L. Carter and H.G. Penman (eds.), Infectious Mononucleosis. p. 64. Oxford: Blackwell, 1969.

33. Fisher, B.D. Neutropenia in infectious mononucleosis. N. Engl. J. Med., 288:633, 1973.

34. Fleisher, G., Lennette, E.T., Henle, G., and Henle, W. Incidence of heterophil antibody responses in children with infectious mononucleosis. J. Ped., 94:723, 1979.

35. Frishman, W., Krause, M.E., Zabkar, J., Brooks, V., Alonso, D. and Dixon, L.M. Infectious mononucleosis and fatal myocarditis. Chest, 72:535, 1977.

36. Gartner, J.G. and Seemayer, T.A. New oncologic association for the Epstein-Barr virus. Am. J. Surg. Pathol., 6:471, 1982.

37. Gerber, P., Nonoyama, M., Lucas, S., Perlin, E. and Goldstein, L.I. Oral excretion of Epstein-Barr virus by healthy subjects and patients with infectious mononucleosis. Lancet, ii:988, 1972.

38. Gervais, F., Wills, A. Leyritz, M., Lebrum, A., and Joncas, J.H. Relative lack of Epstein-Barr virus (EBV) receptors on B cells from persistent EBV seronegative adults. J. Immunol., 126:897, 1981.

39. Glade, P.R. General features of infectious mononucleosis. In: P.R. Glade (ed.), Infectious Mononucleosis. p. 1. Philadelphia: Lippincott, 1972.

40. Gorlieb-Stematski, T. and Glaser, R. Association of Epstein-Barr virus with neurologic diseases. In: R. Glaser and T. Gotlieb-Stematski (eds.), Human Herpes Virus Infections. Clinical Aspects. p. 169. New York: Dekker, 1982.

41. Gowing, N.F.C. Infectious mononucleosis: histopathologic aspects. In: S.C. Sommer (ed.), Pathology Annual. p. 1. New York: Appleton, 1975.

42.   Grose, C., Henle, W., Henle, G., and Feorino, P.M.   Primary
       Epstein-Barr-virus infections in acute neurologic
       diseases. N. Engl. J. Med., 292:392, 1975.
43.   Gutgesell, M.P. Acute airway obstruction in infectious
       mononucleosis. Pediatrics, 47:141, 1971.
44.   Hammond, W.P., Harlan, J.M., and Steinberg, S.E. Severe
       neutropenia in infectious mononucleosis. West. J. Med.,
       131:92, 1979.
45.   Hanto, D.W., Frizzera, G., Purtilo, D.T., Sakamoto, K.,
       Sullivan, J.L., Saemundsen, A.K., Klein, G., Simmons,
       R.L., and Najarian, J.S. Clinical spectrum of
       lymphoproliferative disorders in renal transplant recip-
       ients and evidence for the role of Epstein-Barr virus.
       Cancer Res., 41:4253, 1981.
46.   Harris, J.T. and Ferguson, A.W. Fatal infectious mono-
       nucleosis with liver failure in two sisters. Arch. Dis.
       Child., 43:480, 1968.
47.   Haynes, B.F., Schooley, R.T., Grouse, J.E., Payling-Wright,
       C.R., Dolin, R., and Fauci, A.S. Characterization of
       thymus-derived lymphocyte subsets in acute Epstein-Barr
       virus-induced infectious mononucleosis. J. Immunol.,
       122:699, 1979.
48.   Haynes, B.F., Schooley, R.T., Payling-Wright, C.R., Grouse,
       J.E., Dolin, R., and Fauci, A.S. Emergence of
       suppressor cells of immunoglobulin synthesis during
       acute Epstein-Barr virus induced infectious mono-
       nucleosis. J. Immunol., 123:2095, 1979.
49.   Henle, W., Henle, G., and Horwitz, C.A. Relation of
       Burkitt's tumor-associated herpes-type virus to infec-
       tious mononucleosis. Proc. Natl. Acad. Sci. USA, 59:94,
       1968.
50.   Henle, G. and Henle, W. Observations on childhood infec-
       tions with the Epstein-Barr virus. J. Infect. Dis.,
       121:303, 1970.
51.   Henle, W., Henle, G.E., and Horwitz, C.A.   Epstein-Barr
       virus specific diagnostic tests in infectious mono-
       nucleosis. Hum. Path., 5:551, 1974.
52.   Henle, W., Henle, G., and Lennette, E.T.   The Epstein-Barr
       virus. Sci. Am., 241:48, 1979.
53.   Hoagland, R.J. and Henson, H.M. Splenic rupture in infec-
       tious mononucleosis. Ann. Int. Med., 46:1184, 1957.
54.   Hoagland, R.J. Mononucleosis and heart disease. Am. J.
       Med. Sci., 248:35, 1964.
55.   Hoagland, J.R. Infectious Mononucleosis. New York: Grune
       and Stratton, 1967.
56.   Horwitz, C.A., Henle, W., Henle, G., Palesky, H., Balfour,
       H.H., Jr., Siem, R.A., Borkin, S., and Ward, P.C.
       Heterophile negative infectious mononucleosis and
       mononucleosis-like illnesses. Am. J. Med., 63:947,
       1977.

57. Horwitz, C.A., Henle, W. Henle, G., Penn, G., Hoffman, N., and Ward, P.C. Persistent falsely positive rapid tests for infectious mononucleosis. Am. J. Clin. Pathol., 72:807, 1979.

58. Horwitz, C.A., Henle, W., Henle, G., Polesky, H., and Leonardy, J. Spurious rapid infectious mononucleosis test results in non-infectious mononucleosis sera. Am. J. Clin. Pathol., 78:48, 1982.

59. Ho-Yen, D.O. Autoimmune hemolytic anemia complicating infectious mononucleosis in a patient with hereditary ellipocytosis. Acta Haematol., 59:45, 1978.

60. Hovde, R.F. and Sundberg, R.O. Granulomatous lesions in the bone marrow in infectious mononucleosis. Blood, 5:209, 1950.

61. Hudgins, J.M. Infectious mononucleosis complicated by myocarditis and pericarditis. J. Am. Med. Assoc., 235:2626, 1976.

62. Hutt, L.M., Huang, Y.T., Discomb, H.E., and Pagano, L.S. Enhanced destruction of lymphoid cell lines by peripheral blood leukocytes taken from patients with acute infectious mononucleosis. J. Immunol., 115:243, 1975.

63. Hunt-Fletcher, L.M. The functions of atypical lymphocytes. In: H. Waters, (ed.), The Handbook of Cancer Immunology. Vol. 6, p. 127. Lymphoid Cell Subpopulations: Structure, Function and Interactions. New York: Garland STPM Press, 1981.

64. Jondal, M. and Klein, G. Surface markers on human B and T lymphocytes. II. Presence of Epstein-Barr virus receptors on B lymphocytes. J. Exp. Med., 138:1365, 1973.

65. Jondal, M., Klein, G., Oldstone, M.B.A., Bokish, V., and Hefenof, E. Surface markers on human B and T lymphocytes VIII. Association between complement and Epstein-Barr virus receptors on human lymphoid cells. Scand. J. Immunol., 5:401, 1976.

66. Kano, K. and Milgrom, F. Heterophil antigens and antibodies in medicine. Cur. Top. Microbiol. Immunol., 77:43, 1977.

67. Kemola, E., von Essen, R., Henle, G., and Henle, W. Infectious-mononucleosis-like disease with negative heterophile agglutination test. Clinical features in relation to Epstein-Barr virus and cytomegalovirus antibodies. J. Infect. Dis., 121:608, 1970.

68. Kilpatrick, Z.M. Structural and functional abnormalities of liver in infectious mononucleosis. Arch. Int. Med., 117:47, 1966.

69. Klein, G., Svedmyre, E., Jondal, M., and Persson, P.O. EBV-determined nuclear antigen (EBNA)-positive cells in the peripheral blood of infectious mononucleosis patients. Int. J. Cancer, 17:21, 1976.

70.   Kostinas, J.E. and Cantow, E.F.   Studies on infectious
       mononucleosis.   II.   Autohemolysis.   Am. J. Med. Sci.,
       252:296, 1966.
71.   Koziner, B., Hadler, N., Parillo, J., and Ellman, L.
       Agranulocytosis following infectious mononucleosis.   J.
       Am. Med. Assoc., 225:1235, 1973.
72.   Lee, C.L., Davidsohn, I., and Panczyszyn, O.   Horse aggluti-
       nins in infectious mononucleosis.   II.   The Spot Test.
       Am. J. Clin. Pathol., 49:12, 1968.
73.   Lee, C.L., Zandrew, F., and Davisohn, I.   Horse agglutinins
       in infectious mononucleosis.   I.   Am. J. Clin. Path.,
       49:3, 1968.
74.   Lennette, E.T., Henle, G., Henle, W., and Horowitz, C.A.
       Heterophile antigen in bovine sera detectable by immune
       adherence hemagglutination with infectious mononucleosis
       sera.   Inf. Immun., 19:923, 1978.
75.   Martin, M.F.R.   Atypical infectious mononucleosis with bone
       marrow granuloma and pancytopenia.   Br. Med. J., 2:200,
       1977.
76.   McCurdy, J.A.   Life-threatening complications of infectious
       mononucleosis.   Laryngoscope, 85:1557, 1975.
77.   McKenna, R.W.   Infectious mononucleosis: part 1.
       Morphologic Aspects.   Lab. Med., 10:135, 1979.
78.   Merril, R.H., Barrett, O.N., and Barrett, M.C.   Positive
       monospot test in histiocytic medullary reticulosis.   Am.
       J. Clin. Pathol., 65:407, 1976.
79.   Miller, G., Niederman, J.C., and Andrews, L.L.   Prolonged
       oropharyngeal excretion of Epstein-Barr virus after
       infectious mononucleosis.   N. Engl. J. Med., 288:229,
       1973.
80.   Moir, J.I.   Glandular fever in the Falkland Islands.   Br.
       Med. J., 2:822, 1930.
81.   Mundy, G.R.   Infectious mononucleosis with pulmonary
       parenchymal involvement.   Br. Med. J., 1:219, 1972.
82.   Mir, M.A. and Delamore, I.W.   Aplastic anaemia complicating
       infectious mononucleosis.   Scand. J. Haemat., 11:314,
       1973.
83.   Niederman, J.C., McCallum, R.W., Henle, G., and Henle, W.
       Infectious mononucleosis.   Clinical manifestations in
       relation to EB virus antibodies.   J. Med. Am. Assoc.,
       203:205, 1968.
84.   Nikoskelainen, J., Leikola, J., and Kemola, E.   IgM anti-
       bodies specific for Epstein-Barr virus in infectious
       mononucleosis without heterophile antibodies.   Br. Med.
       J., 4:72, 1974.
85.   Ophoven, J.   Infectious mononucleosis: part 2.   Serologic
       aspects.   Lab. Med., 10:203, 1979.
86.   Pattengale, P.K., Smith, R.W., and Perlin, E.   Atypical
       lymphocytes in acute infectious mononucleosis –

Identification by multiple T and B lymphocyte markers.
N. Engl. J. Med., 291:1145, 1974.

87. Paul, J.R. and Bunnell, W.W. The presence of heterophile
antibodies in infectious mononucleosis. Am. J. Med.
Sci., 183:90, 1932.

88. Penman, H.G. Fatal infectious mononucleosis: a critical
review. J. Clin. Pathol., 23:765, 1970.

89. Pullen, H Wright, N., and Murdoch, J.M. Hypersensitivity
reactions to antibacterial drugs in infectious
mononucleosis. Lancet, ii:1176, 1967.

90. Pullen, H., Wright, N., and Murdoch, J.M. Hypersensitivity
to penicillins. Lancet, i:1090, 1968.

91. Purtilo, D.T., Cassel, C.K., Yang, H.P.S., Harper, R.
Stephenson, S.R., Landing, B.H., and Vawter, G.F. X-
linked recessive progressive combined variable immunodeficiency (Duncan's disease). Lancet, i:935, 1975.

92. Purtilo, D.T. Immunopathology of infectious mononucleosis
and other complications of Epstein-Barr virus infections.
In: S.C. Sommers and P.P. Rosen (eds.), Pathology
Annual. pp. 253-299. New York: Appleton-Century-Croft,
1980.

93. Purtilo, D.T. Immune deficiency predisposing to Epstein-
Barr virus induced lymphoproliferative diseases. The X-
linked lymphoproliferative syndrome as a model. In: G.
Klein and S. Weinhouse (eds.), Advances in Cancer
Research. Vol. 34, pp. 279-312. New York: Academic
Press, 1981.

94. Purtilo, D.T. and Klein, G. (eds.) Symposium on Epstein-Barr
virus-induced lymphoproliferative diseases in immunodeficient patients. Cancer Res., 41:4209, 1981.

95. Purtilo, D.T. and Sakamoto, K. Epstein-Barr virus and
human disease: immune responses determine the clinical
and pathologic expression. Hum. Pathol., 12:677, 1981.

96. Radel, E.G. and Schorr, J.B. Thrombocytopenic purpura with
infectious mononucleosis. J. Pediat., 63:46, 1963.

97. Reitman, M.J., Zirin, J.H., and De Angelis, C.J. Complete
heart block in Epstein-Barr myocarditis. Pediat.,
62:847, 1978.

98. Robinson, J. Mitotic EBNA-positive lymphocytes in
peripheral blood during infectious mononucleosis.
Nature, 287:334, 1980.

99. Royston, I., Sullivan, J.L., Periman, P.O., and Perlin, E.
Cell-mediated immunity to Epstein-Barr virus-transformed
lymphoblastoid cells in acute infectious mononucleosis.
N. Engl. J. Med., 293:1159, 1975.

100. Rutkow, J.M. Rupture of the spleen in infectious mononucleosis. Arch. Surg., 113:718, 19781.

101. Salvador, A.H., Harrison, E.G., and Kyle, R.A.
Lymphadenopathy due to infectious mononucleosis: its

confusion with malignant lymphoma. Cancer, 27:1029,
        1971.

102. Sawyer, R.N., Evans, A.S., Niederman, J.C., and McCallum,
        R.W. Prospective studies on a group of Yale University
        freshman. I. Occurrence of infectious mononucleosis.
        J. Infect. Dis., 123:263, 1971.

103. Schmitz, H. and Scherer, M. IgM antibodies to Epstein-Barr
        virus in infectious mononucleosis. Archiv fur gstamte
        Virusforschung, 37:32, 1972.

104. Shadduck, R.K., Winkelstein, A., Zeigler, Z., Lichtner, J.
        Goldstein, M., Michaels, M., and Rabin, B. Aplastic
        anemia following infectious mononucleosis. Possible
        immune etiology. Exp. Hematol., 7:264, 1979.

105. Shiftan, T.A. and Mendelshohn, J. The circulating
        "atypical" lymphocyte. Hum. Path., 9:51, 1978.

106. Silverstein, A. Steinberg, G., and Nathanson, M. Nervous
        system involvement in infectious mononucleosis - The
        heralding and/or major manifestation. Arch. Neurol.,
        26:353, 1972.

107. Sprunt, T.P. and Evans, F.A. Mononuclear leukocytosis in
        reaction to acute infections ("infectious mono-
        nucleosis"). Bull. Hopkins Hosp., 31:410, 1938.

108. Svedmyr, E., Jondal, M., Henle, W., Weiland, O., Rombo, L.,
        and Klein, G. EBV-specific killer T-cells and serologic
        responses after onset of infectious mononucleosis. J.
        Clin. Lab. Immunol., 1:225, 1978.

109. Tamir, D., Benderly, A., Levy, J., Ben-Parath, E., and
        Vonsover, A. Infectious mononucleosis and Epstein-Barr
        virus in childhood. Pediatric, 53:330, 1974.

110. Tosato, G., Magrath, I., Koski, I., Dooley, N., and Blaese,
        M. Activation of suppressor T cells during Epstein-Barr-
        virus-induced infectious mononucleosis. N. Engl. J.
        Med., 301:1134, 1979.

111. Troxel, D.B., Innella, F., and Cohen, R.J. Infectious mono-
        nucleosis complicated by hemolytic anemia due to anti-i.
        Am. J. Clin. Path., 46:625, 1966.

NASOPHARYNGEAL CARCINOMA

Gerhard R.F. Krueger

Immunopathology Section, Pathology Institute
University of Cologne
5000 Cologne 41, Federal Republic of Germany

INTRODUCTION

Besides Burkitt's lymphoma (BL) nasopharyngeal carcinoma (NPC) represents a unique model for studying the relationships between Epstein-Barr virus (EBV) infection, immune response, and neoplastic transformation. The association of EBV infection and NPC is even closer than in BL: all nonkeratinizing NPC exhibit significantly elevated anti-EBV antibody titers while extra-African BL only sporadically are seropositive.

The association of EBV and NPC was detected by chance when Old and collaborators (1) tested sera from control patients for BL which included NPC cases. Systematic work of Werner and Gertrude Henle (2-6) substantiated EBV infections in NPC. By the Reedman and Klein (7) anti-complement immunofluorescence test EBV nuclear antigen (EBNA) was demonstrated in NPC cells. Zur Hausen and his associates (8) and others (9,10) demonstrated EBV DNA in NPC biopsies. Nucleic acid hybridization studies by Wolf (11,12) proved unequivocally that EBV genome resided in the NPC carcinoma cells and not only in associated lymphoid cells.

Histopathology and Classification of NPC

The nasopharynx is a nearly cylindrical postnasal space with the anterior limit at the choana and the posterior soft palate. The roof is attached to the base of the skull and contains the pharyngeal tonsil. It slopes downward continuously to the posterior wall. The lateral walls include the external orifices of the Eustachian tubes, the torus tubarius, and behind to the roof, Rosenmueller's fossa. The inferior limit of the nasopharynx

is the hypothetical plane of the hard palate. The nasopharyngeal
mucosa in children is pseudostratified columnar ciliated epithelium overlaying well developed lymphoid tissue and containing
scattered sero-mucinous glands. With increasing age (and
apparently recurrent infections) replacement by stratified
squamous epithelium covers up to 60% of the surface. The junction
between columnar and squamous epithelium shows increased cell proliferation and reserve cell hyperplasia. Various degrees of
epithelial atypia may signal precancerous changes or accompany
subepithelial tumor (13-15).

The tumor registry of the German ENT society, notes that 90.5%
are epithelial neoplasms, i.e., carcinomas, and in 9.5% of tumors
from other tissue (e.g. malignant lymphomas and sarcomas) (16)
among malignant tumors in the nasopharynx. About 74% of the carcinomas originate from stratified squamous epithelium and 16.5%
from glandular epithelium. The ratio in other western countries
is similar although adenocarcinomas are usually less frequent (USA
4.0% versus 86.3% squamous cell carcinomas, and in the UK 2.9%
versus 70.2%) (17). Patients from countries with a high incidence
of NPC (see later) such as Tunisia, Colombia, Taiwan and Singapore
show 92-98% of tumors as squamous cell carcinomas (17).

The term nasopharyngeal carcinoma (NPC) refers exclusively to
carcinomas derived from the stratified squamous epithelium. The
separation of this tumor type from all others in the nasopharynx
is justified because of the unique relationships to: EBV infection (see above); apparent genetic predisposition (18-21); and the
implicated co- and carcinogens (22-26). Squamous cell carcinomas
vary, however, in their pathogenetic relation to above factors
according to their degree of differentiation and possibly to the
extent of associated lymphoid stroma. Consequently, NPC is
subclassified into two to three variants (Table 1): according to
the WHO classification (27) into keratinizing squamous cell carcinomas, non-keratinizing carcinomas, and undifferentiated
(anaplastic) carcinomas. The French classification (28) recognizes only two variants: squamous cell carcinoma and undifferentiated carcinoma of nasopharyngeal type (UCNT). The extent of
lymphoid stroma in the tumor tissue is considered important in the
Cologne scheme (29,30). The formulation of this simple and repro-
ducible classification (>80% conformity among 3 and more pathologists) (29,31) from a formerly used terminology identifying up to
13 different entities was possible after the unequivocal
demonstration by Svoboda and collaborators (32) and Perez (33)
that NPC, including the classical lymphoepithelial carcinoma
(SCHMINCKE-REGAUD) originate from the squamous epithelium.
Electron microscopy revealed keratin fibrils, tonofilaments, and
desmosomes even in undifferentiated carcinomas (32,34).
Demonstration by immunofluorescence of keratin antigen in undifferentiated carcinoma cells serves in the differential diagnosis
between NPC and other non-epithelial tumors (35).

Table 1. Histological Classification of Nasopharyngeal Carcinoma

French Scheme	WHO Scheme	Cologne Scheme
(MICHEAU)	(SHANMUGARATNAM)	(KRUEGER & WUSTROW) .
Squamous cell carcinoma	Keratinizing squamous cell carcinoma (Type I, SCC)	Keratinizing squamous cell carcinoma (Type I, SCC)
	Non-keratinizing carcinoma (Type II, NKC)	Non-keratinizing carcinoma (Type IIa, without lymphoid stroma)
		Type IIb, with lymphoid stroma)
Undifferentiated carcinoma of nasopharyngeal type (UCNT)	Undifferentiated (anaplastic) carcinoma (Type III, US)	Undifferentiated carcinoma (UC) (Type IIIa without lymphoid stroma)
		(Type IIIb with lymphoid stroma)

The associated lymphoid stroma in many of these tumors is
reactive or represents residual lymphoepithelial tissue or secondary infiltration. The latter appears probable in some anaplastic
tumors since a selective accumulation of IgA containing B-lymphocytes and T-lymphocytes is noted in the tumor (36,37). Tissue
culture studies (34,38) from NPC biopsies exhibit at least transient growth of epithelial sheets, fibroblasts and lymphoid cells
with blastic transformation. Growth of NPC explants in the nude
mouse confirm that only the epithelial cell is malignant (39,40).

The WHO classification of NPC derived from efforts of
Shanmugaratnam from Singapore and his collaborators (27,41).
They performed detailed epidemiologic, immunovirologic and
clinico-pathologic correlations. The value of this classification
has been confirmed (30,42) and is supported also by serological
data (Table 2). Determinations of anti-EBV antibodies in NPC
patients prove that there are essentially two types of nasopharyngeal carcinomas -- as suggested by the French classification --
well differentiated (keratinizing) squamous cell carcinomas
without apparent relationship to EBV infection and less well differentiated squamous cell carcinomas with a pathogenetic relation
to EBV infection. The amount of associated lymphoid stroma may
differentiate between EBV related and unrelated tumors in the
group of intermediately differentiated carcinomas (NKC of the WHO
classification) (30).

Epidemiology and Genetics of NPC

Detailed epidemiologic studies published in 1976 in "Cancer
Incidence in Five Continents" (43) revealed a characteristic
geographic distribution of NPC which does not correspond, however,
with that of BL. While NPC is rather rare in most countries in
the world with an age-adjusted incidence rate of 1 per 100,000/
year and less, an unusually high incidence occurs among Southern
Chinese and migrants to other countries. They average 5-7/100,000
for females and 10-19/100,000 for males. For certain selected
Chinese dialect groups such as Cantonese the corresponding rates
are even higher (29.4/100,000 for males and 10.8/100,000 for
females) (41). In addition, high incidence rates have been
reported in Greenland Aleuts (8.5 to 12.3/100,000/year) (44) and
in Aleuts from Artic Canada and Alaska (45-47). Certain subtrop-
ical and tropical regions show intermediate incidence rates (about
2-4/100,000/year) in their native populations such as Singapore
(Malays), Hawaii, Thailand, Philippines, Java, Tunisia, Algeria
and Morocco, certain tribes in Kenya, Uganda, and Sudan as well as
natives and mestizos from Colombia (refer to 17,43,44). The data
support the notion of an increased genetic susceptibility in
certain ethnic groups (18). Chan and collaborators (20,21), for
instance, found a strong association of HLA types B17 and Bw 46
with increased risks, and HLA All with decreased risk. The

Table 2. NPC Tumor Types and EBV-Antibody Titers Among 132 Cases

WHO Classification / Cologne Variation (nr. of cases)	Antibody Titers (GMT)					French Classification (nr. of cases)
	EA	VCA	EBNA	CF	IgA/VCA	
SCC (9)	10	100	10	10	10	SCC (35)
NKC Ø Ly (26	45	298	52	25	20	
NKC + Ly (17)	323	961	83	41	208	UCNT (97)
UC Ø Ly (80)	490	1792	188	68	181	
UC + Ly	516	1860	208	81	230	

(Krueger, G.R.F. presented at "Cancer du Naso-pharynx"; Actualites carcinologigues, Institute Gustave- Roussy; Paris, May 1982).
Abbreviations: SCC, squamous cell carcinoma; NKC, nonkeratinizing carcinoma; Ø, without; Ly, lymphoid stroma

combination of HLA A19/B17 and A2/Bw46 were associated with an
even high risk suggesting haplotypes rather than individual
antigens were responsible. While A2 Bw46 is confined to NPC
patients above 30 years of age, A19/B17 is seen in young patients
and B17 correlates with poor survival.

In addition, the association of the DR locus with Chinese NPC
may signal immunogenetic influences (20). Certain immune response
genes are located on chromosome 6 in close association with the
HLA DR locus. Hence, the genetically controlled host responses to
EBV antigens and transformed cells may be altered in the susceptible individuals. In addition, HLA A and B locus antigens probably determined the susceptibility of individuals for carcinogenic
or viral transformation. Studies are needed to test these
hypotheses. The genetic investigations to date have been sporadic
in the non-Chinese populations (48,58). However, Joncas and
associates (58A) have described a Canadian family with NPC, BL,
other lymphoproliferative malignancies, and immune deficiency.
Comprehensive studies of these families comparable to those
performed on families with X-linked lymphoproliferative syndrome
(XLP) may provide immunologic clues to the pathogenesis of NPC.

EBV Immunovirology and Molecular Biology

Extensive immunological and biochemical evidence supports the
etiopathogenic relationships between EBV and NPC (49-51). If
serologic markers indicate the susceptibility for NPC, then
variable antibody titers to EBV-related antigens should be observed in locales having different incidence of NPC. Comparative
international studies correlate (52-56) antibody titers in NPC
patients from low, intermediate, and high incidence regions (Table
3) confirming the value of obtaining antibody titers as indicators
of susceptibility or of populations at risk.

Antibodies to 4 EBV antigens including viral capsid antigen
(VCA), early antigen (EA), soluble complement-fixing antigen (CF),
and nuclear antigen (EBNA) were studied to ascertain their significance. Antibody to VCA indicates the chronology of previous
infection with the virus. The factors determining the titer
(aside from the patient's general immune capacities) are uncertain. Antibodies to EA and VCA antigens, especially IgA anti-EA,
correlate with tumor burden (5,57). The detection of CF antibody
may reflect genetic predisposition in Chinese (59). It does not
correlate with the extent of NPC. Two types of EA expression are
known, diffuse (EA-D) and restricted (EA-R) fluorescent patterns,
suggest that EA is a complex antigen (60). In abortively infected
cells, the D-antigen usually appears before the R-antigen. Their
function during the replicative cycle of EBV is unknown. In BL
antibodies to the R-component of EA are found, NPC patients
possess antibodies to the D-component. IgA antibody response is

Table 3. EBV Antibody Titers in Low, Intermediate and High Populations with NPC

EBV Antigen	Geometric Mean Antibody Titers from:						
	U.S.A. (white)	Germany (W)	France[a]	Tunisia/Algeria (Arabs)	Africa[b] (Black)	Hong Kong (Chinese)	Singapore (Chinese)
IgG VCA	442.3	558.9	752.7	1342.5	1303.6	1059.7	1927.0
EA	77.8	59.6	122.5	202.0	843.8	169.9	277.0
CF	23.0	11.0	97.3	55.8	66.0	70.9	185.0
EBNA	21.2	62.0	64.6	182.5	1673.8	525.2	1643.0
IgA VCA	23.8	26.9	-	32.5	277.5	-	-
NPC Incidence per 10^5/year	0.2-0.5	0.2-0.4	0.2-0.4	1.1-3.0	2.0-4.0	10.2-24.3	7.0-18.4

(m:f)

[a]including Mediterraneans from Southern France
[b]these populations carry a high risk also to develop Burkitt's lymphoma

Table 4.   Review of Major EBV-induced Antigens

Antigen	Source	Structure	Test System
Viral Capsid Antigen	EBV producer lympho-blastic cells	Structural component of viral capsid polypeptide complex of about 160 kD	Immunofluorescence (IF), Immunoperoxi-dase (PAP) of patient's serum against EBV-produc-ing tissue culture cell lines
Early Antigens (EA) diffuse (D) restricted (R)	EBV producer lymphoblastic cells	Virus-induced "non-structural" protein; complex of D and R components (R in cytoplasm, D in nuclei and cytoplasm)	IF and PAP of patient's serum against abortively superinfected non-producer cell lines (e.g. Raji) or BUDR- or IUDR activated non-producer cells
EBV-induced nuclear antigen (EBNA	Non-producer lympho-blastic & epithelial cells (NPC cells)	Virus-induced "non-structural" protein; native 170-200 kD complex (tetramer) of 48-49 kD subunits	Anti-complement immunofluorescence (ACIF) using patient's serum & non-producer cell lines
Soluble antigen (S)	Non-producer cells	apparently identical with EBNA	Complement fixation test with extracts from non-producer cells
Membrane Antigen (MA) complex early (EMA) and late (LMA) forms	EBV producer lympho-blastic cells	Structural components of viral envelopes; proteins & glyco-proteins of 300, 250 170 and 90 kD	Membrane immuno-fluorescence with viable test cells
Lymphocyte-defined Membrane antigen (LYDMA) Antigen for neutr-alizing antibodies (N)	EBV producer and non-producer lympho-blastic cells Infectious EBV	? ?	Lymphocytotoxicity (T-killer cells) for viable test cells Inhibition of EA induction Inhibition of colony formation Inhibition of trans-formation

quite specific for NPC. Similar antibodies are not consistently found in BL or infectious mononucleosis (IM) (for review see Pearson, 1980) (61). Details of these and other antigens are summarized in Table 4.

Data discussed so far strongly implicates EBV as a causative agent of NPC. The structure of the EBV genome is being elaborated (6,62-65). Yet the biological significance of the genome is incompletely understood. It encodes for several RNAs (mRNAs) in abundance which accumulate in polyribosomes and in the cytoplasm of growing transformed cells. Similarly, cytoplasmic RNAs in adenovirus and SV40 infected cells probably participate in RNA processing.

The EBV genome is present in malignant cells in NPC and BL in both circular free form (plasmid or episomal) and as linearly integrated DNA in the host genome (65). Non-malignant B cells from patients with IM, EBV-infected cord blood lymphocytes, and in lymphocytes from healthy individuals with (subclinical) in vivo EBV-infection contain the genome. No obvious differences in the EBV genome in these various disorders have been found.

EBV genomic integration is presumed to be the cause of immortalizing transformed B-lymphoid cells so that they grow as continuous cell cultures. These cell lines express at least one virus-coded antigen such as EBNA (7,67). However, a few human B-lymphoid cell lines lack EBV DNA (68-71). These cells can be infected by transforming virus, express EBNA, and exhibit changes in growth in culture (70,72,73). Since these cells contain only EBV DNA linearly associated with host DNA, the EBV genome probably accounts for their altered growth (74). Whether this finding pertains to transformed (malignant) epithelial cells in NPC (which possess EBNA, yet are EA and VCA negative) remains an open question. These cells grow poorly in tissue culture. NPC cells do not replicate EBV; the virus in the tumor tissue is derived from infected B-lymphoblasts. Passage of carcinoma cells in the nude mouse, however, has demonstrated the production of EBV with transforming activity (75). This indicates that NPC cells contain the complete genome for viral replication.

The unintegrated circular form of the EBV genome is homogeneously preserved in many generations of non-producer cells and may thus be a storage form (inactive) of viral information (65).

The motivated reader is referred to the excellent books "Viral Oncology" edited by George Klein (76) and "The Epstein-Barr Virus" edited by Epstein and Achong (77).

Important questions to be answered include: a) How does EBV enter the epithelial cell?; b) What is the molecular biology of malignant transformation?; and c) How can a transformed cell containing viral surface antigens survive and proliferate? In part, question a. is answered by Volsky and question b. by Sugden elsewhere in this book.

The natural host of EBV is the B-lymphocyte, the bone marrow-derived cell which differentiates (78) to an antibody synthesizing cell. Some of these cells (those with IgM surface immunoglobulin) possess receptors for EBV which are closely related to C3d complement receptors (79,80). Not all cells though with C3d receptors bind EBV (such as macrophages, granulocytes and certain T-cell

subsets) (81) so that probably certain steric features of C3d
receptors on the lymphocyte surface and other structures such as
the HLA-D gene product allow EBV adsorption (82). Following
adsorption to the cell membrane, virus enters the B-lymphocyte by
membrane fusion or by pinocytosis (although the latter process
still leaves the virus extra-cytoplasmically). The virus uncoats,
the nucleocapsid moves to the cell nucleus, and there initiates
transcription after disassociating from the nucleocapsid (83). A
conceptual problem in EBV-induced NPC is that epithelial cells do
not possess receptors for the virus. How does the viral genome
enter the cell? Only exceptionally and under in vitro conditions
can infection by EBV occur, and the mode of infection needs elucidation (91).

Hypothetical mechanisms for the in vivo infection of nasopharyngeal epithelial cells are 1) cell fusion with virus carrying
B-lymphocytes (84) and 2) a carrier-mechanisms for EBV-receptors
to originally receptor-negative cells (87,88). Wolf and collaborators (84) demonstrated that under certain conditions EBV
induces cell fusion; EBV-containing lymphoblastoid cells fused in
confluent cultures with EBV-receptor negative fibroblasts and
human T-lymphocytes form large polykaryocytes. They speculate in
vivo EBV infection of receptorless cells occurs by a similar
process. Elsewhere in this book, Wolf argues the case for his
hypothesis. Lenoir and de The (89) had suggested that syncytium-
forming viruses inhabiting the respiratory tract may mediate
epithelial infection, including paramyxoviruses (i.e., respiratory
syncytial virus). Volsky and coworkers (87,88,90) in elegant
experiments transplanted EBV-receptors to receptorless cells
(including epithelial cells from tonsillar tissue) through fusion
with reconstituted EBV-receptor carrying Sendai virus envelopes.
The results were recently confirmed by Khelifa and Menezes (92).
Sendai virus is a paramyxovirus. Parainfluenza, a member of the
group, causes acute respiratory infections in man. Haas and
collaborators (66) provided evidence that RNA-dependent RNA
polymerase may be present in NPC cells as well as in other tumor
cells. Parainfluenza viruses contain RNA-dependent RNA polymerase. Thus the finding of polymerase in NPC cells may be a
"footprint" of the virus. In summary, EBV susceptibility of
nasopharyngeal epithelial cells is theoretically possible by
EBV-receptor transfer and/or by cell fusion with B-lymphoblasts
harboring EBV.

What is the molecular biology of malignant transformation?
The criteria for malignant transformation of cells include altered
growth behavior with decreased contact inhibition and quasi immortalization of cells in culture; changes in karyotype; membrane
changes in lipid fluidity and receptor availability; acquisition of
new antigens; and limitation of cell differentiation in favor of
cell proliferation.

These features were demonstrated in EBV-transformed cells, primarily in B-lymphoblasts, only to a limited extent in nasopharyngeal epithelium (85,86). However, certain fragments of EBV genome, essential for transformation, are identified as are sequences coding for intracellular virus-related antigens (62,93). What is the significance of the intracellular polypeptides in relation to altered behavior of transformed cells?

In some RNA tumor virus systems an oncogene-coded phosphokinase has been identified which associates with cell membrane bound proteins (94-104) contributing to changes in the cells. (Both, RNA and DNA virus specialists claim that both viruses are completely different as to their mode of cell transformation. · Nevertheless, the biological behavior of the transformed cell (vide supra) is similar. Final steps in cell transformation ought to be comparable, or at least, results obtained in one system can guide research in the other systems.)

Elucidation of biological activities of EBV-induced, intracellular polypeptides is ongoing. For example, studies to identify polypeptides in EBV-transformed and malignant cells and separate them from others observed in normal, functionally activated cells are in progress (66,105,106). Pagano and associates (106) describe two 44kD and 20kD polypeptides in 88% of NPC tissues, the function of which is unknown. Haas (66) identified a cross-reacting 20-25kD polypeptide in several tumors including NPC. They hypothesized that it may be an RNA-dependent RNA polymerase. These data, however, have to be confirmed by specific tests for the enzymatic activity of this polypeptide. RNA polymerase is characterized in certain viruses (see above), virus infected plant cells (107,108), and in rabbit reticulocytes (109). Cytoplasmic RNA-dependent RNA polymerase – whether introduced by a virus or reactivated by viral infection amplifies mRNA enhancing the synthesis of specific proteins independent of the production of multiple gene copies. If such proteins provide growth factors (110,111), the enhanced proliferation of transformed cells will become understood.

How does a transformed cell, that is antigenic, survive and proliferate? Lifelong latency of EBV and permanent seroconversion prevails (112) possibly as a nonproductive latent infection or it is productive, shedding virus from the oro- and nasopharynx (in ca. 20% of healthy seropositive individuals). Both conditions require balanced immune responses.

If primary infection is delayed until adolescence or later, as in the West, about half develop IM (113), a benign, self-limited lymphoproliferative disease. Linder and Purtilo in this volume discuss IM in detail. Only transient immune depression (114,115) occurs in acute IM. Then specific antibodies to EA, VCA, MA, and

activated T-lymphocytes against EBV-transformed lymphoblastoid
cells emerge (116-119) to subdue the virus. Infection in immune
deficient person can cause progressive lymphoproliferation and
death (120-122). Similarly, a defective immune reactivity must be
assumed in patients who develop NPC.

Immune Response and NPC

During the Third International Symposium on NPC (123), evaluation of immune reactivity of NPC patients was recommended including general (tumor- and virus-unrelated) immune reactivity and
specific anti-tumor and anti-viral responses. Also, the immune
response in EBV-infected patients at risk (i.e., before NPC) and
with NPC should be ascertained. None of these investigations have
been done because patients do not seek consultation before symptoms
appear from tumor; many are found at advanced stages. Defective
immune reactivity favors the development of several kinds of
malignancies (124-126). EBV is nearly omnipresent in immunocompromised patients. Specific investigation for immunity to EBV
is needed. Studies can be done in, for example, the People's
Republic of China. Large scale EBV serologic screening is under
way to identify the population at risk for NPC (127). Data of
anti-EBV immunity in precancerous patients is being acquired.
Detailed serological and clinical epidemiological surveys (58,128)
have revealed distinctive patterns of anti-EBV antibody titers in
patients developing NPC compared to BL patients and others with
EBV-unrelated neoplasms (61): while IgG-anti-VCA antibody titers
can be elevated non-specifically, anti-EA antibodies rise in BL
and NPC patients. However, IgA anti-VCA specifically elevates in
NPC-prone patients. Mentioned earlier, antibodies against the
R-component of EA are elevated in BL patients while antibodies
against the D-component appear in NPC patients. These antibody
changes occur prior to the appearance of the tumor indicating a
vigorous immune response against viral antigens. Also immune
response against transformed (malignant) cells and titers against
membrane antigens (e.g. MA and LYDMA in transformed lymphoblasts)
need to be evaluated. Cytotoxic T-lymphocytes reacting against
LYDMA and neutralizing anti-MA antibodies have been described in
NPC (130-132). Specific immune response remains active although
the reaction is probably directed against antigens of transformed
lymphoid cells in NPC patients rather than against malignant
epithelial cells. Levine and collaborators (133) tested the
cell-mediated immunity (lymphocyte stimulation test and leukocyte
migration inhibition test) in NPC patients against EBV-induced
membrane antigen of Raji cells. They observed reactions in
seropositive healthy individuals as well. Two advanced NPC
patients undergoing chemotherapy did not react. However, the
antigen used was derived from a lymphoblastoid cell line and not
from epithelial cells. These limitations apply to the evaluation
of various skin tests in NPC patients (134,135). Pope et al. have

demonstrated HLA-restricted cytotoxic T-cells specific for autologous lymphoblastoid cell lines in seropositive patients, and discussed their significance in NPC.

Demonstration of specific immune responses against NPC cells require identification of a specific antigen on these cells, or cross-reactivity of antibodies against lymphoblast membrane antigens with epithelial antigens. When skin tests were done with antigens from NPC-derived HKLy-28 cell lines, a significantly higher percentage of NPC patients reacted than control lymphoma patients (136).

Referring to the general, EBV-independent immune status in NPC, both hyporesponsive and normoresponsive patients have been identified using skin tests (Tuberculin, SK/SD, DNCB) with the degree of hyporeactivity correlating to the clinical stage of the disease (138-140).

Thus the data available regarding the immune status of NPC patients do not allow conclusions about the postulated immune deficiency. Primary EBV infection probably occurs during childhood. Reactivation due to unknown factors occurs in adulthood in those developing NPC. Reactivation patterns of high antibody titers against EBV-related antigens mark persons at risk. Changes

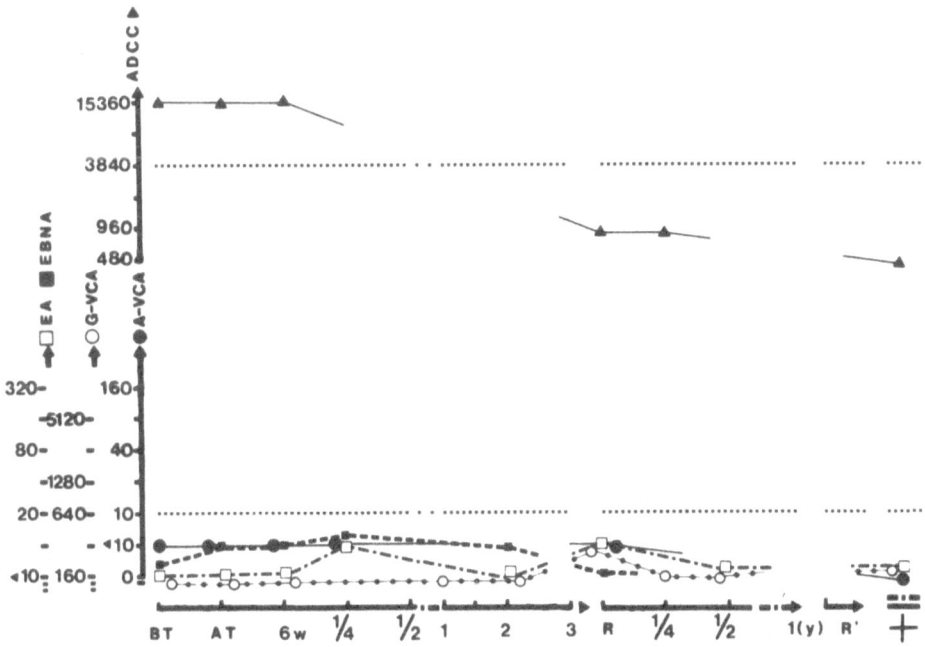

Fig. 1. Correlation of EBV-serology to the clinical course (SCC/NKC 1).

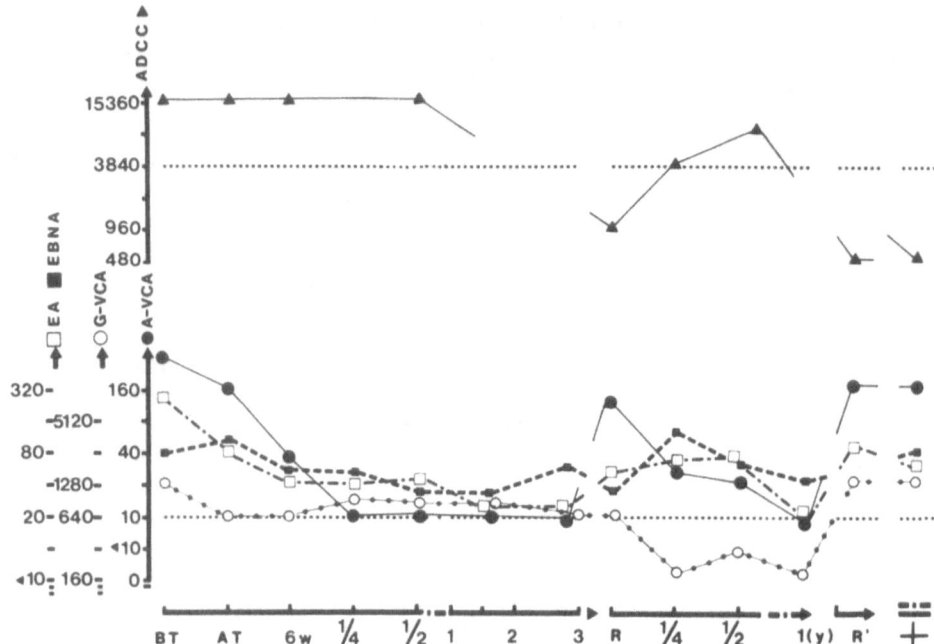

Fig. 2. Correlation of EBV-serology to the clinical course (UC
         2).

in immune responses during the evolution of NPC according to tumor
stage, regression or recurrence is clinically relevant and may
reflect tumor growth and host immune defense.

Serological longitudinal studies of NPC patients reveal patterns of antibodies in WHO Type II (NKC) and III (UC) tumors.
Type I (SCC) squamous cell carcinoma is not apparently related to
EBV infection (Figures 1 and 2) (30,141,140). When WHO's classification scheme for tumor staging (142) is applied, antibody
titers to VCA and EA correlate with NPC stage, i.e., increasing
tumor masses enhance the antibody response against virus-induced
antigens (in lymphoblastic cells admixed with the tumor) (57,143,
146). This finding concurs well with IgA-containing B-lymphocytes
accumulating in undifferentiated (WHO Type III) NPC tissue (144).
Moreover, the IgA antibody reacts specifically with VCA (145).
This correlation with the tumor burden does not apply to anti-
EBNA antibodies, i.e., to antibodies against an antigen present
within carcinoma cells.

The ADCC test (antibody-dependent cellular cytotoxicity) is
significantly elevated in patients with BL and NPC (147,148),
however, elevated titers also occur in healthy individuals and in
patients with various neoplasms (140,149). Hence initial titers
in NPC are of lesser prognostic significance (although patients

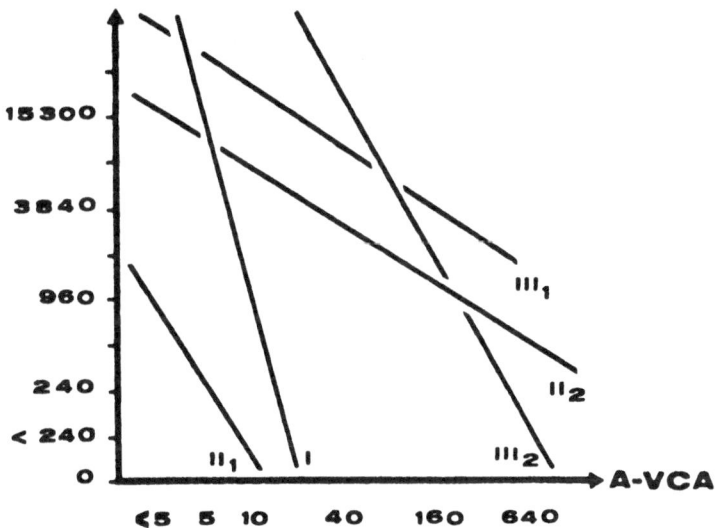

Fig. 3. Correlation of IgA anti-VCA and ADCC titers in
         nasopharyngeal carcinoma (numbers refer to histological
         types; see Table 1).

with high initial ADCC titers have better survival than those with
low initial titers). Prognostic information is gained from
follow-up studies (See Figures 1 and 2) as well as from correlations of ADCC test results with IgA anti-VCA titers (Figures 3 and

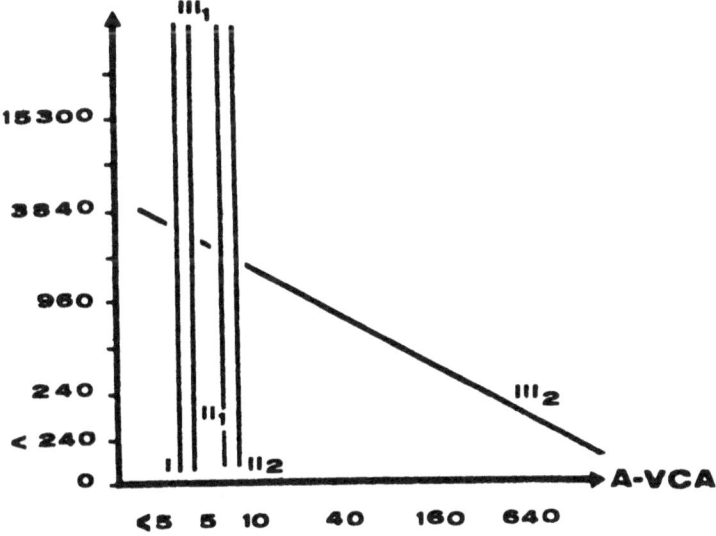

Fig. 4. Correlation of IgA anti-VCA and ADCC titers in meso- and
         hypopharyngeal carcinomas.

4). A decrease in ADCC titers and an accompanying increase of the
IgA anti-VCA titers signal progression. In complete remissions
(clinically defined), ADCC titers return to high initial values
and IgA anti-VCA decrease to insignificant levels. Renewed reversal of these titers signal recurrent NPC.

I must emphasize that these tests for anti-tumor immune
response are against lymphoblast antigens rather than against carcinoma cell antigens. In addition, ADCC tests are performed with
sera from NPC patients using foreign lymphocytes. The studies are
limited by a lack of NPC cell targets. The patients' lymphocytes
should be included in the ADCC test. Pope et al. (137) reported
HLA-restricted cytotoxic T-killer cells in the blood of seropositive patients which reacted with syngeneic transformed lymphoblasts.

ADCC and IgA anti-VCA titers show an inverse relationship in
NPC patients suggesting that IgA antibodies may actually inhibit
the ADCC reaction (150) (Table 5). Thus the specific IgA antibody
against virus-induced capsid antigen apparently interferes with
the cellular immune response directed against the tumor. Locally
secreted IgA antibody in the tumor tissue might favor rather than
inhibit tumor growth. In this context circulating immune

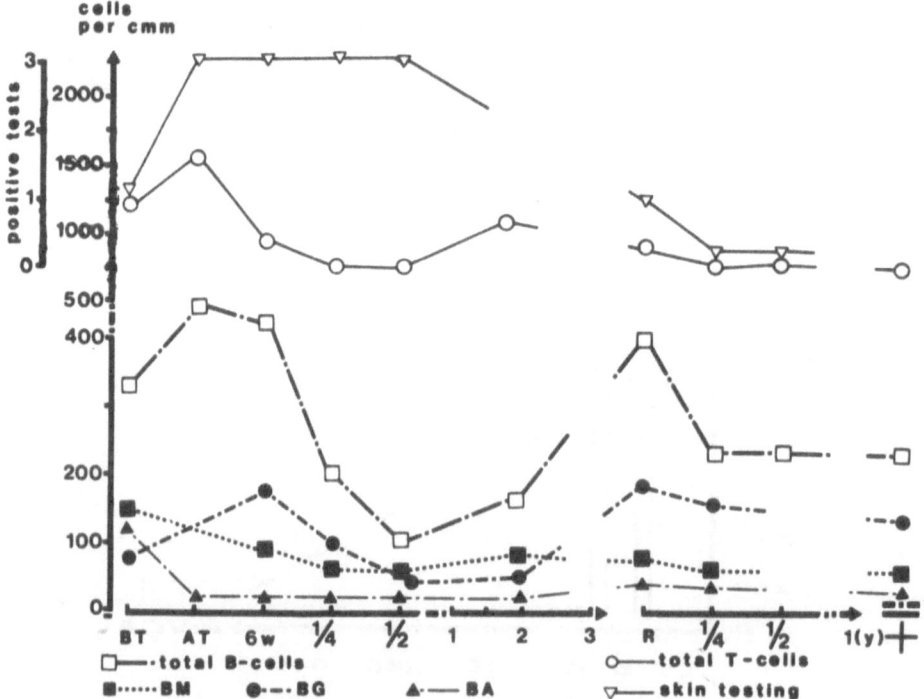

Fig. 5. Correlation of non-EBV related tests to the clinical
         course (SCC/NKC 1).

Table 5. The Effect of the Immunoglobulin Fractions Isolated from the NPC Sera and Other Controls on Antigen-Induced Blastogenesis.

Source of serum	Serum IgA antibody titer	Serum/immuno-globulin fraction[a]	Lymphocyte stimulation[b]			
			EB-Virus		Soluble antigen	
			CPM	% Inhibition	CPM	% Inhibition
Control	<10	serum	32,818	0	35,274	0
		IgG	26,224	20	33,338	7
		IgM	32,536	0	47,054	0
		IgA	28,744	24	30,418	14
Undifferentiated NPC patient[c]	640	IgG	37,813	0	41,961	0
		IgM	39,613	0	40,605	0
		IgA	5,302	87	4,118	89
NPC patient in remission	10	IgG	29,718	10	34,796	4
		IgM	37,903	0	40,663	0
		IgA	37,160	18	39,147	0
Other head & neck cancer patients	<10	IgG	30,895	6	34,611	0
		IgM	29,854	10	31,058	0
		IgA	29,554	10	30,085	0

a Immunoglobulins were fractionated from 1-2 mls of sera by $ZnSO_4$ precipitation procedure.
b The serum and the immunoglobulin fractions were tested for the presence of the blocking factor as described in Table 2.
c Immunoglobulin fractions were isolated from 4 NPC sera and only the IgA fraction inhibited the EBV-specific lymphocyte stimulation (range of the percent inhibition was 65-95). (From Sundar, S.K. et al. Int. J. Cancer 29:497, 1982.)

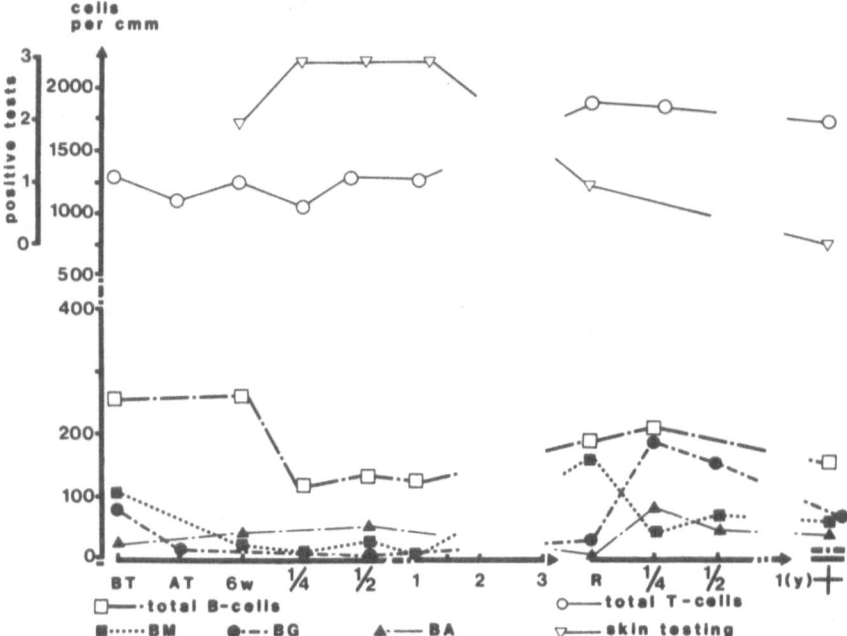

Fig. 6.   Correlation of non-EBV related tests to the clinical
          course (NKC 2).

complexes were demonstrated in NPC patients (151) which probably
suppress anti-MA immunity. Finally, when various aspects of nonspecific, EBV-unrelated immunoreactivity were investigated in NPC
patients (139,140), a decreased response in delayed type hypersensitivity skin reactions was observed depending on the tumor mass
(Figures 5-7).

SUMMARY AND CONCLUSIONS

     NPC and BL are models of viral-induced malignancies. The
pathogenic relationship of this tumor to EBV infection appears
stronger than in BL. Cofactors of the carcinogenesis - genetically determined susceptibility and exogenous chemicals - could
impair specific immune responses and allow the transformed epithelial cells to grow. Perhaps certain antibodies against EBV-
induced antigens interfere with the effective cell-mediated immune
response against transformed (malignant) epithelial cells. The
natural hosts for EBV are B lymphocytes. Transfection of epithelial cells theoretically occurs due to fusion of infected B
lymphocytes with epithelial cells or when EBV receptors are
transferred to receptorless epithelial cells by cooperation with
fusigenic viruses. The molecular biology of epithelial cell

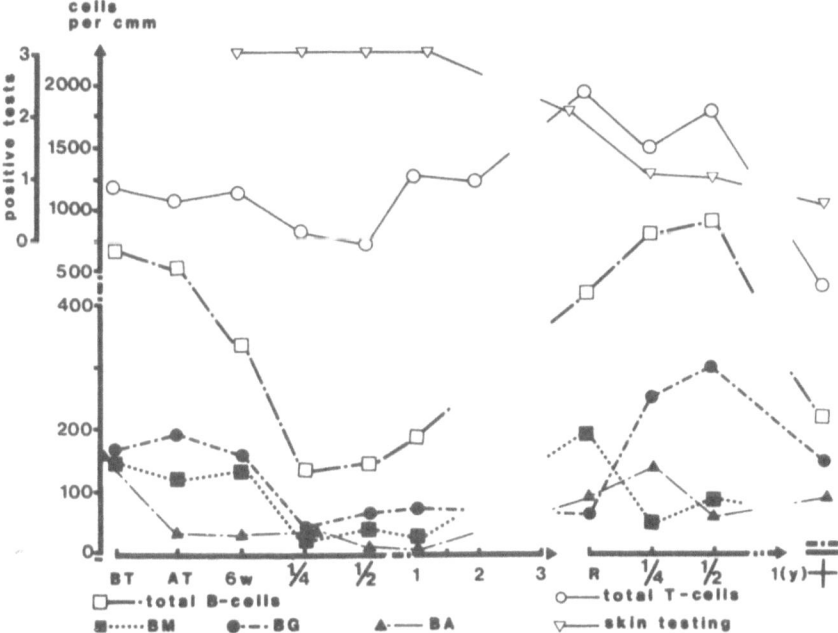

Fig. 7.   Correlation of non-EBV related tests to the clinical
          course (UC 2).

transformation by EBV is unknown. Preliminary observations
suggest that virus-coded, polypeptides in the 20-25 kD range may
alter growth of carcinoma cells.

REFERENCES

1.   Old, J.L., Boyse, E.A., Oettgen, H.F., de Harven, E.,
       Geering, G., Williamson, B., and Clifford, P.
       Precipitating antibody in human serum to an antigen pres-
       ent in cultured Burkitt's lymphoma cells. Proc. Natl.
       Acad. Sci. (USA), 56:1699, 1966.
2.   Henle, G. and Henle, W. Immunofluorescence in cells derived
       from Burkitt's lymphoma. J. Bact., 91:1248, 1966.
3.   Henle, W., Henle, G., Ho, H.C., Burtin, P., Cachin, Y.,
       Clifford, P., de Schryver, Cl., de Thé, G., Diehl, V.,
       and Klein, G. Antibodies to Epstein-Barr virus in
       nasopharyngeal carcinoma, other head and neck neoplasms
       and control groups. J. Natl. Cancer Inst., 44:225,
       1970.
4.   Henle, G., Henle, W., and Klein, G. Demonstration of two
       distinct components in the early antigen complex of
       Epstein-Barr virus infected cells. Int. J. Cancer,
       8:272, 1971.

5.   Henle, W., Ho, H.D., Henle, G., and Kwan, H.C.   Antibodies
        to Epstein-Barr virus-related antigens in nasopharyngeal
        carcinoma, comparison of active cases of long term sur-
        vivors. J. Natl. Cancer Inst., 51:361, 1973.

6.   Henle, G. and Henle, W. Epstein-Barr virus-specific IgA serum
        antibodies as an outstanding feature of nasopharyngeal
        carcinoma. Int. J. Cancer, 17:1, 1976.

7.   Reedman, B.M. and Klein, G. Cellular localization of an
        Epstein-Barr virus (EBV)-associated complement-fixing
        antigen in producer and non-producer lymphoblastoid cell
        lines. Int. J. Cancer, 11:499, 1973.

8.   zur Hausen, H., Schulte-Holthausen, H., Klein, G., Henle,
        W., Henle, G., Clifford, P., and Santesson, L.
        EB-virus DNA in biopsies of Burkitt tumors and
        anaplastic carcinomas of the nasopharynx. Nature,
        228:1056, 1970.

9.   Nonoyama, M., Huang, C.H., Pagano, J.S., Klein, G., and
        Singh, S. DNA of Epstein-Barr virus detected in tissue
        of Burkitt's lymphoma and nasopharyngeal carcinoma.
        Proc. Natl. Acad. Sci. (USA), 70:3265, 1973.

10.   Andersson-Anvret, M., Forsby, N., Klein, G., and Henle, W.
        Studies on the occurrence of Epstein-Barr virus DNA in
        nasopharyngeal carcinomas, in comparison with tumors of
        other head and neck regions. Int. J. Cancer, 20:486,
        1977.

11.   Wolf, H., zur Hausen, H., and Becker, V. EB viral genomes in
        epithelial nasopharyngeal carcinoma cells. Nature New
        Biol., 244:245, 1973.

12.   Wolfe, H., zur Hausen, H., Klein, G., Becker, V., Henle, G.,
        and Henle, W. Attempts to detect virus-specific DNA se-
        quences in human tumors. III. Epstein-Barr virus DNA
        in nonlymphoid nasopharyngeal carcinoma cells. Med.
        Microbiol. Immunol., 161:15, 1975.

13.   Prasad, U. Significance of metaplastic transformation in
        the pathogenesis of nasopharyngeal carcinoma. Clinical,
        histopathological, and ultrastructural studies. In: E.
        Grundmann, G.R.F. Krueger, and D.V. Ablashi (eds.),
        Nasopharyngeal Carcinoma. Cancer Campaign. Vol. 5, pp.
        31-39. New York: Gustav Fischer Verlag-Stuttgart, 1981.

14.   Prathap, K., Prasad, U., and Ablashi, D.V. The pathology of
        nasopharyngeal carcinoma in Malaysians. In: IVth
        Internatl. Symposium NPC. Kuala Lumpur, Malaysia, 1982;
        in print.

15.   Yin, S.Y. Study on the histogenesis of nasopharyngeal car-
        cinoma (NPC). In: IVth Internatl. Symposium NPC.
        Kuala Lumpur, Malaysia, 1982; in print.

16.   Krueger, G.R.F. and Hirano, T. Special procedures for the
        differential diagnosis of nasopharyngeal carcinoma. In:
        IVth Internatl. Symposium NPC. Kuala Lumpur, Malaysia,
        1982; in print.

28. Micheau, C., Rilke, F., and Pilotti, S. Proposal for a new
     histopathological classification of the carcinomas of
     the nasopharynx. Tumori., 64:513, 1978.
29. Krueger, G.R.F. and Wustrow, J. Current histological
     classification of nasopharyngeal carcinoma (NPC) at
     Cologne University. In: E. Grundmann, G.R.F. Krueger,
     and D.V. Ablashi (eds.), Nasopharyngeal Carcinoma.
     Cancer Campaign. Vol. 5, pp. 11-15. New York: Gustav
     Fischer Verlag-Stuttgart, 1981.
30. Krueger, G.R.F., Kottaridis, S.D., Wolf, H., Ablashi, D.V.,
     Sesterhenn, K., and Bertram, G. Histological types of
     nasopharyngeal carcinoma as compared to EBV serology.
     Anticancer Research, 1:187, 1981.
31. Costa, J. The histopathological diagnosis of nasopharyngeal
     carcinoma. In: E. Grundmann, G.R.F. Krueger, and D.V.
     Ablashi (eds.). Nasopharyngeal Carcinoma. Cancer
     Campaign. Vol. 5, pp. 7-10. New York: Gustav Fischer
     Verlag-Stuttgart, 1981.
32. Svoboda, D.J., Kirchner, F.R., and Shanmugaratnam, K. The
     fine structure of nasopharyngeal carcinomas. In: C.S.
     Muir and K. Shanmugaratnam (eds.), Cancer of the
     Nasopharynx. UICC Monograph Series, Vol. 1, pp.
     163-171. Copenhagen: Munksgaard, 1967.
33. Perez, C.A., Ackerman, L.V., Mill, W.B., Ogura, J.H., and
     Powers, W.E. Cancer of the nasopharynx: factors
     influencing prognosis. Cancer, 24:1, 1969.
34. Gazzolo, L., de Thé, G., Vuillaume, M., and Ho, H.C.
     Nasopharyngeal carcinoma. II. Ultrastructure of normal
     mucosa, tumor biopsies, and subsequent epithelial growth
     in vitro. J. Natl. Cancer Inst., 48(1):73, 1972.
35. Sesterhenn, J., Sesterhenn, K., Hyams, V., Krueger, G.R.F.,
     and Langloos, B.G. Demonstration of keratin-antigens in
     undifferentiated carcinomas of the nasopharyngeal type
     and malignant lymphomas – a contribution ot practical
     differential diagnosis. In: IVth Internatl. Symposium
     NPC. Kuala Lumpur, Malaysia, 1982, in print.
36. Wustrow, J., Karpinski, A., Haas, W., Krueger, G.R.F.,
     Bertram, G., and Sesterhenn, K. Correlation of histo-
     logical NPC tumor types with local and peripheral T-
     and B-cell values. In: E. Grundmann, G.R.F. Krueger,
     and D.V. Ablashi (eds.), Nasopharyngeal Carcinoma.
     Cancer Campaign. Vol. 5, pp. 193-199. New York: Gustav
     Fischer Verlag-Stuttgart, 1981.
37. Jondal, M. and Klein, G. Classification of lymphocytes in
     nasopharyngeal carcinoma (NPC) biopsies. Biomedicine,
     23:163, 1975.
38. de Thé, G., Ho, H.C., Kwan, H.C., Desgranges, C., and Favre,
     M.C. Nasopharyngeal carcinoma (NPC). I. Types of
     cultures derived from tumour biopsies and non-tumorous
     tissues of Chinese patients with special reference to

lymphoblastoid transformation. Int. J. Cancer, 6:189, 1970.

39. Klein, G., Giovanella, B.C., Lindahl, T., Fialkow, P.J., Singh, S., and Stehlin, J. Direct evidence for the presence of Epstein-Barr virus DNA and nuclear antigen in malignant epithelial cells from patients with anaplastic carcinoma of the nasopharynx. Proc. Natl. Acad. Sci. (USA), 71:4737, 1974.

40. Wustrow, J. personal communication, 1980.

41. Shanmugaratnam, K., Cahn, S.H., de Thé, G., Goh, J.E.H., Khor, T.H., Simons, M.J., and Tye, C.Y. Histopathology of nasopharyngeal carcinoma. Correlations with epidemiology survival rates and other biological characteristics. Cancer, 44:1029, 1979.

42. Weiland, L. Clinical pathology: current status. In: IVth Internatl. Sympos. NPC. Kuala Lumpur, Malaysia, 1982; in print.

43. Waterhouse, J., Muir, C., Correa, P., and Powell, J. (eds.). Cancer Incidence in Five Continents. IARC Scientific Publ. Vol. III, No. 15. Lyon, 1976.

44. Nielsen, N.H., Mikkelsen, F., and Hart-Hansen, J.P. Nasopharyngeal cancer in Greenland. The incidence in an Artic Eskimo population. Acta Path. Microbiol. Scand. Sect. A., 85:850, 1977.

45. Blot, W.J., Lanier, A., Fraumeni, J.F., and Bender, T.R. Cancer mortality among Alaskan natives, 1960-1969. J. Natl. Cancer Inst., 55:547, 1975.

46. Mallen, R.W. and Shandro, W.G. Nasopharyngeal carcinoma in Eskimos. Canad. J. Otolaryng., 3:175, 1974.

47. Schaefer, J., Hildes, J.A., Medd, L.M., and Cameron, D.G. The changing pattern of neoplastic disease in Canadian Eskimos. Canad. Med. Ass., 112:1399, 1975.

48. Krueger, J., Ieromnimon, V., and Dahr, W. Frequencies of HLA antigens in patients with NPC. In: E. Grundmann, G.R.F. Krueger, and D.V. Ablashi (eds.), Nasopharyngeal Carcinoma. Cancer Campaign. Vol. 5, pp. 201-203. New York: Gustav Fischer Verlag-Stuttgart, 1981.

49. Klein, G. The Epstein-Barr virus. In: A.S. Kaplan (ed.), The Herpesviruses. pp. 521-555. New York: Academic Press, 1973.

50. de Thé, G. Role of Epstein-Barr virus in human diseases: infectious mononucleosis, Burkitt's lymphoma, and nasopharyngeal carcinoma. In: G. Klein (ed.), Viral Oncology. pp. 769-797. New York: Raven Press, 1980.

51. Henle, W. and Henle, G. The association of Epstein-Barr virus with nasopharyngeal carcinoma. In: E. Grundmann, G.R.F. Krueger, and D.V. Ablashi (eds.), Nasopharyngeal Carcinoma. Cancer Campaign. Vol. 5, pp. 1-6. New York: Gustav Fischer Verlag-Stuttgart, 1981.

52. Levine, P.H., Wallen, W.C., Ablashi, D.V., Granlund, D.J., and Connelly, R. Comparative studies on immunity to EBV-associated antigens in NPC patients in North America, Tunisia, France and Hong Kong. Int. J. Cancer, 20:332, 1977.

53. Levine, P.H., Lamelin, J.P., and Stevens, D.A. Cell mediated immunity, Epstein-Barr virus and nasopharyngeal carcinoma. In: G. de The and Y. Ito (eds.), Nasopharyngeal Carcinoma: Etiology and Control. Vol. 20, pp. 483-494. Lyon: IARC Publ., 1978.

54. Ablashi, D.V., Easton, J.M., Levine, P.H., Krueger, G.R.F., and Connelly, R. Immunological comparison of nasopharyngeal carcinoma and Burkitt's lymphoma from relatively high and low-risk populations. In: L. Severi (ed.), Tumours of Early Life in Man and Animals. VIth Perugia Quadrennial International Conference on Cancer, pp. 195-210. Preugia, Italy, 1977.

55. Ebbesen, P., Levine, P.H., Connelly, R., Walker, S., and Mestre, M. Case-control study of antibodies to Epstein-Barr viral capsid antigen and early antigen in Greenland Eskimos and Caucasian controls living in Greenland and Denmark. In: E. Grundmann, G.R.F. Krueger, and D.V. Ablashi (eds.)., Nasopharyngeal Carcinoma. Cancer Campaign. Vol. 5, pp. 119-123. New York: Gustav Fischer Verlag-Stuttgart, 1981.

56. Armstrong, G.R., Ablashi, D.V., Pearson, G.R., Krueger, G., Easton, J.M., Bouguermouth, A., Allal, L., Prasad, U., and Connelly, R. Comparison of Epstein-Barr virus antigens in nasopharyngeal carcinoma from intermediate and low risk populations. In: E. Grundmann, G.R.F. Krueger, and D.V. Ablashi (eds.), Nasopharyngeal Carcinoma. Cancer Campaign. Vol. 5, pp. 169-178. New York: Gustav Fischer Verlag-Stuttgart, 1981.

57. Ho, H.C., Lau, W.H., Kwan, H.C., Chan, C.L., Au, G.K.H., Saw, D., and de Thé, G. Diagnostic and prognostic serological markers in nasopharyngeal carcinoma (NPC). In: E. Grundmann, G.R.F. Krueger, and D.V. Ablashi (eds.), Nasopharyngeal Carcinoma. Cancer Campaign. Vol. 5, pp. 219-224. New York: Gustav Fischer Verlag-Stuttgart, 1981.

58. Levine, P.H., Chan, S.H., Terasaki, P., and Hewetson, J. Studies on HLA antigens and EBV antibodies: implications for the prevention of nasopharyngeal carcinoma. In: E. Grundmann, G.R.F. Krueger, and D.V. Ablashi (eds.), Nasopharyngeal Carcinoma. Cancer Campaign. Vol. 5 pp. 247-253. New York: Gustav Fischer Verlag-Stuttgart, 1981.

58A. Joncas, J., Seeley, J., Purtilo, D.T., Ghibu, F.M., Lichaa, H., Robillard, L., Alfieri, C., Rioux, E., and Montplatsir, S. Immunological defect in a family with multiple nasopharyngeal carcinoma (NPC) and Burkitt's lymphoma (BL). In: D. Yohn (ed.), Comparative Leukemia and Related Diseases. pp. 561-562. New York: Elsevier North-Holland, 1982.

59.   de Thé, G., Day, N.E., Geser, A. et al. Seroepidemiology of the Epstein-Barr virus: preliminary analysis of an international study - a review. In: G. de The, M.A. Epstein and H. zur Hausen (eds.), Oncogenesis and Herpesviruses. Part 2, pp. 3-16. II. Internatl. Agency for Research on Cancer, Lyon, 1975.

60.   Henle, G., Henle, W., and Klein, G. Demonstration of two distinct components in the early antigen complex of Epstein-Barr virus infected cells. Int. J. Cancer, 8: 272, 1971.

61.   Pearson, G.R. Epstein-Barr virus: immunology. In: G. Klein (ed.), Viral Oncology. pp. 739-767. New York: Raven Press, 1980.

62.   Kieff, E., Dambaugh, T., Heller, M., King, W., van Santen, V., and Cheung, A. Structure and function of the Epstein-Barr virus genome: a brief overview. In: E. Grundmann, G.R.F. Krueger, and D.V. Ablashi (eds.), Nasopharyngeal Carcinoma. Cancer Campaign. Vol. 5 pp. 87-94. New York: Gustav Fischer Verlag-Stuttgart, 1981.

63.   Kieff, E. Virology: current status. In: IVth Internatl. Sympos. NPC. Kuala Lumpur, Malaysia, 1982; in print.

64.   Bornkamm, G.W. and Desgranges, C. The Epstein-Barr virus genome: structural organization and its detection in nasopharyngeal carcinoma. In: Actualites carcinoloquques. Institut Gustave-Roussy. "Cancer du naso-pharynx." Paris, 1982.

65.   Adams, A. Molecular biology of the Epstein-Barr virus. In: G. Klein (ed.), Viral Oncology. pp. 683-711. New York: Raven Press, 1980.

66.   Haas, W., Krueger, G.R.F., and Vix, M. Further attempts to search for retrovirus related antigens in nasopharyngeal carcinomas and in other neoplasms. In: IVth Internatl. Sympos. NPC. Kuala Lumpur, Malaysia in print, 1982.

67.   Lindahl, T., Klein, G., Reedman, B.M., Johansson, B., and Singh, S. Relationship between Epstein-Barr virus (EBV) DNA and the EBV-determined nuclear antigen (EBNA) in Burkitt lymphoma biopsies and other lymphoproliferative malignancies. Int. J. Cancer, 13:764, 1974.

68.   Epstein, A.L., Henle, W., Henle, G., Hewetson, J.F., and Kaplan, H.S. Surface marker characteristics and Epstein-Barr virus studies of two established North American Burkitt's lymphoma cell lines. Proc. Natl. Acad. Sci. (USA), 73:228, 1976.

69.   Andersson, M. and Lindahl, T. Epstein-Barr virus DNA in human lymphoid cell lines: in vitro conversion. Virology, 73:96, 1976.

70. Klein, G., Giovanella, B., Westman, A., Stehlin, J.S., and
     Mumford, D. An EBV-genome-negative cell line
     established from an American Burkitt lymphoma; receptor
     characteristics, EBV-infectibility, and permanent con-
     version into EBV-positive sublines by in vitro infec-
     tion. Intervirology, 5:319, 1974.
71. Klein, G., Lindahl, T., Jondal, M., Leibold, W., Menezes,
     J., Nilsson, K., and Sundstrom, C. Continuous lymphoid
     cell lines with characteristics of B-cells (bone-marrow-
     derived), lacking the Epstein-Barr virus genome and
     derived from three human lymphomas. Proc. Natl. Acad.
     Sci. USA, 71:3283, 1974.
72. Steinitz, M. and Klein, G. Comparison between growth charac-
     teristics of an Epstein-Barr virus (EBV)-genome-negative
     lymphoma line and its EBV-converted subline in vitro.
     Proc. Natl. Acad. Sci. USA, 72:3518, 1975.
73. Steinitz, M. and Klein, G. Epstein-Barr virus (EBV)-induced
     change in the saturation sensitivity and serum depen-
     dence of established EBV-negative lymphoma lines in
     vitro. Virology, 70:570, 1976.
74. Andersson-Anvret, M. and Lindahl, T. Integrated viral DNA
     sequences in EB virus-converted human lymphoma lines. J.
     Virol. 25:710, 1978.
75. Trumper, P.A., Epstein, M.A., Giovanella, B.C., and Finerty,
     S. Isolation of infectious EB virus from the epithelial
     tumour cells of nasopharyngeal carcinoma. Int. J.
     Cancer, 20:655, 1977.
76. Viral Oncology. G. Klein (ed.). New York: Raven Press,
     1980.
77. The Epstein-Barr Virus. M.A. Epstein, and B.G. Achong
     (eds.). Berlin-Heidelberg-New York: Springer-Verlag,
     1979.
78. Greaves, M.F., Owen, J.J., and Raff, M.C. T- and
     B-lymphocytes: properties and roles in immune response.
     Excerpta Medica Amsterdam, 1973.
79. Jondal, M. and Klein, G. Surface markers on human B- and T-
     lymphocytes. II. Presence of Epstein-Barr virus recep-
     tors on B-lymphocytes. J. Exp. Med., 138:1365, 1973.
80. Klein, G., Yefenof, E., Falk, K., and Westman, A.
     Relationship between Epstein-Barr virus (EBV)-production
     and the loss of EBV receptor/complement receptor complex
     in a series of sublines derived from the same original
     Burkitt's lymphoma. Int. J. Cancer, 21:552, 1978.
81. Einhorn, L., Steinitz, M., Yefenof, E., Ernberg, I., Bakacs,
     T., and Klein, G. Epstein-Barr virus (EBV) receptors,
     complement receptors, and EBV-infectivity of different
     lymphocyte fractions of human peripheral blood. II.
     Epstein-Barr virus studies. Cell. Immunol., 35:43, 1978.
82. Orr, H., Fuks, A., Kaufmann, J. Lancet, D. et al. Structural
     studies of the membrane associated products of the human

major histocompatibility complex. In: C.M. Fenoglio and
D.W. King (eds.), Advances in Pathobiology: Cell
Membranes. New York: Intercontinental Medical Book,
1978.

83. Strominger, J.L. and Thorley-Lawson, D. Early events in
transformation of human lymphocytes by the virus. In:
M.A. Epstein and B.G. Achong (eds.), The Epstein-Barr
virus. Chapter 9. Berlin-Heidelberg-New York: Springer
Verlag, 1979.

84. Wolf, H., Bayliss, G.J., and Wilmes, E. Biological proper-
ties of Epstein-Barr virus. In: E. Grundmann, G.R.F.
Krueger, and D.V. Ablashi (eds.), Nasopharyngeal
Carcinoma. Cancer Campaign. Vol. 5 pp. 101-109. New
York: Gustav Fischer Verlag-Stuttgart, 1981.

85. Pope, J.H. Transformation by the virus in vitro. In: M.A.
Epstein, and B.G. Achong (eds.), The Epstein-Barr Virus.
Chapter 10. Berlin-Heidelberg-New York: Springer Verlag,
1979.

86. Huang, D.P., Ho, H.C., Ng, M.H., and Lui, M. Possible
transformation of nasopharyngeal epithelial cells in
culture with Epstein-Barr virus from B985-8 cells. Br.
J. Cancer, 35:630, 1977.

87. Volsky, D.J., Shapiro, I.M., and Klein, G. Transfer of
Epstein-Barr virus receptors to receptor-negative cell
permits virus penetration and antigen expression. Proc.
Natl. Acad. Sci. USA, 77:9:5453, 1980.

88. Volsky, D.J., Klein, G., Volsky, B., and Shapiro, I.M.
Production of infectious Epstein-Barr virus in mouse
lymphocytes. Nature, 293;5831:399, 1981.

89. Lenoir, G. and de The, G. Epstein-Barr virus epithelial
cell interaction and its implication in the etiology of
nasopharyngeal carcinoma. In: G. de The, and Y. Ito
(eds.), Nasopharyngeal Carcinoma: Etiology and Control.
p. 377. Lyon: IARC.

90. Volsky, D.J. and Shapiro, I.M. Infection of normal human
epithelial cells by Epstein-Barr virus (EBV) following
transplantation of EBV receptors onto epithelial cell
surface. In: IVth Internatl. Sympos. NPC. Kuala
Lumpur, Malaysia, 1982; in print.

91. Glaser, R. The infection of epithelial cells with
Epstein-Barr virus. In: IVth Internatl. Sympos. NPC.
Kuala Lumpur, Malaysia, 1982; in print.

92. Khelifa, R. and Menezes, J. A model study of Epstein-Barr
virus (EBV) penetration into EBV receptor-negative cells.
In: IVth Internatl. Sympos. NPC. Kuala Lumpur, Malaysia,
1982; in print.

93. Pagano, J.S., Raab-Traub, N., Feighny, R., and Pearson, G.
EBV expression in nasopharyngeal carcinoma. In: IVth
Internatl Sympos. NPC. Kuala Lumpur, Malaysia, 1982; in
print.

94. Collett, M.S. and Erikson, R.L. Protein kinase activity associated with the avian sarcoma virus src gene product. Proc. Natl. Acad. Sci. USA, 75:4:2021, 1978.

95. Sen, A. and Todaro, G.J. A murine sarcoma virus-associated protein kinase: interaction with actin and microtubular protein. Cell., 17:347, 1979.

96. Barnekow, A., Boschek, B.C., Ziemiecki, A., and Bauer, H. Detection of src-gene product pp60^{src} and its associated protein kinase on the surface of Rouse-sarcoma-virus-transformed cells. Viochem. Soc. Trans., 8:735, 1980.

97. Erikson, E. and Erikson, R.L. Identification of a cellular protein substrate phosphorylated by the Avian sarcoma virus-transforming gene product. Cell., 21:829, 1980.

98. Hunter, T. and Sefton, B.M. Transforming gene product of Rous sarcoma virus phosphorylates tyrosine. Proc. Natl. Acad. Sci. USA 77:3:1311, 1980.

99. Courtneidge, S.A., Levinson, A.D., and Bishop, J.M. The protein encoded by the transforming gene of avian sarcoma virus (pp60^{src}) and a homologous protein in normal cells (pp60$^{proto-src}$) are associated with the plasma membrane. Proc. Natl. Acad. Sci. USA, 77:7:3783, 1980.

100. Spector, M., O'Neal, S., and Racker, E. Phosphorylation of the subunit of Na$^+$K$^+$-ATPase in Ehrlich ascites tumor by a membrane-bound protein kinase. J. Biol. Chem. 255:18:8370, 1980.

101. Senger, D.R., Wirth, D.F., and Hynes, R.O. Transformation-specific secreted phosphoproteins. Nature, 286:619, 1980.

102. Sharp, P.A. Summary: molecular biology of viral oncogenes. Cold Spring Harbor Sympos. Quant Biol., 44:1305, 1980.

103. Newmark, P. Tyrosine phosphorylation and oncogenes. Nature, 292:15, 1981.

104. Spector, M., Pepinsky, R.B., Vogt, V.M., and Racker, E. A mouse homolog to the Avian sarcoma virus src protein is a member of a protein kinase cascade. Cell., 25:9, 1981.

105. Nonoyama, M., Casareale, D., Tanaka, A., and Smith, M. Macromolecular events during blastogenic transformation of B-lymphocytes with Epstein-Barr virus. In: IVth Internatl. Sympos. NPC. Kuala Lumpur, Malaysia, 1982; in print.

106. Pagano, J.S., Raab-Traub, N., Fleighny, R. and Pearson, G. EBV expression in nasopharyngeal carcinoma. In: IVth Internatl. Sympos. NPC. Kuala Lumpur, Malaysia, 1982; in print.

107. Fraenkel-Conrat, H. RNA polymerase from tobacco necrosis virus infected and uninfected tobacco. Purification of the membrane-associated enzyme. Virology, 72:23, 1976.

108. LeRoy, C., Stussi-Garaud, C., and Hirth, L. RNA-dependent RNA polymerase in uninfected and in Alfalfa Mosaic virus-infected tobacco plants. Virology, 82:48, 1977.

109. Downey, K.M., Byrnes, J.J., Jurmark, B.S., and So, A.G.
       Reticulocyte RNA-dependent RNA polymerase. Proc. Natl.
       Acad. Sci. USA, 70:12:3400, 1973.
110. Todaro, G.J., Fryling, C.H., and deLarco, J.E. Transforming
       growth factors produced by certain human tumor cells:
       polypeptides that interact with epidermal growth factor
       receptors. Proc. Natl. Acad. Sci. USA, 77:9:5258, 1980.
111. Roberts, A.B., Lamb, L.C., Newton, D.L., Sporn, M.B.,
       deLarco, J.E., and Todaro, G.J. Transforming growth
       factors: isolation of polypeptides from virally and
       chemically transformed cells by acid/ethanol extraction.
       Proc. Natl. Acad. Sci. USA, 77:6:3494, 1980.
112. Epstein, M.A. and Achong, B.G. Introduction: discovery and
       general biology of the virus. In: M.A. Epstein and B.G.
       Achong (eds.), The Epstein-Barr Virus. Chapter 1.
       Berlin-Heidelberg-New York: Springer Verlag, 1979.
113. University Health Physicians and PHLS Laboratories.
       Infectious mononucleosis and its relationship to EB
       virus antibody. Br. J. Med., IV:643, 1971.
114. Haider, S., Soutino, M.D., and Emond, R.T.D. Tuberculin
       anergy and infectious mononucleosis. Lancet, ii:74,
       1973.
115. Mangi, R.J., Niederman, J.C., Kelleher, J.E. Jr., Dwyer,
       J.M., Evans, A.S., and Kanto, F.S. Depression of cell
       mediated immunity during acute infectious mononucleosis.
       N. Engl. J. Med., 291:1149, 1974.
116. Henle, G. and Henle, W. Serum IgA antibodies of
       Epstein-Barr virus (EBV)-related antigens. A new
       feature of nasopharyngeal carcinoma. Bibl. Haematol.,
       43:322, 1975.
117. Hutt, L.M., Huang, Y.T., Dascomb, H.E., and Pagano, J.S.
       Enhanced destruction of lymphoid cell lines by
       peripheral blood leukocytes taken from patients with
       acute infectious mononucleosis. J. Immunol., 115:243,
       1975.
118. Royston, I., Sullivan, J.L., Perlman, P.O., and Perlin, E.
       Cell mediated immunity to Epstein-Barr virus-transformed
       lymphoblastoid cells in acute infectious mononucleosis.
       N. Engl. J. Med., 293:1159, 1977.
119. Svedmyr, E. and Jondal, M. Cytotoxic effector cells specif-
       ic for B-cell lines transformed by Epstein-Barr virus
       are present within patients with infectious mono-
       nucleosis. Proc. Natl. Acad. Sci. USA, 72:1622, 1975.
120. Purtilo, D.T., Sakamoto, K., Saemundsen, A.K., Sullivan,
       J.L., Synnerholm, A.C., Andersson-Anvret, M., Pritchard,
       J., Sloper, C., Sieff, C., Pincott, J., Pachman, L.,
       Rich, K., Cruzi, F., Cornet, J., Collins, R., Barnes,
       N., Knight, J., Sandstedt, B., and Klein, G.
       Documentation of Epstein-Barr virus infection in immuno-
       deficient patients with life-threatening lymphoproli-

ferative diseases by clinical, virological, and immunopathological studies. Cancer Res., 41:4226, 1981.

121. Saemundsen, A.K., Purtilo, D.T., Sakamoto, K., Sullivan, J.L., Synnerholm, A.C., Hanto, D., Simmons, R., Anvret, M., Collins, R., and Klein, G. Documentation of Epstein-Barr virus infection in immunodeficient patients with life-threatening lymphoproliferative diseases by Epstein-Barr virus complementary RNA/DNA and viral DNA/DNA hybridization. Cancer Res., 41:4237, 1981.

122. Purtilo, D.T. X-linked lymphoproliferative syndrome: an immunodeficiency disorder with acquired agammaglobulin-emia, fatal infectious mononucleosis or malignant lymphoma following infection by Epstein-Barr virus. Arch. Pathol. Lab. Med., 105:119, 1981.

123. Krueger, G.R.F. and Chan, S.H. Session IVb: non virus-related immunologic data on NPC. In: E. Grundmann, G.R.F. Krueger, and D.V. Ablashi (eds.), Nasopharyngeal Carcinoma. Cancer Campaign. Vol. 5 pp. 324-325. New York: Gustav Fischer Verlag-Stuttgart, 1981.

124. Symposium on Epstein-Barr virus-induced lymphoproliferative diseases in immunodeficient patients. G. Klein and D.T. Purtilo (eds.), Cancer Res., 41:4209, 1981.

125. Penn, I. Allograft Transplant Cancer Registry. In: D.T. Purtilo (ed.), Immune Deficiency and Cancer: Epstein-Barr Virus and Lymphoproliferative Malignancies. New York: Plenum Press, 1983.

126. Penn, I. Malignancies associated with immunosuppressive or cytotoxic therapy. Surgery, 83:492, 1978.

127. Chen-Chuan, L., Jian-Jing, C., and Wan-Jun, L. Early detection of NPC by mass screening and nasopharyngeal mucosal hyperplastic lesion (NPHL). In: IVth Internatl. Sympos. NPC, Kuala Lumpur, Malaysia, in print, 1982.

128. de Thé, G., Desgranges, C., Zeng, Y., Wang, P.C., Bornkamm, G.W., Zhu, J.S., and Shang, M. Search for precancerous lesions and EBV markers in the nasopharynx of IgA positive individuals. In: E. Grundmann, G.R.F. Krueger, and D.V. Ablashi (eds.), Nasopharyngeal Carcinoma. Cancer Campaign. Vol. 5 pp. 111-117. New York: Gustav Fischer Verlag-Stuttgart, 1981.

129. Ho, J.H., Kwan, H.C., Ng, M.H., and de Thé, G. Serum IgA antibodies to Epstein-Barr viral capsid antigen preceding symptoms of nasopharyngeal carcinoma. Lancet, 1:436, 1978.

130. Jondal, M., Svedmyr, E., and Klein, E. Killer T-cells in a Burkitt's lymphoma biopsy. Nature, 225:405, 1975.

131. Klein, E., Svedmyr, E., Jondal, M. and Vanky, F. Functional studies on tumor-infiltrating lymphocytes in man. Isr. J. Med. Sci., 13:747, 1977.

132. de Schryver, A., Rosen, A., Gunven, P., and Klein, G. Comparison between two antibody populations in the EBV

system: anti-MA versus neutralizing antibody activity.
Int. J. Cancer, 17:8, 1976.

133. Levine, P.H., Pizza, G., Cannon, G., Ablashi, D.V.,
     Armstrong, G., and Viza, D. Cell-mediated immunity to
     Epstein-Barr virus-associated membrane antigens in
     patients with nasopharyngeal carcinoma. In: E.
     Grundmann, G.R.F. Krueger, and D.V. Ablashi (eds.),
     Nasopharyngeal Carcinoma. Cancer Campaign. Vol. 5, pp.
     137-144. New York: Gustav Fischer Verlag-Stuttgart,
     1981.

134. Nkrumah, F.K., Herberman, R., Biggar, R.M., and Perkins,
     J.V. Sequential evaluation of cutaneous delayed hyper-
     sensitivity responses to recall and lymphoid cell line
     antigens in Burkitt's lymphoma. Int. J. Cancer, 20:6,
     1977.

135. Levine, P.H., Ho, J.H.C., Nkrumah, F.K., Perlman, P.,
     Mauroli, N., Cannon, G., Middleton, M.B., Perkins,
     J.V., and Herberman, R. Delayed hypersensitivity reac-
     tions of cancer patients to antigens of lymphoid cell
     lines. Int. J. Cancer, 22:400, 1978.

136. Levine, P.H., de Thé, G., Brugere, J., Schwaab, G.,
     Mouroli, N., Herberman, R.B., Ambrosioni, J.C., and
     Rebol, P. Immunity to antigens associated with a cell
     line derived from nasopharyngeal cancer (NPC) in
     on-Chinese NPC patients. Int. J. Cancer, 17:155, 1976.

137. Pope, J.H. Specificity of the cytotoxic T-cell response to
     EBV virus in vitro. In: IVth Internatl. Sympos. NPC.
     Kuala Lumpur, Malaysia, 1982; in print.

138. Chan, S.H., Chew, T.S., Goh, E.H., Simons, M.J., and
     Shanmugaratnam, K. Impaired general cell-mediated
     immune functions in vivo and in vitro in patients with
     nasopharyngeal carcinoma. Int. J. Cancer, 18:139, 1976.

139. Sesterhenn, K., Bertram, G., and Wustrow, F. Skin testing
     in NPC patients. In: E. Grundmann, G.R.F. Krueger, and
     D.V. Ablashi (eds.), Nasopharyngeal Carcinoma. Cancer
     Campaign. Vol. 5, pp. 179-191. New York: Gustav Fischer
     Verlag-Stuttgart, 1981.

140. Bertram, G., Pearson, G.R., Faggioni, A. et al. Long-term
     survey of EBV-serology and non-EBV related tests in
     correlation to the clinical course. In: IVth Internatl.
     Sympos. NPC. Kuala Lumpur, Malaysia, 1982; in print.

141. Micheau, C., de Thé, G., Orofiamma, B., Schwaab, G.,
     Brugere, J., Tursz, T., Sancho-Garnier, H., and
     Cachin, Y. Practical value of classifying NPC in two
     major microscopical types. In: E. Grundmann, G.R.F.
     Krueger, and D.V. Ablashi (eds.), Nasopharyngeal
     Carcinoma. Cancer Campaign. Vol. 5, pp. 51-57. New
     York: Gustav Fischer Verlag-Stuttgart, 1981.

142. Ho, J.H.C. Stage classification of nasopharyngeal carcinoma:
     a review. In: G. de The and Y. Ito (eds.), IARC

Scientific Publ. Vol. 20, pp. 99-113. Lyon: IARC, 1978.

143. de Thé, G., Ho, J.H.C., Ablashi, D.V., Day, N.E., Macario, A.J.L., Martin-Berthelson, M.Cl., Pearson, G., and Sohier, R. Nasopharyngeal carcinoma. IX. Antibodies to EBNA and correlation with response to other EBV antigens in Chinese patients. Int. J. Cancer, 16:713, 1974.

144. Wustrow, J., Karpinski, A., Haas, W., Krueger, G.R.F., Bertram, G., and Sesterhenn, K. Correlation of histological NPC tumor types with local and peripheral T- and B-cell values. In: E. Grundmann, G.R.F. Krueger, and D.V. Ablashi (eds.), Nasopharyngeal Carcinoma. Cancer Campaign. Vol. 5, pp. 193-199. New York: Gustav Fischer Verlag-Stuttgart, 1981.

145. Desgranges, C., Li, J.Y., and de Thé, G. EBV-specific secretory IgA saliva of NPC patients. Presence of secretory piece in epithelial malignant cells. Int. J. Cancer, 20:881, 1977.

146. Pearson, G.R., Weiland, L.F., Neel III, H.G., Taylor, W., Goepfert, H., Huang, A., Hyams, V., Lanier, A., Levine, L., Pilch, B., Henle, G., and Henle, W. Evaluation of antibodies to the Epstein-Barr virus (EBV) in the diagnosis of American nasopharyngeal carcinoma. In: E. Grundmann, G.R.F. Krueger, and D.V. Ablashi (eds.), Nasopharyngeal Carcinoma. Cancer Campaign. Vol. 5, pp. 231-236. New York: Gustav Fischer Verlag-Stuttgart, 1981.

147 Pearson, G.R., Johansson, B., and Klein, G. Antibody-dependent cellular cytotoxicity against Epstein-Barr virus-associated antigens in African patients with nasopharyngeal carcinoma. Int. J. Cancer, 22:120, 1978.

148. Chan, S.H., Levine, P.H., de The, G., Mulroney, S.E., Lauoue, M.F., Glen, S.P.P., Goh, E.H., Khor, T.H., and Connelly, R.R. A comparison of the prognostic values of antibody-dependent lymphocyte cytotoxicity and other EBV antibody assays in Chinese patients with nasopharyngeal carcinoma. Int. J. Cancer, 23:181, 1979.

149. Bertram, G., Pearson, G.R., Faggioni, A., Armstrong, G., Krueger, G.R.F., and Ablashi, D.V. The nasopharyngeal carcinoma (NPC): prognostic estimation of antibody-dependent-cellular-cytotoxicity (ADCC). Arch. Otorhinolaryngol., 231:768, 1981.

150. Sundar, K.S., Ablashi, D.V., Kamaraju, L.S., Levine, P.H., Fagguni, A., Armstrong, G.R., Pearson, G.R., Krueger, G.R.F., Hewetson, J.F., Bertram, G., Sesterhenn, K., and Menezes, J. Sera from patients with undifferentiated nasopharyngeal carcinoma contain a factor which abrogates specific Epstein-Barr virus antigen-induced lymphocytes responses. Int. J. Cancer, 29:407, 1982.

151. Heimer, R. and Klein, G. Circulating immune complexes in
        sera of patients with Burkitt's lymphoma and
        nasopharyngeal carcinoma. Int. J. Cancer, 18:310, 1976.

BURKITT'S LYMPHOMA

James Linder and
David T. Purtilo

Department of Pathology and Laboratory Medicine
University of Nebraska Medical Center
Omaha, NE

INTRODUCTION

In this review of Burkitt's lymphoma, we discuss recent
clinical and pathological advances in the understanding of this
unique malignancy. Burkitt's lymphoma (BL) has been the subject
of intense investigation ever since Burkitt's classic description
in 1958 (18). The lively interest in this lymphoma stems from
climatological and geographical distribution which had suggested a
mosquito-vectored virus as the etiologic agent (20,21,49). The
subsequent discovery of the Epstein-Barr virus (EBV) in cultured
BL cells gave credence to this view (38). Virologists continue
to study this herpesvirus as a model for viral-induced oncogenesis
(23,39,66,145). Second, the exquisite sensitivity of this tumor
to chemotherapy suggested a potential for cure. This plus the
pioneering work regarding chemotherapy of acute lymphocytic leukemias by the prominent pathologist, Sidney Farber, has provided
impetus for modern chemotherapy programs. Finally, BL is unique
in its histopathologic, immunologic, and cytogenetic attributes.
The surface markers studies of BL have demonstrated arrested
lymphocyte differentiation. Other cancers are viewed also in the
context of blocked autogeny.

We address etiologic, clinical and pathologic attributes of
Burkitt's lymphoma. Space limitations prevent us from discussing
all subjects in detail, however, we have endeavored to provide an
update. The monograph by Burkitt and Wright remains an invaluable
resource (22).

CLINICAL FEATURES

African Burkitt's Lymphoma

In the early 1900's, Cook, Smith, Elmes, and others observed tumors in jaws of African children (56). Denis Burkitt brought attention to this tumor outside the African continent and noted the association between the jaw "sarcomas" and similar visceral tumors (18). His observations were corroborated and amplified by O'Connor and Davies, and Brew and Jackson in studies of malignant lymphomas in Uganda and Nigeria, respectively (56). Subsequent work defined the clinical features of Burkitt's lymphoma and the distribution of tumor (19,87,90,93).

The spectrum of presenting clinical features of 557 cases of Burkitt's lymphoma seen in Kampala from 1950 to 1965 are enu-

Table 1.   Main presenting features of African Burkitt's Lymphoma in Uganda - 1950 to 1965*

Clinical Feature	No.	%
Jaw tumors	306	55
Single jaw tumor	145	26
Multiple jaw tumors	119	21.5
All 4 quadrants of jaw involved	42	7.5
Abdominal swelling	139	25
Ovarian tumors[a]	70	38
Testicular tumors[b]	14	3.8
Paraplegia	38	6.8
Bone tumors other than jaw	37	6.7
Femur	18	3.2
Tibia	7	1.2
Humerus	4	0.7
Others	11	2.0
Tumor of the thyroid	24	4.3
Tumor of salivary glands	17	3.0
Enlargement of superficial lymph nodes	29	5.2
Cervical nodes	19	3.4
Inguinal nodes	9	1.6
Others	1	0.2
Tumors of the breast	9	1.6
Others	9	1.6

[a]Percentages based on the number of females in the series.
[b]Percentages based on the number of males in the series.
*Adapted from Wright, D.H.: Burkitt's lymphoma: A review of the pathology, immunology and possible etiologic factors. Path. Ann. 5:337-363, 1971.

merated in Table 1 (128). The jaws, the most frequent site, were involved in virtually all patients, followed by abdominal tumors in 25%. In subsequent studies, from 1967 to 1977, involvement of jaw occurred in 72% of cases and abdomen 56%; in addition, 30% had central nervous system (CNS) involvement (96). Based on these data and other experiences the following observations can be made.

The mandible and maxilla are involved at approximately equal frequency. The tumor presents as a large expansile mass distorting facial structures (Figure 1). Orbital involvement with exophthalmos or ophthalmoplegia affects approximately 18% of patients, secondary to direct extension of maxillary tumor.

Lymphoma involves CNS in approximately one-third of cases (96,134). Intracranial extension of facial tumors proceeds along cranial nerves and soft tissues, or by hematogenous spread. The manifestion of CNS involvement are protean. Paraplegia occurs in 15% of patients, by bulky retroperitoneal tumor directly compressing the spinal cord, or compromising its vascular supply. Patients may exhibit cranial nerve palsies, increased intracranial pressure, or meningeal signs. These symptoms are often the harbinger of relapse in treated patients (139).

Massive ascites usually portends abdominal tumor (1,45,63, 100). Lymphoma in the mesentary bowel wall may cause obstruction or trigger intussusception. Lymphoma may extend to multiple abdominal organs and peritoneal surfaces before being recognized.

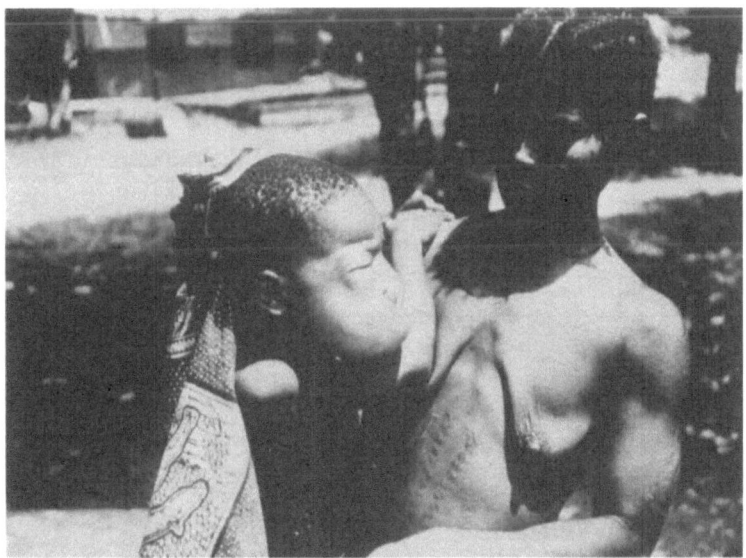

Fig. 1. Burkitt's lymphoma of jaw in a young African male.

This reflects the difficulty of identifying early abdominal
involvement and the rapid growth rate (doubling time 18-24 hours)
of BL (57,141).

Autopsy series in the early 1960's showed approximately 50%
had tumor in the jaw, gastrointestinal tract or endocrine glands
with only 8% involving CNS (127).   In contrast, in chemotherapy
eras from 1964-1967 and 1968-1971 a progressive decrease in residual jaw or visceral tumors emerged (121).   Concomitantly, CNS
involvement developed.   This observations mirrored longer survival, and chemotherapy protocols ineffective in the CNS, which
provides a sanctuary for tumor.

Non-Africa Burkitt's lymphoma

A search was begun in the 1960's for BL in the United States
and other countries.   Pediatric files covering a 40 year period at
the Armed Forces Institute of Pathology uncovered 20 out of 148
cases of malignant lymphoma showing histologic and clinical
features compatible with BL (89).   Additional American cases have
been identified and studied through the American Burkitt's
Lymphoma Registry (2,3,28,67,142,144).   Sporadic cases have been
reported worldwide (1,4,42,63).   Table 2 compares the African and
non-African patients.   The histology and response to chemotherapy
of the American and African tumors is similar.   However, the mode
of presentation differs.   American patients more frequently have
abdominal rather than jaw lymphoma.   Although the proportion of
African patients presenting with abdominal tumor is increasing
(13).   American patients are older at presentation than African
counterparts.   The mean age is 12 years with nearly one-third over
age 15.   While African patients have peak incidence at approximately 7 years.   Involvement of the bone marrow is more common in

Table 2.   Comparison of Burkitt's Lymphoma in
African and Non-African Children

Feature	African	Non-African
Distribution	Endemic	Non-endemic
Mean age	7 years	13 years
Histopathology	Identical	Identical
Chromosome abnormalities	t(8;14, 2, 22)	t(8;14, 2, 22)
Anti-EBV antibodies	All high titer	Rare
EBV genome	90-97%	15-20%
Bone marrow involvement	Rare	31%
Response to chemotherapy	Excellent	Excellent

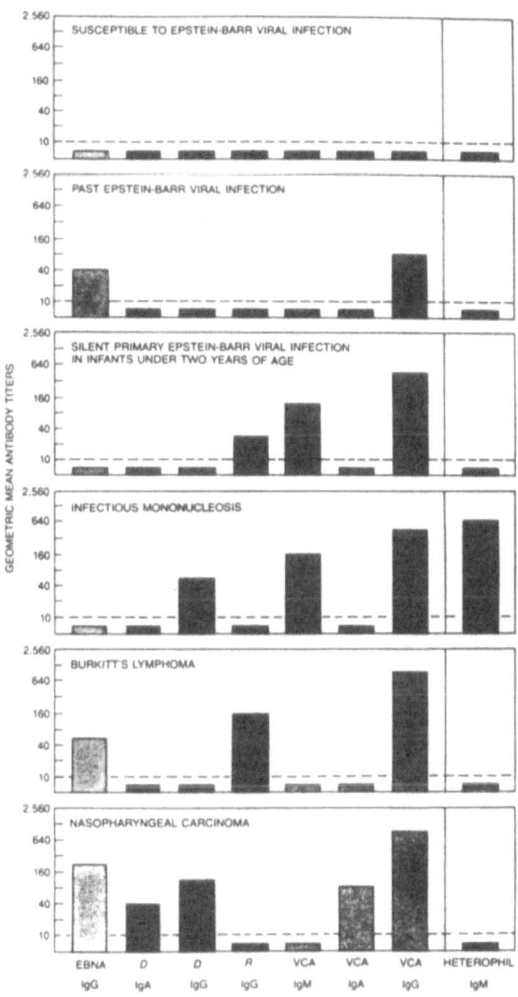

Fig. 2.   Pattern of antibodies to the Epstein-Barr virus differ
          significantly in the various diseases associated with the
          virus. Susceptible individuals lack antibody while those
          with past infections exhibit anti-EBNA and VCA IgG.
          Acute infections have anti-VCA IgM. African Burkitt's
          lymphoma patients have high titer antibodies, as do
          patients with nasopharyngeal carcinoma. (EBNA =
          Epstein-Barr nuclear-associated antigen; D, R = diffuse
          or restricted early antigen; VCA = viral capsid antigen)
          (From: Henle, W. et al. The Epstein-Barr virus. Sci.
          Am. 241:48, 1979. Copyright© (1983) by Scientific
          American, Inc. All rights reserved).

non-African patients (26,117,119). A leukemic phase of Burkitt's lymphoma, analogous to the L_3 type of lymphocytic leukemia in the French-American-British (FAB) classification may occur in American patients. Significant differents in association between EBV and BL on the two continents is seen. Serologic evidence of EBV infection is present in virtually all cases of African Burkitt's lymphoma, while less common in American patients (Figure 2) (52,54,69). Moreover, EBV genome is found in nearly all (i.e., 90-97%) of African cases, whereas the genome is found in only 15-20% of non-African cases (29,46,95).

Staging

Owing to the unusual predilection for extranodal tissues, the classic staging on non-Hodgkin's lymphoma has been modified for BL (Table 3) (142). Stages A through D indicate increasing tumor burden. Stage AR describes patients who have undergone surgical resection of intraabdominal tumor prior to chemotherapy. Adequate staging requires thorough physical examination, radiologic studies (36) (i.e., intravenous pyelography, skeletal, and computerized tomography), bone marrow aspiration, and cytologic examination of cerebral spinal fluid. Patients with BL often show elevated B-aminoisobutyric acid in urine and lactate dehydrogenase (LDH) in serum (16,58). The level of LDH measures tumor burden and predicts chemotherapy response.

Treatment

The explosive growth of BL is unique and renders it exquisitely sensitive to chemotherapy. The growth fraction approaches 100%, and the doubling time is less than 24 hrs (57,141). This feature mandates prompt and accurate diagnosis and treatment. Early studies showed 157 and 192 Ugandan patients responding to high dose cyclosphosphamide (148), while other protocols employed

Table 3. Clinical Stages of Burkitt's Lymphoma

Stage	Extent of Tumor
A	Single extra-abdominal site
B	Multiple extra-abdominal sites
C	Intra-abdominal tumor
D	Intra-abdominal tumor, with extra-abdominal tumor
AR	Stage C, but with more than 90% of tumor surgically resected

methotrexate alone (92). However, cyclophosphamide is the drug of choice (136,138,142). Other anti-metabolite agents, including methotrexate, cytosine arabinoside, and vincristine have been incorporated into multi-agent protocols which improve initial remissions and lessen relapse (Table 4) (88,94,146). Excellent response rates with all protocols is seen. The combination of cyclophosphamide, vincristine and methotrexate is advantageous in achieving complete response and low relapse rates in American patients (147).

A blemish in the management has been failure to develop adequate CNS prophylaxis. Protocols employing prophylactic intrathecal methotrexate and cranio-spinal irradiation have not uniformly lessened the occurrence of meningeal lymphoma (137). A recent study combining chemotherapy and intrathecal methotrexate lowered the risk of very late relapses (74).

Relapses in Burkitt's lymphoma occur equally in either of two patterns (12,86,139). Early relapses, occurring less than 12 weeks after the induction of remission most likely represents regrowth of the original tumor. In these cases, drug resistance is common and patients have a poorer prognosis than relapses occurring 12 weeks after the induction of remission. Late relapses may represent a second clone of tumor, distinct from the primary lesion. This hypothesis is supported by finding different G6PD isoenzyme types in primary and recurrent lymphoma of a young girl (41).

Surgery is required for diagnosis, and is a useful adjunct in the management since resection of greater than 90% of the tumor bulk doubles survival, independent of other prognostic factors (72).

The role of radiotherapy in the treatment of Burkitt's lymphoma is unclear. Because the tumor is usually multicentric, radiotherapy is not a practical solitary mode of treatment. Abdominal and CNS radiotherapy has been attempted to minimize relapse. Regrettably, this adjunctive therapy has not been beneficial.

The high responsiveness to chemotherapy is paralleled by a very favorable survival rate. Individuals with stage A or B disease respond well to chemotherapy and have 5 year survival rates ranging from 67 to 82%. Patients with C and D stages have survival rates of 50% and 15%, respectively. As mentioned earlier, the survival of the high stage patients may be dramatically improved by surgically debulking the tumor. Aside from stage, favorable prognoses are associated with young age, females, and high titers of antibody directed against the viral capsid antigen (VCA) of EBV (51). The survival rates, response to che-

Table 4. Results of Treatment Regimens for Burkitt's Lymphoma*

Site of Trial	Regimen**	Ref.	Evaluable	Complete Response	Partial Response	Relapse/Complete Response
				No. of Patients†		
Africa	CTX	94	18	15(83)	3	7/15(47)
	CTX	88	42	34(81)	8	21/34(62)
	CTX	138	79	74(94)	5	46/74(62)
	COM	94	19	16(84)	3	10/16(32)
	CVA	88	31	29(94)	2	9/29(31)
	TRIKE	140	22	21(95)	1	12/21(57)
United States	COM	146	27	27(100)	0	13/27(48)
	COMP	146	37	35(95)	2	15/35(43)
	CHOMP	74	25	22(88)	3	5/22(23)

** CTX denotes cyclophosphamide; COM, cyclophosphamide/vincristine/
methotrexate, CVA cyclophosphamide/vincristine/cytarabine, TRIKE
Cyclophosphamide alternating with vincristine/methotrexate and cytarabine,
COMP COM plus prednisolone, and CHOMP COMP plus doxorubicin and intermittent
high-dose methotrexate.

† Figures in parentheses denote percentages

* Adapted from Ziegler, J.L. Burkitt's lymphoma. N. Engl. J. Med., 305:735,
1981.

motherapy, and long term prognoses of American and African
patients is similar (149).

The rapid growth of BL may cause several complications. Head
and neck tumor involvement may compromise respiratory or vascular
channels. Abdominal lymphoma may obstruct the bowel, or induce
intussusception. Large retroperitoneal tumors may compress
ureters, resulting in hydronephrosis and renal failure. The blood
supply to the spinal cord may be compromised, or direct cord
compression can occur. Because of the exquisite sensitivity to
chemotherapeutic agents, massive tumor necrosis can occur at the
onset of therapy. Release of large amounts of potassium, uric
acid and other metabolites produces the Tumor Lysis Syndrome
(24,27). Acute renal failure due to uric acid nephropathy is a
life-threatening manifestation of this syndrome. Adequate hydra-
tion and alkalinization of the urine can obviate this complication. Potassium-wasting diuretics and oral exchange resins help
to manage the hyperkalemia and hyperphosphatemia.

Hematopathology

Proper tissue preparation is essential for the diagnosis of
BL. For histopathologic sections, tissue must be sectioned, 2-3
mm, and placed in adequate amounts of buffered formalin or other
fixative. Fixation is the most important step in the preparation
of histologic sections. Subsequent processing cannot restore
tissue destroyed by poor fixation. The technical aspects of lymph
node processing have been recently reviewed. Thorough immunologic
and virologic examination of lymph node requires tissue be frozen
at -70°C for determining surface immunoglobulin or specific
markers for T- and B-lymphocytes by using monoclonal antibodies.
Frozen tissue may also be probed for specific viral antigens,
viral DNA or RNA. Such studies may aid in understanding of the
etiology of malignant lymphomas. Touch imprints are useful for
enzyme histochemistry, and for identification of subtle cytoplasmic features such as lipid vacuoles. Portions of tissue should be
fixed in glutaraldehyde or other suitable preservatives in the
event that ultrastructural studies are indicated. Considering the
high frequency of chromosomal abnormalities in malignant lymphomas, samples of freshly explanted tumor should be studied by
karyotyping.

Light Microscopy

The striking appearance of BL in jaws of African children
prompted some clinicians to regard it as a clinical syndrome
rather than a distinct entity. Support for this view came from
observations that tumors of varied histogenesis and behavior
mimicked the clinical presentation. Prospective studies in the
1960's however, proved that characteristic histologic features of

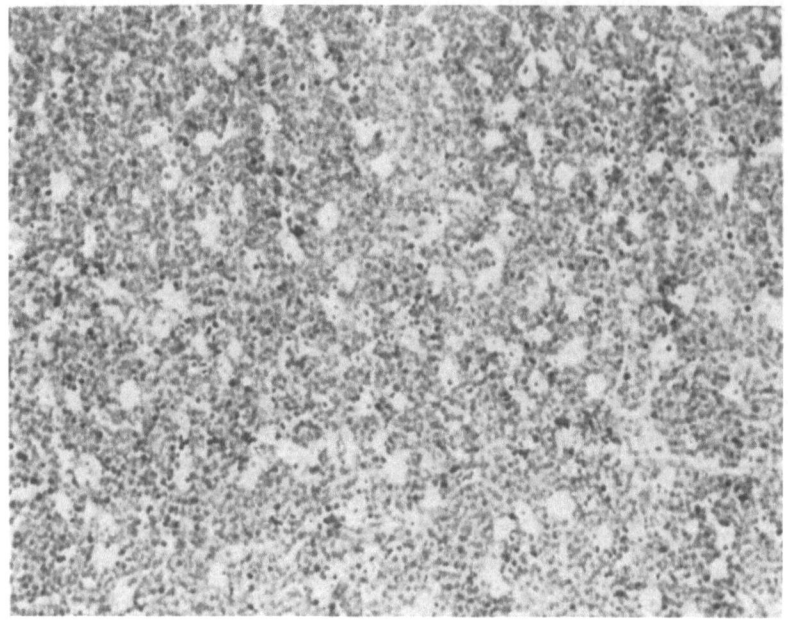

Fig. 3. Burkitt's lymphoma with monotonous small lymphocytes
with interspersed macrophages.

BL could be defined and that neoplasms with these histologic
features had a unique clinical course and responsiveness to
chemotherapy (34). A select group of hematopathologists, under
the auspices of the World Health Organization (WHO), developed
diagnostic criteria for BL in 1969 (5). Histologically, BL is
expansile and nodular rather than diffusely infiltrating. At
scanning magnification the tumor appears as a monotonous growth of
darkly staining uniform round cells, with large clear cells
interspersed throughout. Macrophages ingesting cellular debris
from necrosis of the rapidly growing tumor produces the so-called
"starry sky" pattern (Figure 3). Mitoses are numerous and prominent.

The malignant cells measure 8 to 10 micrometers in diameter in
tissue section. The nucleus is round to oval and has a prominent
nuclear membrane. Chromatin is coarse, reticulated, and irregularly distributed. Two to five nucleoli are usually present
(Figure 4) and may be more prominent at the center of the tumor
where fixation is suboptimal. The nucleus occupies nearly the
entire volume of the cell. The narrow rim of cytoplasm is moderately basophilic and vacuolated. The quantity of the supporting
stroma depends on the tissue involved. Usually, tumor masses have
scanty reticular support.

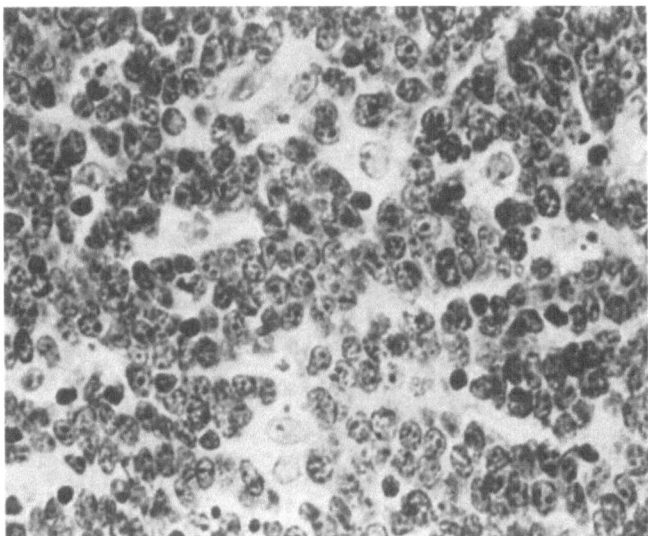

Fig. 4. Photomicrograph of small lymphoid cells of Burkitt's
         lymphoma. Note the oval nuclei with coarse chromatin
         and two to five nucleoli. Hematoxylin and eosin X450.

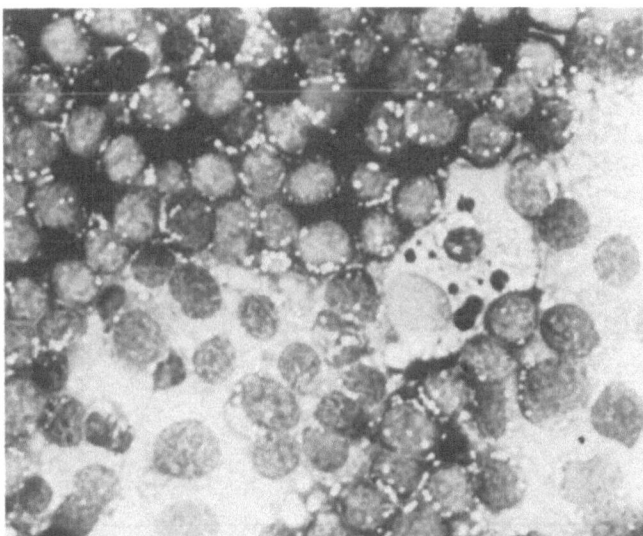

Fig. 5. Photomicrograph of imprint preparation of Burkitt's
         lymphoma reveals prominent cytoplasmic basophilia and
         lipid vacuoles. A macrophage with ingested cellular
         debris is present. Wright's-Giemsa stain, X970.

Table 5.   Cytologic Features of Burkitt's Lymphoma

Uniform lymphoid cells 12 um to 25 um in diameter
Round to oval nuclei
Coarse nuclear chromatin with clear parachromatin
One to five nucleoli per cell
High nuclear:cytoplasm ratio
Amphophilic cytoplasm
Cytoplasmic lipid vacuoles

Air-dried Romanovsky or Wright-Giemsa stained imprints of BL show several characteristic features (Figure 5) (Table 5) (99). The cells are usually larger than in tissue section, i.e., 8 to 24 micrometers in diameter. Cytoplasmic basophilia and lipid vacuoles are prominent. These vacuoles stain with both Sudan Black B and Oil-Red O. Sudanophilia is intense near areas of

Table 6.   Comparison of Cytochemical Properties of
            Burkitt's Lymphoma, Acute Lymphocytic
            Leukemia and Lymphoblastic Lymphoma

Method	Burkitt's Lymphoma	Acute Lymphocytic Leukemia	Lymphoblastic Lymphoma
Oil-Red-O/ Sudan Black B	+++	−	−
Periodic Acid Schiff	+̲	++	+
Methyl Green Pyronin	++	−	−
Alkaline Phosphatase	+̲	+̲	+̲
Acid Phosphatase	−	+̲	+
Alphanaphthyl Acetate esterase	−	−	+
Terminal deoxytransferase	−	+	+

Key: −   = negative
         +̲   = weakly positive
         +   = moderately positive
         ++   = moderate to strongly positive
         +++   = strongly positive (most cells)

degeneration. Macrophages may be stuffed with fat globules, and phagocytized debris. Tumor cells generally are not periodic acid Schiff (PAS) reactive. The cytoplasm has intense pyrinophilia with methyl green pyronin due to an abundance of ribonucleic acid. Alkaline phosphatase, acid phosphatase, esterase, and 5' nucleotidase are lacking in BL, however, sensitive methods can detect acid phosphatase in some cells. Cytochemical properties are sometimes useful in differential diagnosis, Table 6.

Immunohistochemistry

During the 1960's, knowledge of the immune system mushroomed. Simultaneously, immunologic techniques were applied to study malignant lymphomas, allowing stages of lymphocyte differentiation to be defined (10,73). Classification schemes based on the immunologic characteristics, as well as the histology of lymphomas naturally developed.

Production of monoclonal IgM by cultured BL cells lines and surface immunoglobulin on free lymphoma cells in more than 85% of cases has been demonstrated (48,64,75,135). Cytoplasmic immunoglobulin is difficult to demonstrate. Other B-cell markers on BL cells include receptors for C3d, EBV, peanut agglutinin, Fc fragments, and Ia antigen (HLA DR) (112). BL binds monoclonal antibodies specific for B-lymphocytes (118) but do not express T-

Table 7. Comparison of Immunologic Characteristics of
Burkitt's Lymphoma, Acute Lymphocytic Leukemia,
and Lymphoblastic Lymphomas

Marker	Burkitt's Lymphoma	Acute Lymphocytic Leukemia	Lymphoblastic Lymphoma
SIg	+(IgM)	-*	-
EAC	+	+	-
Ia	+	Rare+	-
E-Rosette Receptor	-	-	+
CALLA	rare+	Many+	-

Comments:	SIg	= Surface immunoglobulin
	EAC	= Erythrocyte Activated Complement Receptor
	Ia	= HLADR
	CALLA	= Common Acute Lymphocytic Leukemia Antigen
	* Except for Burkitt's Leukemia	

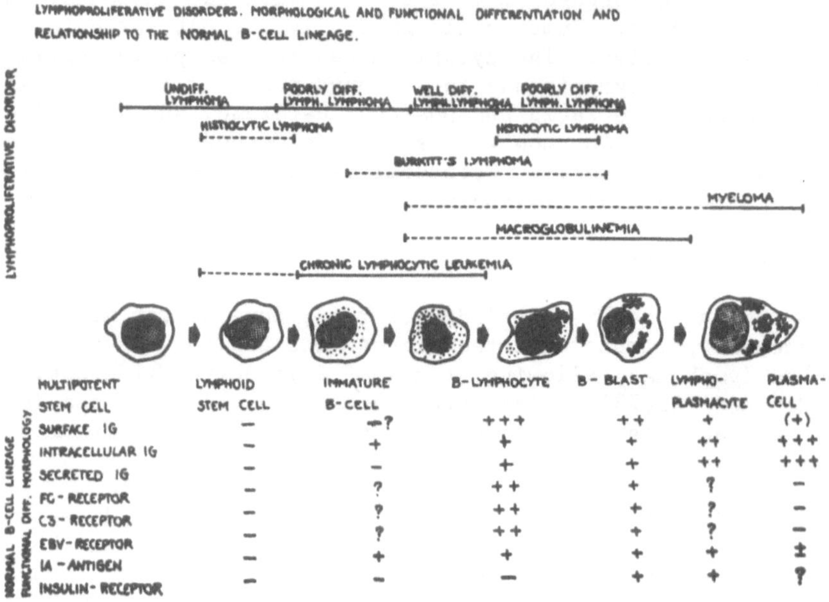

LYMPHOPROLIFERATIVE DISORDERS. MORPHOLOGICAL AND FUNCTIONAL DIFFERENTIATION AND
RELATIONSHIP TO THE NORMAL B-CELL LINEAGE.

Fig. 6.   Burkitt lymphoma cells are intermediate in differen-
          tiation with features of early, and mature B lymphocytes.
          Published with permission of Anders Rosen.

lymphocyte antigens OKT3, OKT4, OKT8 and OKT11. Rare cases exhibit the common ALL antigen. Regrettably, no prognostic significance has been derived from these marker studies. However, they
may aid in differential diagnosis (Table 7).

     These features confirm the origin of BL from B-lymphocytes
(14). In the context that malignant lymphomas are disorders of
lymphoid differentiation, BL cells are frozen at an early stage of
differentiation, just beyond the pre-B-cell. The tumor cells will
differentiate slightly when treated with phorbol esters. Insulin
and other receptors can be induced, but basically the cells are
frozen in an immature state (Figure 6).

Electron Microscopy of Burkitt's Lymphoma

     Primitive monomorphism mirroring the tissue sections in
including oval nuclei, which may have nuclear pockets or invagina-
tions characteristic of lymphoma cells are seen in electron
micrographs (37,62). The nuclear membrane is distinct and
overlies condensed chromatin. One or more nucleoli are present.
The cytoplasm is relatively simple, containing scattered
mitochondria, polyribosomes and scant glycogen. Lipid vacuoles
are seen in 13 to 30% of cells. The surface of cells may have

small projections corresponding to cytoplasmic ruffles viewed by scanning electron microscopy (68).

Extensive ultrastructural studies on biopsies have not definitively identified viral particles. Epstein and colleagues worked five years before finding viral particles. Only after explanted tumor was grown in culture did the virus form particles demonstrable by electron microscopy. Immune surveillance _in vivo_ may block formation of viral particles.

Classification

The World Health Organization in 1969 designated Burkitt's lymphoma as a "malignant lymphoma, undifferentiated, Burkitt's type" (5). The widely used Rappaport classification simply refers to this neoplasm as "Burkitt's tumor." In the Lukes-Collins classification scheme, Burkitt's lymphoma is a follicular center cell (FCC) lymphoma of a "small, non-cleaved type." The New International Formulation of Non-Hodgkin's Malignant Lymphomas classifies this neoplasm as a "malignant lymphoma, small non-cleaved cell, Burkitt type." Whichever classification scheme is used, it is prudent to include the term "Burkitt's lymphoma" to alert clinicians to necessity for prompt treatment.

Cytogenetics

Significant technical advances have facilitated cytogenetic study of hematologic malignancies. Sandberg summarizes these advances elsewhere in this book. The consistent findings of chromosomal deletions or reciprocal translocations in lymphomas have provoked interest (110,131). Subgroups with specific chromosome abnormalities may have different responses to treatment (132). Furthermore, translocations might be a pathogenetic mechanism in these tumors.

The chromosomal abnormalities in BL have been extensively studied after the description of marker chromosome 14q+ (76). In most cases, translocation occurs between chromosomes 8 and 14 [t(8;14) (q24:q32)] (61,77,111,133). Initially the t(8;14) was thought to be specific for BL. However, reciprocal translocations between chromosome 8 and chromosomes 2 or 22 also occur, suggesting that 8q- may be the specific change in BL, rather than 14q+ (Figure 7) (7,9,8,17,55,82,124). This viewpoint is supported by the observation that a 14q+ anomaly occurs in many other histologic types of malignant lymphoma (78,106). In a recent report 55 of 128 non-Hodgkin's, non-Burkitt's lymphomas expressed a 14q+ anomaly (111). The donor chromosomes translocated include chromosomes 1, 8, 10, 11, 14, and 18 (33,43,44,79,131,133). The 14q+ translocation has also been found in mycosis fungoides, multiple myeloma, and Hodgkin's disease (111). This translocation may be

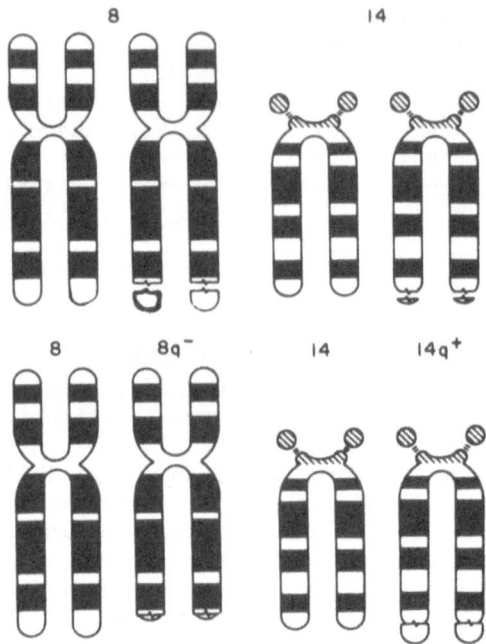

Fig. 7.   In Burkitt's lymphoma cells the terminal region of chro-
          mosome 8 (top left) exchanges with the terminal segment
          of chromosome 14 (top left) to form altered chromosomes
          8q- and 14q+.   The translocated portion of chromosome 8
          harbors the myc oncogene, which may play a role in B
          lymphocyte transformation (80).   (From: Merz, B. Migrant
          oncogene-Burkitt's lymphoma link. J. Am. Med. Assoc.,
          248:2424, 1982.   "Copyright 1982, American Medical
          Association.")

due to instability of the genetic locus coding for heavy chain of
immunoglobulin located at the distal region of the long arm of
chromosome 14.   Besides translocations, numerical changes of chromosomes 3, 7 and X, and morphologic abnormalities of chromosomes
2, 8 and 11 occur in BL (6,7,8).   Similar chromosomal abnormalities typify the L_3 type B-cell acute lymphoblastic leukemia
(81,85,107,115) in the FAB classification, suggesting that this
leukemia and BL are manifestations of the same malignancy (71).

    The specific chromosomal translocations in BL has tempted
Rowley (109) to speculate that they are instrumental to malignant
transformation of cells.   She noted that the loci for genes at the
sites on chromosomes 14, 2 and 22 code for heavy chain, kappa
light chain, and lambda light chain, respectively.   These sites on
these chromosomes are frequently reciprocally translocated with
chromosome 8 in Burkitt's lymphoma.   Genes adjacent to the immu-

noglobulin locus, or the immunoglobulin locus itself may promote
proliferation (Figure 7). Activation of the myc oncogenes on
chromosome 8 at the reattachment point is thought to turn-on cell
proliferation (80). This hypothesis is being investigated.

Differential Diagnosis

Aside from BL, the differential diagnoses of bulky jaw tumors
includes a variety of small-cell tumors, benign and malignant bone
tumors, and disorders of the hematopoietic system that are morphologically similar to Burkitt's lymphoma.

Embryonal rhabdomyosarcomas of the face and jaw may be grossly
indistinguishable from the jaw tumor of BL. Identification of
spindle cells and rhabdomyoblasts with cross-striations and PAS
positivity establishes the diagnosis. Ewing's sarcoma uncommonly
involves the jaw (79,80). The nuclei of Ewing's sarcoma have
finely-dispersed chromatin which imparts a ground-glass appearance, in contrast to the coarse, reticulated chromatin of BL. The
cells of Ewing's sarcoma have less cytoplasm, and contain abundant
glycogen.

Retinoblastoma and neuroblastoma often occur as orbital tumors
in children. In both, tumor cells may form rosettes while
Burkitt's lymphoma cells do not, and the tumors differ in their
touch-imprint morphology. Neuroblastomas, and nephroblastomas
(Wilms' tumors) in the abdomen can simulate BL.

Benign jaw lesions to be distinguished from BL, include
ossifying fibroma, adamantinoma, dental cysts, and osteomyelitis
(70,127).

Several hematopoietic tumors may have histologic appearance
similar to BL, including acute lymphoblastic leukemia; malignant
lymphoma, poorly differentiated lymphocytic type; malignant
lymphoma, histiocytic type; acute myeloblastic leukemia; and
follicular center cell lymphoma of childhood. These tumors may
have a "starry sky" pattern, or tumor cells with cytoplasmic
vacuoles mimicking BL (25). In a recent critical review of 24
cases of "Burkitt's lymphoma", for example, 9 were actually immunoblastic sarcomas. The major source of confusion was a "starry
sky" pattern.

Acute lymphoblastic leukemia is distinguished from BL by
nuclear clefts, delicate nuclear chromatin, less conspicuous
nucleoli, less intense cytoplasmic pyrinophilia and PAS-positive
granules (Table 6, 7). Immunologic marker studies are an
excellent method to distinguish these diseases. Acute lymphoblastic lymphoma of childhood expresses T-lymphocyte markers, in
contrast to the B-lymphocyte markers of BL (47).

Malignant lymphoma, histiocytic type, generally has more
cytoplasm, larger, more pleomorphic nuclei and more prominent
nucleoli than cells of BL. Lipid vacuoles can occur in the
cytoplasm of histiocytic lymphomas, but they tend to be larger
than those of BL cells.

The variability of nuclear shape of the poorly differentiated
lymphocytic lymphoma distinguishes this tumor from BL. The cells
of poorly differentiated lymphocytic lymphoma have prominent
nuclear clefts and grooves, with coarse irregularly distributed
chromatin. These cells lack the cytoplasmic pyrinophilia of BL.

Acute myeloblastic leukemia rarely presents as a chloroma of
the soft tissues of the face. Usually a concomitant leukemic picture is present, which facilitates differentiation from Burkitt's
lymphoma. Positive reactions with the naphthol-AS-D chloracetate
esterase reaction reveals the granulocytic origin of these tumors.

Malignant lymphomas with a follicular growth pattern are unusual in childhood. Although individual cells may resemble BL,
the follicular architecture, the presence of cytopplasmic immunoglobulin, and the nuclear cleavages in some cells permits differentiation from BL (129).

Epidemiology and Etiology

In endemic areas of Africa, such as Kenya and Uganda, BL is
the most common malignancy of childhood, approaching 10/100,000/
year. In tropical Africa the tumor is most common in warm, moist
areas and is absent in the mountains. Such a distribution is
consistent with a mosquito-vectored virus, similar to yellow fever
(20). Early studies of BL also demonstrated space-time clustering, giving credence to an infectious etiology, particularly in
the West Nile district of Uganda (83,84). In the United States
clustering of BL has also been observed (59,65). More recent
studies, however, have pointed out the difficulty of interpreting
space-time clustering (114).

The search for a potential etiologic agent came to fruition in
1966 when Epstein, Achong and Barr discovered a herpes-like virus
(what is now the Epstein-Barr virus [EBV]) in a Burkitt's lymphoma
cell line (38). This fostered much investigation on the link between EBV and BL. No study, however, has yet to conclusively prove
EBV as the etiologic agent of BL. EBV viral genome has been found
by DNA hybridization techniques in 88 of 90 biopsies from Uganda
and Kenya patients, with 6 to 133 genome equivalents per tumor
cell. In contrast, American Burkitt's lymphoma infrequently
(8-17% of cases) harbors EBV genome (150,151).

Seroepidemiological studies in endemic areas reveal EBV infec-

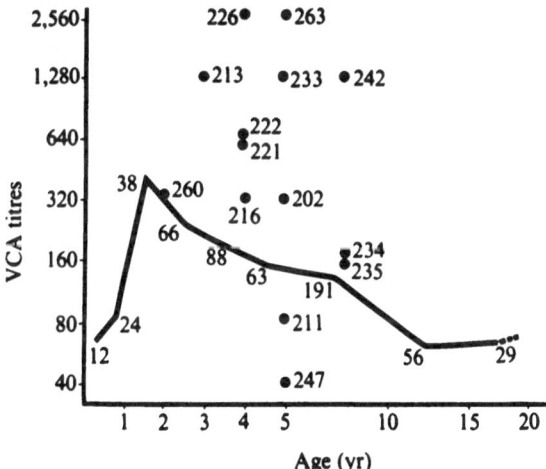

Fig. 8.   Viral capsid antibody titers in sera collected from BL
          cases (), before tumor manifestation compared with
          antibody titers in a random sample of the population
          in the study area (-). Numbers against the solid line
          indicate number of sera tested in the random sample.
          (From: de The, G. et al. Epidemiological evidence for
          causal relationship between Epstein-Barr virus and
          Burkitt lymphoma from Ugandan prospective study. Nature,
          274:756, 1978. Published with permission of Nature.)

tion occurs early so that by age 2 years, nearly 80% of African
children have anti-EBV viral capsid antigen (52). In contrast,
only 10 to 20% of 2 year old Americans are EBV seropositive.
Although EBV infection is ubiquitous in African children, a marked
difference in the titer of anti-VCA antibody is found in children
destined to develop BL (Figure 8) (31). In a retrospective study,
the mean geometric titer of 139 patients was 1:275, while controls
were only 1:37. High anti-VCA titer has been reported in an
American infant with Burkitt's lymphoma (123). But most studies
of American cases have failed to demonstrate association of high
titer anti-EBV and BL. Elevated anti-EBV titers have been
observed in Hodgkin's disease, and likely reflects acquired immunodeficiency (40).

     The low incidence of BL, relative to the high prevalence of
EBV infection, suggests that if EBV is etiologic for this
lymphoma, it is one among several factors. Consider for a moment
the effects of EBV infection on the immune system itself, and the
potential role of immune deficiency in lymphomagenesis. EBV is a
potent stimulator of lymphocytes, both _in vitro_ and _in vivo_,
transforming B-cells into immortalized cell lines and during
infectious mononucleosis inducing polyclonal proliferation of B-

lymphocytes. Such proliferation provides a setting for spawning a malignant clone of B-lymphocytes. The crucial event could be a 8q- chromosomal translocation that occurs randomly. The specific translocation could endow the cell with the BL phenotype, freeing it from immunoregulatory surveillance.

The distribution of BL in areas of holoendemic malaria prompted Burkitt and O'Connor to postulate chronic malaria as an etiologic cofactor (20,60,91). Malarial infection induces intense lymphoid proliferation (98,120,126,130). Children with Falsiparum malaria have lymphocytes that can undergo spontaneous lymphocyte transformation (97). Moreover, experimental studies reveal a higher prev-alence of lymphomas in animals infected with a malarial parasite (125). Supporting this notion is the reduced occurence of BL after successful malaria eradication, and in individuals with sickle cell trait who have a relative immunity to malaria.

A pathogenetic mechanism incorporating these observations has been proposed by Klein involving at least three steps: 1) human B-lymphocytes are immortalized by EBV; 2) a co-factor, either malaria or the underlying EBV infection stimulates B-cells to chronically proliferate and 3) a random by specific cytogenetic event, such as a 8-14q+ translocation endows a clone of cells with a growth advantage by providing escape from immunologic regula-tion. This clone of cells expands to become Burkitt's lymphoma (15).

This model is consistent with the epidemologic differences in African and American Burkitt's lymphoma. The lymphomas on these two continents have identical histologic, immunologic, and che-motherapeutic sensitivities suggesting origin in B-cells fixed at the same undifferentiated stage. In the United States and other countries where the immunostimulatory effects of EBV and malarial infection are uncommon, the incidence of BL is low. Whereas in areas of endemic malaria and childhood EBV infection, the B-cells are likely subjected to intense polyclonal stimulation, increasing chances for malignancy. Such a model need not employ genetic dif-ferences in populations, or the participation of other viruses. However, as Lynch notes elsewhere in this volume, familial BL has been described.

Further supporting an abnormal immunoregulation as a cofactor in the genesis of Burkitt's lymphoma is the occurrence of BL in males with the X-linked lymphoproliferative syndrome (XLP) (101-104,108). These males have defective T-lymphocyte functions, and are susceptible to developing polyclonal B-lymphocyte prolif-erations after EBV infection (101,103,104). Renal transplant recipients, who require immunosuppression are also prone to devel-oping lymphomas (50). Burkitt's lymphoma has also been described

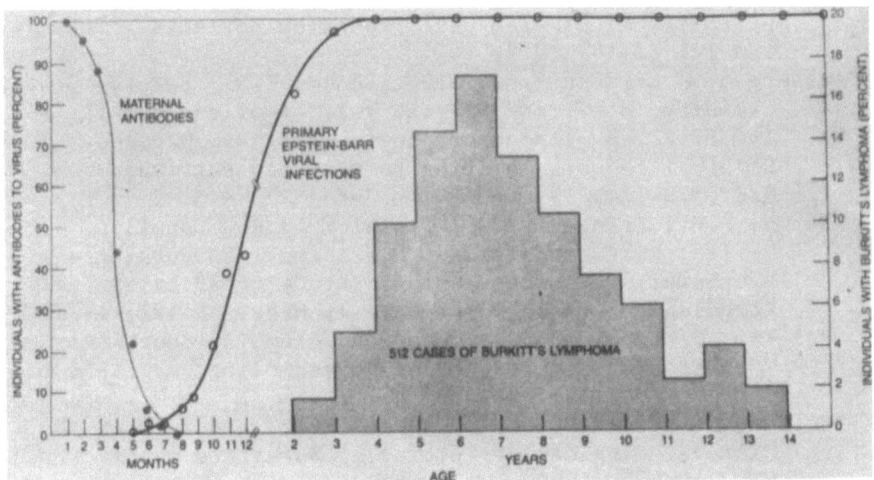

Fig. 9. Antibody to EBV occurs in high-titer in African Burkitt's
lymphoma patients near the peak age of incidence.
(From: Henle, W. et al. The Epstein-Barr virus. Sci.
Am. 241:48, 1979. Copyright© (1983) Scientific American,
Inc. All rights reserved.)

in homosexual males with the acquired immunodeficiency syndrome
(32). These males exhibit profound immunoregulatory disturbances
and reactivation of EBV (116).

SUMMARY AND CONCLUSIONS

     The African child at risk for BL has disturbed immunoregula-
tion due to EBV infection, chronic malaria, and malnutrition
(30,105,122). Intestinal parasitism and chronic measles infection
may further exacerbate malnutrition and impair immunity (35).
Males develop BL twice as often as do females, possibly due to
relative inferiority of immunity to EBV (102). These factors may
be additive in producing immune deficiency in the African child,
reflected by two years of increasing viral burden in children who
develop BL in the West Nile (Figure 9) (31). Prevention of immune
deficiency may lessen the occurrence of BL. Investigation of
chromosomal rearrangements, oncogenes and their gene products
promises to give insight into the molecular events triggering this
and other lymphomas.

REFERENCES

   1. Al-Attar, A., Al-Mondhiry, H., Al-Bahrani, Z., and

Al-Saleen, T. Burkitt's lymphoma in Iraq. Clinical and pathological studies of forty-seven patients. Int. J. Cancer, 23:14, 1979.

2.   Arseneau, J.C., Canellos, G.P., Banks, P.M., Berard, C.W., Gralnick, H.R., and DeVita, V.T. American Burkitt's lymphoma: a clinicopathologic study of 30 cases. I. Clinical factors relating to proposed survival. Am. J. Med., 58:314, 1975.

3.   Banks, P.M., Arsenau, J.C., Gralnick, H.R., Canellos, G.P., DeVita, V.T., and Berard, C.W. American Burkitt's Lymphoma: a clinicopathologic study of 30 cases. II. Pathologic correlations. Am. J. Med., 58:322, 1975.

4.   Beltran, G. Childhood lymphoma in Colombia, South America. With special mention of cases resembling Burkitt's tumor. Cancer, 19:1124, 1966.

5.   Berard, C., O'Conor, G.T., Thomas, L.B., and Torloni, H. Histopathological definition of Burkitt's tumor. Bull. WHO, 40:601, 1969.

6.   Berger, R., Bernhelm, A., Fellous, M., and Brouet, J-C. Cytogenetic study of a European Burkitt's lymphoma cell line. J. Nat. Cancer Inst., 62:1187, 1979.

7.   Berger, R., Bernheim, A., Weh, H.J., Flandrin, G., Daniel, M.T., Brouet, J-C., and Colbert, N. A new translocation in Burkitt's tumor cells. Hum. Genet., 53:111, 1979.

8.   Berger, R., Bernheim, A., Flandrin, G., Daniel, M.-T, Schaison, B., Brouet, J.C., and Bernard, J. Transloca- tion t(8;14) dans la leuceme lymphoblastigne de type Burkitt. Nouv. Presse Med., 8:81, 1979.

9.   Bertrand, S., Berger, R., Philip, T., Bernheim, A., Bryon, P.-A., Bertoglio, J., Dore, J.F., Brunat-Mentigny, M., and Lenoir, G.M. Variant translocation in a non-endemic case of Burkitt's lymphoma: t(8;22) in an Epstein-Barr virus negative tumor and in a derived cell line. Eur. J. Cancer, 17:577, 1981.

10. Bhan, A.K., Nadler, L.M., Stashenko, P., McCluskey, R.T., and Schlossman, S.F. Stages of B-cell differentiation in human lymphoid tissue. J. Exp. Med., 154:737, 1981.

11. Biggar, R.J., Henle, W., Fleisher, G., Bocker, Jorg, Lennette, E.T., and Henle, G. Primary Epstein-Barr virus infections in African infants. I. Decline of maternal antibodies and time of infection. Int. J. Cancer, 22:239, 1978.

12. Biggar, R.J., Nkrumah, F.K., Henle, W., and Levine, P.H. Very late relapses in patients with Burkitt's lymphoma: clinical and serologic studies. J. Natl. Cancer Inst., 66:439, 1981.

13. Biggar, R.J., Nkrumah, F.K., Neeguaye, J., and Levine, P.H. Changes in presenting tumor site of Burkitt's lymphoma in Ghana, West Africa, 1965-1978. Br. J. Cancer, 43:632, 1981.

14.   Binder, R.A., Jencks, J.A., Chun, B., and Rath, C.E. "B"
      cell origin of malignant cells in a case of American
      Burkitt's lymphoma. Cancer, 36:161, 1975.

15.   Bird, A.G. and Britton, S. The relationship between
      Epstein-Barr virus and lymphoma. Sem. Hematol., 19:285,
      1982.

16.   Blatt, J., Reaman, G., and Poplack, D.G. Biochemical
      markers in lymphoid malignancy. N. Engl. J. Med.,
      303:918, 1980.

17.   Bornkamm, G.W., Kaduk, B., Kachel, G., Schneider, U.,
      Fresen, K.O., Schwanitz, G., and Hermanek, P. Epstein-
      Barr virus-positive Burkitt's lymphoma in a German woman
      during pregnancy. Blut, 40:167, 1980.

18.   Burkitt, D. A sarcoma involving the jaws in African
      children. Br. J. Surg., 46:218, 1958.

19.   Burkitt, D. and O'Conor, G.T. Malignant lymphoma in
      African children. I. A clinical syndrome. Cancer,
      14:258, 1961.

20.   Burkitt, D. A children's cancer development dependent upon
      climactic factors. Nature, 194:232, 1962.

21.   Burkitt, D. Determining the climatic limitations of a
      children's cancer common in Africa. Br. Med. J.,
      2:1019, 1962.

22.   Burkitt, D.P. and Wright, D.H. Burkitt's Lymphoma,
      Livingstone, Edinburgh, 1970.

23.   Burkitt, D.P. Oncogenic viruses and their tumours. Proc.
      R. Soc. Med., 64:909, 1971.

24.   Cadman, E.C., Lundberg, W.B., and Bertino, J.R.
      Hyperphosphatemia and hypocalcemia accompanying rapid
      cell lysis in a patient with Burkitt's lymphoma and
      Burkitt cell leukemia. Am. J. Med., 62:283, 1977.

25.   Castella, A., Davey, F.R., Kurec, A.S., and Nelson, D.A.
      The presence of Burkitt-like cells in non-Burkitt's
      neoplasms. Cancer, 50:1764, 1982.

26.   Cehreli, C. and Niyazi, T. Burkitt's lymphoma cell leuke-
      mia in a Turkish boy. Cancer, 36:1444, 1975.

27.   Cohen, L.F., Balow, J.E., Magrath, I.J., Poplack, D.G., and
      Ziegler, J.L. Acute tumor lysis syndrome. A review of
      37 patients with Burkitt's lymphoma. Am. J. Med.,
      68:486, 1980.

28.   Cohen, M.H., Bennett, J.M., Berard, C.W., Ziegler, J.L.,
      Vogel, C.L., Sheagren, J.N., and Carbone, P.P.
      Burkitt's tumor in the United States. Cancer, 23:1259,
      1969.

29.   Dambaugh, T., Nkrumah, F.K., Biggar, R.J., and Kieff, E.
      Epstein-Barr virus RNA in Burkitt tumor tissue. Cell,
      16:313, 1979.

30.   de The, G. Is Burkitt's lymphoma related to perinatal
      infection by Epstein-Barr virus? Lancet, 1:335, 1977.

31.   de The, G., Geser, A., Day, N.E., Tukei, P.M., Williams,
      E.H., Beri, D.P., Smith, P.G., Dean, A.G., Bornkamm,
      G.W., Feorino, P., and Henle, W. Epidemiological evi-
      dence for causal relationship between Epstein-Barr virus
      and Burkitt lymphoma from Ugandan prospective study.
      Nature, 274:756, 1978.
32.   Doll, D.C. and List, A.F. Burkitt's lymphoma in a homo-
      sexual. Lancet, i:1026, 1982.
33.   Douglass, E., Magrath, I.T., Lee, E.C., and Whang-Peng, J.
      Cytogenetic studies in non-African Burkitt lymphoma.
      Blood, 55:148, 1980.
34.   Dorfman, R.F. Diagnosis of Burkitt's tumor in the United
      States. Cancer, 21:563, 1968.
35.   Dossetor, J., Whittle, H.C., and Greenwood, B.M. Persistent
      measles infection in malnourished children. Br. Med. J.,
      1:1633, 1977.
36.   Dunnick, N.R., Reaman, G.H., Head, G.L., Shawker, T.H., and
      Ziegler, J.L. Radiographic manifestations of Burkitt's
      lymphoma in American patients. Am. J. Radiology, 132:1,
      1979.
37.   Epstein, M.A. and Herdson, P.B. Cellular degeneration
      associated with characteristic nuclear fine structural
      changes in the cells from two cases of Burkitt's
      malignant lymphoma syndrome. Brit. J. Cancer, 17:56,
      1963.
38.   Epstein, M.A., Achong, B.G., and Barr, Y.M. Virus particles
      in cultured lymphoblasts from Burkitt's malignant
      lymphoma. Lancet, i:702, 1964.
39.   Epstein, M.A. Epstein-Barr virus as the cause of a human
      cancer. Nature, 274:740, 1978.
40.   Evans, A.S. and Comstock, G.W. Presence of elevated anti-
      body titers to Epstein-Barr virus before Hodgkin's
      disease. Lancet, i:1183, 1981.
41.   Fialkow, P.J., Klein, G., and Clifford, P. Second malignant
      clone underlying a Burkitt-tumor exacerbation. Lancet,
      ii:629, 1972.
42.   Fiorentio, M., Palu, G., Sperandio, P., Vinanti, O., DeBeis,
      P., Realdi, G., and Pennelli, N. Non-African sporatic
      Burkitt's lymphoma in Italian patients. Eur. J. Cancer,
      44:15, 1978.
43.   Fleischmann, E.W. and Prigogina, E.L. Karyotype peculiari-
      ties of malignant lymphoma. Hum. Genet., 35:269, 1977.
44.   Fukuhara, S., Rowley, J.D., Variakojis, D., and Golomb, M.
      Chromosome abnormalities in poorly differentiated lympho-
      cytic lymphoma. Cancer Res., 39:3119, 1979.
45.   Griere, J.W. and Binder, R.A. Burkitt's lymphoma involving
      the ovary and jaw. Obstet. Gynecol., 48:635, 1976.
46.   Gravell, M., Levine, P.H., McIntyre, R.F., Land V.J., and
      Pagano, J.S. Epstein-Barr virus in an American patient
      with Burkitt's lymphoma: detection of viral genome in

tumor tissue and establishment of a tumor-derived cell
line (NAB). J. Natl. Cancer Inst., $\underline{56}$:701, 1976.

47. Grogan, R.M., Warnke, R.A., and Kaplan, H.S. A comparative
study of Burkitt's and non-Burkitt's "Undifferentiated"
malignant lymphoma: immunologic, cytochemical,
ultrastructural, cytologic, histopathologic, clinical
and cell culture features. Cancer, $\underline{49}$:1817, 1982.

48. Grunven, P., Klein, G., Klein, E., Norin, T., and Singh, S.
Surface immunoglobulin on Burkitt's lymphoma biopsy
cells from 91 patients. Int. J. Cancer, $\underline{25}$:711, 1980.

49. Haddow, A.J. Epidemiologic evidence suggesting an infective
element in the etiology. In: D. P. Burkitt and D. H.
Wright, D.H. (eds.), Burkitt's Lymphoma. pp. 198-209.
Edinburgh: Churchill Livingstone, 1970.

50. Hanto, D.W., Frizzera, G., Purtilo, D.T., Sakamoto, K.,
Sullivan, J.L., Saemundsen, A.K., Klein, G., Simmons,
R.L., and Najarian, J.S. Clinical spectrum of
lymphoproliferative disorders in renal transplant recip-
ients and evidence for the role of Epstein-Barr virus.
Cancer Res., $\underline{41}$:4253, 1981.

51. Henle, W., Henle, G., Grunven, P., Klein, G., Clifford, P.,
and Singh, S. Patterns of antibodies to Epstein-Barr
virus induced early antigens in Burkitt's lymphoma:
comparison of dying patients with long term survivors.
J. Natl. Cancer Inst., $\underline{50}$:1163, 1973.

52. Henle, W., Henle, G., and Lennette, E.T. The Epstein-Barr
virus. Sci. Am., $\underline{241}$:48, 1979.

53. Hillman, E.A., Charamella, L.H., Temple, M.J., and Elser,
J.E. Biological characterization of an Epstein-Barr
nuclear antigen-positive American Burkitt's tumor-
derived cell line. Cancer Res., $\underline{37}$:4546, 1977.

54. Hirschaut, Y., Cohen, M.H., and Stevens, D.A. Epstein-Barr
virus antibodies in American and African Burkitt's
lymphoma. Lancet, $\underline{ii}$:114, 1973.

55. Hubner, K.R. and Littlefield, G. Burkitt lymphoma in three
American children. Clinical and cytogenetic observations. Am. J. Dis. Child., $\underline{129}$:1219, 1975.

56. Hutt, M.S.R. Introduction and historical background in
Burkitt's lymphoma. In: D.P. Burkitt and D.H. Wright,
(eds.), Burkitt's Lymphoma. pp. 1-5. Edinburgh:
Livingstone, 1970.

57. Iversen, O.H., Iversen, U., Ziegler, J.L., and Bluming, A.Z.
Cell kinetics in Burkitt's lymphoma. Eur. J. Cancer,
$\underline{10}$:155, 1974.

58. Jacobs, S.A., Lakings, D.B., Gehrke, C.W., Anderson, T.,
Ziegler, J.L., and Waalkes, T.P. Biochemical markers in
Burkitt's lymphoma. Lancet, $\underline{ii}$:309, 1976.

59. Judson, S.C., Henle, W., and Henle, G. A cluster of
Epstein-Barr virus associated American Burkitt's lymphoma.
N. Engl. J. Med., $\underline{297}$:464, 1977.

60. Kafuko, G.W. and Burkitt, D.P. Burkitt's lymphoma and
     malaria. Int. J. Cancer, 6:1, 1970.
61. Kaiser-McCaw, B., Epstein, A.L., Kaplan, H.S., and Hecht, F.
     Chromosome 14 translocations in African and North
     American Burkitt's lymphoma. Int. J. Cancer, 19:482,
     1977.
62. Katayama, I., Uehara, H., Gleser, R.A., and Weintraub, L.
     The value of electron microscopy in the diagnosis of
     Burkitt's lymphoma. Am. J. Clin. Pathol., 61:540,
     1974.
63. Kerndrup, G. and Pallesen, G. A clinicopathological study
     of 13 Danish cases of Burkitt's lymphoma. Scand. J.
     Haematol., 27:99, 1982.
64. Klein, E., Eskeland, T., Inoue, M., Strom, R., and
     Johansson, B. Surface immunoglobulin-moieties on
     lymphoid cells. Exp. Cell. Res., 62:133, 1970.
65. Levine, P.H., Sandler, G., Komp, D.M., O'Conor, G.T., and
     O'Connor, D.M. Simultaneous occurrence of "American
     Burkitt's lymphoma" in neighbors. N. Engl. J. Med.,
     288:562, 1973.
66. Levine, P.H. Evidence for a role of the Epstein-Barr virus
     in the etiology of human lymphoma. Biomedicine, 20:86,
     1974.
67. Levine, P.H., Cho, B.R., Connelly, R.R., Berard, C.W.,
     O'Conor, G.T., Dorfman, R.F., Easton, J.M., and DeVita,
     V.T. The American Burkitt's lymphoma registry: a
     progress report. Ann. Int. Med., 83:31, 1975.
68. Lewinski, U.H., Gafter, U., Klein, B., and Djaldetti, M.
     Transmission and scanning electron microscopy study on
     Burkitt-like leukemia. Arch. Pathol. Lab. Med.,
     103:558, 1979.
69. Lindahl, T. Klein, G., Reedman, B.M., Johansson, B., and
     Singh, S. Relationship between Epstein-Barr virus (EBV)
     DNA and EBV-determined nuclear antigen (EBNA) in Burkitt
     lymphoma biopsies and other lymphoproliferative malignan-
     cies. Int. J. Cancer, 13:764, 1974.
70. Mace, M.C. Oral African histoplasmosis resembling Burkitt's
     lymphoma. Oral Surg., 46:407, 1978.
71. MacMahon, B. Epidemiologic aspects of acute leukemia and
     Burkitt's tumor. Cancer, 21:558, 1968.
72. Magrath, I.T., Lwanga, S., Carswell, W., and Harrison, N.
     Surgical reduction of tumor bulk in management of ab-
     dominal Burkitt's lymphoma. Br. Med. J., 2:308, 1974.
73. Magrath, I.T. Lymphocyte differentiation: an essential
     basis for the comprehension of lymphoid neoplasia. J.
     Natl. Cancer Inst., 67:501, 1981.
74. Magrath, I.T., Spiegel, R.J., Edwards, B.K., and Janus, C.
     Improved results of chemotherapy in young patients with
     Burkitt's (BL), undifferentiated (UL) and lymphoblastic

lymphomas (LL). Proc. Am. Assoc. Cancer Res. Am. Soc. Clin. Oncol., 22:520, 1981 (abstract).

75. Mann, R.B., Jaffe, E.S., Braylan, R.C., Nanba, K., Frank, M.M., Ziegler, J.L., and Berard, C.W. Non-endemic Burkitt's lymphoma. A B-cell tumor related to germinal centers. N. Engl. J. Med., 295:685, 1976.

76. Manolov, G. and Manolova, Y. Marker Band in one chromosome 14 from Burkitt lymphomas. Nature, 237:33, 1972.

77. Manolova, Y., Manolov, G., Kielen, J., Levan, A., and Klein, G. Genesis of the 14q+ marker in Burkitt's lymphoma. Hereditas, 90:5, 1979.

78. Mark, J., Ekedahl, C., and Hagman, A. Origin of the translocated segment of the 14q+ plus 2 marker in non-Burkitt lymphomas. Hum. Genet., 36:277, 1977.

79. Mark, J., Ekedahl, C., and Dahlenfors, R. Characteristics of the banding patterns in non-Hodgkin and non-Burkitt lymphomas. Hereditas, 88:229, 1978.

80. Merz, B. Migrant oncogene-Burkitt's lymphoma link. J. Am. Med. Assoc., 248:2424, 1982.

81. Mitelman, F., Andersson-Anvret, M., Brandt, L., Catovsky, D., Klein, G., Manolov, G., Manolova, Y., Mark-Vendel, E., and Nilsson, P.G. Reciprocal 8;14 translocation in EBV-negative B-cell acute lymphocytic leukemia with Burkitt-type cells. Int. J. Cancer, 24:27, 1979.

82. Miyoshi, I., Hiraki, S. Kimura, I., Miyamoto, K., and Sato, J. 2/8 translocation in a Japanese Burkitt's lymphoma. Experientia, 35:742, 1979.

83. Morrow, R.H., Pike, M.C., and Smith, P.G. Further studies of space-time clustering of Burkitt's lymphoma in Uganda. Br. J. Cancer, 35:668, 1977.

84. Morrow, R.H., Pike, M.C., Smith, P.G., Ziegler, J.L., Kisuule, A. Burkitt's lymphoma: a time-space cluster of cases in Bawamba County of Uganda. Br. Med. J., 2:491, 1971.

85. Nassar, V.H., Jacobs, J., Mirra, S.S., Pandya, K.J., Schwartz, S. and Benett, J.M. Burkitt cell leukemia following therapy for Hodgkin's disease. Am. J. Hematol., 12:73, 1982.

86. Nkrumah, F.K. and Perkins, I.V. Relapse in Burkitt's lymphoma. Int. J. Cancer, 17:455, 1976.

87. Nkrumah, F.K. and Perkins, I.V. Burkitt's lymphoma. A clinical study of 110 patients. Cancer, 37:671, 1976.

88. Nkrumah, F.K., Perkins, I.V., and Biggar, R.J. Combination chemotherapy in abdominal Burkitt's lymphoma. Cancer, 40:1410, 1977.

89. O'Conor, G.T., Rappaport, H., and Smith, E.B. Childhood lymphoma resembling "Burkitt tumor" in the United States. Cancer, 18:411, 1965.

90. O'Conor, G.T. Malignant lymphoma in African children. II. A pathologic entity. Cancer, 14:270, 1961.

91.   O'Conor, G.T.   Persistent immunologic stimulation as a fac-
      tor in oncogenesis, with special reference to Burkitt's
      tumor. Am. J. Med., 48:279, 1970.
92.   Oettgen, H.F., Burkitt, D., and Burchenal, J.H. Malignant
      lymphoma involving the jaw in African children: treat-
      ment with methotrexate. Cancer, 16:616, 1963.
93.   Olson, C.W., Smith, J.H., Testerman, N. Bastin, J.-P., and
      Frazer, H. Burkitt's tumor in the demographic republic
      of the Congo. Cancer, 23:740, 1969.
94.   Olweny, C.L.M., Kaongole-Mbidde, E., Kaddu-Mukasa, A.,
      Atine, I, Owor, R., Lwanga, S., Carswell, W., and
      Magrath, I.T. Treatment of Burkitt's lymphoma: ran-
      domized clinical trial of a single agent versus com-
      bination chemotherapy. Int. J. Cancer, 17:436, 1976.
95.   Olweny, C.L.M., Atine, I., Kaddu-Mukasa, A., Owor, R.,
      Anderson-Anvret, M., Klein, G., Henle, W., and de The,
      G. Epstein-Barr virus genome studies in Burkitt's and
      non-Burkitt's lymphomas in Uganda. J. Natl. Cancer
      Inst., 58:1191, 1977.
96.   Olweny, C.L.M., Katongole-Mbidde, E., Otim, D., Lwanga,
      S.K., Magrath, I.T., and Ziegler, J.L. Long-term
      experience with Burkitt's lymphoma in Uganda. Int. J.
      Cancer, 26:261, 1980.
97.   Osunkoya, B.O., Williams, A.I.O., and Reddy, S. Spontaneous
      lymphocyte transformation in leukocyte cultures of
      children with falciparum malaria. Trop. Geogr. Med.,
      24:157, 1972.
98.   Osunkoya, B.O. Immunopathology of human malaria. Israel J.
      Med. Sci., 14:617, 1978.
99.   Owings, R.M. and Oyama, A.A. Imprint cytology in the rapid
      diagnosis of Burkitt's lymphoma. A case report. Acta
      Cytologica, 26:331, 1982.
100. Pitts, J.R. and Cowley, A. Non-African Burkitt lymphoma
      presenting as dysphagia. Post. Med. J., 53:276, 1977.
101   Purtilo, D.T., Deflorio, D., Hutt, L.M., Bhawan, J., Yang,
      J.P.S., Otto, R., and Edwards, W. Variable phenotypic
      expression of an X-linked recessive lymphoproliferative
      syndrome. N. Engl. J. Med., 297:1077, 1977.
102. Purtilo, D.T. Szymanski, F., Bhawana, J., Yang, J.P.S.,
      Hutt, L.M., Boto, W., DeNicola, L., Maier, R., and
      Thorley-Lawson, D. Epstein-Barr virus infection in the
      X-linked recessive lymphoproliferative syndrome.
      Lancet, 1:798, 1978.
103. Purtilo, D.T. Epstein-Barr-virus-induced oncogenesis in
      immune-deficient individuals. Lancet, 1:300, 1980.
104. Purtilo, D.T. X-linked lymphoproliferative syndrome: an
      immunodeficiency disorder with acquired agammaglobu-
      linemia, fatal infectious mononucleosis or malignant
      lymphoma. Arch. Pathol. Lab. Med., 105:119, 1981.

105. Purtilo, D.T. Nutritional considerations in the epide-
        miology of lymphoma. In: C.E. Butterworth and M.
        Hutchinson (eds.), Nutritional Factors in Induction and
        Maintenance of Malignancy. New York: Academic Press,
        1983.
106. Reves, B.R. and Pickup, B.L. The chromosome changes in
        non-Burkitt lymphomas. Human. Genet., 53:349, 1980.
107. Roos, G., Nordenson, I., Osterman, B., Jorpes, P., and
        Rudolphi, O. Patient with acute B-cell leukemia of
        Burkitt's type (L3) and marker chromosomes including an
        (8;14) translocation. Leukemia Res., 6:27, 1982.
108. Rosen, F.S. Lymphoma, immunodeficiency and the Epstein-Barr
        virus. N. Engl. J. Med., 297:1120, 1977.
109. Rowley, J.D. Indentification of the constant chromosome
        regions involved in human hematologic malignant disease.
        Science, 215:749, 1982.
110. Sandberg, A.A. The Chromosomes in Human Cancer and
        Leukemia. New York: Elsevier North-Holland, 1980.
111. Sandberg, A.A. Chromosomes changes in the lymphomas. Hum.
        Pathol., 12:531, 1981.
112. Schlossman, S.F., Chess, L., Humphreys, R.E., and
        Strominger, J.L. Distribution of Ia-like molecules on
        the surface of normal and leukemic human cells. Proc.
        Nat. Acad. Sci. USA, 73:1288, 1976.
113. Scully, R.E., Galdabini, J.J., and McNeely, B.U. Case
        records of the Massachusetts General Hospital, 302:389,
        1980.
114. Siemiajycki, J., Brubaker, G., and Geser, A. Space-time
        clustering and Burkitt's lymphoma in east Africa: analy-
        sis of recent data and a new look at old data. Int. J.
        Cancer, 25:197, 1980.
115. Slater, R.M., Philip, P., Badsberg, E., Behrendt, H.,
        Hansen, N.E., and van Heerde, P. A 14q+ chromosome in a
        B-cell acute lymphocytic leukemia and a leukemic non-
        endemic Burkitt lymphoma. Int. J. Cancer, 23:639, 1979.
116. Sonnabend, J., Witkin, S., and Purtilo, D.T. Acquired
        immunodeficiency syndrome, opportunistic infections and
        malignancies in male homosexuals. A hypothesis of
        etiologic factors in pathogenesis. J. Am. Med. Assoc.,
        249:2370, 1983.
117. Stansfield, D. Haematological findings in African children
        in Uganda with malignant lymphoma. Brit. J. Cancer,
        15:41, 1961.
118. Stashenko, P., Nadler, L.M., Hardy,R., and Schlossman, S.F.
        Expression of cell surface markers after human B lympho-
        cyte activation. Proc. Natl. Acad. Sci. USA, 78:3848,
        1981.
119. Stevens, D.A., O'Conor, G.T., Levine, P.H., and Rosen, R.B.
        Acute leukemia with "Burkitt's lymphoma cells" and
        Burkitt's lymphoma. Simultaneous onset in American

siblings: description of a new entity. Ann. Int. Med.,
        76:967, 1972.

120.   Taylor, D.W. and Siddigni, W.A. Recent advances in
        malarial immunity. In: W.P. Creger, C.H. Coggins, and
        E.W. Hancock (eds.), Ann. Review of Medicine, 33:69,
        1982.

121.   Templeton, A.C. Changing pattern of residual tumor in
        Burkitt lymphoma. Findings at autopsy. Arch. Pathol.
        Lab. Med., 100:503, 1976.

122.   Upaohyaya, K.C., Verma, I.C., and Ghai, O.P. Chromosomal
        aberrations in protein-calorie malnutrition. Lancet,
        ii:704, 1975.

123.   Valsamis, M.P., Levine, P.H., Rapin, I., Santorineou, M.,
        and Shulman, K. Primary intracranial Burkitt's lymphoma
        in an infant. Cancer, 37:1500, 1976.

124.   Van Den Berghe, H., Parloir, C., Gosseye, S., Englebienne,
        V., Cornu, G., and Sokal. Variant translocation in
        Burkitt lymphoma. Cancer Genet. Cytogenet., 1:9, 1979.

125.   Wedderburn, N. Effects of concurrent malarial infection on
        development of virus-induced lymphoma in BALB/c mice.
        Lancet, ii:1114, 1970.

126.   Wells, R.A., Pavanada, K., Zolyomi, S., Permpanich, B., and
        MacDermott, R.P. Loss of circulating T-lymphocytes with
        normal levels of B and "null" lymphocytes in Thai adults
        with malaria. Clin. Exp. Immunol., 35:202, 1979.

127.   Wright, D.H. Gross distribution and hematology. In: D.P.
        Burkitt and D.H. Wright (eds.), Burkitt's Lymphoma. pp.
        64-81. Edinburgh: Churchill Livingstone, 1970.

128.   Wright, D.H. Burkitt's lymphoma: a review of the patholo-
        gy, immunology and possible etiologic factors. Pathol.
        Ann., 6:337, 1971.

129.   Wright, D.H. and Isaacson, P. Follicular center cell
        lymphoma of childhood: a report of three cases and a
        discussion of its relationship to Burkitt's lymphoma.
        Cancer, 47:915, 1981.

130.   Wyler, D.J. Peripheral lymphocyte subpopulations in human
        falciparum malaria. Clin. Exp. Immunol., 23:471, 1976.

131.   Yunis, J.J. Specific fine chromosomal defects in cancer:
        an overview. Hum. Pathol., 12:503, 1981.

132.   Yunis, J.J. Chromosomes and cancer: new nomenclature and
        future directions. Hum. Pathol., 12:494, 1981.

133.   Zech, L., Haglund, U., Nilsson, K., and Klein, G.
        Characteristic chromosomal abnormalities in biopsies and
        lymphoid-cell lines from patients with Burkitt and
        non-Burkitt lymphomas. Int. J. Cancer, 17:47, 1976.

134.   Ziegler, J.L., Bluming, A.Z., Morrow, R.H., Fass, L., and
        Carhone, P.P. Central nervous system involvement in
        Burkitt's lymphoma. Blood, 36:718, 1970.

135.   Ziegler, J.L., Cohen, M.H., Morrow, R.H., Kyalwazi, S.K.,

and Carbone, P.P. Immunologic studies in Burkitt's
lymphoma. Cancer, 25:734, 1970.

136. Ziegler, J.L., Morrow, R.H. Jr., Fass, L., Kyalwazi, S.J.,
      and Carbone, P.P. Treatment of Burkitt's lymphoma with
      cyclophosphamide. Cancer, 26:474, 1970.

137. Ziegler, J.L. and Bluming, A.Z. Intrathecal chemotherapy
      in Burkitt's lymphoma. Br. Med. J., 3:508, 1971.

138. Ziegler, J.L. Chemotherapy of Burkitt's lymphoma. Cancer,
      30:1534, 1972.

139. Ziegler, J.L., Bluming, A.Z., Fass, L., and Morrow, R.H.,
      Jr. Relapse patterns in Burkitt's lymphoma. Cancer
      Res., 32:1267, 1972.

140. Ziegler, J.L., Bluming, A.Z., Magrath, I.T., and Carbone,
      P.O. Intensive chemotherapy in patients with generalized
      Burkitt's lymphoma. Int. J. Cancer, 10:254, 1972.

141. Ziegler, J.L., Bluming, A.Z., Fass, L., Morrow, R.H., and
      Iversen, O.H. Burkitt's lymphoma cell kinetics treat-
      ment and immunology. In: R.M.N. Dutcher and L.
      Chirco-Bianchi (eds.), Unifying Concepts of Leukemia.
      No. 39, pp. 1046-1052. Basel: Karger, 1973.

142. Ziegler, J.L. and Magrath, I.T. Burkitt's lymphoma.
      Pathobiol. Ann., 4:129, 1974.

143. Ziegler, J.L., Andersson, M., Klein, G., and Henle, W.
      Detection of Epstein-Barr virus DNA in American
      Burkitt's lymphoma. Int. J. Cancer, 17:701, 1976.

144. Ziegler, J.L. Treatment results of 54 American patients
      with Burkitt's lymphoma are similar to the African
      patients. N. Engl. J. Med., 297:75, 1977.

145. Ziegler, J.L., Magrath, I.T., Gerber, P., and Levine, P.H.
      Epstein-Barr virus and human malignancy. Ann. Intern.
      Med., 86:323, 1977.

146. Ziegler, J.L., Magrath, I.T., Deisseroth, A.B., Glaubiger,
      D.L., Kent, H.C., Pizzo, P.A., Poplack, D.G., and
      Levine, A.S. Combined modality treatment of Burkitt's
      lymphoma. Cancer Treat. Rep., 62:2031, 1978.

147. Ziegler, J.L. Management of Burkitt's lymphoma: an update.
      Cancer Treat. Rev., 6:95, 1979.

148. Ziegler, J.L., Magrath, I.T., and Olweny, C.L.M. Cure of
      Burkitt's lymphoma. Ten-year follow-up of 157 Ugandan
      patients. Lancet, ii:936, 1979.

149. Ziegler, J.L. Burkitt's lymphoma. N. Engl. J. Med.,
      305:735, 1981.

150. zur Hausen, H. and Schulte-Holthausen, H. Presence of EB
      virus nucleic acid homology in a "virus-free" line of
      Burkitt tumour cells. Nature (London), 227:245, 1970.

151. zur Hausen, H. Epstein-Barr virus in human tumor cells.
      In: G.W. Richter and M.A. Epstein (eds.),
      International Review of Experimental Pathology. Vol. 11,
      pp. 233-258. New York: Academic Press, 1972.

HEMATOPATHOLOGY OF X-LINKED LYMPHOPROLIFERATIVE SYNDROME

David T. Purtilo

Department of Pathology and Laboratory Medicine
Eppley Institute for Research in Cancer and Allied
Diseases
University of Nebraska Medical Center
42nd & Dewey Avenue
Omaha NE 68105

INTRODUCTION

Recognition of the X-linked lymphoproliferative syndrome
(XLP) as a discrete entity emerged during the early 1970's. This
immunodeficiency syndrome results from inherited susceptibility to
Epstein-Barr virus (EBV). It is manifested by a variety of
aproliferative (aplastic anemia, red cell aplasia, agranulocytosis, acquired hypo- or agammaglobulinemia) and lymphoproliferative phenotypes (fatal or chronic infectious mononucleosis, B cell
lymphomas, and pseudolymphoma). I aim to: 1) provide a historical description of the events leading to the present definition of
the syndrome; 2) portray morphological manifestations of the major
phenotypes of XLP; and 3) briefly consider other potential
oncogenic viruses which may provoke opportunistic malignancies in
individuals with acquired or inherited immunodeficiency.

Cottom and Hambleton (1) probably reported the initial family
with XLP in an abstract 1969. They wrote manuscripts regarding
maternally related males who had experienced infectious mononucleosis (IM) followed by malignant lymphoma and hypogammaglobulinemia. Both short and long versions of these manuscripts
were rejected for publication (personal communication with
Cottom). The reviewers were unable to appreciate the significance
of the events because the boys had succumbed prior to the discovery that EBV caused IM and possibly lymphoma.

Three discoveries during one decade have elucidated viral induced lymphoproliferative diseases. In 1958, Denis Burkitt defined Burkitt's lymphoma in tropical Africa (2); infectious viral particles were identified by electron microscopy in cultured BL cells in 1964 (3); and in 1968 the Henles discovered that EBV causes IM (4).

In 1969 an 8 year-old Duncan child died of IM. His brother had also succumbed to IM, however, a diagnosis of acute lympho-cytic leukemia was made. At autopsy, the thymus gland was markedly depleted as were T-dependent regions in lymph nodes and spleen. In contrast, B cell compartments were overrun by immunoblasts, lymphocytes, and plasma cells.

In 1969 the author moved to Minneapolis where Robert Good was pioneering in the study of immunodeficiency. Gatti and Good (5) had described a high frequency of malignancy in individuals with immunodeficiency. Predominant among these malignancies is malignant B cell lymphomas. About the same time, Starzl and Penn (6) had reported a high frequency of malignant lymphomas in renal transplant recipients.

In 1973 a third brother in the Duncan kindred had succumbed to IM. Initially, males in the family were described as experiencing fatal IM with familial lymphohistiocytosis (7). Further study revealed maternally related half-brothers who had succumbed to B cell lymphoma following chronic IM and another cousin had IM followed by agammaglobulinemia (Figure 1). Following review of the clinical, laboratory, and morphologic findings and pedigree, we coined the term X-linked recessive progressive combined

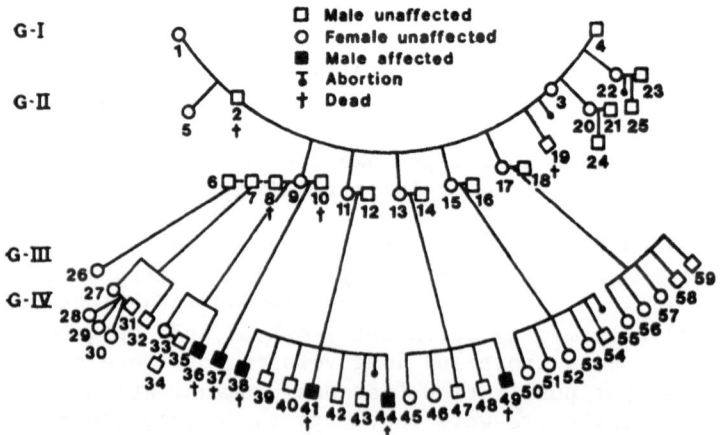

Fig. 1. Pedigree of the Duncan family with X-linked lymphopro-
         liferative syndrome (published with the permission of the
         Lancet).

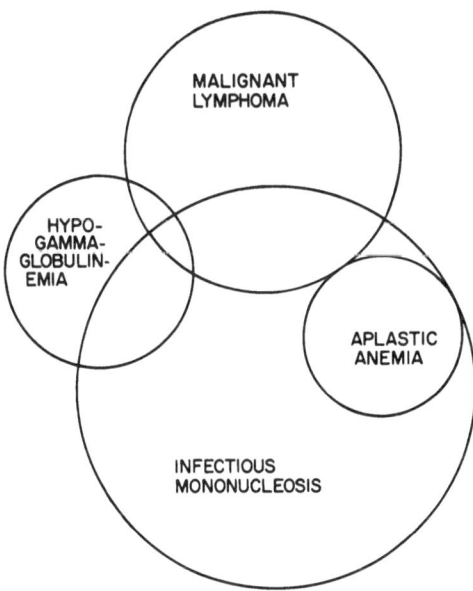

Fig. 2.   Venn diagram summarizes the overlap and the relative frequency of the initial 100 cases of X-linked lymphoproliferative syndrome in our registry. (From: Purtilo, D.T.
et al. Epstein-Barr virus-induced diseases in boys with
the X-linked lymphoproliferative syndrome (XLP). Am. J.
Med., 73:49, 1982.)

variable immunodeficiency disease (Duncan's disease) (8). The
eponym, Duncan was applied since the generic name was cumbersome.
An additional family was found. Eighteen affected males were
found with identical phenotypes to the Duncan kindred (9).

Thus in 1977, the disorder was redefined as the X-linked
lymphoproliferative syndrome (XLP) and a hypothesis was developed
to explain the variable phenotypic expression (11).

In 1978 a registry of XLP and laboratory were developed to
define diagnostic criteria, investigate the immunopathogenesis, and
provide consultation and referrals for study (11). The XLP
Registry has allowed us to determine the frequency of the major
phenotypes, their overlap in a given patient, and the chronologi-
cal sequences of the diseases resulting from EBV infections
(Figure 2). Fatal IM, by far, is the most common expression of
XLP, i.e., two-thirds of the cases (12). Death results frequently
from massive liver failure and associated hemorrhage and/or
encephalopathy. Aplastic anemia also frequently occurs as a
complication of IM and opportunistic infections ensue. Note in
Figure 2 that hypogammaglobulinemia and aplastic anemia are

Table 1.   Diagnostic Criteria of X-Linked
Lymphoproliferative Syndrome

---

1. Phenotypes of fatal or chronic infectious mononucleosis (IM),
    acquired agammaglobulinemia, immune deficiency with elevated
    IgM, red cell aplasia, neutropenia, aplastic anemia, pseudo-
    lymphoma or B cell lymphoma in males from three months to 25
    years of age.

2. Involvement of two or more maternally related males by the
    above phenotypes.

3. Documentation of Epstein-Barr virus infection and failure to
    mount anti-EB nuclear-associated antigen (EBNA) antibody
    response.

4. Mothers of affected males usually (but not always) show ele-
    vated EBV-specific antibody titers, i.e., anti-viral capsid
    antigen (VCA) or IgG, IgA, or IgM isotypes, anti-early antigen
    (EA) antibodies.

5. Birth defects (i.e., heart and brain especially) can occur in
    female as well as male children born of carrier females.

---

mutually exclusive phenotypes. This suggests that different immu-
nopathogenetic mechanisms are responsible for them. Hypogammaglobulinemia generally followed IM, however in several cases
studied propsectively, IM occurred after hypogammaglobulinemia.
Thirty-five patients developed malignant B cell lymphoma. The
vast majority (26 of 35) occurred in the terminal ileum. Extranodal localization was nearly always evident.

Diagnosis of XLP requires documentation of several key findings (13) (Table 1). Inheritance is always X-linked recessive.
Family history and review of clinical materials and microscopical
slides are mandatory. Phenotypes after infection by EBV occur
after 3 months of age (i.e., after maternal antibody dissipates).
The oldest living patient is 25 years of age. In addition to the
phenotypes displayed in Figure 2, dysgammaglobulinemia, agranulocytosis, red cell aplasia, and an apparently increased frequency
of birth defects especially involving the heart in females and
males have been found in the kindreds with XLP. Female carriers
of XLP rarely, if ever, manifest untoward responses to EBV.
Hodgkin's lymphoma has not occurred after EBV infection in
affected boys.

With acute IM, heterophile determinations may or may not be
strongly positive, however, Monospot® determinations usually react

positively (12). EBV-specific serology reveals variable immunodeficient responses: some infected males mount IgM anti-viral capsid antigen (VCA) and anti-early antigen (EA) responses (14).
Other infected males are apparently entirely anergic, i.e., no EBV
antibodies are detectable. Virtually all XLP patients infected
with EBV lack anti-EB nuclear-associated antigen (EBNA). In
contrast, carrier females usually show partial immunodeficiency to
EBV and have paradoxically elevated anti-VCA and EA titers (15).
Please see the accompanying chapter by Harada et al.

Given that immune deficient individuals may lack the capacity
to produce antibody responses to the virus, then special measures
are required for documentation of EBV infection. Obtaining throat
washings and transforming cord B cells; development of spontaneous
lymphoblastoid EBNA-positive cell lines; and performing in situ
EBV DNA hybridization and vDNA/DNA and cRNA/DNA hybridization
reveals EBV genome in biopsy or autopsy derived tissue samples
(16,17).

Identification of males at risk for XLP has been possible by
challenging the subjects with ϕX174. The children who have XLP
mount normal primary IgM anti-ϕX174 antibodies. However, they
fail to switch from IgM to IgG antibodies on secondary challenge
(18). Normal siblings can be ascertained by their demonstrating
normal responses to ϕX174 or more readily by demonstrating anti-
EBNA of titers of 1:20 or greater (12,14).

The differential diagnosis of XLP requires exclusion of non-
inherited fatal IM, aplastic anemia, acquired hypogammaglobulinemia, or malignant B cell lymphoma (13). Various types of
histiocytosis can be misdiagnosed. This can be achieved by
pedigree analysis and specific immunological studies for EBV.
Additional disorders sometimes confused with XLP are listed (Table
2).

Hematopathology of XLP

Hematopathological findings in the acute IM phenotype of XLP
frequently include the presence of numerous atypical (plasmacytoid) lymphocytes in peripheral blood. Concurrently, polyclonal
elevation in serum immunoglobulin levels are found. Electron
microscopy studies have revealed that many of these cells show
dilated endoplasmic reticulum cisternae suggestive of plasma
cells. However, marking of several IM cases with monoclonal antibodies has revealed increased numbers of T8 (suppressor/lytic)
cells. Thus the cellular population in the blood is probably
variable in individual patients. Most of the patients will mount
an atypical lymphocytosis (Figure 3). Decreased numbers of circulating erythrocytes, neutrophils and platelets are variously
seen.

Table 2. Syndromes Requiring Differential Diagnosis from the X-Linked Recessive Lymphoproliferative Syndrome

Syndrome	Inheritance	Involvement of		Opportunistic Lymphoma	Infectious Mononucleosis	Comments
		T cells	B cells			
Severe combined	XR,AR	+	+	Rare	-	Death during infancy
Agammaglobulinemia	XR	-	-	Rare	-	Lack surface Ig cells
Wiskott-Aldrich	XR	+ progressive	-	15%	-	Platelet defects
Hyper IgM	XR	?	-	Uncommon	-	-
Selective IgM deficiency	XR(?)	?	+	7%	-	Elevated IgG, IgA
Lymphoproliferative	XR	+ progressive	+	35%	67%	Variable B-cell phenotypes
Chronic granulomatous disease	XL,AR	-	(?) hypergamma-globulinemia	-	-	Granulocyte defect
Ataxia-telangectasia	AR	+	+	Occasionally 14q chromosome	EBV antibody elevation	Ataxia and telangectasia
Familial malignant lymphomas	AR,AD	+	+ proliferation	Associated immunodeficiency	-	Various phenotypes
Fatal infectious mononucleosis	Sporadic(?)	?	?	?	100%	Diverse complications
Chediak-Higashi	AR	?	+	Pseudolymphoma	?	Hypopigmentation, giant lysosomes

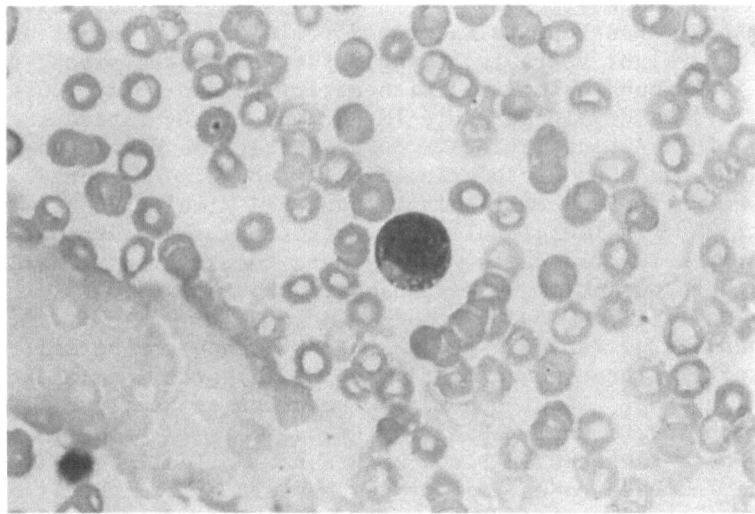

Fig. 3.   Photomicrograph of peripheral blood smear of patient with
          X-linked lymphoproliferative syndrome with the infectious
          mononucleosis phenotype.   Note the plasmacytoid lympho-
          cyte.   Wright's Giemsa, X970.

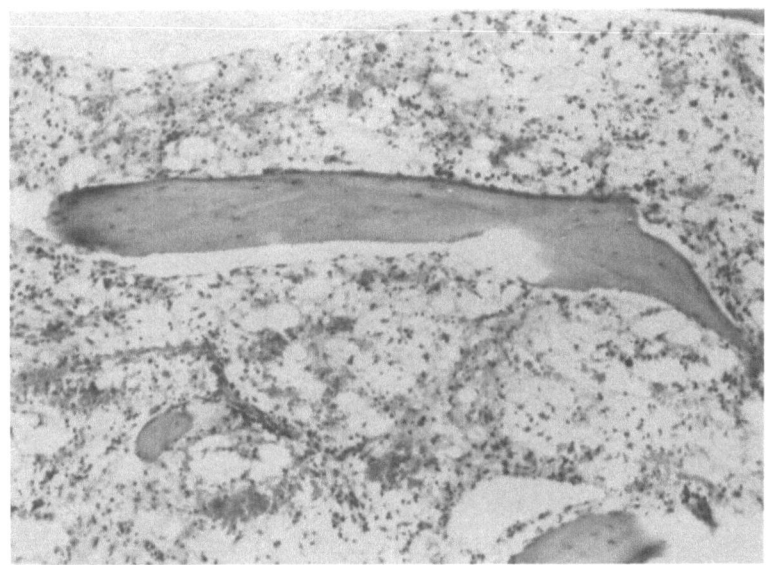

Fig. 4.   Photomicrograph of bone marrow displaying aplastic anemia
          in a patient with X-linked lymphoproliferative syndrome
          and infectious mononucleosis.   Hematoxylin and eosin
          X450.

In one long-term survivor in the Duncan kindred, persistent
mild absolute neutropenia was noted following EBV infection in
1974 (19). Eight years following infection by the virus, red cell
aplasia was found associated with anti-i autoantibody (20).
Thereafter, he developed acute IM accompanied by marked increased
numbers of T8 subpopulations. Subsequently, he developed agammaglobulinemia and no circulating B cells could be detected.
Abatement of the red cell aplasia occurred simultaneously with the
acquisition of agammaglobulinemia suggesting that autoantibodies
were suppressing red cells. Allogeneic bone marrow transplantation restored in immune responses to EBV in 1983.

Bone marrow early in the IM phenotype appears normal. After
approximately three weeks of florid IM, aplastic anemia can be
seen (Figure 2). This bone marrow suppression usually is found in
those with severe mono hepatitis (Figure 4). In other instances,
pancytopneia is noted in blood with a paradoxically cellular bone
marrow. In these cases histiocytes appear to be markedly activated (Figure 5) and erythro- and nucleophagocytosis is evident.
Late in the IM phenotype the bone marrow may be replaced by mononuclear cells having plasmacytoid features.

Death is often due to <u>Staphylococcus</u> <u>aureus</u> or candida septi-
cemia in individuals with aplastic anemia.

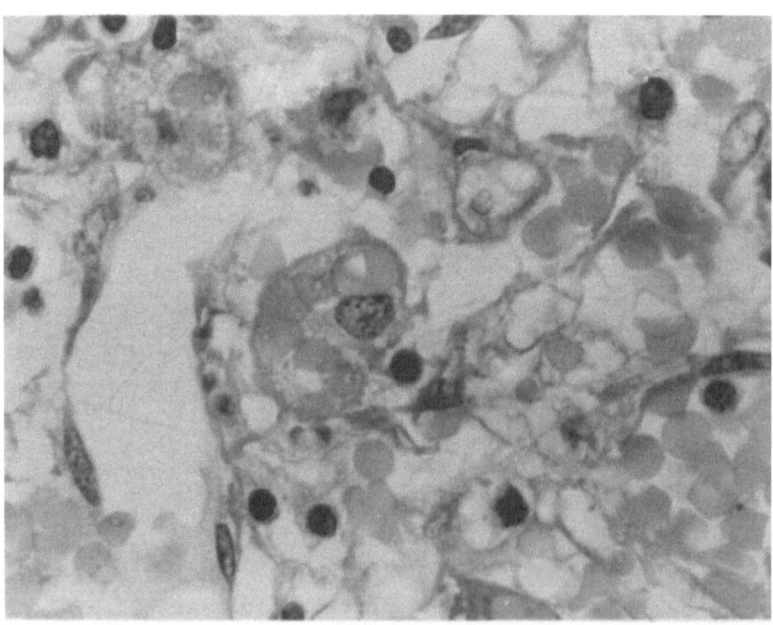

Fig. 5.   Photomicrograph of bone marrow showing reactive histiocytes from a patient with X-linked lymphoproliferative
syndrome. Hematoxylin and eosin X970.

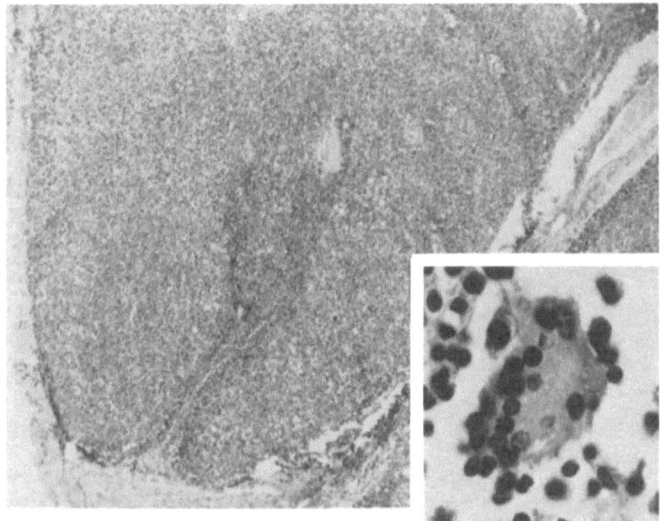

Fig. 6. Photomicrograph of thymus gland of patient dying in the
         second week of infectious mononucleosis. Hematoxylin and
         eosin X100. A multi-nucleated giant cell (inset)
         apparently destroyed thymic Hassall's epithelium.
         Hematoxylin and eosin, X970.

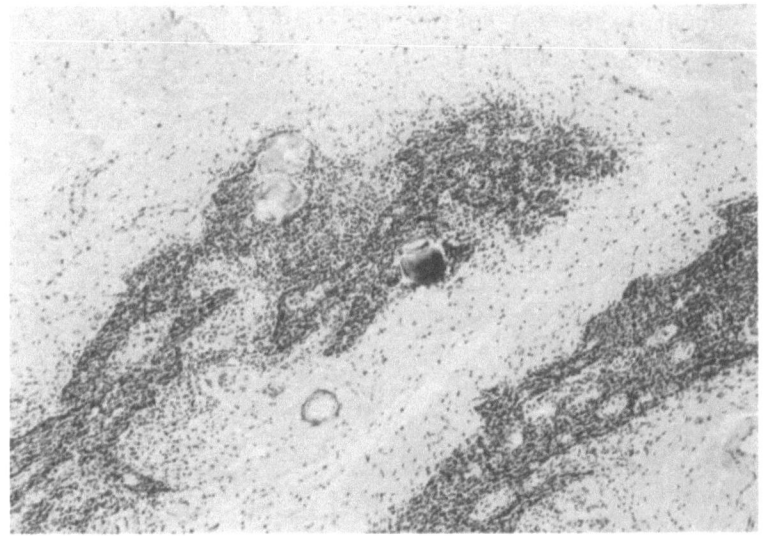

Fig. 7. Photomicrograph of thymus gland of patient succumbing to
         infectious mononucleosis and the X-linked lymphoprolifer-
         ative syndrome in the fourth week. The thymus gland is
         markedly depleted of thymocytes and calcified Hassall's
         epithelium are found. Hematoxylin and eosin, X100.

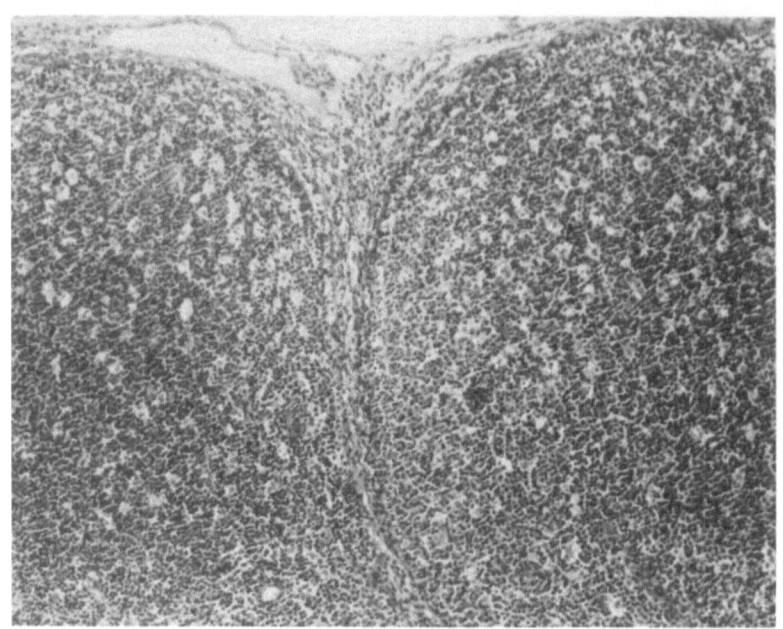

Fig. 8.   Photomicrograph of lymph node from patient with the
          infectious mononucleosis phenotype of X-linked lymphopro-
          liferative syndrome. The node is hyperplastic.
          Hematoxylin and eosin, X200 (published with the per-
          mission of Lancet).

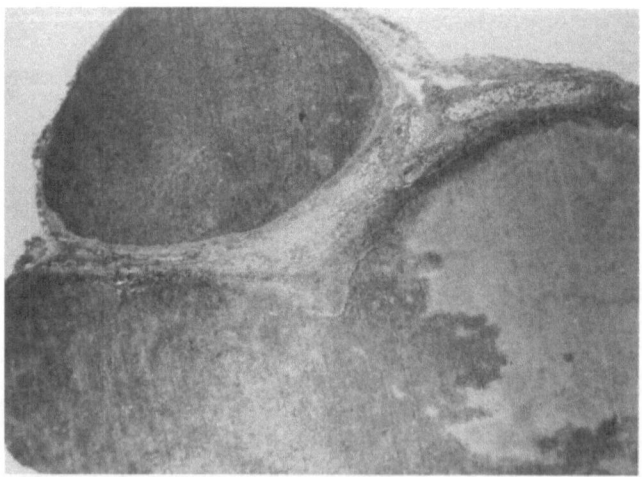

Fig. 9.   Photomicrograph of lymph node displaying extensive focal
          necrosis. The patient had infectious mononucleosis and
          succumbed to massive liver failure. Hematoxylin and
          eosin, X250.

Destruction of thymic epithelium due to EBV infection in boys with this syndrome may be responsible for the progressive character of the immune deficiency (12). Biphasic changes in the appearance of the thymus gland are found. Thymus gland shows immunoblastic proliferation with plasmacytoid cellular infiltrates during the initial two weeks of IM. Within three to four weeks, Hassall's thymic epithelium can be destroyed by multinucleated giant cells (Figure 6). This is found in experimental graft-versus-host disease in mice (21). Later, calcified epithelium or no corpuscles can be found (Figure 7). Beyond three weeks the thymus gland becomes depleted of thymocytes and may become invaded by B cells and plasma cells. Simultaneously, T cell dependent regions in the spleen and lymph nodes become depleted.

Lymph nodes also vary in appearance with time. Initially, extensive immunoblastic proliferation effaces lymphoid follicles and compresses sinuses (Figure 8). Focal to wide-spread necrosis can be seen, especially in lymph nodes. Perhaps such patients acquire agammaglobulinemia (Figure 9). After the initial week of illness, polyclonal B cell proliferation with differentiation to plasma cells is evident in many of the lymph nodes. Concurrently, serum levels of IgM, IgG, and IgA often become increased in a polyclonal fashion. Those who die after a few weeks of IM show depletion of thymus-dependent regions of lymph node and spleen.

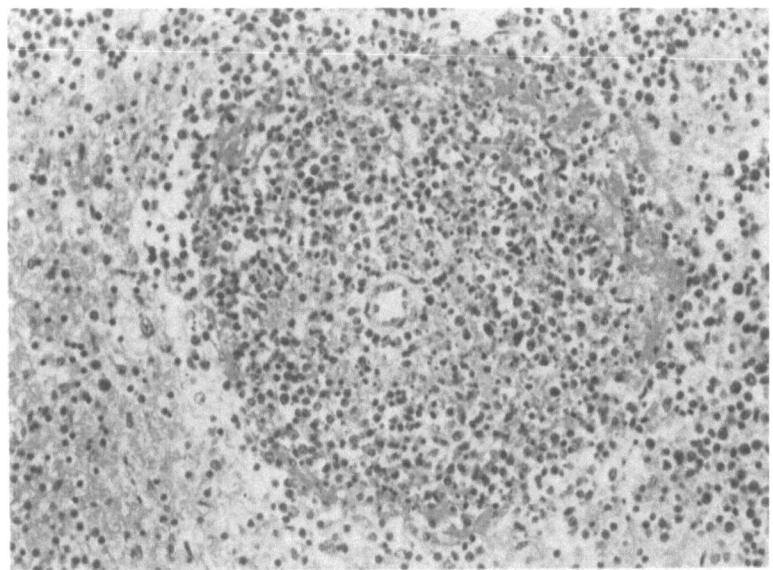

Fig. 10. Photomicrograph of spleen of patient succumbing to infectious mononucleosis phenotypes of XLP. The lymphoid
sheath displayed marked necrosis. Hematoxylin and eosin,
X110.

Erythrophagocytosis and activated macrophages are usually seen in
the hematopoietic organs.

The spleen generally increases in size progressively with
time. It weighs 3 to 5 fold above normal. The increase in size
is apparently due to lymphoid proliferation; infiltration, and
also congestion. The splenic T cell lymphoid sheath often shows
extensive necrosis early on (Figure 10). This is a feature of
acute graft-versus-host disease (22). Later, plasma cells and
their precursors invade this site. Subendothelial and capsular
invasion by the cells is often present. Erythrophagocytosis is
frequently prominent. Long-term survivors may show depletion of
the lymphoid sheath.

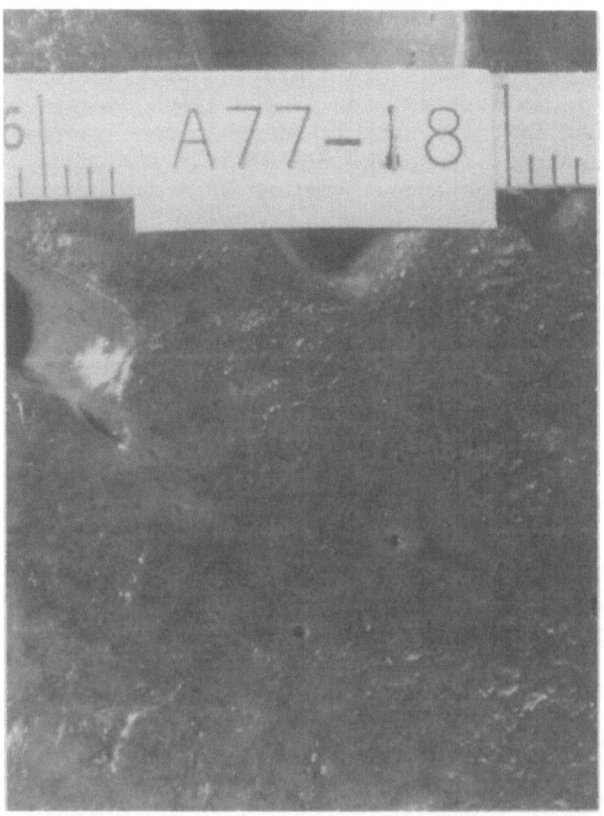

Fig. 11. Gross photo of liver from patient with infectious mono-
         nucleosis phenotype of XLP sustaining massive liver
         failure. Note the variegated pattern which is due to
         necrosis.

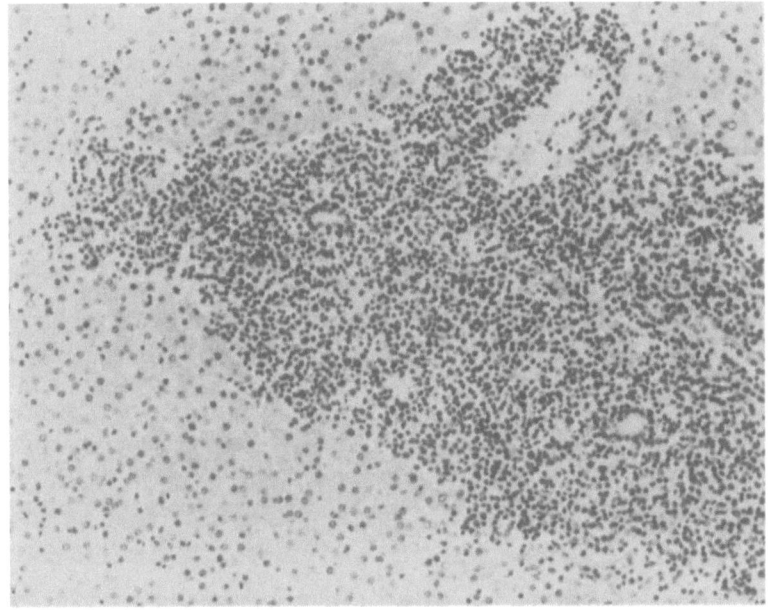

Fig. 12 Photomicrograph of liver shown in Figure 11. A periportal lymphoid infiltrate is seen and the hepatocytes are
necrotic. Hematoxylin and eosin, X450.

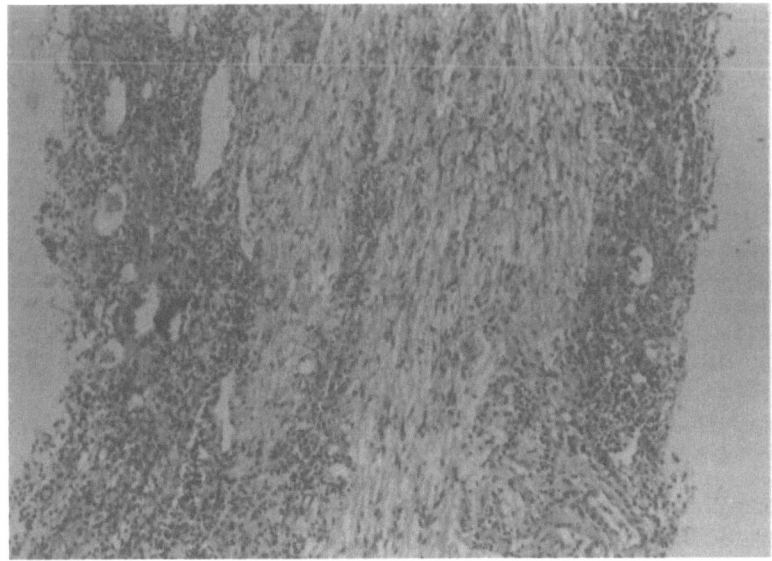

Fig. 13. Photomicrograph of neurohypophysis infiltrated by
lymphoid cells. Hematoxylin and eosin, X450.

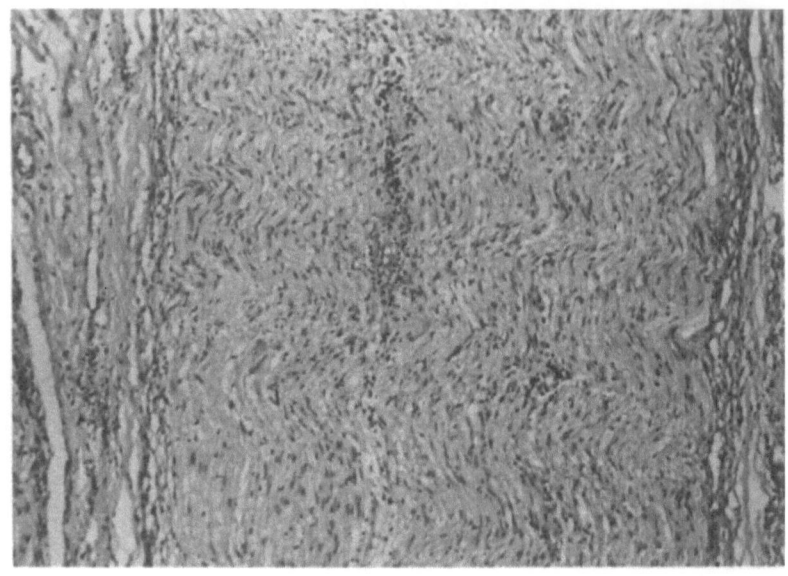

Fig. 14. Photomicrograph of sciatic nerve showing infiltrate by
lymphoid cells. The patient had the infectious
mononucleosis phenotype of XLP. Hematoxylin and eosin
X250.

The proliferating B cells often disseminate throughout the
body into perivascular spaces of brain, peribronchiolar regions of
lung, periportal zones of liver, heart, and other organs producing
necrosis. Disseminated infiltration is not generally found in the
individuals with malignant lymphoma phenotypes, suggesting the
cells of the IM phenotype are different with regards to their
migratory capabilities.

Massive hepatic necrosis is frequently found in the IM phenotype (Figures 11,12). Failure to recognize that EBV can produce
massive hepatic necrosis has frequently lead to misdiagnosis of
viral hepatitis (23). The visceral and central nervous system
infiltrates by atypical lymphocytes are often accompanied by
histiocytes. Hence, the misdiagnosis of lymphohistiocytosis has
been a common event. Infiltration of the neurohypophysis (Figure
13) provokes secretory defects of anti-diuretic hormone and
infiltrate into peripheral nerves (Figure 14) has been associated
with neurological deficits.

Malignant lymphomas have always been of the B cell type.
Never has Hodgkin's disease occurred. Regrettably, cell surface
or intracytoplasmic marking studies and cytogenetic evaluation
have not been possible to ascertain whether the tumors are mono-
or polyclonal. Likely, there is a spectrum of lymphoproliferative

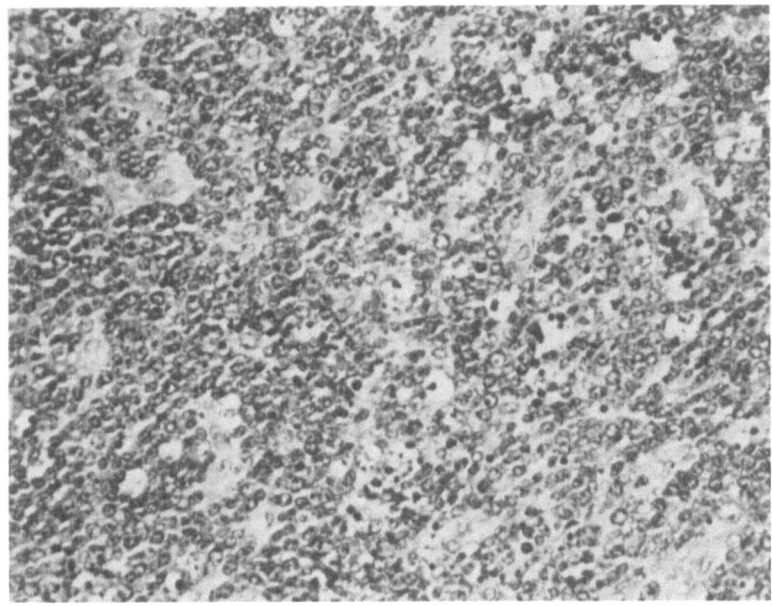

Fig. 15. Photomicrograph of small malignant lymphoma involving
        terminal ileum. Hematoxylin and eosin X250. The tumor
        had infiltrated through the wall.

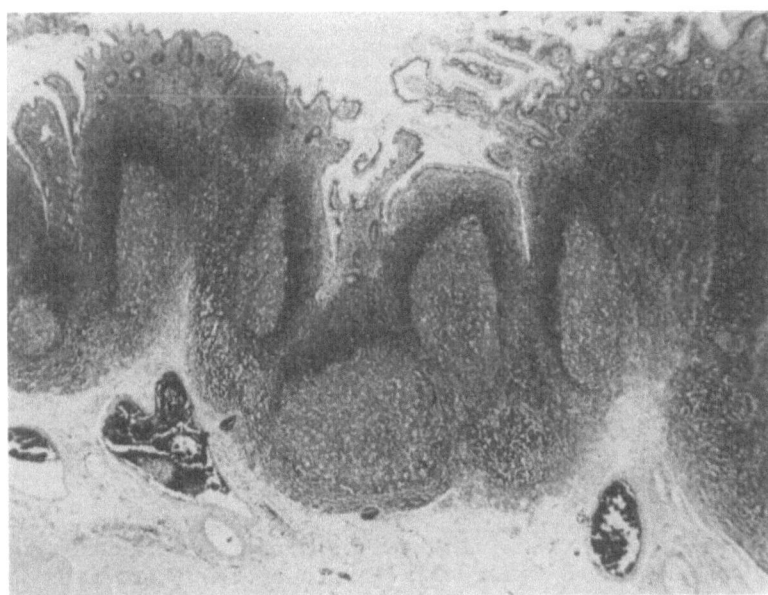

Fig. 16. Photomicrograph of ileum from patient of Figure 15. Note
        the markedly expanded germinal centers. Hematoxylin and
        eosin X250.

disease from polyclonal to monoclonal. The tumors which are
homogeneous in morphology (Figures 15 and 16) are likely monoclonal, presumably due to their being frozen in one phase of
differentiation by a genetic alteration. Important distinctions
are possible between the fatal IM phenotype of XLP and malignant
lymphoma. The lymphomas localize as masses of locally infiltrating immature lymphoid tissue. They do not usually disseminate
throughout the body. However, the dissemination is found in fatal
IM. Twenty-six of 35 malignant lymphomas were localized to the
terminal ileum (12). Other less frequent extranodal sites include
colon, brain, liver, kidneys, lung, thymus and bone marrow.
Involvement of lymph nodes is uncommon. Classification of the
lymphomas by the Rappaport system (24) suggests that the majority
are histiocytic lymphomas and Burkitt lymphoma is also found
(so-called histiocytic lymphomas are actually B cell lymphomas in
patients with XLP).

    The B cell lymphomas most frequently arise without antecedent
IM (Figure 2). IM can follow the malignant lymphoma phenotype.
Several individuals have developed life-threatening EBV infections
years following successful treatment of their malignant lymphomas
(Figure 17). We have hypothesized that conversion from the IM to
malignant lymphoma phenotype occurs due to a cytogenetic error
(25) and that the various phenotypes are in the individuals immune
responses at a given moment.

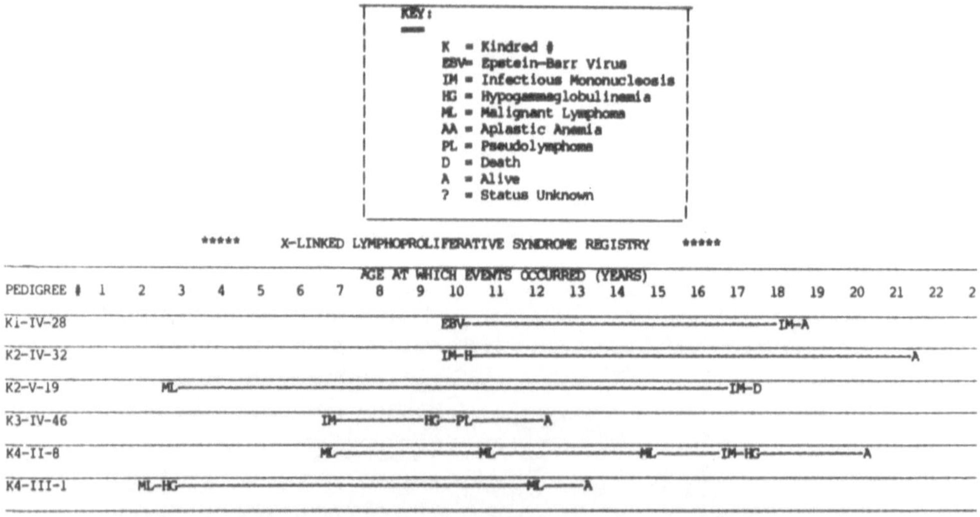

```
KEY:
                    K  = Kindred #
                    EBV= Epstein-Barr Virus
                    IM = Infectious Mononucleosis
                    HG = Hypogammaglobulinemia
                    ML = Malignant Lymphoma
                    AA = Aplastic Anemia
                    PL = Pseudolymphoma
                    D  = Death
                    A  = Alive
                    ?  = Status Unknown
```

*****   X-LINKED LYMPHOPROLIFERATIVE SYNDROME REGISTRY   *****

PEDIGREE #	AGE AT WHICH EVENTS OCCURRED (YEARS)
	1 2 3 4 5 6 7 8 9 10 11 12 13 14 15 16 17 18 19 20 21 22 2
K1-IV-28	EBV————————————————————IM-A
K2-IV-32	IM-H———————————————————————————A
K2-V-19	ML————————————————————————IM-D
K3-IV-46	IM————HG—PL————A
K4-II-8	ML———————ML————————ML————IM-HG————A
K4-III-1	ML-HG——————————————ML———A

Fig. 17. Displayed is a representative group of patients in the
         XLP Registry. Note the changes of the phenotypes with
         time. (From: Purtilo, D.T. et al. Epstein-Barr virus-
         induced diseases in boys with the X-linked lymphopro-
         liferative syndrome (XLP). Am. J. Med., 73:49, 1982.)

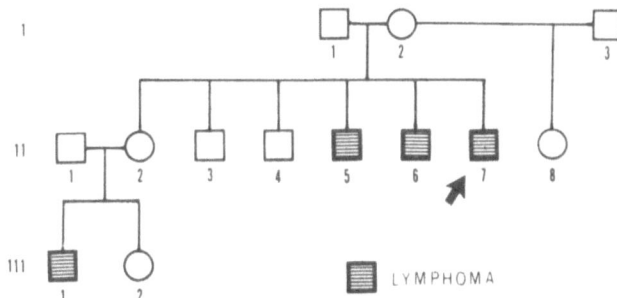

Fig. 18. Pedigree of family with X-linked lymphoproliferative
syndrome. Patient II-IV had died of "infectious
hepatitis." (From: Mauer, H. et al. Cancer 37:
2224, 1976.)

CONCLUSIONS

     Studies of XLP during the past eight years have demonstrated
an XLP locus on the X chromosome which accounts for a variety of
diseases following EBV. The prospective and retrospective studies
of families with the syndrome indicate that the clinical and
pathological outcome of EBV infections are determined by individual immune responses. This is evident in the family shown in
Figures 18 and 19.

     The predominance of males with malignant B cell lymphoma in
childhood may be accounted for, in part, due to XLP (26). A
rational basis for prevention and treatment of males with XLP has
been established by offering genetic counseling, providing antiviral therapy with Acyclovir® and interferon; giving immunotherapy
(i.e., gammaglobulin containing high titer EBV antibodies), and
potentially correcting immunity with bone marrow transplantation.
Immune reconstitution has already been achieved by bone marrow
transplantation in one patient with XLP.

     The role of immune deficiency in EBV-induced oncogenesis is
being documented in studies of XLP (27-28). This provides insight
regarding etiology of lymphoma in renal transplant recipients who
develop phenotypes similar to XLP, many of the patients have been
shown to have aberrant or deficient immune responses to the virus
and EBV genome has been found in the lymphomas and tissues
(16,17). Elsewhere in this book, chapters by Hanto and Bieber and
their colleagues document EBV as an etiological factor of lymphomas in renal and cardiac transplant recipients, respectively. A
variety of other patients with inherited or acquired immune deficiency have also been evaluated for EBV and many of their tumors
have contained the virus (17).

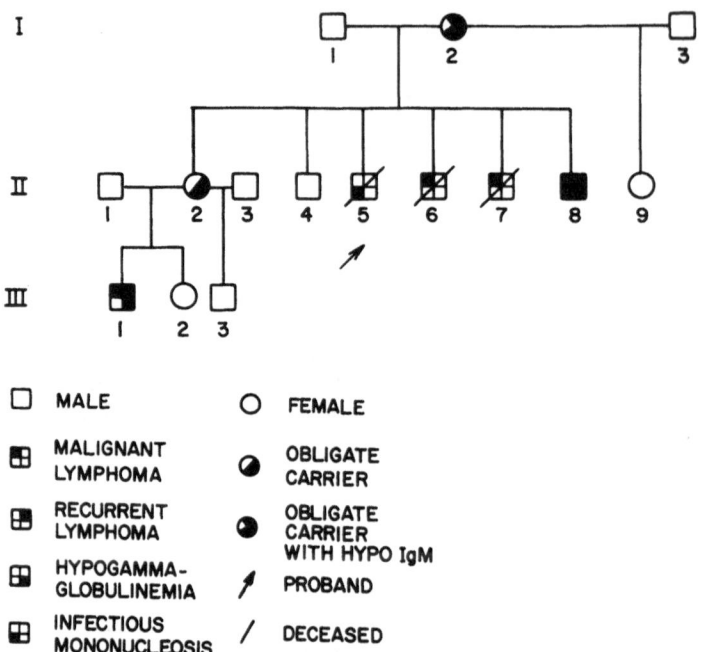

Fig. 19. Pedigree and phenotypes from the family displayed in
         Figure 18. Restudy of the family revealed that the
         patient thought to have succumbed to viral hepatitis in
         fact had infectious mononucleosis hepatitis with massive
         liver failure. XLP has been diagnosed in the family.

What role does immune deficiency play in other malignancies?
XLP and EBV-induced lymphoproliferative diseases due to the
underlying immune deficiency are providing a model for understanding mechanisms of viral oncogenesis. Elsewhere in this book,
Penn summarizes malignancies found in renal transplant recipients.
These may be due to ubiquitous viruses (30). For example,
Kaposi's sarcoma may be due to a cytomegalovirus (31). This virus
has been isolated recently in Kaposi's sarcoma in tissues from
patients with the acquired immune deficiency syndrome. Human
papilloma virus may be responsible for some squamous cell carcinomas (32). Males tend to become chronic carriers of hepatitis B
virus (HBV) and have a much higher frequency of hepatocellular
carcinoma than due females (33). Co-factors such as alcohol or
aflatoxins may be important in hepatocarcinogenesis induced by
HBV. Finally, Ziegler et al. (34) have identified EBV genome in
malignant B cell lymphomas in male homosexual patients with
acquired immunodeficiency syndrome (AIDS). The chapter by
Sonnabend et al. explores the relationship between EBV and
lymphomas in males with AIDS (35).

Empirical observations of malignancies in individuals with inherited or acquired immune deficiency point to a number of viruses and neoplasms that may have a viral basis. Worldwide, large numbers of patients may experience potentially preventable viral oncogenesis, i.e., nasopharyngeal carcinoma, Burkitt lymphoma, Kaposi's sarcoma, and hepatocellular carcinoma are examples. Tumors not seen in increased frequency in immune deficient patients probably are not generally caused by ubiquitous viruses.

Finally, longitudinal studies of individuals at risk for XLP and follow-up evaluation using laboratory testable hypothesis have elucidated the role of EBV in lymphoproliferative diseases. Long-term follow-up studies of individuals enrolled in a registry have proven useful for determining mechanisms of viral oncogenesis.

REFERENCES

1. Hambleton, G. and Cottom, D.G. Familial lymphoma. Proc. R. Soc. Med., 62:1095, 1965.
2. Burkitt, D.P. A sarcoma involving the jaws in African children. Br. J. Surg., 46:218, 1958.
3. Epstein, M.A., Achong, B.G., and Barr, Y.M. Virus particles in cultured lymphoblasts from Burkitt's lymphoma. Lancet, 1:702, 1964.
4. Henle, W., Henle, G., and Lennette, E.L. The Epstein-Barr virus. Sci. Am., 24:48, 1979.
5. Gatti, R.A. and Good, R.A. Occurrence of malignancy in immunodeficiency diseases. Cancer, 28:89, 1971.
6. Penn, I., Hammond, W., Brettschneider, L., and Starzl, T.E. Malignant lymphomas in transplanation patients. Transplant. Proc., 1:106, 1969.
7. Purtilo, D.T., Cassel, C., and Yang, J.P.S. Fatal infectious mononucleosis in familial lymphohistiocytosis. N. Engl. J. Med., 291:736, 1974.
8. Purtilo, D.T., Yang, J.P.S., Cassel, C.K., Harper, P., Stephenson, S.R., Landing, B.H., and Vawter, G.F. X-linked recessive progressive combined variable immunodeficiency (Duncan's disease). Lancet, 1:935, 1975.
9. Purtilo, D.T., DeFlorio, D., Hutt, L.M., Bhawan, J., Yang, J.P.S., Otto, R. and Edwards, W. Variable phenotypic expression of an X-linked recessive lymphoproliferative syndrome. N. Engl. J. Med., 297:1077, 1977.
10. Purtilo, D.T. Hypothesis: pathogenesis and phenotypes of an X-linked recessive lymphoproliferative syndrome. Lancet, ii:882, 1976.
11. Hamilton, J.K., Paquin, L.A., Sullivan, J.L., Maurer, H.S., Cruzi, P.G., Provisor, A.J., Steuber, C.P., Hawkins, E., Yawn, D., Cornet, J., Clausen, K., Finkelstein, G.Z.,

Landing, B., Grunnet, M., and Purtilo, D.T.   X-linked
Lymphoproliferative Syndrome Registry report.   J. Pedi.,
96:669, 1980.

12.   Purtilo, D.T., Sakamoto, K., Barnabei, V., Seeley, J.,
Bechtold, T., Rogers, G., Yetz, J., and Harada, S.
Epstein-Barr virus-induced diseases in boys with the X-
linked lymphoproliferative syndrome (XLP).   Update on
studies of the registry.   Am. J. Med., 73:49, 1982.

13.   Purtilo, D.T., Paquin, L.A., DeFlorio, D., Virzi, F., and
Sukhuja, R.   Immunodiagnosis and immunopathogenesis of
the X-linked recessive lymphoproliferative syndrome.
Sem. Hematol., 16:309, 1979.

14.   Sakamoto, K., Freed, H., and Purtilo, D.T.   Antibody responses to Epstein-Barr virus in families with the X-
linked lymphoproliferative syndrome.   J. Immunol.,
125:921, 1980.

15.   Sakamoto, K., Seeley, J.K., Lindsten, T., Sexton, J., Yetz,
J., Ballow, M., and Purtilo, D.T.   Abnormal anti-Epstein-
Barr virus antibodies in carriers of the X-linked
lymphoproliferative syndrome andin females at risk.   J.
Immunol., 128:904, 1982.

16.   Purtilo, D.T., Sakamoto, K., Saemundsen, A.K., Sullivan,
J.L., Synnerholm, A.C., Andersson-Anvret, M., Pritchard,
J., Sloper, C, Sieff, C., Pincott, J., Pachman, L.,
Rich, K., Cruzi, F., Cornet, J., Collins, R., Barnes,
N., Knight, J., Sandstedt, B., and Klein, G.
Documentation of Epstein-Barr virus infection in immuno-
deficient patients with life-threatening lymphoproli-
ferative disease by clinical, virological and
immunopathological studies.   Cancer Res., 41:4226, 1981.

17.   Saemundsen, A.K., Purtilo, D.T., Sakamoto, K., Sullivan,
J.L., Synnerholm, A.C., Hanto, D., Simmons, R., Anvret,
M., Collins, R., and Klein, G.   Documentation of
Epstein-Barr virus infection in immunodeficient patients
with life-threatening lymphoproliferative diseases by
Epstein-Barr virus complementary RNA/DNA and viral
DNA/DNA hybridization.   Cancer Res., 41:4237, 1981.

18.   Ochs, H.D., Sullivan, J.L., Wedgewood, R.J., Seeley, J.K.,
Sakamoto, K., and Purtilo, D.T.   X-linked lymphoproliferative syndrome: abnormal antibody responses to bacteriophage ØX174.   In: R. Wedgewood and F. Rosen
(eds.), Primary Immunodeficiency Diseases.   New York:
Alan R. Liss, in press.

19.   Purtilo, D.T., Hutt, L.M., Allegra, S., Cassel, C., Yang,
J.P.S., and Rosen, F.S.   Immunodeficiency to the
Epstein-Barr virus in the X-linked recessive lymphoproliferative syndrome.   Clin. Immunol. Immunopath.,
9:147, 1978.

20.   Purtilo, D.T., Zelkowitz, L., Harada, S., Brooks, C.D.,
Bechtold, T., Saemundsen, A.K., Lipscomb, H., Yetz, J.,

and Rogers, G. Delayed onset of infectious mononucleosis associated with acquired agammaglobulinemia
and red cell aplasia. Submitted for publication.

21. Seemayer, T.A., Lapp, W.S., and Bolande, R.P. Thymic
Involution in murine graft-versus-host reaction. Amer.
J. Pathol., 88:119, 1977.

22. Kersey, J.H., Meuwissen, H.J., and Good, R.A. Graft versus
host reactions following transplantation of allogeneic
hematopoietic cells. Hum. Path., 2:389, 1971.

23. Maurer, H.S., Gotoff, S.P., Allen, L., and Bolan, J.
Malignant lymphoma of the small intestine in multiple
family members. Association with an immunologic deficiency. Cancer, 37:2224, 1976.

24.
25. Purtilo, D.T. Immune deficiency predisposing to
Epstein-Barr virus-induced lymphoproliferative diseases:
the X-linked lymphoproliferative syndrome as a model.
In: G. Klein and S. Weinhouse (eds.), Advances in Cancer
Research. Vol. 34, pp. 279-312. New York: Academic
Press, 1980.

26. Purtilo, D.T. Opportunistic non-Hodgkin's lymphoma in X-
linked recessive immunodeficiency and lymphoproliferative
syndromes. Sem. Oncol., 4:335, 1977.

27. Harada, S., Sakamoto, K., Seeley, J.K., Lindsten, T.,
Rogers, G., Pearson, G., and Purtilo, D.T. Immune
deficiency in the X-linked lymphoproliferative syndrome.
I. Epstein-Barr virus-specific defects. J. Immunol.,
129:2532, 1982.

28. Lindsten, T., Seeley, J.K., Sakamoto, K., Yetz, J., Harada,
S., Bechtold, T., Rogers, G., and Purtilo, D.T. Immune
deficiency in the X-linked lymphoproliferative syndrome.
II. Immunoregulatory T cell defects. J. Immunol., 129:
2536, 1982.

29. Harada, S., Bechtold, T., and Purtilo, D.T. Cell-mediated
immunity to Epstein-Barr virus (EBV) and natural killer
(NK)-cell activity in X-linked lymphoproliferative
syndrome. Int. J. Cancer, 216:739, 1982.

30. Linder, J. and Purtilo, D.T. Oncological consequences of
impaired immune surveillance against ubiquitous viruses.

31. Drew, W.L., Conant, M.A., Miner, R.C., Huang, E.S., Ziegler,
J.L., Groundwater, J.R., Gullett, J.H., Volberding, P.,
Abrams, D.I., Mintz, L. Cytomegalovirus and Kaposi's
sarcoma in young homosexual men. Lancet, ii:125, 1982.

32. Purtilo, D.T. Viruses, tumors, and immune deficiency.
Lancet, 1:684, 1982.

33. Deinhardt, F., Gust, I.D. Viral hepatitis. Bull WHO,
60:661, 1982.

34. Ziegler, J., Drew, W.L., Miner, R.C., Mintz, L., Rosenbaum,
E., Gershow, J., Casavant, C., Yamamoto, K., Lennette,
E.T., Greenspan, J., Shillitoe, E., and Beckstead, J.

The outbreak of Burkitt's-like lymphoma in homosexual
men. Lancet, ii:631, 1982.

35.   Sonnabend, J., Witkin, S.S., and Purtilo, D.T. Acquired
immunodeficiency syndrome, opportunistic infections, and
malignancies in male homosexuals. A hypothesis of
etiologic factors in pathogenesis. J. Am. Med. Assoc.,
249:2370, 1983.

RESPONSES TO EPSTEIN-BARR VIRUS IN IMMUNE DEFICIENT PATIENTS

Shinji Harada, Eiji Tatsumi, Helen
Lipscomb and David T. Purtilo

Department of Pathology & Laboratory Medicine
University of Nebraska Medical Center
Omaha, NE 68105

INTRODUCTION

Two decades have passed since Epstein-Barr virus (EBV) was
described (1) and yet new diseases continue to be attributed to
the virus. Debates initiated in the early 1960's are ongoing
regarding the role of the virus in Burkitt lymphoma (BL), and
nasopharyngeal carcinoma (NPC). Recently, the opportunistic
malignant lymphomas (ML) occurring in immune deficient individuals
have provided new puzzles. Questions remaining to be answered are
whether latent virus is activated in B cells transformed by other
agents or alternatively, does the virus infect the malignant B
cell after transformation owing to the presence of viral receptors
on the cell. Attention has also been directed to find oncogenic
and benign strains of the virus. In our view, underlying
inherited or environmentally induced immune deficiency is important in determining the outcome of EBV infections.

Here we describe inherited and acquired immune deficiency
disorders and the immune responses (or lack of) associated with
life-threatening EBV infection. The X-linked lymphoproliferative
syndrome (XLP) serves as a model for studying the impact of this
virus in lymphomagenesis in immune deficient individuals (2). A
compelling case is presented that an individual's immune competence at a given time is the major determinant of the clinical
expression of primary or reactivated EBV infections. Owing to the
unique site of EBV infections (i.e., B cell) and dependence on
activation of normal immunoregulatory mechanisms to cope with the

virus, immune deficient patients can develop progressive life-
threatening lymphoproliferative diseases. Secondly, immunosuppressed (i.e., patients with lymphoid or other malignancies) can
reactivate EBV leading to opportunistic malignant lymphomas.

EBV Cycle and Normal Immune Responses

The virus is restricted to B cell infection due to the

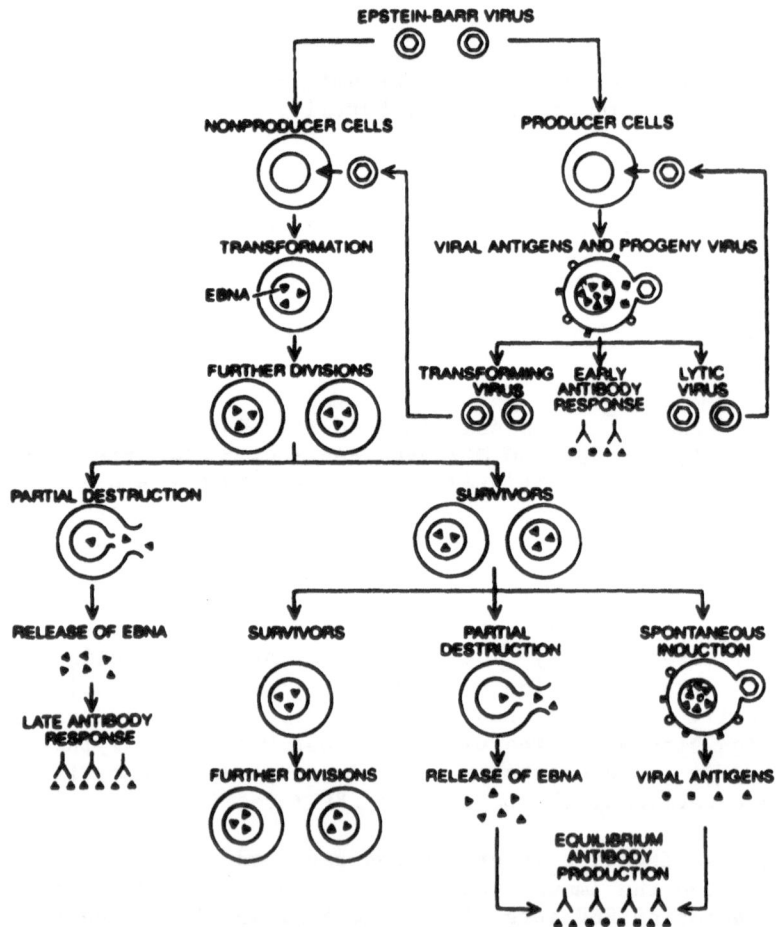

Fig. 1. Molecular events occurring when EBV infects B cells.
         Productive or nonproductive (lytic) pathways may be
         pursued. (From: Henle, W., Henle, G., and Lennette, E.T.
         Epstein-Barr virus. Sci. Am. 241:48-59, 1979. Copyright©
         (1983) by Scientific American, Inc. All rights
         reserved.)

presence of viral receptor on this cell. Elsewhere in this volume
Volsky describes transplantation of EBV receptors and infection of
unnatural host cells including oral epithelial cells.

   When the virus infects the B cell, it pursues one of two pathways. The initial transforming antigen elaborated by the virus is
EB nuclear-associated antigen (EBNA). Cells blocking the viral
cycle at EBNA translation are capable of unlimited proliferation
and latency is established (Figure 1). An alternate pathway leads
to the death of the cell. The virus advances in the cycle and
expresses early antigen (EA) and then synthesis can proceed to
viral capsid antigen (VCA) (3). Finally, lysis of the cell occurs
and viral particles are liberated to infect other B cells or it is
excreted in the saliva. Other articles in this volume by Roubal,
Krueger, and Volsky discuss these molecular and cellular events
more extensively.

   The vast majority of individuals become infected by EBV during
early childhood. Silent seroconversion supervenes to establish
life-long latency. However, in individuals in middle and upper
socioeconomic classes the children do not become infected.
Infectious mononucleosis (IM) occurs in approximately one-half to
two-thirds of individuals becoming infected in their teens or
early twenties (4). The clinical manifestations of infectious
mononucleosis are the result of polyclonal B cell transformation

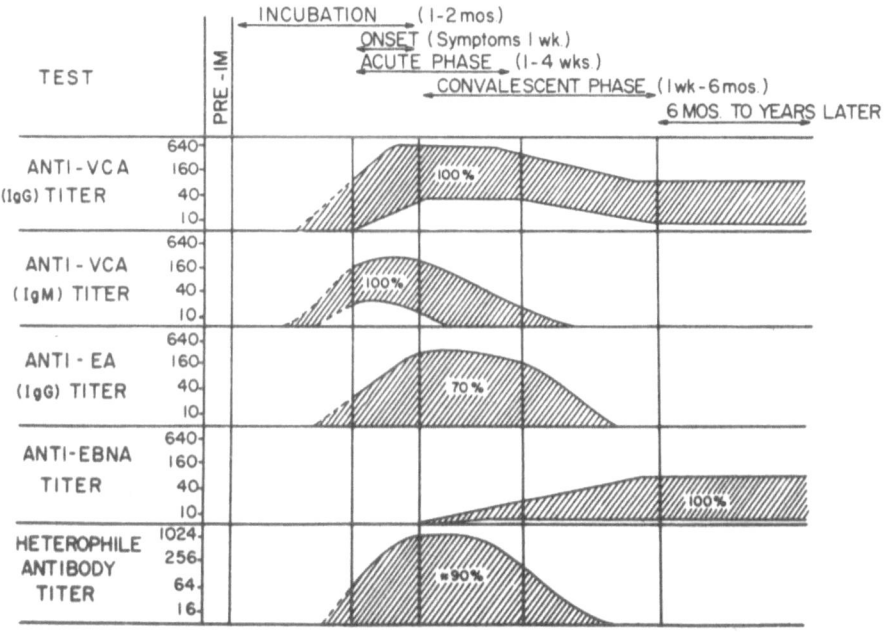

Fig. 2. Chronologic events in acute EBV infection to con-
         valescence.

and an explosive counter response by T cells. Enlargement of tonsils, lymph nodes and spleen along with lymphocytosis are manifestations of this immune struggle. The peripheral blood displays
atypical lymphocytosis. Marking of the subpopulations of lymphoid
cells in the peripheral blood by monoclonal antibodies reveal the
dominant cell to be a suppressor T cell (OKT8) population (5).
Only a few percent of B cells can be shown to be EBNA positive
(6,7). Concurrently, antibodies form against viral antigens to
neutralize spread of virus and arm antibody-dependent cellular
cytotoxicity (ADCC).

     Assessment of EBV-specific antibody responses can demonstrate
the phase of illness (Figure 2). Linder and Purtilo, elsewhere in
this monograph, describe immune responses in infectious mononucleosis. Life-long latency can be documented in approximately
85 to 95% of the population (8).

     If an individual does not mount cytotoxic T cell responses,
the B cells can continue proliferating unabated; vital organs are
infiltrated and damaged. Purtilo has illustrated destruction of
tissues by infiltrating lymphoid cells in the accompanying chapter
and elsewhere (9). Comprehensive studies of the X-linked
lymphoproliferative syndrome (XLP) are providing an understanding
of the role of this virus in lymphoproliferative diseases in
immune deficient patients.

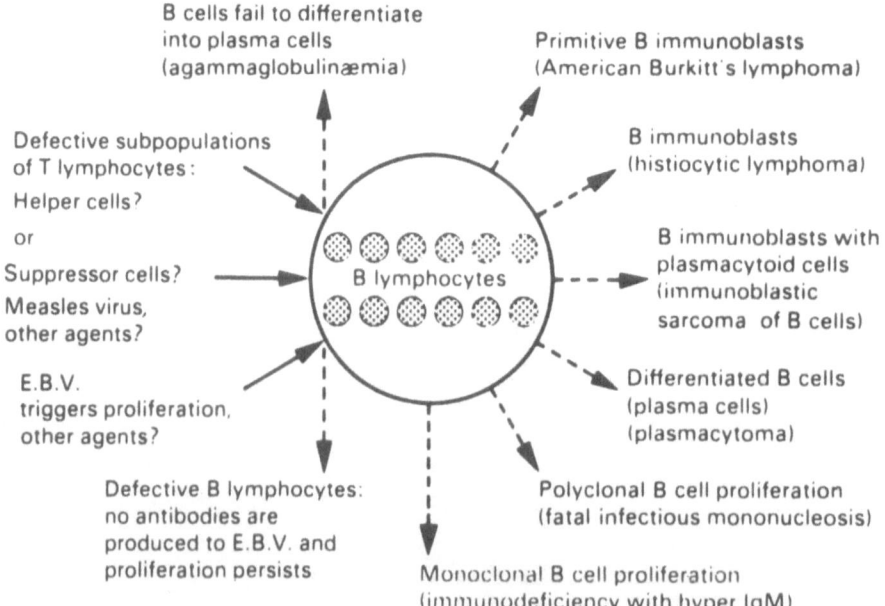

Fig. 3. Hypothesis regarding pathogenesis of phenotypes of XLP.
         (From: Purtilo, D.T. et al. Lancet ii:882, 1976.)

Immunopathology of X-linked Lymphoproliferative Syndrome

XLP is manifested by a defect on the X chromosome - the lymphoproliferative control locus (10). Following EBV infection, a variety of phenotypes can be seen. These have been grouped into two major categories: aproliferative and lymphoproliferative. The aproliferative expressions of EBV infection in these immune deficient individuals consist of acquired agammaglobulinemia, agranulocytosis, red cell aplasia, and aplastic anemia (11). The lymphoproliferative phenotypes consist of chronic or fatal IM, pseudolymphoma, and malignant B cell lymphomas. Hodgkin's disease has never occurred in these patients. Moreover, the mothers have not manifested these phenotypes.

In 1976, we reasoned that T cell regulation of B cells might explain the diverse diseases following EBV infection in XLP (12). We had considered that the lymphoproliferative phenotypes of IM and B cell lymphomas might occur in the males due to defective suppressor T cell function. Previous viral infection such as Rubeola seem to contribute to progressive impairment of suppressor T cell function, in certain patients prior to EBV triggering of B cell lymphoproliferation (Figure 3). Defects in helper T cell functions or excessive suppressor activity might cause agammaglobulinemia. Prior to discussing the results of testing of this hypothesis, diagnostic determinations necessary for diagnosing EBV infections in immune deficient patients are provided.

Diagnosis of EBV Infection in Immunodeficient Patients

Difficulties may arise in diagnosing EBV infections in immune deficient individuals due to the patient's inability to produce heterophil or EBV-specific antibodies. Individuals with primary immune deficiency who develop a primary EBV infection may have too low antibody titer responses. In contrast, individuals who become immune suppressed after EBV latency has been established will usually show elevated antibody titers.

Despite the immune deficiency of XLP, Monospot® (Ortho Diagnostics, Raritan, NJ), reactivity and low to moderate heterophil titers are produced in the IM phenotype. EBV-specific antibody responses to VCA of IgM class appear in acute infection and IgG isotype of anti-VCA persist in remote infection (13). Invariably the involved males lack the T cell function required to produce anti-EB nuclear-associated antigen. Routine diagnostic findings include atypical lymphocytosis (i.e., plasmacytoid lymphocytes) and polyclonal elevation of serum Ig in males.

Specific determinations to document virus in males lacking EBV antibody production include: transformation of cord B cells

Table 1.   Immune Competence in X-linked
Lymphoproliferative Syndrome

Normal

1.   White blood differential counts when not acutely infected
are normal.
2.   Numbers of OKT3, IA, HNK1, and surface Ig positive cells
are normal.
3.   Lymphocyte proliferative responses to mitogens (PHA, PWM,
and EBV) are normal to slightly reduced.
4.   Primary immune response to ØX174 in vivo of IgM is normal.
5.   IgM production of EBV-transformed B cell lines is normal.
6.   Serum immunoglobulin levels pre EBV infection are often
normal.

Defects

1.   Incomplete EBV-specific antibody production: no
anti-EBNA.
2.   Poor or reduced activity of EBV-specific memory T cells.
3.   Abnormal levels and ratios of OKT4 and OKT8 cells.
4.   Poor polyclonal Ig production by lymphoblastoid cell lines
in vitro.
5.   Deficient secondary response to ØX174 in vivo: no
IgM ———> IgG switch.
6.   Acquired natural killer cell activity post EBV infection.
7.   Thymic epithelial destruction post EBV infection.

---

by throat washings; development of spontaneous lymphoblastoid cell
lines which are EBNA positive from peripheral blood or lymphoid
organ; and use of complementary RNA/DNA or viral DNA/DNA as
molecular probes in tissues or tumor homogenates (14,15) (Table
1).   To date all males diagnosed with XLP who have been evaluated
contain significant numbers of EBV genomes in biopsy or autopsy
derived tissue specimens (14).

Study of approximately 18 males surviving XLP has demonstrated
variable immune responses to the virus (16).   Immune responses
appear to determine the phenotypic expressions: different strains
of virus do not seem to exist.   This virus has been such a successful parasite that mutation is unlikely to have occurred.   We
have sought to identify EBV-specific and general immunoregulatory
defects in surviving males with the syndrome.

Normal Immune Functions in XLP

The adjective, variable, was carefully chosen in describing the phenotypic expression of XLP (17). Summarized in Table 1 are the variable immune capacities of XLP patients. Many normal immune functions are present in males with XLP. The white blood cell differential count is normal when the viral infection is inactive (16). Enumeration of subsets of lymphoid cells in peripheral blood using monoclonal antibodies in cytofluorography reveals normal numbers of cells bearing OKT3 or T11 (pan-T cells), a positive, surface Ig positive, and HNK1 subsets (18). Proliferative responses to phytohemagglutinin, pokeweed mitogen and EBV are also relatively normal. The primary antibody responses of the IgM isotype to intravenous challenge by bacteriophage ØX174 are relatively normal in vivo (19). The EBV-transformed B cell lines of the patients produce normal quantities of IgM in vitro (20).

Importantly, patients with XLP are not generally vulnerable to a variety of infectious agents that are incapable of infecting the immune system itself. Other herpesviruses such as varicella-zoster, herpes hominus, and cytomegalovirus have not been opportunistic in XLP. The immune response of patients with XLP is adequate to cope with these virus infecting cells outside of the immune system but not to EBV which infects within the immune system.

Table 2. Defective Immune Responses in X-Linked Lymphoproliferative Syndrome (XLP) and Males at Risk

Abnormal Immune Function	Controls	XLP	Males at Risk
Lack of anti-EBNA is VCA (+) individuals	0/20	11/11	3/9
EBV-specific T memory defect	0/10	6/8	3/3+
No IgM ———> IgG switch in ØX174 response*	0/?	5/5?	3/3+
Abnormal OKT4/OKT8 subset ratio	0/20	8/11	5/15
Hypogammaglobulinemia**	0/29	19/11	0/15
Low natural killer activity	0/20	4/9	0/12

*Individual values were considered abnormal if they fell outside of 2 S.D. of the control mean.
**Outside the standard range for their age group.
+The at risk males tested are 3 of the VCA+ EBNA negative donors, i.e., individuals #1, 2, and 3.

Defective Immune Responses in XLP

    XLP patients fail to mount anti-EBNA antibody responses (13).
Patients at risk for XLP who are capable of producing anti-EBNA
titer above 1:20 do not have the syndrome (Table 2). Another
EBV-specific defect in XLP is failure of memory T cells to clone
and become cytotoxic against autologous EBV infected cell lines in
vitro (21) (Figure 4). Lymphocytes challenged by extracts of
lymphoblastoid cell lines carrying EBV antigens cannot inhibit
leukocyte migration (22). Lymphocytes challenged by mitogens
in vitro showed deficient polyclonal Ig production. Defective
switching in vivo from IgM to IgG antibody in response to
ØX174 on secondary challenge is evidence of XLP (19). The
majority, but not all patients with XLP, exhibit defective natural
killer cell activity against K562 (23). Inversion of the ratio of
OKT4 (helper/inducer)/T8 (lytic/suppressor) populations is found
following EBV infection in survivors of XLP (16) (Table 2). At
necropsy, thymic epithelium is damaged or destroyed in most individuals succumbing to IM (24). The accompanying chapter by
Purtilo illustrates the destruction of thymus gland. Concomitantly the thymus-dependent regions in lymph nodes and spleen

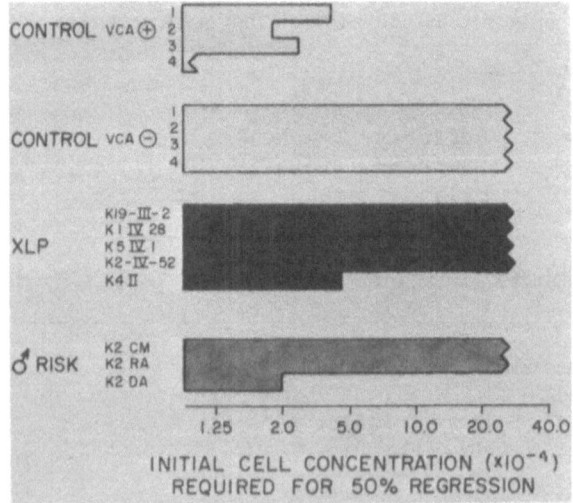

Fig. 4. Defective memory T cell function is found in X-linked
         lymphoproliferative syndrome in the B lymphoblastoid cell
         outgrowth inhibition assay. Seronegative individuals
         form lymphoblastoid cell lines on infection, whereas
         seropositive individuals activate memory T cells and
         abrogate the lymphoblastoid cell line outgrowth.
         Patients with XLP behave frequently as seronegative indi-
         viduals due to their immune defects.

are depleted. Diagnosis of males at risk for XLP prior to infection by the virus is difficult, but possible.

Detection of Affected Males at Risk for XLP

Prospective studies of males at risk for XLP have focused on
male infants born to mothers with previously affected sons or
whose maternally related relatives had phenotypes of XLP. No
obvious evidence clinically of immune deficiency is found usually
prior to EBV infection. Immunologic evaluation of the blood
reveals normal natural killer cell activity, normal immunoglobulin
levels, seronegativity for EBV, normal lymphoproliferative responses to mitogens in vitro, and relatively normal T4/T8 ratios (20).

The index of suspicion for XLP is increased when elevated
antibody titers to EBV are found in a mother of a boy, i.e., elevated and persisting anti-VCA of IgG, IgA, or IgM isotypes, and
anti-EA antibodies are found in most obligate carriers of XLP
(25,26). We have proposed that the antibodies continue to
increase following EBV infection to compensate for T cell defects
until a immune-virus detente is achieved. The female carriers
possess approximately 50% normal lymphocytes presuming that inactivation of X chromosomes occurs randomly during lyonization. No
females have developed phenotypes of XLP.

Seeley et al. (20) have studied and compared nineteen at risk
males with ten affected males. The males at risk were divided
into three categories according to their anti-VCA and EBNA titers
(Table 2). Four individuals positive for VCA had failed during a
two year period to produce antibody to EBNA, a pattern found in
XLP patients. Nine developed normal anti-EBNA titers. Six had no
detectable antibodies to EA and EBNA antigens, indicating they had
not yet been infected by the virus.

We had demonstrated that males at risk have normal numbers of
circulating T and B cells; however, the majority of XLP patients
have reversed ratios of T4/T8. The at risk males tended to show
this defect which also correlated with a lack of anti-EBNA production.

Three boys at risk for XLP were immunized with bacteriophage
ØX174. All cleared the phage normally and produced measurable
antibodies (19,20). The primary antibody response was markedly
depressed in all three individuals. The titers following a second
injection of phage were low for subjects 2 and 3 and within the
normal range for another boy (Figure 5). However, all 3 of the
boys failed to switch from IgM to IgG antibody production on
secondary challenge (Figure 6). In contrast, ten normal male
controls showed approximately 25 to 78% IgG antibody response.

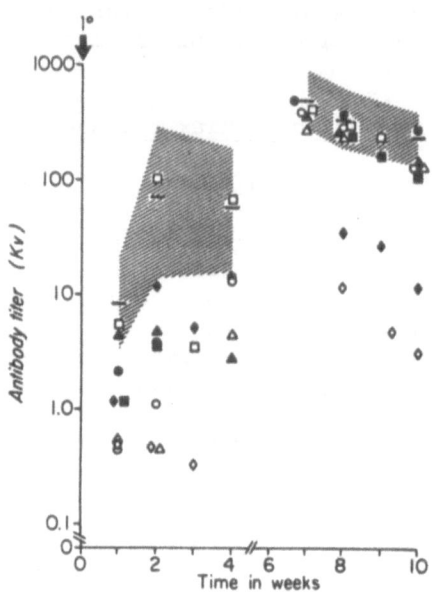

Fig. 5.   Primary (1°) and secondary (2°) antibody responses to
          bacteriophage ØX174. The Kv of each individual patient
          is indicated by a symbol. 2 XLP patients have chronic
          infectious mononucleosis (□, ●); 3 have hypogam-
          maglobulinemia (△ , ▲, ○); and 3 are at risk for XLP
          (□ ,◇, ◆). the range of Kv's from normal male
          controls are indicated by the hatched area, the geometric
          mean by the horizontal bar. (From: Ochs, H.D., Sullivan,
          J.L., Wedgwood, R.J., Seeley, J.K., Sakamoto, K., and
          Purtilo, D.T. X-linked lymphoproliferative syndrome:
          abnormal antibody responses to bacteriophage ØX174. In:
          R.J. Wedgewood and F. Rosen (eds.), Primary Immuno-
          deficiency Diseases. BD:OAS 19(3):1983. New York:
          Alan R. Liss for the March of Dimes Birth Defects
          Foundation.)

     Natural killer cell activity (NK) against K562 and other NK
sensitive human target cells is thought to help explain immune
surveillance against malignancies. Previously, we have demonstrated that NK activity is deficient in most but not all affected
males (23,27). However, NK function in males at risk was within
the normal range even for EBNA negative individuals (Figure 7)
(20). Thus we conclude that the NK defect is not the ultimate
deterrent of lymphoproliferation and that in XLP this defect is an
acquired phenomenon.

     EBV-specific memory function has been assayed using the tech-
nique of Rickinson (28) wherein T cell cytotoxicity against

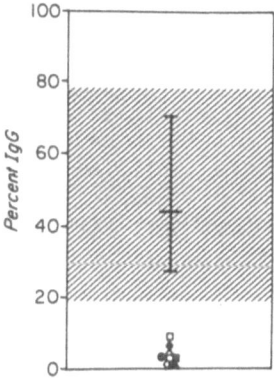

Fig. 6. Percent IgG of the antibody to bacteriophage ØX174 at 2
weeks post 2° immunization. The geometric mean of 10
normal male controls is indicated by the horizontal bar,
the 66% confidence limit by the vertical bar, and the
range by the hatched area. (From: Ochs, H.D., Sullivan,
J.L., Wedgwood, R.J., Seeley, J.K., Sakamoto, K., and
Purtilo, D.T. X-linked lymphoproliferative syndrome:
abnormal antibody responses to bacteriophage ØX174. In:
R.J. Wedgewood and F. Rosen (eds.), Primary
Immunodeficiency Diseases. BD:OAS 19(3):1983. New York:
Alan R. Liss for the March of Dimes Birth Defects
Foundation.)

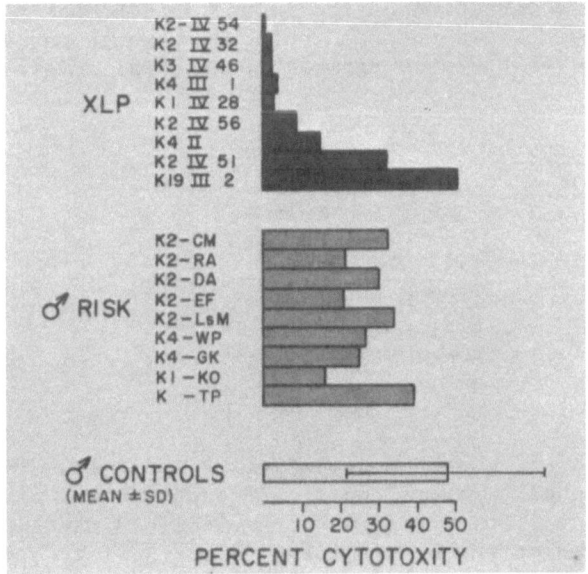

Fig. 7. Natural killer cell activity of at risk males with XLP.
Compared to known patients with XLP. The majority of
established XLP patients have NK defects, whereas those
at risk do not.

autologous EBV infected B cells is assayed. B cells from all
donors when infected with EBV will proliferate indefinitely. A
cell line can be established in seronegative individuals.
However, in the presence of sufficient sensitized T cells from
seropositive donors, the initial B cell proliferation at two weeks
post infection is completely abolished by week four. Even in high
cell numbers of seronegative T cells there is a failure to induce
regression. Lymphocytes from most XLP patients (Figure 4) fail to
inhibit outgrowth regression.

In summary, approximately one-fourth of apparently healthy
males at risk for developing XLP share two of the four immune
abnormalities of XLP. This implies failure to produce anti-EBNA
titers and the abnormal T cell subset balance may be due to primary congenital immune defects. Alternatively, secondary immune
defects are due to abnormal host immune responses to EBV. The NK
deficiency and hypogammaglobulinemia observed in patients with XLP
may be acquired as the disease progresses.

Many questions remain to be answered regarding molecular
aspects of XLP. Evaluation of purine degradation enzymes in red
cells of XLP patients has failed to disclose defects. Similarly,
efforts to identify microtubular aberrations in lymphoid cells
have been unrewarding. To be explored are changes in concentrations and subtypes of thymic hormonal factors, interferon and
leukotrienes. These are being measured sequentially following EBV
infection while progression of the immune defect continues. A
cluster of genes resides on the X chromosome which may lead to
immune deficiency: Bruton's agammaglobulinemia, severe combined

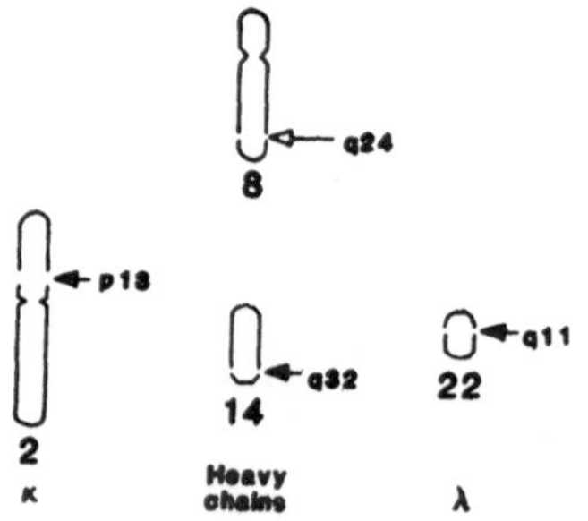

Fig. 8.   Breakpoints on chromosomes 14, 22 and 2 are at loci for
          heavy chain, lambda chain, and kappa chain, respectively.
          Translocation to recipient chromosome 8 may activate an
          oncogene at the breakpoint. (From: Rowley, J.D. Identi-
          fication of the constant chromosome regions involved in
          human hematologic malignant disease. Science
          216:749-751, 1982. Copyright© 1983 by the American
          Association for the Advancement of Science.)

immune deficiency, XLP, Wiskott-Aldrich syndrome, and immunodeficiency with hyper IgM (29). Are these disorders due to mutations in regulatory of structural genes? Where do they map on the X chromosome? These questions remain to be answered.

Another important question concerns clonality of EBV driven B cell proliferation. How is it possible to convert polyclonal B cell proliferation to monoclonality in XLP and related lymphoproliferative disorders? Using the model of African Burkitt lymphoma (30), we speculate that specific cytogenetic alterations occur between chromosomes (Figure 8) at breakpoints at genetic loci for coding for Ig on chromosomes 14, 22, and 2. Potentially in genetically activated B cells, being driven by EBV, the gene loci may become fragile sites. Reciprocal translocation from these three chromosomes to sites on the long arm of chromosome 8 occur and determine the Ig phenotype of the lymphoma. Rowley (31) and others have postulated that the transposition of loci coding for Ig synthesis to a specific break point on the long arm of chromosome 8 may activate an oncogene at this site, thereby promoting oncogenesis. The cell receiving this specific translocation would be endowed with the capacity to escape immunoregulatory and other control mechanisms. We are testing this hypothesis prospectively with XLP.

Several laboratories are now exploring the role of EBV in lymphoproliferative disorders in individuals with inherited and acquired immunodeficiency syndromes. The results of these studies point to EBV as a major etiologic factor in lymphomagenesis in immune deficient individuals.

EBV Induced Lymphomagenesis in Immune Deficiency

We have pursued studies to determine the potential contribution of EBV in lymphoproliferative malignancies in individuals with acquired or inherited immunodeficiencies. Unexplained, thus far, is the high frequency of malignant non-Hodgkin's lymphoma in individuals with immune deficiency (32). The frequency of malignancy ranges from 0.7% in Bruton's agammaglobulinemia to 35% in XLP. Patients with Bruton's may lack EBV receptors and be protected from lymphoma whereas the immunoregulatory defects of XLP make these persons very vulnerable. The finding of EBV genome in lymphoproliferative malignancies with ataxia-telangiectasia (33) and selective IgM deficiency (34) suggest that other immunodeficient patients ought be evaluated for EBV. A variety of other lethal EBV induced diseases have been associated with a variety of immune defects. EBV genome has been documented in the tissues, by molecular hybridization studies, in patients with XLP, common variable immunodeficiency (14,15), and in the Chediak-Higashi syndrome (K. McClain - personal communication).

Allograft recipients show a high frequency of malignant B-cell lymphoproliferative diseases (35). Elsewhere in this book, Penn describes cancer in immunodeficient transplant recipients. Hodgkin's disease is underrepresented in frequency in these patients, suggesting that EBV is not a direct etiologic agent of this malignancy. EBV genome has to date been found in all lymphomas in renal transplant recipients (RTR) examined by EBV molecular hybridization techniques (15). Following primary infection young RTR may succumb to a disseminated fatal IM-like disease. The antibody responses to the virus are similar to XLP (i.e., low titer antibodies and lack of anti-EBNA). In contrast, older RTR reactivate latent EBV, show high titer antibodies, and tend to develop localized lymphomas (36). Occasionally, cytogenetic conversion from polyclonality to monoclonality is observed in RTR (37). Hanto et al. provide a detailed description of these events elsewhere in this volume. Bieber from Stanford decribes EBV genome in malignant lymphomas in cardiac transplant recipients in this volume (30). Polyclonal EBV carrying lymphoproliferative diseases have been found in individuals receiving cultured thymic epithelium for reconstitution of severe combined immune deficiency (39). Only rarely do bone marrow transplant recipients develop EBV carrying lymphomas (40). This paucity of lymphomas in bone marrow allograft recipients compared to renal and cardiac recipients may be due to their being subjected to only a brief burst of immune suppression as compared to the other allograft recipients. Also, suppressor T-cells may be activated in bone marrow transplant patients and these cells provide adequate surveillance against EBV (41).

Individuals receiving cytoxic immunosuppressive therapy for malignancies can become immune deficient and life-threatening EBV-induced lymphoproliferative diseases can arise (42). We have studied a young male in remission for acute lymphoblastic leukemia who had acquired an immune defect analogous to those seen in XLP. He had succumbed to profound proliferation of gut-associated lymphoid tissues (43). Given the latent presence of EBV in most adults, certain immunosuppressing conditions may reactivate EBV; rarely fatal illness results. However, more commonly the immune system adapts to establish a detente with the virus. Various unexplained clinical signs of the basic underlying disease (i.e., cancer or autoimmune disorder) might be attributed to reactivation of EBV. This hypothesis can be tested.

The profound promiscuity practiced by a subgroup of male homosexuals may lead to the acquired immunodeficiency syndrome (AIDS). Exposure to multiple allogeneic sperm and cytomegalovirus provoke immune responses which impair cytotoxic T-cell surveillance against infectious agents and reactivate EBV (44). These men are at high risk for developing autoimmune disturbances, opportunistic infections, Kaposi's sarcoma and non-Hodgkin's lymphoma. EBV

genome has been identified in two B-cell lymphomas from AIDS
patients (45). Sonnabend and collaborators discuss their hypothesis regarding AIDS in a chapter in this book

    Owing to changing lifestyles; the introduction of antibiotics
and other therapies to support children with primary immunodeficiencies and the use of new immunosuppressive agents for
allografting organs and treating malignancies and autoimmune
disorders with cytotoxic drugs, an increasing number of patients
with acquired immunodeficiency who are vulnerable to EBV-induced
life-threatening diseases can be anticipated. Knowledge regarding
the immunopathogenesis of EBV induced diseases in immune deficient
patients will facilitate developing rational strategies for preventing immunodeficiency or enhancing immune competence by providing immunotherapy and treating with new anti-viral agents.

SUMMARY AND CONCLUSIONS

    Information regarding the development of diverse diseases
associated with Epstein-Barr virus in immunodeficient patients has
been gained by studying males and their families with the X-linked
lymphoproliferative syndrome (XLP). Multiple immune defenses normally protect against the ubiquitous EBV. Depending on the type
and degree of inherited or acquired immunodeficiency, EBV may more
or less be capable of inducing a variety of diseases. Multiple
methods may be needed to document EBV in the immune deficient
individual. Rational approaches to prevention and intervention in
EBV induced diseases in immune compromised individuals are being
developed.

REFERENCES

1.   Epstein, M.A., Achong, B.G., and Barr, Y.M. Virus particles
        in cultured lymphoblasts from Burkitt's Lymphoma.
        Lancet, 1:702-703, 1964.
2.   Purtilo, D.T. X-linked lymphoproliferative syndrome: an
        immunodeficiency disorder with acquired agam-
        maglobulinemia, fatal infectious mononucleosis or
        malignant lymphoma. Arch. Path. Lab. Med., 106:119,
        1981.
3.   Henle, W., Henle, G., and Lennette, E.T. Epstein-Barr virus.
        Sci. Am., 241:48, 1979.
4.   Niederman, J.C. Prevalence, incidence and persistence of EB
        virus antibody in young adults. N. Engl. J. Med.,
        282:361, 1970.
5.   Tosato, G., Magrath, I., Koski, I., Dooley, N., and Blaese,
        M. Activation of suppressor T cells during
        Epstein-Barr-virus-induced infectious mononucleosis. N.
        Engl. J. Med., 301:1133, 1979.

6. Klein, G., Svedmyr, E., Jondal, M., and Persson, P.O.
    EBV-determined nuclear antigen (EBNA)-positive cells in
    the peripheral blood of infectious mononucleosis
    patients. Int. J. Cancer, 17:21, 1976.

7. Robinson, J.E., Smith, D., and Niederman, J. Plasmacytic
    differentiation of circulating Epstein-Barr virus-
    infected B lymphocytes during acute infectious mono-
    nucleosis. J. Exp. Med., 153:235, 1980.

8. Epstein-Barr Virus. Editors, M.A. Epstein and B. Achong,
    Springer-Verlag, Berlin, 1979.

9. Purtilo, D.T. Immunopathology of infectious mononucleosis
    and other complications of Epstein-Barr virus infections.
    In: S.C. Sommers and P.P. Rosen (eds.), Pathology
    Annual, 1980. pp. 253-299. New York: Appleton-Century-
    Crofts, 1980.

10. Purtilo, D.T., DeFlorio, D., Hutt, L.M., Bhawan, J., Yang,
    J.P.S., Otto, R., and Edwards, W. Variable phenotypic
    expression of an X-linked recessive lymphoproliferative
    syndrome. N. Engl. J. Med., 297:1077, 1977.

11. Purtilo, D.T., Paquin, L.A., DeFlorio, D., Virzi, F., and
    Sukhuja, R. Immunodiagnosis and immunopathogenesis of
    the X-linked recessive lymphoproliferative syndrome.
    Sem. Hematol., 16:309, 1979.

12. Purtilo, D.T. Hypothesis: pathogenesis and phenotypes of
    an X-linked recessive lymphoproliferative syndrome.
    Lancet, ii:882, 1976.

13. Purtilo, D.T., Sakamoto, K., Barnabei, V., Seeley, J.,
    Bechtold, T., Rogers, G., Yetz, J., and Harada, S.
    Epstein-Barr virus-induced diseases in males with the X-
    linked lymphoproliferative syndrome (XLP). Am. J. Med.,
    73:49, 1982.

14. Purtilo, D.T., Sakamoto, K., Saemundsen, A.K., Sullivan,
    J.L., Synnerholm, A.C., Andersson-Anvret, M., Pritchard,
    J., Sloper, C., Sieff, Collins, R., Barnes, N., Knight,
    J., Sandstedt, B., and Klein, G. Documentation of
    Epstein-Barr virus infection in immunodeficient patients
    with life-threatening lymphoproliferative disease by
    clinical, virological and immunopathological studies.
    Cancer Res., 41:4226, 1981.

15. Saemundsen, A.K., Purtilo, D.T., Sakamoto, K., Sullivan,
    J.L., Synnerholm, A.C., Hanto, D., Simmons, R., Anvret,
    M., Collins, R., and Klein, G. Documentation of
    Epstein-Barr virus infection in immunodeficient patients
    with life-threatening lymphoproliferative diseases by
    Epstein-Barr virus complementary RNA/DNA and viral
    DNA/DNA hybridization. Cancer Res., 41:4237, 1981.

16. Seeley, J.K., Sakamoto, K., Ip, S., Hansen, P., and Purtilo,
    D.T. Abnormal subsets in the X-linked lymphoprolifer-
    ative syndrome. J. Immunol., 127:2618, 1981.

17. Purtilo, D.T., Yang, J.P.S., Cassel, C.K., Harper, P.,
     Stephenson, S.R., Landing, B.H. and Vawter, G.F. X-
     linked recessive progressive combined variable immunode-
     ficiency (Duncan's disease). Lancet, 1:935, 1975.
18. Lindsten, T., Seeley, J.K., Sakamoto, K., Yetz, J., Harada,
     S., Bechtold, T., Rogers, G., and Purtilo, D.T. Immune
     deficiency in the X-linked lymphoproliferative syndrome.
     II. Immunoregulatory T cell defects. J. Immunol.,
     129:2536, 1982.
19. Ochs, H.D., Sullivan, J.L., Wedgewood, R.J., Seeley, J.K.,
     Sakamoto, K., and Purtilo, D.T. X-linked lymphoprolifer-
     ative syndrome: abnormal antibody responses to bac-
     teriophage ØX174. In: R. Wedgewood and F. Rosen (eds.),
     Primary Immunodeficiency Diseases. New York: Alan R
     Liss, 1983.
20. Seeley, J.K., Harada, S., Bechtold, T., Ochs, H.D.,
     Wedgewood, R.J., Sakamoto, K., Lindsten, T., Yetz, J.,
     and Purtilo, D.T. Primary and acquired immune defects
     in X-linked lymphoproliferative syndrome. In prepara-
     tion.
21. Harada, S., Bechtold, T., and Purtilo, D.T. Comparison of
     long-term T-cell-mediated immunity to Epstein-Barr virus
     and NK cell-activity in obligate carrier females and
     males with the X-linked lymphoproliferative syndrome.
     Int. J. Cancer, 216:739, 1982.
22. Szigeti, R., Masucci, M.G., Henle, W., Henle, G, Purtilo,
     D.T., and Klein, G. Effects of different EBV-determined
     antigens (EBNA, EA and VCA) on mononucleosis and certain
     immunodeficiencies. Clin. Immunol. Immunopath., 22:128,
     1982.
23. Sullivan, J.L., Byron, K., Brewster, F., and Purtilo, D.T.
     Deficient natural killer cell activity in the X-linked
     lymphoproliferative syndrome. Science, 210:543, 1981.
24. Purtilo, D.T. Immune deficiency predisposing to Epstein-Barr
     virus-induced lymphoproliferative diseases: the X-
     linked lymphoproliferative syndrome as a model. In: G.
     Klein and S. Weinhouse (eds.), Advances in Cancer
     Research. Vol. 34, pp. 279-312. New York: Academic
     Press, 1980.
25. Sakamoto, K., Freed, H., and Purtilo, D.T. Antibody re-
     sponses to Epstein-Barr virus in families with the X-
     linked lymphoproliferative syndrome. J. Immunol.,
     125:921, 1980.
26. Sakamoto, K., Seeley, J.K., Lindsten, T., Sexton, J., Yetz,
     J., Ballow, M., and Purtilo, D.T. Abnormal anti-
     Epstein-Barr virus antibodies in carriers of the X-
     linked lymphoproliferative syndrome and in females at
     risk. J. Immunol., 128:904, 1982.

27.   Seeley, J.K., Bechtold, T., Lindsten, T., and Purtilo, D.T.
      NK deficiency in X-linked lymphoproliferative syndrome.
      In: R.B. Herberman (ed.), Natural Cell Mediated
      Immunity 1982. Vol. 2, pp. 1211-1218. New York:
      Academic Press, 1982.

28.   Rickinson, A.B., Moss, D.J., Wallace, L.E., Rowe, M., Misko,
      I.S., Epstein, M.A., and Pope, J.H. Long-term T-cell-
      mediated immunity to Epstein-Barr virus. Cancer Res.,
      41:4216, 1981.

29.   Purtilo, D.T. and Sullivan, J.L. Immunological bases for
      superior survival of females. Am. J. Dis. Child.,
      133:1251, 1979.

30.   Klein, G. Lymphoma development in mice and humans: diver-
      sity of initiation is followed by convergent cytogenetic
      evolution. Proc. Natl. Acad. Sci., 76:2442, 1979.

31.   Rowley, J.D. Identification of the constant chromosome
      regions involved in human hematologic malignant disease.
      Science, 216:794, 1982.

32.   Kersey, J.H. and Spector, B.D. Immune deficiency disease.
      In: J. F. Fraumeni, Jr. (ed.), Persons at High Risk of
      Cancer: An Approach to Cancer Etiology and Control. pp.
      55-67. New York: Academic Press, 1975.

33.   Saemundsen, A.K. Epstein-Barr virus-carrying lymphoma in a
      patient with ataxia-telangiectasia. Brit. Med. J.,
      282:425, 1981.

34.   Purtilo, D.T., Liao, S.A., Sakamoto, K., Snyder, L.M.,
      DeFlorio, D., Bhawan, J., Paquin, L.A., Yang, J.P.S.,
      Hutt-Fletcher, L.M., Muralidharan, K., Raffa, P.,
      Saemundsen, A.K., and Klein, G. Diverse familial
      malignant tumors and Epstein-Barr virus. Cancer Res.,
      41:4248, 1981.

35.   Penn, I. Depressed immunity and the development of cancer.
      Clin. Exp. Immunol., 46:459-474, 1981.

36.   Hanto, D.W., Frizzera, G., Purtilo, D.T., Sakamoto, K.,
      Sullivan, J.L., Saemundsen, A.K., Klein, G., Simmons,
      R.L., and Najarian, J.S. Clinical spectrum of
      lymphoproliferative disorders in renal transplant recip-
      ients and evidence for the role of Epstein-Barr virus.
      Cancer Res., 41:4253, 1981.

37.   Hanto, D.W., Frizzera, G., Gajl-Peczalska, K.J., Sakamoto,
      K., Purtilo, D.T., Balfour, H.H., Simmons, R.L., and
      Najarian, J.S. Epstein-Barr virus-induced B-cell lym-
      phoma after renal transplantation: Acyclovir therapy
      and transition from polyclonal to monoclonal B-cell pro-
      liferation. N. Engl. J. Med., 306:913, 1982.

38.   Bieber, C. Lymphoma in cardiac transplant recipients asso-
      ciated with cyclosporin A, prednisone, and anti-thymocyte
      globulin (ATG). In: D.T. Purtilo (ed.), Immune
      Deficiency and Cancer: Epstein-Barr Virus and
      Lymphoproliferative Malignancies. New York: Plenum
      Press, in press.

39.   Reece, E.R., Gartner, J.G., Seemayer, T.A., Joncas, J.H. and
      Pagano, J.S. Epstein-Barr virus in a malignant lympho-
      proliferative disorder of B cells occurring after thymic
      epithelial transplantation for combined immunodefi-
      ciency. Cancer Res., 41:4243, 1981.
40.   Schubach, W.H., Hackman, R., Neiman, P.E., Miller, G.,
      Thomas, E.D. Blood, in press.
41.   Fox, R., McMillan, R., Spruce, W., Tani, P., and Mason, D.
      Analysis of T lymphocytes after bone marrow transplan-
      tation using monoclonal antibodies. Blood, 60:578,
      1982.
42.   Look, A.T., Naegle, R.F., Calihan, T., Herrod, H.G., and
      Henle, W. Fatal Epstein-Barr virus infection in a child
      with acute lymphoblastic leukemia in remission. Cancer
      Res., 41:4280, 1981.
43.   Hardy, C., Harada, S., Lubin, B., Sanger, W., von Schmidt,
      B., Yetz, J., Saemundsen, A.K., Feusner, J., Lennette,
      E., Linder, J., Seeley, J.K., and Purtilo, D.T.
      Epstein-Barr virus (EBV) induced lymphoproliferation
      complicating acute lymphoblastic leukemia. J. Peds., in
      press.
44.   Sonnabend, J., Witkin, S.S., and Purtilo, D.T. Acquired
      immunodeficiency syndrome (AIDS), opportunistic infec-
      tions and malignancies in male homosexuals. A hypothe-
      sis of etiologic factors in pathogenesis. J. Am. Med.
      Assoc., 249:2370, 1983.
45.   Zeigler, J.L., Wagner, G., and Greenspan, J.S. Diffuse,
      Undifferentiated, non-Hodgkin's lymphoma in homosexual
      male - United States. Morbidity and Mortality Weekly
      Report, 31:277, 1982.

IMMUNODEFICIENCY TO EPSTEIN-BARR VIRUS IN CHEDIAK-HIGASHI SYNDROME

Fernando Merino

Institute for Scientific Investigation

Caracas, Venezuela

INTRODUCTION

In 1943 Bequez (4) described three patients of the same family affected by autosomal recessive process characterized by albinism, pale hair, lymphadenomegaly, hepatosplenomegaly, lympho-monocytosis, and thrombocytopenia (Figure 1). Death was due to bone marrow failure. Large intracytoplasmatic azurophilic granules in polymorphonuclear neutrophils and lymphocytes were seen. Based on the symptoms, "Downey-McKinley" cells, and a positive Paul Bunnell reaction in one case, Cesar postulated that infectious mononucleosis (IM) "an organism in the patient lacking host defenses, was the reason...for the bone marrow failure."

Similar reports by Steinbrinck in 1948 (82), and detailed hematological studies by Chediak in 1952 (13), and cases from Higashi in 1954 (31), further defined this entity. It incorrectly was designated the Chediak-Higashi syndrome by Sato (76). However, incorrect the designation, convention forces us to use the term.

The Chediak-Higashi syndrome (CHS) does not show racial restriction. The majority of reports are individual cases, however a cluster is found in Andean mountains in Venezuela (65). We have estimated an incidence of more than 1 case per 10,000 newborns a year, in comparison to the estimated world frequency of 1 case per 1,000,000 newborns. This cluster is probably the result of a "founder effect" which was brought about by the geographic isolation, and a tendency of inbreeding of these populations. Supporting this view is the index of high consanguinity among the inhabitants.

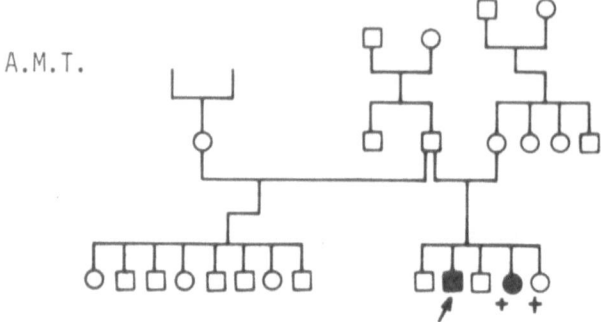

Fig. 1.   Family study of Chediak-Higashi patient from Venezuela.
          Blackened areas represent the CHS cases.

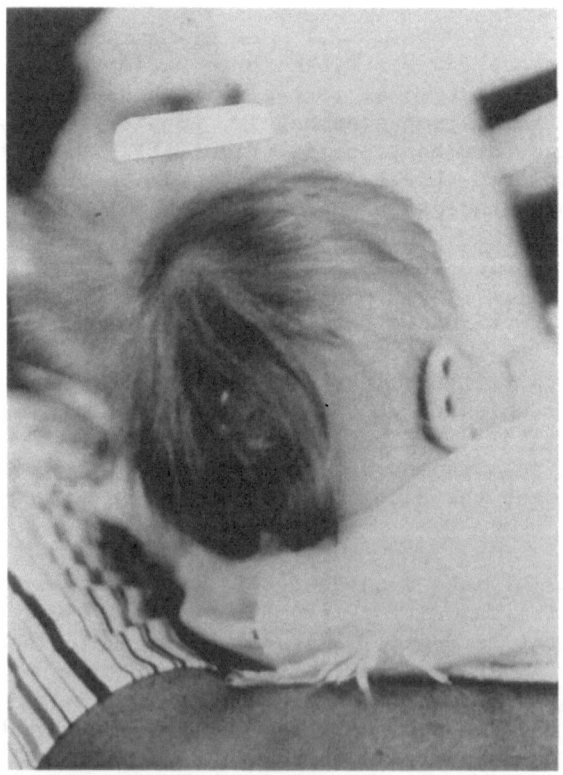

Fig. 2.   Note the pale gray hair of the child with Chediak-Higashi
          syndrome in contrast to black hair of the mother.

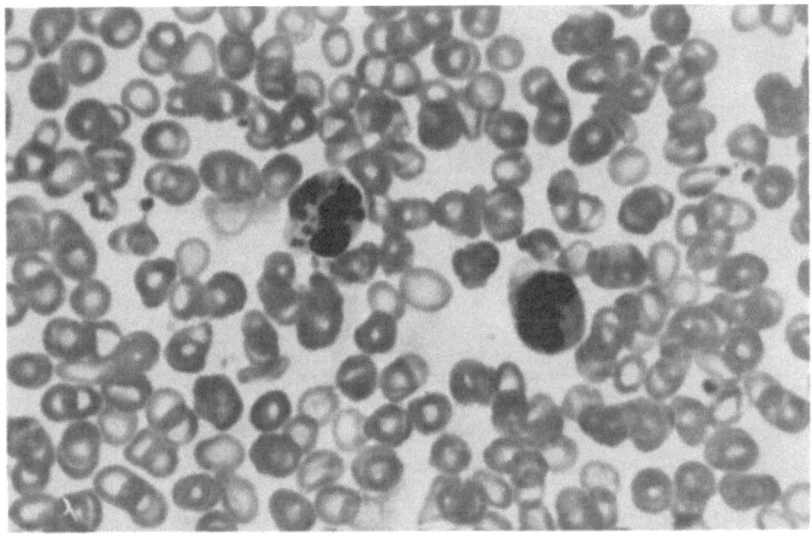

Fig. 3.   Photomicrograph of lymphocytes and a polymorphonuclear
          neutrophil of a Chediak-Higashi patient. Typical
          large azurophilic cytoplasmic granulations can be
          observed. Wrights stain, X450.

Manifestations of CHS

     The clinical features of the CHS were described by Beguez (4).
Rare adults with CHS have also been described. Ash-gray hair,
partial albinism (Figure 2), increased susceptibility to infectious agents, hepatosplenomegaly, lymph node enlargement, and
hemorrhagic disorders are found. Two phases are being defined in
the natural history of the syndrome.

     The initial phase is marked by high susceptibility to skin,
respiratory tract, and ear infections. The second phase, called
the accelerated phase, is characterized by a lymphoproliferative,
"lymphoma" or "lymphoma-like" disorder. Moderately enlarged lymph
nodes, hepatosplenomegaly, ecchymoses and petechiae are generalized. Death of the patients commonly occurs within the first
years of life.

     Hallmarks of CHS are the large azurophilic granules in the
cytoplasm of polymorphonuclear neutrophils (PMN) and lymphocytes
(Figure 3) and partial albinism (Figure 2). The intracytoplasmic
granules have also been described in kidney, neurons, peripheral
glia, etc. These are abnormal lysosomes (31,93). They form in
the bone marrow through fusion of azurophilic granules (67,70).

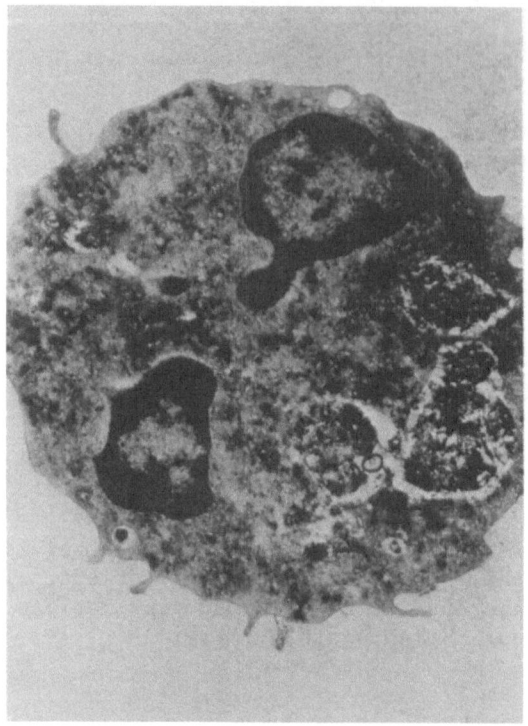

Fig. 4.   Electron micrograph of neutrophil from a patient with
          Chediak-Higashi syndrome.   Note the giant lysosomes
          X5000.

     Electron microscopy studies reveal that the granules are
surrounded by a unit membrane (Figure 4).   The internal structure
is composed of membranous or myelin-like material undergoing
internal destruction from autodigestion by hydrolytic enzymes
(93,94,97).

Inheritance

     Beguez stated that CHS was an autosomic recessive entity.
Blume and Wolff (7) confirmed this interpretation.   However, con-
sanguineous marriages were only present in 48% of the cases.   This
has also been observed in a previous series of 14 cases in
Venezuela and in the cases we are studying.

     No chromosomal abnormalities have been described in most cases
where karyotypes have been performed (21,43,54,84,88).   However,
Say et al. (76) have reported partial monosomy of chromosome 21 in
a case and Salmanca-Gomez et al. (74) described polymorphism in

chromosome #1. Rosenszajn et al. (69) described abnormalities
consisting of chromatid and chromosomal breakage, elongated chromosomes, heteropycnotic gaps, and a tetraploid cell. They
interpreted chromosomal changes to be due to the liberation of
deoxyribonuclease by the giant lysosomes. Detailed studies must
be performed in large number of patients using banding technique
before concluding no chromosomal alterations are found in CHS.

Abnormal DNA repair mechanisms has been described by Tanaka et
al. (86,87) in CHS cells. They have shown that EBV transformed
lymphoblastoid cell lines from CHS show increased sensitivity to
ultraviolet light and 4-nitroquinoline 1-oxide, but no unscheduled
DNA synthesis is found after UV irradiation. Conversion of low
to high molecular-weight DNA was slow, indicative of a defective
post-replication repair. Thus they have tried to explain the high
risk of cancer in these patients.

The Large Azurophilic Cytoplasmic Granules

The ultrastructural features of the three different types of
cytoplasmic granules have recently been reviewed by White and
Clawson (99): 1) giant lysosomes containing acid phosphatase and
myeloperoxidase activity, possibly arising by fusion of small
azurophilic lysosomes in the marrow promyelocytes and metamyelo-
cytes; 2) giant secondary lysosomes enlarging through all stages
of neutrophil maturation, and growing in peripheral blood granulocytes by continuous fusion with other large granules, and with
normal azurophilic granules, secondary lysosomes and cytoplasmic
constituents; and 3) a type developing as a result of cytoplasmic
sequestration. This is postulated to arise from leakage of
lysosomes from the huge organelles.

The CHS Polymorphonuclear Neutrophil (PMN) in CHS

The susceptibility to pyogenic infections results from altered
function of the PMN. An abnormal inflammatory response, due to
defective leukocyte migration and reduced chemotactic response,
altered adherent properties, and bactericidal capacities in the
PMN has been demonstrated. This reduced bactericidal capacity is
the result of an altered degranulation capacity and defective
phagolysosome formation. In contrast, the phagocytic activity is
well preserved (8,11,14,15,18,20,25,58,69,73,78,91,99,100). The
exocytosis process by these granulocytes is defective (101).

The basic defect in the PMN is not known. However, altered
lysosome-phagosome fusion is due to abnormal membrane assembly of
microtubules, or in membrane-microtubule interaction. Their PMN
spontaneously form concanavalin A (con A)-like caps (51,52). This
membrane alteration results from defective microtubule assembly.
It is corrected by cholinergic agonists increasing intracellular

cGMP levels. The spontaneous con A-like cap formation is
corrected by Levamisole or ascorbic acid (12,20).

Boxer et al. (12) has shown that centrioles in PMN were normal
in structure and virtually no microtubules were detected in the
centriolar region of either untreated or con A treated cells.
However, White and Clawson (98) report no significant differences
in centriole associated microtubules in the mononuclear cells.

A high rate of tubulin tyrosylation and its reduction by
ascorbate, indicating an altered state or function of tubulin/
microtubules, in the CHS granulocytes has been described (49).
They also reported a reduction in particulate protease which
digests tubulin.

Microtubular function is regulated by cyclic nucleotides.
Thus, alterations in the levels of cyclic nucleotides might be
associated with defective function. High levels of cAMP in CHS
PMN, but normal of cGMP have been described (11,91). In both
cases cAMP levels were reduced by ascorbate. Gallin et al. (25),
however, did not observe abnormalities in cAMP or cGMP levels. In
vitro treatment of CHS cells with agents modifying intracellular
levels of cyclic nucleotides improve degranulation (10), bactericidal capacity (10,73), leukocyte migration (18), chemotaxis
(10,73,91), and adherence properties (11).

Skin fibroblasts show abnormally low rates of vinblastine-
induced microtubular paracrystal formation (32). Similar results
were reported by Iseki et al. (34) suggesting that microtubules
cause defective association with cellular membranes. Ostlund et
al. (53) reported that fibroblasts have a marked perinuclear localization of the lysosomes, but after colchicine treatment peripheral dispersion develops. Gross alteration in the microtubules
was not apparent. The CHS defect is associated with the lysosomal
membrane or is due to the lysosomal membrane-microtubule interaction.

Clinical trials to increase the phagocytic capacity have been
performed. After ascorbic acid, stimulation of leukocyte cGMP,
normal or improved degranulation, bactericidal activity, adherence
properties, and reduction in the cAMP levels was observed. Oral
administration of ascorbic acid produced a 5 fold stimulation of
microtubule assembly and the number of centriole-associated microtubules increased (8,11,73,91). However, Galli et al. (25) have
shown that ascorbic acid therapy does not improve mononuclear
migration and chemotaxis in the skin window response. Similarly,
ascorbic acid therapy did not improve bactericidal capacity.
Ascorbate did not prevent the accelerated phase (73) or cause a
clinical improvement or severity of infections (61). Ascorbic
acid does not improve the platelet abnormality (91), lymphocyte

mitogenic responses (25,91) or the antibody-dependent cell-
mediated cytotoxicity (91).

Spin label electron resonance spectrometry studies reveal high
membrane fluidity which is not altered by changing the ratio of
intracellular cyclic nucleotides. The PMN membrane fluidity
abnormalities and microtubule disfunction probably are not related
(27). Abnormal membrane fluidity has also been reported in
erythrocyte membranes of CHS patients. Hence a generalized
membrane disorder has been proposed (33).

A decrease in the content of myeloperoxidase and B-
glucuronidase, but normal of chatepsin, muramidase and basic
phosphatase has been quantitated in CHS (10,35,39,100). Moreover,
granulocytes have low or undetectable elastase (90) and there is a
marked reduction of a-mannoside, a-galactoside and a-fucoside
activity (85). In CHS lymphocytes, B-glucuronidase and a-
mannoside were decreased. Nishi et al. (50) have detected a high
zinc concentration in granulocytes, plasma, erythrocytes and
lymphocytes of the patients.

Platelet Anomalies

Petechiae, ecchymoses and prolonged bleeding time is due to
altered platelet function. Ultrastructural studies show abnormal
cytoplasmic granules in a few circulating platelets (59,95,99) and
in bone marrow megakaryocytes (59), and reduced amounts of dense
bodies in cytoplasm (16,91). The altered platelet function is
considered a storage pool disorder (9,91). Defect in microtubule
assembly may cause the platelet anomaly whereas cyclic nucleotide
levels are at normal levels (91,96). The basic defect in platelet
function remains to be established.

Host Defense Mechanisms

The only clinically significant, immune perturbation in CHS
patients is the abnormal bactericidal function of PMNS. Most previous reports have not revealed alterations in immune mechanisms.
However, absence of the natural killer (NK) and antibody-dependent
cell mediated cytotoxicity (ADCC) has been described (28,42,46,
91). The clinical significance is unclear.

Clearance rates of aggregated 125-I human albumin was normal
in two CHS cases (7). Serum immunoglobulins have been normal to
increased (7,20,38,44,66,88). However IgG was low and IgA and IgM
levels decreased in the accelerated phase (7). We have also made
this observation. Isoagglutinin titers, antiviral and antibacterial antibodies, and in vivo antibody response to S. typhosa (7)
or to vaccines has been normal (20). Skin reaction to PPD, mumps,

Table 1. Percent of Peripheral Blood T, B, and NK
          Lymphocytes in Chediak-Higashi Patients

Patient	WBC	T	B	NK
A.M.T.	10500	96	16	15
E.J.G.	11250	60	31	32
W.L.G.	7250	76	9	39
J.R.	18850	33	16	6
Y.V.	5050	49	6	nd
W.R.C.	9800	83	19	16
Normal	4-9000	55-80	6-20	6-14

WBC: White blood cell count/mm3. T cells are
spontaneous rosette forming cells with sheep
erythrocytes. B cells were determined by
fluorescence microscopy surface immunoglobulin
using a polyvalent anti-immunoglobulin serum.
NK cells are defined as the positive staining
OKM1 monoclonal antibody lymphocytes after the
elution of gradient purified lymphocytes in a
nylon wool column and determined in a
cytofluorograph.

candida, tricophyton, histoplasma and varidase antigens, have been
normal (7,20,91) and sensitization to DNCB has been successful
(7,85).

Peripheral blood T and B lymphocyte populations were normal in
several studies (20,25,91), but reduced in others (89). In two of
six of our patients, E rosette forming cells were low and slightly
high in the other (Table 1). Similar T cell values were obtained
using monoclonal OKT3 antibody (for pan T lymphocytes). However,
an increase in numbers of OKT8 (suppressor/cytotoxic) cells, a
reduction of OKT4 (helper) cells, and an increased of OKIa1
(Ia-like reactive cells) were observed (47) (Table 2).

In vitro responses of T and B cells to various stimuli have
been normal. Leukocyte migration inhibition in response to PPD
and, in vitro lymphotoxin production by PHA was normal too
(18,20,25,41,54,62). Monocyte-mediated lymphocytoxicity has been
essentially normal (41,91).

Table 2. Number/mm^3 of Peripheral Blood Lymphocyte Subsets Characterized by Monoclonal Reagents in Chediak-Higashi Patients

Patient	OKT4		OKT8		R 4/8	Ia1	
	Percent	N°/mm^3	Percent	N°/mm^3		Percent	N°/mm^3
AMT	32	1848	54	3118	1.7	19	772
EJG	27	1609	72	4293	2.7	29	1951
JR	30	1384	55	2539	1.8	20	2577
WLG	25	1288	33	1508	1.3	26	1317
WRC	30	1781	55	3265	1.8	34	3970

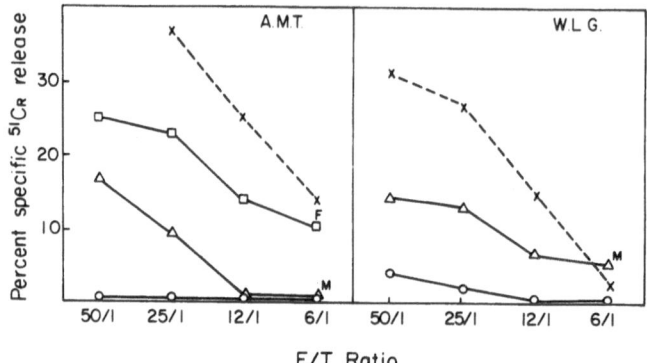

Fig. 5.   Natural killer cell activity in two CHS patients (open
          circles). WLG was an 8 month old boy, and AMT a 13 year
          old girl. None of them were in the accelerated phase.
          (M) is the mother, (F) the father. Dashed line is a
          healthy control subject.

        Roder et al. (28,42,68) demonstrated decreased natural killer
(NK) and antibody dependent-cellular cytotoxicity due to a functional defect and not to an absence of NK cells. We have confirmed these findings (65) (Figure 5). Normal numbers of NK cells
in peripheral blood were found by staining with monoclonal HNK-1
(1) or OKM-1 after nylon wool elution (Table 1). Abo et al. (1)
described the HNK-1 monoclonal antibody positive cells to be
lymphocytes having large cytoplasmic granules. Our observations
indicate that there is no relationship between the clinical stage
of the patient and the NK and ADCC deficiency. The NK defect
occurs prior to the onset of the accelerated or lymphoma-like
phase. In contrast, the NK defect in X-linked lymphoproliferative
syndrome is acquired after EBV infection [see the chapter by
Harada for details].

        These studies indicate that T cells and their subsets in
peripheral blood are present in abnormal numbers. B cells seem to
be present in normal numbers and function is normal. However,
longitudinal studies during the disease have not been performed.
The relevance of the changes in T lymphocytes and subsets, remains
to be determined. The CHS-like mouse model, the beige mouse, in
addition to the NK defect shows impaired T cell responses (77).

        The morphological alterations observed in lymphoid organs can
be of importance and the lymphocyte depletion in lymphoid organs
is probably accompanied by a deficit in the immunological capacity. This contention is supported by finding lower serum immunoglobulin levels in patients in the accelerated phase.

The granulocyte platelets, NK and ADCC defects could be phenotypic expressions of CHS gene stemming from membrane or microtubule assembly defects.

Accelerated Phase of Lymphoproliferation

In 1964 Kritzler et al. (43) recognized two stages of the
disease: "the course of the disease may be rapidly progressive
from birth or may be relatively quiescent for years before an
accelerated terminal phase begins" which is characterized by hepatomegaly, splenomegaly, lymphadenopathy, thrombocytopenia, anemia
and less frequently jaundice and neurological manifestations.
Histological examination shows a lymphohistiocytic infiltration in
almost all organs. Because of the clinical signs, the lymphoid
infiltration, and death this process has been diagnosed as
malignant or pseudolymphoma. However, other authors have
diagnosed a reactive proliferative disorder (44).

In our recently reported series of 14 cases, typical clinical
findings were observed including hepatosplenomegaly, hemorrhagic
disorders, and anemia. Post-mortem examination in three cases
revealed mixed lymphoid infiltrates which were not malignant.
Noteworthy, jaundice almost always preceded the development of
lymphoproliferation, i.e., an episode of fever, jaundice, hepatosplenomegaly, moderate lymph node enlargement, occasionally
hemorrhage and then death occurred within days to years.

A review of the literature does not support the lymphoproliferation to be a malignant lymphoma. In the first description of
the infiltrating cells, Donohue and Bain (22) indicated that they
were presumably lymphocytes and that in no way resembled leukemic
infiltration.

The classification of the infiltration by others as a
malignant lymphoma was based on 5 cases (19,24,26,37,58,92).
These authors described their morphological findings in a lymph
node as similar to malignant histiocytosis. However, the
infiltrating cells and the lymphoid organ morphology was very
variable.

Efrati and Jones in 1957 (24) described total destruction of
lymph node architecture replaced by "hyperchromatic cells with a
small amount of basophilic cytoplasm and round or oval nuclei with
fairly prominent nucleoli." The infiltrating cells in the tissues
were described as "lymphosarcoma" or "tumor cells." Page et al.
(58) in 1962 described a case reporting: "a cervical lymph node
biopsy revealed malignant lymphoma." Histological examination at
autopsy of tissues revealed "immature lymphoid cells and
histiocytes" which destroyed architecture. Dent et al. (19)
described "extensive infiltration of viscera by immature lymphoid

cells and histiocytes." White et al. (92) also described two cases one of which was also described by Page et al. (58). In the second they found "lymphomatous involvement of lymph nodes, spleen, liver and other organs." Gillon et al. (26) reported "The histological picture of lymphosarcoma."

Evidence against malignant lymphoma has been documented in 15 different reports (3,5,21,29,35,44,45,47,54,56,75,80,81). The infiltrating cells have been described as "large mononuclear cells with copious amounts of cytoplasm", medium-sized lymphocytes, and plasma cells. In lymphoid organs, atrophy, lymphocyte depletion, loss of germinal centers, replacement by histocytes with phagocytosis, erythrophagocytosis and leukophagocytosis is seen (17,35, 44,56,75). The morphological findings have been interpreted as due to a reactive process (44,75) or resembling those of infectious mononucleosis (35,56).

In our series of CHS lymphocyte and histiocytic cells infiltrated almost all tissues, severe lymphocytic depletion in lymphoid organs and a marked histiocytic proliferation was associated with erythrophagocytosis. The infiltrating cells were not immature and malignant, but mature.

I concluded the lymphoproliferative phase is characterized not only by infiltration of the tissues of the body by mature lymphocytes and histiocytes, but also by changes in the lymphoid organs consisting of atrophy of the thymus, moderate or severe depletion of lymphocytes in lymph nodes and follicles of spleen, loss of germinal centers and histiocytic proliferation and activation. Krueger and associates (44) have described absence of thymic epithelium in CHS.

The difference in the histological findings are attributable to the variability in the natural history of the disease. For example, the time of onset and duration of the accelerated phase. Variable expression might be due to the first stage being dominated by an intense lymphoproliferation of differentiated lymphocytes and histiocytes. As the disease progress, bone marrow, thymus, lymph nodes, and spleen become depleted. Histiocytic proliferation and activation associated with erythro- and leukophagocytosis, lymphoid proliferation and depletion may emerge from the same etiological agent. No malignant transformation occurs.

Using electron microscopy White et al. (92) have described the virus-like particles in leukocytes of two patients composed of an inner dense nucleoid, a membrane-like capsule, and having diameters from 65 to 75 mu. Similar virus-like particles were described by Dent et al. (19). Long-term cultivation of peripheral blood lymphocytes (6) or spleen cells (19) of CHS patients has been achieved (23). Reticular arrays of 22 mu in the rough endoplasmic reticulum were observed in the lymphoid cell line similar to those in established cell lines from IM patients. However, malignant features in the cultured cells could have been acquired during long term cultivation.

Infectious Mononucleosis in CHS

The possibility of the lymphoproliferative disorder of CHS being a form of IM had been suggested by Beguez: he had postulated that IM caused marrow failure due to defective host defenses (4). Others (35,56) interpreted morphological findings as being compatible with IM. Padgett postulated: "Perhaps mononucleosis prepares the way for bacterial invasion of the already inadequate host defense mechanism. Perhaps mononucleosis in the initial attack or after one or two exacerbations kills CHS children though it does not kill normal children" (55).

Blume and Wolff (7) discarded the possibility of IM in their report of two cases with accelerated disease who had high titer anti-EBV antibodies and positive heterophile antibodies. The presence of EBV antibody in more than 80% of normal children detracted from these findings, however, they did not report the titers. Paul-Bunnell antibodies have been reported in other cases (4,24,36,45) but not in all (2,35,37,54).

Unusually high antibody responses to EBV in children with CHS were studied over a period of a year and a half (46). Two cases were in the accelerated phase. Two of the patients were seronegative but two had high titers against viral capsid antigen (VCA), to the restricted component (R) of early antigen (EA) complex and to EBV nuclear-associated antigen (EBNA). No antibodies to the diffuse component (D) of the EBV-induced early antigen complex were detected. This pattern is seen in Burkitt's lymphoma and rarely in other conditions. Seropositive patients had the accelerated phase with hepatosplenomegaly and lymphadenopathy. Seroconversion transpired in the other two patients giving a serological pattern similar to the other two cases. When anti-EBV antibodies were detected, enlargement of liver, spleen and lymph nodes, and hemorrhagic problems became evident. One patient died shortly afterward. Postmortem examination revealed widespread lymphoproliferation. Negative Monospot® tests were found before and during the accelerated phase. A hepatitis/mononucleosis-like episode was recorded in both cases prior to seroconversion consisting of moderate lymphadenomegaly, jaundice, hepatosplenomegaly, and with abnormal tests of liver function.

These results implied associations between infection by EBV and the lymphoproliferation. However, studies indicating that EBV-infected B cells were proliferating were incomplete. In our recent series of cases, we found no increase in the number of B cells. Atypical mononuclear cells in peripheral blood can also be observed in CHS patients (16,24,35,72) and, before the accelerated phase, the hepatitis/mononucleosis-like episode, and the appearance of anti-EBV antibodies.

EBV could cause the lymphoproliferative phase in the CHS patients. The histological observations in tissues of one of our cases who had high titer anti-EBV antibodies support this speculation. Previously reported histopathological findings were compatible with EBV-induced lymphoproliferation. Thus, I postulate that fatal or chronic mononucleosis was responsible for lymphoproliferation. This lymphoproliferative disorder and its association to EBV needs further clarification.

SUMMARY AND CONCLUSIONS

Immune deficiency in CHS is likely due to the lysosomal defect. The novel immune deficiency in the Chediak-Higashi patients consists of a marked reduction of NK and ADCC cell activity (Figure 4). The NK defect can be observed at a very early age preceding the onset of the lymphoproliferative process.

A possible relationship between the NK deficiency and the control of the EBV infection in the CHS patients has been suggested (46). Owing to the immune deficiency, I postulate that primary EBV infection provokes a smoldering disease. Evidence supporting this view is the unusually high anti-EBV antibody titers which are probably the consequence of NK deficiency. However, NK cells are not vital as the first line of defense against primary EB viral infection.

A unique deficiency of NK cells in both CHS and the beige mouse (63) is found. Impaired cytotoxic T lymphocytes (CTL) have recently been described in the beige mouse indicating T cell defects due to the CHS gene (77). But in CHS, no alteration of the T cell function has been found when measuring responses to mitogen, antigen or allogeneic lymphocyte in vitro. These studies are incomplete. For example, memory T cells against autologous lymphoblastoid cell lines carrying EBV have not been done. Imbalance in immunoregulatory subsets are found in CHS patients including a marked increase in the OKT8 (suppressor/cytotoxic) subpopulation, decreased numbers of E rosette forming cells, and a reduction in Ty cells (47,89). Krueger et al. (44) described absence of thymic epithelium in CHS patients analogous to patients with XLP who have T cell defects and succumb to EBV-induced B cell lymphoproliferation. CHS patients and Aleutian mink have similar genetic defects. They are susceptible to Aleutian virus which induces a marked lymphoproliferation with infiltration of plasma cells in tissues and hypergammaglobulinemia. The CHS anomaly in

minks probably alters their defense against this virus (55,57).
In the beige model, however, such natural occurring susceptibility
to a particular viral infection has not been documented. It is
tempting to speculate on the possibility of an abnormal response
to polyoma virus, a mouse ubiquitous naturally occurring virus
causing neoplasm mainly in immunodeficient mice (41).

ACKNOWLEDGEMENTS

The experimental results herein described are the product of
the collaborative work with Drs. Pedro Ramirez-Duque, (Hospital
Central, San Cristobal, Venezuela), Werner Henle (The Children
Hospital, Philadelphia, PA, U.S.A.), Gunnar Klein, George Klein
(Intitute Tumor Biology, Stockholm, Sweden) and David Purtilo
(University of Nebraska Medical Center, Omaha, Nebraska, U.S.A.).
The assistance and collaboration of Mrs. Carmen Amesty, Marilena
Biondo and Rosa Maldonado is greatly acknowledged.

REFERENCES

1. Abo, T., Roder, J.C., Abo, W., Cooper, M.D., and Balch, C.M.
    Natural killer (HNK-1+) cells in Chediak-Higashi patients
    are present in normal numbers but are abnormal in func-
    tion and morphology. J. Clin. Invest., 70:193, 1982.
2. Balsano, V., Arena, F., and Amato, G. Un caso di sindrome
    di Begues Cesar-Steinbrinck-Chediak Higashi. Minerva
    Pediat., 19:780, 1967.
3. Bedoya, V., Grimley, P.M., and Duque, O. Chediak-Higashi
    syndrome. Arch. Pathol., 88:340-349, 1969.
4. Bequez Cesar, A. Neutropenia cronica maligna familiar con
    granulaciones atipicas de lose leucocitos. Bol. Soc.
    Cubana Pediat., 15:900, 1943.
5. Bernard, J., Bessis, M., Seligman, N.N., Chassigneux, J.,
    and Chome, J. Un cas de maladie de Chediak-Steinbrinck-
    Higashi. Presse Med., 68:563, 1960.
6. Blume, R.S., Glade, P.R., Gralnick, H.R., Chessin, L.N.,
    Haase, A.T., and Wolff, S.M. The Chediak-Higashi
    syndrome: continuous suspension cultures derived from
    peripheral blood. Blood, 33:821, 1969.
7. Blume, R.S. and Wolff, S.M. The Chediak-Higashi syndrome:
    studies in four patients and a review of the literature.
    Medicine, 51:247, 1972.
8. Boxer, L., Watanabe, A.M., Rister, M., Besch, H.R., Allen,
    J., and Baehner, R.L. Correction of leukocyte function
    in Chediak-Higashi syndrome by ascorbate. N. Engl. J.
    Med., 295:1041, 1976.
9. Boxer, G.J., Holmsen, H., Robkin, L., Bang, N.U., Boxer,
    L.A. and Baehner, R.L. Abnormal platelet function in

Chediak-Higashi syndrome. Brit. J. Hemaet., 35:521, 1977.

10. Boxer, L.A., Rister, M., Allen, J., and Baehner, R.L. Improvement of Chediak-Higashi leukocyte function by cyclic guanosine monophosphate. Blood, 49:9, 1977.

11. Boxer, L.A., Allen, J.M., Watanabe, A.M., Besch, H.R., and Baehner, R.L. Role of microtubules in granulocyte adherence. Blood, 51:1045, 1978.

12. Boxer, L.A., Albertini, D.F., Baehner, R.L., and Oliver, J. M. Impaired microtubule assembly and polymorphonuclear leucocyte function in the Chediak-Higashi syndrome correctable by ascorbic acid. Brit. J. Hemaet., 43:207, 1979.

13. Chediak, M. Novelle anomalie leucocytaire de caractere constitutionnel et familial. Rev. Hemat., 7:362, 1952.

14. Clawson C.C., White, J.G., and Repine, J.E. The Chediak-Higashi syndrome. Evidence that defective leukotaxis is primarly due to an impediment by giant granules. Am. J. Pathol., 92:745, 1978.

15. Clawson, C.C., Repine, J.E., and White, J.G. The Chediak-Higashi syndrome. Quantitation of a deficiency in maximal bactericidal capacity. Am. J. Pathol., 94:539, 1979.

16. Costa, J.L., Fauci, A.S., and Wolff, S.M. A platelet abnormality in the Chediak-Higashi syndrome of man. Blood, 48:517, 1976.

17. De Bastos, O. and Resende Barros, O. Sindrome de Bequez Cesar-Steinbrinck-Chediak-Higashi. Sangre, 5:367, 1960.

18. De Beer, H.A., Anderson, R., and Findlay, G.H. Chediak-Higashi syndrome in a 'black' child. S. Afr. Med. J., 60:108, 1981.

19. Dent, P.B., Fish, L.A., White, J.G., and Good, R.A. Chediak-Higashi syndrome. Observations on the nature of the associated malignancy. Lab. Invest., 15:1634, 1966.

20. Deprez, P., Laurent, R., Griscelli, C., Buriot, D., and Agache, P. La maladie de Chediak-Higashi. A propos d'une nouvelle observation. Ann. Dermatol. Venereol., 105:841, 1978.

21. Dondo Lescano, F., Ferreyra, M.E., and Seoane, M. Enfermedad de Chediak-Higashi. Presentacion de dos casos. Prensa Med. Arg., 56:127, 1969.

22. Donohue, W.L. and Bain, H.W. Chediak-Higashi syndrome. A lethal familial disease with anomalous inclusions in the leukocytes and constitution stigmata: report of a case with necropsy. Pediatrics, 20:416, 1957.

23. Douglas, S.D., Blume, R.S., Glade, P.R., Chessin, L.N., and Wolff, S.M. Fine structure of continuous long term lymphoid cell cultures from a Chediak-Higashi patient and heterozygote. Lab. Invest., 21:225, 1969.

24. Efrati, P. and Jonas, W. Chediak's anomaly of leukocytes in malignant lymphoma associated with leukemic manifestations: case report with necropsy. Blood, 13:1063, 1958.
25. Gallin, J.I., Elin, R.J., Hubert, R.T., Fauci, A.S., Kaliner, M.A., and Wolff, S.M. Efficacy of ascorbic acid in Chediak-Higashi syndrome (CHS): studies in humans and mice. Blood, 53:226, 1979.
26. Gillon, J.R., Pease, G.L., and Mills, S.D. Chediak-Higashi anomaly of the leukocytes: report of a case. Proc. Mayo Clin., 35:635, 1960.
27. Haak, R.A., Ingraham, L.M., Baehner, R.L., and Boxer, L.A. Membrane fluidity in human and mouse Chediak-Higashi leukocytes. J. Clin. Invest., 64:138, 1979.
28. Haliotis, T., Roder, J., Klein, M., Ortaldo, J., Fauci, A.S., and Herberman, R.B. Chediak-Higashi gene in humans. I. Impairment of natural-killer function. J. Exp. Med., 151:1039, 1980.
29. Hansson, H., Linell, F., Nilsson, L.R., Soderhjelm, L., and Undritz, U. Die Chediak-Steinbrinck-anomalie resp. erblich-konstitutionelle risengranulation (granulagiganten) der leukozyyten in Nordschweden. Folia Haematol., 3:152, 1959.
30. Herberman, R.B. Natural killer cells. Hosp. Pract., 17:9, 1982.
31. Higashi, O. Congenital gigantism of peroxidase granules. The first case ever reported of qualitative abnormity of peroxidase. Tohuku J. Exp. Med., 59:315, 1954.
32. Hinds, K. and Dane, B.S. Microtubular defect in Chediak-Higashi syndrome. Lancet, ii:146, 1976.
33. Ingraham, L.M., Burns, C.P., Boxer, L.A., Baehner, R.L., and Haak, R.A. Fluidity properties and lipid composition of erythrocyte membranes in Chediak-Higashi syndrome. J. Cell Biol., 89:510, 1981.
34. Iseki, S., Ebina, T., and Ishida, N. Mode of paracrystal formation in Chediak-Higashi fibroblasts. Lancet, i:1409, 1979.
35. Ito, J., Tokumaru, M., and Okazaki, T. Chediak-Higashi syndrome: report of case with autopsy and electron microscopic studies. Acta Path. Jap., 22:755, 1972.
36. Janini, P., Pinto Lima, X., Franca, H.H., Tricta, F., and Tannos, D. Sobre tres casos de anomalia leucocitaria identica a la descrita pos Bequez Cesar, Steinbrinck, Chediak, Higashi y Sato. Sangre, 8:138, 1963.
37. Kearny, P.J., Swift, P.G.F., Brow, N.J., and Savage, D.C.L. The Chediak-Higashi syndrome in a boy of Irish parents. J. Irish Med. Assoc., 72:22, 1979.
38. Khan, A., Hill, J.M., Loeb, E., MacLellan, A., and Hill, N.A. Management of Chediak-Higashi syndrome with transfer factor. Am. J. Dis. Child., 126:797, 1973.

39.   Kimball, H.R., Ford, G.H., and Wolff, S.M. Lysosomal
      enzymes in normal and Chediak-Higashi blood leukocytes.
      J. Lab. Clin. Med., 86:616, 1975.

40.   Klein, G. and Purtilo, D. Symposium on Epstein-Barr virus-
      induced diseases in immunodeficient patients. Cancer
      Res., 41:4209, 1981.

41.   Klein, G. Lymphoma development in mice and humans:
      diversity of initiation is followed by convergent cyto-
      genetic evolution. Proc. Natl. Acad. Sci. USA,
      76:2442, 1979.

42.   Klein, M., Roder, J., Haliotis, T., Korec, S., Jett, J.R.,
      Herberman, R.B., Katz, P., and Fauci, A.S. Chediak-
      Higashi gene in humans. II. The selectivity of the
      defect in natural-killer and antibody-dependent cell-
      mediated cytotoxicity function. J. Exp. Med., 151:1049,
      1980.

43.   Kritzler, R.A., Terner, J.Y., Lindenbaun, J., Magidson, J.,
      Williams, R., Preisig, R., and Phillips, G. Chediak-
      Higashi syndrome. Cytologic and serum lipid obser-
      vations in a case and family. Am. J. Med., 36:583,
      1964.

44.   Krueger, G.R.F., Bedoya, V., and Grimley, P.M.
      Lymphoreticular tissue lesions in Steinbrinck-Chediak-
      Higashi syndrome. Virchows Arch. Abt. A. Path. Anat.,
      353:273, 1971.

45.   Maggi, R., Gutierrez, E., Penalber, J., and DiMenna, A.,
      Roccotagliata, M., Matera, F., Etchegaray, E., and
      Millan, J. Sindrome de Bequez Cesar-Chediak-Higashi.
      Arch. Arg. Pediat., 48:323, 1957.

46.   Merino, F., Klein, G., Henle, W., Ramirez-Duque, P.,
      Forsgren, M., and Amesty, C. Elevated antibody titers
      to Epstein-Barr virus and low natural killer cell acti-
      vity in patients with Chediak-Higashi syndrome. Clin.
      Immunol. Immunopathol., in press.

47.   Merino, F., Lipscomb, J., Amesty, C., and Purtilo, D.
      Lymphocyte subsets in Chediak-Higashi syndrome patients.
      Immunol. Letters, 6:81, 1983.

48.   Moran, T.J. and Estevez, J.M. Chediak-Higashi disease.
      Morphological studies of a patient and her family. Arch.
      Pathol., 88:329, 1969.

49.   Nath, J., Flavin, M., and Gallin, J.I. Tubulin tyrosylation
      in normal and Chediak-Higashi syndrome neutrophils. J.
      Cell. Biol., 87:256a, 1980.

50.   Nishi, Y., Sawano, K., Kagosaki, Y., Tanaka, Y., Kobayashi,
      Y., and Usui, T. High plasma, erythrocyte, lymphocytic
      and granulocyte zinc concentrations in a patient with
      the Chediak-Higashi syndrome. Eur. J. Pediatr., 134:9,
      1980.

51. Oliver, J.M. Impaired microtubule function correctable by cyclic GMP and cholinergic agonists in the Chediak-Higashi syndrome. Am. J. Pathol., 85:395, 1976.

52. Oliver, J.M. and Zurier, R.B. Correction of characteristic abnormalities of microtubule function and granule morphology in Chediak-Higashi syndrome with colinergic agonists. J. Clin. Invest., 57:1239, 1976.

53. Ostlund, R.E., Tucker, R.W., Leung, J.T., Okun, N., and Williamson, J.R. The cytoskeleton in Chediak-Higashi syndrome fibroblasts. Blood, 56:806, 1980.

54. Pachioli, R., Caramia, G., and DiBattista, C. L'anomalia di Beguez-Steinbrinck-Chediak-Higashi. Rassegna sintetica e descrizione di un caso. Minerva Pediatr., 22:368, 1970.

55. Padgett, G.A. The Chediak-Higashi syndrome. Adv. Vet. Sci., 12:239, 1968.

56. Padgett, G.A., Reiquam, C.W., Gorham, J.R., Henson, J.B., and O'Mary, C.C. Comparative studies of the Chediak-Higashi syndrome. Pathology Am. J. Pathol., 51:553, 1967.

57. Padgett, G.A., Reiquam, C.W., Henson, J.B., and Gorham, J.R. Comparative studies of susceptibility to infection in the Chediak-Higashi syndrome. J. Path. Bact., 95:509, 1968.

58. Page, A.R., Berendez, H., Warner, J., and Good, R.A. The Chediak-Higashi syndrome. Blood, 20:330, 1962.

59. Parmley, R.T., Poon, M.-C., Crist, W.M., and Malluh, A. Giant platelet granules in a child with the Chediak-Higashi syndrome. Am. J. Hematol., 6:51, 1979.

60. Pierini, D.D., Turro, D., Torales, E., and Piantanida, J.J. Chediak-Higashi disease. Arch. Arg. Dermatol., 19:143, 1969.

61. Prchal, J.T., Crist, W.M., Malluh, A., Tauxe, W.N. and Carroll, A.J. A new glucose-6-phosphate dehydrogenase deficient variant in a patient with Chediak-Higashi syndrome. Blood, 56:476, 1980.

62. Prieur, A.-M., Griscelli, C., and Gaugillard, F. Lymphotoxin (LT) production by lymphocytes from children with primary immunodeficiency disease. Clin. Immunol. Immunopathol., 10:468, 1978.

63. Prieur, D.J. and Collier, L.L. Animal model: Chediak-Higashi syndrome of animals. Am. J. Pathol., 90:533, 1978.

64. Purtilo, D.T. Immunopathology of infectious mononucleosis and other complications of Epstein-Barr virus infections. Pathol. Ann., 15:253, 1980.

65. Ramirez-Duque, P., Arends, T., and Merino, F. Chediak-Higashi syndrome: description of a cluster in a Venezuelan Andean isolated region. J. Medicine, in press.

66. Ratto, L.-A., Hliba, E., Yatorno, C.-E., and Rupil, A.
     Sindrome de Chediak-Higashi-Steinbrinck. Estudio hema-
     tologico y ultraestructural. Sangre, 22:263, 1977.
67. Rausch, P.G., Pryzwansky, K.B., and Spitnagel, J.K.
     Immunocytochemical identification of azurophilic and
     specific granule markers in the giant granules of
     Chediak-Higashi neutrophils. N. Engl. J. Med., 298:693,
     1978.
68. Roder, J.C., Haliotis, T., Klein, M., Korec, S., Jett, J.R.,
     Ortaldo, J., Herberman, R.B., Katz, P., and Fauci, A.S.
     A new immunodeficiency disorder in humans involving NK
     cells. Nature, 284:553, 1980.
69. Root, R.K., Rosenthal, A.S., and Balestra, D.J. Abnormal
     bactericidal, metabolic and lysosomal functions of
     Chediak-Higashi syndrome leukocytes. J. Clin. Invest.,
     51:649, 1972.
70. Rosenszajn, L.A., Ben David, E., and Bar Sela, S. Large
     granules and lysosomal fusion in human Chediak-Higashi
     white blood cells. Acta Haemat., 57:279, 1977.
71. Rosenzajn, L.N., Radnai, J., Tatarski, A., and Benderlei, A.
     Blood cell culture and chromosomal findings in Chediak-
     Higashi syndrome. Israel J. Med. Sci., 5:1087, 1969.
72. Sadan, N., Yaffe, D., Rosensjan, L., Adar, H., Soroker, B.,
     and Efrati, P. Cytochemical and genetic studies in four
     cases of Chediak-Higashi-Steinbrinck syndrome. Acta
     Haemat., 34:20, 1965.
73. Saitoh, H., Komiyama, A., Narose, N., Morosawa, H., and
     Akabane, T. Development of the accelerated phase during
     ascorbic acid therapy in Chediak-Higashi syndrome and
     efficacy of colchicine on its management. Br. J.
     Haemat., 48:79, 1981.
74. Salamanca-Gomez, F., Salazar-Mallen, M., and Amezcu, M.E.
     Chromosome one polymorphism in a girl with the
     Chediak-Higashi syndrome. Acta Cytologica, 22:402,
     1978.
75. Saraiva, L.G., Azevedo, M., Correa, J.M., Carvalho, G., and
     Prospero, J.D. Anomalous panleukocytic granulation.
     Blood, 14:112, 1959.
76. Sato, A. Chediak-Higashi's disease, preliminary report.
     Probable identity of Chediak's and Higashi's diseases.
     Tohuku J. Exp. Med., 60:22, 1954.
77. Saxena, R.K., Saxena, Q.B., and Adler, W.H. Defective T-
     cell responses in beige mutant mice. Nature, 295:240,
     1982.
78. Sawano, K., Sakono, T., Kagosaki, Y., Yoshimitsu, H.,
     Miyake, Y., Kobayashi, Y. and Usui, T. Chemotaxis of
     granulocytes in Chediak-Higashi syndrome with agarose
     plate and filter chamber methods. Hiroshima J. Med.
     Sci., 28:107, 1979.

79. Say, B., Tuncbilek, E, Yamack, B., and Balci, S. An unusual chromosomal aberration in a case of Chediak-Higashi syndrome. J. Med. Genet., 7:417, 1970.

80. Sheramata, W., Kott, S., and Cyr, D.P. The Chediak-Higashi-Steinbrinck syndrome. Presentation of three cases with features resembling spinocerebellar degeneration. Arch. Neurol., 25:289, 1971.

81. Spencer, W.H. and Hogan, M.J. Ocular manifestations of Chediak-Higashi syndrome. Report of a case with histopathological examination of ocular tissues. Am. J. Ophtal., 50:1197, 1960.

82. Steinbrinck, W. Uber eine neue granulationsanomalie der leukocyten. Dtsch. Arch. Klin. Med., 193:577, 1948.

83. Stossel, T.P., Root, R.K., and Vaughan, M. Phagocytosis in chronic granulomatosis disease and the Chediak-Higashi syndrome. N. Engl. J. Med., 286:120, 1972.

84. Tan, C., Etcubanas, E., Leiberman, P., Isenberg, H., King, O., and Murphy, M.L. Chediak-Higashi syndrome in a child with Hodgkin's disease. Am. J. Dis. Child., 121:135, 1971.

85. Tanaka, T. Chediak-Higashi syndrome: abnormal lysosomal enzymal levels in granulocytes of patients and family members. Pediat. Res., 14:901, 1980.

86. Tanaka, T. and Orii, T. High sensitivity but normal DNA-repair activity after UV irradiation in Epstein-Barr-transformed lymphoblastoid cell lines for Chediak-Higashi syndrome. Mutation Res., 72:143, 1980.

87. Tanaka, H., Ito, T., and Orii, T. DNA repair mechanisms in Chediak-Higashi syndrome cells. J. Inher. Metab. Dis., 5:65, 1982.

88. Tay, C.H., Lopez, C.G., and Lazarus, A.R. The Chediak-Higashi syndrome. Med. J. Aust., 2:1027, 1970.

89. Van de Griend, R.J., Astaldi, A., de Bruin, H.G., and Weening, R.S. T cells in Chediak-Higashi syndrome. N. Engl. J. Med., 306:1368, 1982.

90. Vasalli, J.-D., Granelli-Piperno, A., Griscelli, C., and Reich, E. Specific protease deficiency in polymorphonuclear leukocytes of Chediak-Higashi syndrome and beige mice. J. Exp. Med., 147:1285, 1978.

91. Weening, R.S., Schoorel, E.P., Vanschaik, M.L.J., Voetman, A.A., Bot, A.A.M., Batenburg-Plenter, A.M., Willems, Ch., Zeijlemaker, W.P., and Astaldi, A. Effect of ascorbate on abnormal neutrophil, platelet, and lymphocyte function in a patient with the Chediak-Higashi syndrome. Blood, 57:856, 1981.

92. White, J.G. Virus-like particles in the peripheral blood cells of two patients with Chediak-Higashi syndrome. Cancer, 19:877, 1966.

93. White, J.G. The Chediak-Higashi syndrome: a possible lysosomal disease. Blood, 28:143, 1966.

94.   White, J.G.   The Chediak-Higashi syndrome: cytoplasmic
       sequestration in circulating leukocytes.   Blood,
       29:4335, 1967.
95.   White, J.G.   Platelet microtubules and giant granules in the
       Chediak-Higashi syndrome.   Am. J. Med. Tech., 44:273,
       1978.
96.   White, J.G. and Gerrard, J.M.   The ultrastructure of defec-
       tive human platelets.   Mol. Cell. Biochem., 21:109,
       1978.
97.   White, J.G. and Clawson, C.C.   The Chediak-Higashi syndrome.
       Ring-shaped lysosomes in circulating monocytes.   Am. J.
       Pathol., 96:781, 1979.
98.   White, J.G. and Clawson, C.C.   The Chediak-Higashi syndrome:
       microtubules in monocytes and lymphocytes.   Am. J.
       Hematol., 7:349, 1979.
99.   White, J.G. and Clawson, C.C.   The Chediak-Higashi syndrome:
       the nature of the giant neutrophil granules and their
       interactions with cytoplasm and foreign particles.   I,
       II, III.   Am. J. Pathol., 98:151, 1980.
100.   Wolff, S.M., Dale, D.C., Clark, R.A., Root, K., and Kimball,
       H.R.   The Chediak-Higashi syndrome: studies of host de-
       fenses.   Ann. Int. Med., 76:293, 1972.
101.   Zabucchi, G., Cramer, R., Soranzo, M.R., Tamaro, P., and
       Panizon, F.   Biochemical studies on the leukocytes in
       Chediak-Higashi syndrome.   Acta Haemat., 58:50, 1977.

EXPRESSION OF VIRUS-ASSOCIATED FUNCTIONS IN CELLS TRANSFORMED
IN VITRO BY EPSTEIN-BARR VIRUS: EPSTEIN-BARR VIRUS CELL SURFACE
ANTIGEN AND VIRUS-RELEASE FROM TRANSFORMED CELLS

Bill Sugden

McArdle Laboratory
University of Wisconsin
Madison, WI   53706

INTRODUCTION

Epstein-Barr virus (EBV) infects resting human B lymphocytes
in vitro and induces up to 10% of the infected cells to proliferate as measured in a clonal transformation assay (1-5). This
virus also infects B lymphocytes in vivo; up to 20% of the
peripheral B cells in patients with infectious mononucleosis (IM)
express an EBV-associated nuclear antigen, EBNA (6). When
peripheral lymphocytes from IM patients are collected and cloned
directly in soft agar, some B cells are found to proliferate
indefinitely and to express EBNA (7). Although it is not known
that virus infections in vitro and in vivo are functionally
equivalent, no differences between B cells infected in vitro and
in vivo have yet been identified once the cells are studied in
vitro. We have studied cells transformed by EBV in vitro with the
hope that such studies will help to define characteristics of some
of the cells infected by EBV in vivo. The advantage of studying
cells transformed in vitro is that we can chart their history from
their exposure to EBV to the time of study.

The expression of EBV-associated functions in transformed
human cells can be conveniently divided into three categories: 1.
common viral functions expressed intracellularly; 2. common
virus-associated functions expressed at the cell surface; and 3.
viral maturation functions which are expressed rarely. These
categories are a reflection of many studies of EBV-transformed
cells carried out by many researchers.

The first general observation to be drawn from these studies
is that only a limited set of viral genes are expressed in cells

transformed in vitro (8,9), although all of the viral DNA is
usually present in these cells (10). Only 10 to 20% of the viral
DNA is transcribed (9), the predominant transcripts are small,
non-polyadenylated RNAs (9,11), and the only identified protein
currently assumed to be virally encoded in these cells is EBNA
(8).

     The second general observation to be noted is that EBV-
transformed cells generally do not express cell surface antigens
recognized by antisera from patients with EBV-related diseases.
On the other hand, they do express some structure, often referred
to as LYDMA, which serves as the recognition target for specific,
T cell mediated cytotoxicity (12-20). Recently a cell surface
protein present on all cells transformed in vitro by EBV has been
described which is detected by monoclonal antibodies (21-24).
This protein is a candidate for LYDMA.

     The third general observation is that consistent with the
immortalized phenotype of EBV-transformed cells virus is released
rarely by these cells (10,25,26) and therefore late viral functions cannot generally be detected in them (24). The efficiency
of release of EBV by EBV-transformed adult cells is unknown. This
cell type is the only virus reservoir thought to be present in
most infected people.

     I shall describe our studies on the last two categories of
EBV-associated functions expressed in transformed cells; that is,
our work on a virally associated, cell surface antigen and on the
release of infectious virus from these cells. I shall attempt to
relate the extent to which the study of these functions expressed
in cells transformed in vitro can inform us about their infected
analogues in vivo. These virally associated functions are likely
to play a role in the course of EBV infections in vivo.

Epstein-Barr Virus Cell Surface Antigen (EBVCS)

     We have generated five hybridomas whose antibodies detect
determinants on EBV-transformed cells but not on primary human B-
lymphocytes (21, unpublished observations). Three other groups
have isolated monoclonal antibodies with similar specificities
(22-24). Of all the cell lines tested, only those carrying EBV
express these determinants at detectable levels (21-24).
EBV-positive Burkitt's lymphoma cell lines, however, often express
these determinants at reduced levels (21,23). We have not
detected binding of the five monoclonal antibodies to any primary
cells not infected with EBV (21). Thorley-Lawson and his
colleagues (26a) have observed weak binding of their antibody to
cells from patients with chronic lymphocytic leukemia and to cells
in some regions of normal human lymph nodes. So long as the cells
tested are not infected with EBV (which seems likely but see (27))

the antigen detected by all of these antibodies is likely to be induced by infection with EBV, but not encoded by the virus. We term this antigen EBVCS.

EBVCS is a predominant cell surface antigen on cell lines established by transformation with EBV in vitro. To measure the level of EBVCS per cell the five monoclonal antibodies were labelled metabolically (28), purified, and bound at increasing concentrations to clones of EBV-transformed cells. Saturation binding levels were achieved at 2×10^5 to 4×10^6 molecules per cell (28a). This level of binding at saturation indicates that there are approximately 10^6 molecules of EBVCS per transformed cell. Similarly, about 10^6 molecules of HLA-A,B,C are expressed on these cell types (29).

EBVCS is a protein with an approximate molecular weight of 47,000 D (21-24). To determine the mass of EBVCS surface proteins of EBV-transformed cells we first labelled cells with $[^{125}I]$ NaI, lactoperoxidase, and H_2O_2. These proteins had specific activities of 10^5 to 10^6 cpm per microgram. The labelled proteins were dissolved, immunoprecipitated with the five mono-clonal antibodies, and the immunoprecipitates resolved on poly-acrylamide gels containing SDS. Four of the five immunopre-cipitates resolved into a single band with an apparent molecular weight of 47,000 D. The fifth gave no signal although this antibody competes for the binding of one of the antibodies which does specifically immunoprecipitate a signal at 47,000 D (28a). The apparent molecular weight of EBVCS is close to that found for the heavy chain of HLA-A and B molecules (30).

The similarities between the numbers of molecules and their sizes for EBVCS and HLA-A,B,C has prompted us to determine whether these molecules are related. We labelled cell surface proteins, solubilized them, and immunoprecipitated the lysates either with a pool of anti-EBVCS antibodies or with monoclonal antibodies to HLA-A,B,C (PA2.6) and to $\beta 2$-microglobulin (BBM.1) (31). That these immunoprecipitations were complete was determined by reprecipitating aliquots of the first supernatants with the same reagents. The supernatant remaining after immunoprecipitation with anti-EBVCS was then immunoprecipitated with anti-HLA and anti-$\beta 2$ microglobulin; similarly, the reciprocal experiment was performed. In each case pre-clearing with one set of antibodies failed to remove the antigens detected by the second set (28a). We conclude EBVCS is not associated with $\beta 2$-microglobulin; that is, it is not a Type 1 major histocompatibility antigen. Within the limits set by the monoclonal antibodies used, therefore, EBVCS is not antigenically related to HLA-A,B,C determinants.

EBVCS is a predominant cell surface antigen induced by infection with EBV, and it is not associated with $\beta 2$-microglobulin.

Is it LYDMA? Is it the structure recognized by those cytotoxic T
cells thought to be specific for autologous, EBV-transformed
cells? Two experiments have been published in which the cytotoxicity of uncloned T cells directed against autologous EBV-
transformed cells was not blocked by two antibodies presumably
directed against EBVCS (22,23). The potential heterogeneity of
cytotoxic T cells makes these experiments difficult to interpret.
Ideally, similar experiments will be done using many clones of
specific, cytotoxic T cells and many anti-EBVCS antibodies. A
more compelling experimental approach to associate or dissociate
EBVCS with or from LYDMA would be to select mutants of EBV which
fail to induce EBVCS or variants of EBV-transformed cells which
fail to express EBVCS. EBVCS-positive and -negative cell clones
established after transformation of cells from the same donor
could be tested for their ability both to stimulate autologous,
specific, cytotoxic T cell clones and to serve as targets for such
cells. Use of all combinations of EBVCS-positive and -negative
cells should indicate if EBVCS is functionally equivalent to
LYDMA.

With the goal of generating reagents which could be used to
select EBVCS-negative, EBV-transformed cells and might possibly be
of therapeutic value, we have conjugated the toxic A-chain of ricin
(RTA) to three of the anti-EBVCS antibodies. RTA when introduced
into cells inhibits protein synthesis and kills the cells (32).
One method of introducing RTA is by coupling it to a molecule
which has a high affinity for a cell surface moiety and which
after binding is endocytosed. For example, Cawley et al. (33)
have coupled the RTA to epidermal growth factor (EGF) and found
that the conjugate is toxic for EGF-receptor-positive cells at
concentrations of 10^{-9} molar.

RTA was separated from the galactose binding moiety of ricin
using β-mercaptoethanol and sepharose column chromatography (33).
RTA was then coupled to anti-EBVCS antibodies which had been
purified on Sephacryl-200 columns using the bifunctional coupling
reagent, N-succinimidyl-3(2-pyridyldithio)-propionate, (33) and
the conjugates purified on Sephacryl-200 columns. Each conjugate
contained approximately one RTA chain per 150,000 D of immunoglobulin.

None of the anti-EBVCS-RTA conjugates showed detectable cytotoxicity at concentrations up to 5 micrograms/ml for the EBV-
negative cell lines tested. These lines included three EBV-
negative Burkitt's lymphomas and one T cell lymphoma. One
conjugate, an IgM which has the highest affinity of all the
antibodies tested, was non-toxic for most of the EBV-transformed
cells tested. One of the IgG conjugates tested was toxic for
EBV-transformed cells only at moderate concentrations (1
microgram/ml), while the other IgG conjugate was toxic at concen-

trations between 20 and 200 picrograms per ml. In experiments in
which the conjugates were toxic for EBV-transformed cells different clones of cells were killed differentially. In general, cells
stopped dividing in two to four days and the cell numbers declined
to undetectable levels over the course of two to three weeks.

That conjugates of RTA with different anti-EBVCS antibodies
have different toxicities for different EBV-transformed cell
clones indicates that any therapeutic use of these reagents awaits
much study. However, the most toxic conjugate can probably be
used to select EBVCS-negative, EBV-transformed cells in vitro.
One explanation for the varied toxicity of these anti-EBVCS-RTA
conjugates may lie in the half-life of EBVCS at the cell surface.
We have found that in cells treated with tunicamycin EBVCS has a
half-life several times shorter than that of HLA (28a). If EBVCS
has a short half-life on normal cell surfaces, then different
anti-EBVCS antibodies may promote antigen shedding and concomitantly decrease their endocytosis.

Release of Infectious EBV by EBV-transformed B Lymphocytes

A second set of viral functions whose expression in transformed cells should affect the course of EBV infection in vivo are
those required for maturation and release of infectious progeny.
In patients with nasopharyngeal carcinoma, EBV is found in the
epithelial tumor cells (34) and in patients with a variety of
lymphoid tumors apparently not associated with EBV, EBNA is
expressed in some Ig-negative lymphoid cells (27). However, in
normal donors the only cells known to be infected with EBV are B
lymphoblasts. No analogue to the feather follicle which permits
efficient replication of the otherwise lymphotropic Marek's
disease virus in chickens (35,36) has yet been found for EBV in
people. If EBV infection spreads in vivo in part by recruitment,
then based on our present knowledge the transformed lymphoblast is
the only candidate for the source of EBV needed for recruitment.

We have measured the release of infectious EBV from cells isolated from the peripheral blood of seronegative donors of 18 to 25
years of age after infection of those cells with EBV in vitro.
Similar studies have been performed using neonatal B lymphocytes
(26), but such cells behave differently than do adult B lymphocytes
when infected with EBV (37). To measure the release of infectious
EBV, we have used an adaptation of our clonal transformation assay
(4). EBV-transformed cells to be tested were irradiated with 4000
rads of gamma rays, incubated for 24 to 60 hours with either a
100-fold excess of seronegative lymphocytes or a 1- to 5-fold
excess of purified, seronegative B lymphocytes, and plated as
single cells in agarose over a human fibroblast feeder layer (4).
Proliferating clones were scored 28 to 35 days after seeding.
Control experiments were performed which indicate that no clones

Table 1.   Release of Infectious EBV from Clones of
EBV-transformed Cells

Clones Tested	Co-Cultivated clones observed per $2x10^4$ cells tested	
	Tested at Cell Generation 15-20[a]	Tested at Cell Generation 20-30[b]
JO-L B1	0	–
JO-L C2	0	–
JO-L C3	7	0
JO-H A2	0	–
JO-H A3	80	15
JO-H A4	20	–
JO-H B1	0	–
JO-H C4	0	–
JO-H C5	0	–
TH-L A2	30	125
TH-L A3	0	–
TH-L B1	0	–
TH-L B2	0	–
TH-L B4	1	–
TH-L B5	0	–
TH-L C1	20	–
TH-L C2	0	–
TH-L C4	130	150
TH-L D3	40	175
TH-L D4	15	50
TH-H A3	0	–
TH-H A4	0	–
TH-H B5	0	–
TH-H C6	1	0
TH-H D3	0	–
B95-8[c]	200	800

$1x10^4$ - $5x10^4$ clone cells were lethally irradiated and
incubated with a 100-fold excess of seronegative lymphocytes for (a) 24-36 hrs or (b) 60 hrs. These cells were
then plated in agarose over a feeder layer and rescued
clones were counted 4-5 weeks later. JO and TH are two
seronegative donors used to establish the clones.
Postscript L indicates that the clones arose after exposure of 100 seronegative lymphocytes to 1 particle of EBV.
Postscript H indicates that the clones arose after exposure of 1 seronegative lymphocyte to $3x10^4$ particles of
EBV. (c) B95-8 cells are included in each set of co-
cultivation experiments as a positive control and provide
a standard for the reproducibility of the co-cultivation
protocol.

grew when only the gamma-irradiated, EBV-transformed cells were
plated and that when EBV-neutralizing antisera was added to the
co-cultivation the number of proliferating clones was reduced by
95%.   The sensitivity of the assay was measured by co-cultivating
gamma-irradiated B95-8 cells, which release infectious EBV
relatively efficiently (38), with seronegative lymphocytes and

plating the co-cultivated cells. For each viral capsid antigen positive B95-8 cell tested, between 0.5 and 2 proliferating clones were scored.

In a series of experiments 25 clones of EBV-transformed cells were tested (Table 1). The clones were established from two seronegative donors after exposure of lymphocytes to low (less than one virus particle per cell) or to high (3×10^4 particles per cell) multiplicities of infection. Forty percent of the clones released detectable levels of infectious EBV when only 2×10^4 cells of each were tested 15 to 20 cell generations after the cells were infected. Most of these clones (80%) continued to release virus at comparable levels after another 10 generations in culture. In general, the efficiency of release was found to be independent of the donor and of the multiplicity of infection used to transform the cells. Finally, between 30 and 60% of the clones that did release detectable levels of EBV did so within an order of magnitude of the level that the producer cell line, B95-8, did (Table 1).

In a second series of experiments, mass populations of infected B lymphocytes were tested to measure how soon after infection those cells released infectious EBV (Table 2). No released, infectious virus was detected until 10 days after infections although in different experiments cells were tested at 3,4,7, and 8 days after infection. This 10-day period represents approximately 5 cell generations for the transformed cells (39). By 21 days after infection or 10 cell generations the transformed cells released as much EBV as found for the average of the clones tested between 15 and 30 generations after transformation (Table 1).

When the data from Tables 1 and 2 are viewed together they indicate that by 10 cell generations after transformation, EBV-transformed, adult human lymphoblasts release virus such that for each 1000 transformed cells co-cultivated, one clone of proliferating cells would be scored among the indicator lymphocytes. The measured cloning efficiency for our assay is about 3% (4). Therefore, in vitro each 24 hours 30 transformed cells can release enough infectious EBV to recruit approximately one newly infected cell.

Possible Roles for EBVCS and for the Release of Virus from Lymphoblasts in Affecting the Course of EBV Infections In Vivo

There are two weak bits of circumstantial evidence that indicate EBVCS may play a role in the host's cellular immune response to EBV infection. The first is that EBVCS is the only presently identified candidate for LYDMA, the target recognized by specific, cytotoxic T cells. This apparent evidence, if it simply

Table 2. Release of Infectious EBV by Mass Cultures as a Function of Time After Infection

Experiment	TFU per cell	Days after infection that co-cultivation was begun	Duration of co-cultivation (hr)	Number of infected cells co-cultivated	Number of cells per 1000 infected cells that grew as clones at the time of co-cultivation	Number of clones arising from co-cultivation of 10^5 irradiated infected cells with B lymphocytes	
						−AB	+AB
1	1–2	3	48	9×10^5	25	0	
2	1–2	4	48	2×10^6	100	0	0
	1–2	8	48	2×10^6	140	0	0
	1–2	12	48	2×10^6	150	11	0
3	1–2	7	24	1.5×10^5	60	0	
4	10	10	48	5.5×10^5	80	5	
5	10	7	48	2×10^5	8	0	0
	10	14	48	2×10^5	17	5	0
	10	21	48	1.5×10^5	17	130	7

B lymphocytes were exposed to EBV at either 1 or 10 transforming units per cell, incubated overnight, washed two times, and incubated 37°C. From 3 to 21 days later aliquots of infected cells were plated in agarose over feeder layers to measure the number of cells transformed (column 6). Another aliquot (column 5) was irradiated with 4000 rads of gamma-rays, mixed with a 1–5 fold excess of purified, indicator B lymphocytes for 24 or 48 hours in the presence (+AB) or absence (−AB) of neutralizing antibodies, and plated in agarose. Clones arising by infection of indicator B lymphocytes with virus released by the irradiated, infected cells were scored after five weeks (column 7).

reflects our ignorance, is no evidence at all. The second bit of
evidence is that EBVCS is usually expressed at reduced levels on
Burkitt's lymphoma cell lines relative to other EBV-transformed
cells (21,23). If the earliest infected progenitor cell which
gave rise to a tumor expressed EBVCS at normal levels, then it
seems likely that the observed, diminished expression on the tumor
cell lines indicates that the diminished expression of EBVCS on
some cells gave a selective growth advantage to those cells. This
hypothetical case is consistent with EBVCS being involved in
recognition by the immune response of the host. Those cells which
escape the response give rise to Burkitt's lymphoma.

There is one experiment that is inconsistent with EBVCS being
LYDMA. Two anti-EBVCS monoclonal antibodies fail to block
specific killing of autologous EBV-transformed cells (22,23).
These experiments were performed using cloned T cells and must be
repeated with cloned effector populations. In addition, blocking
of virally associated T cell mediated cytotoxicity is unexpectedly
difficult to achieve in examples which are much better understood
than is immunity to EBV infections (40).

Although the role of EBVCS in affecting the course of infection in vivo is now merely speculative, the role played by
lymphoid release of EBV is more certain. However, the magnitude
of this role is not now known. Given that primary B lymphocytes
infected in vivo behave similarly to those we infect in vitro,
EBV-transformed lymphocytes will release some infectious virus
which will recruit more infected cells. The extent of this
recruitment will obviously be affected by the host's immune
response and, in particular, will be blocked by virus-neutralizing
antibodies. In general, the time course of development of
neutralizing antibodies to EBV during primary infection has not
been studied. If we assume that the appearance of antibodies to
membrane antigen is equivalent to the appearance of neutralizing
antibodies (24), then the titer of neutralizing antibodies peak in
IM patients soon after the onset of the illness (41). This
humoral response should limit recruitment in vivo resulting from
EBV released from infected lymphoblasts. A failure to mount a
humoral response to EBV-associated antigens (42), however, might
elevate the role of virus release and subsequent recruitment of
more cells to being a major influence during the course of
infection in such immunocompromised hosts.

ACKNOWLEDGEMENTS

This work was supported by the National Cancer Institute
grants CA-09135, CA-22443, and CA-07175 and an American Cancer
Society Faculty Research Award FRA-203.

REFERENCES

1. Pope, J.H., Horne, M.K., and Scott, W. Transformation of
    foetal human leukocytes in vitro by filtrates of a human
    leukaemic cell line containing herpes-like virus. Int.
    J. Cancer, 3:857, 1968.
2. Pattengale, P.K., Smith, R.W., and Gerber, P. Selective
    transformation of B lymphocytes by EB virus. Lancet,
    ii:93, 1973.
3. Yamamoto, N. and Hinuma, Y. Clonal transformation of human
    leukocytes by Epstein-Barr virus in soft agar. Int. J.
    Cancer, 17:191, 1976.
4. Sugden, B. and Mark, W. Clonal transformation of adult
    human leukocytes by Epstein-Barr virus. J. Virol.,
    23:503, 1977.
5. Henderson, E., Miller, G., Robinson, J., and Heston, L.
    Efficiency of transformation of lymphocytes by
    Epstein-Barr virus. Virology, 76:152, 1977.
6. Robinson, J.E., Smith, D., and Niederman, J. Plasmacytic
    differentiation of circulating Epstein-Barr virus-
    infected B lymphocytes during acute infectious mono-
    nucleosis. J. Exp. Med., 153:235, 1981.
7. Hinuma, Y. and Katsuki, T. Colonies of EBNA-positive cells
    in soft agar from peripheral leukocytes of infectious
    mononucleosis patients. Int. J. Cancer, 21:426, 1978.
8. Reedman, B.M. and Klein, G. Cellular localization of an
    Epstein-Barr virus (EBV)-associated complement-fixing
    antigen in producer and non-producer lymphoblastoid cell
    lines. Int. J. Cancer, 11:499, 1973.
9. van Santen, V., Cheung, A., and Kieff, E. Epstein-Barr virus
    RNA. VII. Size and direction of transcription of virus-
    specific cytoplasmic RNAs in a transformed cell line.
    Proc. Natl. Acad. Sci. USA, 78:1930, 1981.
10. Kintner, C. and Sugden, B. Conservation and progressive
    methylation of Epstein-Barr virus DNA sequences in
    transformed cells. J. Virol., 38:305, 1981.
11. Lerner, M.R., Andrews, N.C., Miller, G., and Steitz, J.A.
    Two small RNAs encoded by Epstein-Barr virus and
    complexed with protein are precipitated by antibodies
    from patients with systemic lupus erythematosus. Proc.
    Natl. Acad. Sci. USA, 78:805, 1981.
12. Svedmyr, E. and Jondal, M. Cytotoxic effector cells specif-
    ic for B cell lines transformed by Epstein-Barr virus are
    present in patients with infectious mononucleosis. Proc.
    Natl. Acad. Sci. USA, 72:1622, 1975.
13. Royston, I., Sullivan, J.L., Periman, P.O., and Perlin, E.
    Cell-mediated immunity to Epstein-Barr-virus-transformed
    lymphoblastoid cells in acute infectious mononucleosis.
    N. Engl. J. Med., 293:1159, 1975.

14. Svedmyr, E., Jondal, M., Henle, W., Weiland, O., Rombo, L.,
     and Klein, G. EBV-specific killer T cells and serologic
     responses after onset of infectious mononucleosis. J.
     Clin. Lab. Immunol., 1:225, 1978.
15. Sugamura, K. and Hinuma, Y. In vitro induction of cyto-
     toxic T lymphocytes specific for Epstein-Barr virus-
     transformed cells: kinetics of autologous restimulation.
     J. Immunol., 124:1045, 1980.
16. Tanaka, Y., Sugamura, K., Hinuma, Y., Sato, H., and Okochi,
     K. Memory of Epstein-Barr virus-specific cytotoxic T
     cells in normal seropositive adults as revealed by an in
     vitro restimulation method. J. Immunol., 125:1426,
     1980.
17. Misko, I.S., Moss, D.J., and Pope, J.H. HLA antigen-related
     restriction of T lymphocyte cytotoxicity to Epstein-Barr
     virus. Proc. Natl. Acad. Sci. USA, 77:4247, 1980.
18. Tsoukas, C.D., Fox, R.I., Slovin, S.F., Carson, D.A.,
     Pellegrino, M., Fong, S., Pasquali, J.-L., Ferrone, S.,
     Kung, P., and Vaughan, J.H. T lymphocyte-mediated cyto-
     toxicity against autologous EBV-genome-bearing B cells.
     J. Immunol., 126:1742, 1981.
19. Rickinson, A.B., Moss, D.J., Allen, D.J., Wallace, L.E.,
     Rowe, M., and Epstein, M.A. Reactivation of Epstein-Barr
     virus-specific cytotoxic T cells by in vitro stimulation
     with autologous lymphoblastoid cell line. Int. J.
     Cancer, 27:593, 1981.
20. Lipinski, M., Fridman, W.H., Tursz, T., Vincent, C., Pious,
     D., and Fellous, M. Absence of allogeneic restriction in
     human T-cell-mediated cytotoxicity to Epstein-Barr virus-
     infected target cells. J. Exp. Med., 150:1310, 1979.
21. Kintner, C. and Sugden, B. Identification of determinants
     unique to the surfaces of cells transformed by
     Epstein-Barr virus. Nature, 294:458, 1981.
22. Slovin, S.F., Frisman, D.M., Tsoukas, C.D., Royston, I.,
     Baird, S.M., Wormsley, S.B., Carson, D.A., and Vaughan,
     J.H. Membrane antigen on Epstein-Barr virus-infected
     human B cells recognized by a monoclonal antibody.
     Proc. Natl. Acad. Sci. USA, 79:2649, 1982.
23. Rowe, M., Hildreth, J.E.K., Rickinson, A.B., and Epstein,
     M.A. Monoclonal antibodies to Epstein-Barr virus-
     induced, transformation-associated cell surface
     antigens: binding patterns and effect upon virus-
     specific T cell cytotoxicity. Int. J. Cancer, 29:373,
     1982.
24. Thorley-Lawson, D.A., Edson, C.M., and Geilinger, K.
     Epstein-Barr virus antigens - a challenge to modern bio-
     chemistry. In: G. Klein and S. Weinhouse (eds.),
     Advances in Cancer Research. Vol. 36, pp. 295-348. New
     York: Academic Press, 1982.

25. Sugden, B., Phelps, M., and Domoradzki, J. Epstein-Barr virus DNA is amplified in transformed lymphocytes. J. Virol., 31:590, 1979.

26. Wilson, G. and Miller, G. Recovery of Epstein-Barr virus from nonproducer neonatal human lymphoid cell transformants. Virology, 95:351, 1979.

26a. Thorley-Lawson, D.A., Schooley, R.T., Bhan, A.K., and Nadler, L.M. Epstein-Barr virus superinduces a new human B cell differentiation antigen (B-last-1) expressed on transformed cells. Cell, 30:415, 1982.

27. Fu, S.M. and Hurley, J.N. Human cell lines containing Epstein-Barr virus but distinct from the common B cell lymphoblastoid lines. Proc. Natl. Acad. Sci. USA, 76:6637, 1979.

28. Galfre, G. and Milstein, C. Preparation of monoclonal antibodies: strategies and procedures. In: J.J. Langone and H. van Vunakis (eds.), Method in Enzymology. Vol. 73, pp. 3-46. New York: Academic Press, 1981.

28a. Sugden, B. and Metzenberg, S. Characterization of an antigen whose cell surface expression is induced by infection with Epstein-Barr virus. J. Virol., 46:800, 1983.

29. Parham, P., Barnstable, C.J., and Bodmer, W.F. Use of monoclonal antibody (W6/32) in structural studies of HLA-A,B,C antigens. J. Immunol., 123:342, 1979.

30. Strominger, J.L., Mann, D.L., Parham, P., Robb, R., Springer, T., and Terhorst, C. Structure of HLA-A and B antigens isolated from cultured human lymphocytes. Cold Spring Harbor Symp. Quant. Biol., 41:323, 1977.

31. Brodsky, F.M., Parham, P., Barnstable, C.J., Crumpton, M.J., and Bodmer, W.F. Monoclonal antibodies for analysis of the HLA system. Immunological Rev., 47:3, 1979.

32. Olsnes, S., Fernandez-Puentes, C., Carrasco, L., and Vasques, D. Ribosome inactivation by the toxic lectins abrin and ricin. Kinetics of the enzymic activity of the toxic A-chains. Eur. J. Biochem., 60:281, 1975.

33. Cawley, D.B., Herschman, H.R., Gilliland, D.G., and Collier, R.J. Epidermal growth factor - toxin A chain conjugates: EGF-ricin A is a potent toxin while EGF-diphtheria fragment A is nontoxic. Cell, 22:563, 1980.

34. Klein, G., Giovanella, B.C., Lindahl, T., Fialkow, P.J., Singh, S., and Stehlin, J.S. Direct evidence for the presence of Epstein-Barr virus DNA and nuclear antigen in malignant epithelial cells from patients with poorly differentiated carcinoma of nasopharynx. Proc. Natl. Acad. Sci. USA, 71:4737, 1974.

35. Calnek, B.W. and Hitchner, S.B. Localization of viral antigen in chickens infected with Marek's disease herpesvirus. J. Natl. Cancer Inst., 43:935, 1969.

36. Nazerran, K. and Witter, R.L. Cell-free transmission and
     in vivo replication of Marek's disease virus. J.
     Virol., 5:388, 1970.

37. Andersson, U., Bird, A.G., Britton, S., and Palacios, R.
     Humoral and cellular immunity studied at the cell level
     from birth to two years of age. Immunological Rev.,
     57:5, 1981.

38. Miller, G. and Lipman, M. Release of infectious Epstein-
     Barr virus by transformed marmoset leukocytes. Proc.
     Natl. Acad. Sci. USA, 70:190, 1973.

39. Mark, W.H. Transformation of adult human lymphocytes in
     vitro by Epstein-Barr virus. Doctoral thesis,
     University of Wisconsin, Madison, 1981.

40. Zinkernagel, R.M. and Rosenthal, K.L. Experiments and
     speculation on anti-viral specificity of T and B cells.
     Immunological Rev., 58:131, 1981.

41. Henle, W. and Henle, G. Seroepidemiology of the virus.
     In: M.A. Epstein and B.G. Achong (eds.), The
     Epstein-Barr Virus. pp. 61-78. Berlin: Springer-
     Verlag, 1979.

42. Purtilo, D.T., Sakamoto, K., Saemundsen, A.K., Sullivan,
     J.L., Synnerholm, A-C., Anvret, M., Pritchard, J.,
     Sloper, C., Seiff, C., Pincott, J., Pachman, L., Rich,
     K., Cruzi, F., Cornet, J., Collins, R., Barnes, N.,
     Knight, J., Sandstedt, B., and Klein, G. Documentation
     of Epstein-Barr virus in immunodeficient patients with
     life-threatening lymphoproliferative diseases by clini-
     cal, virological and immunopathological studies. Cancer
     Res., 41:4226, 1981.

IN VITRO MODULATION OF EPSTEIN-BARR VIRUS-CARRYING LYMPHOBLASTOID

CELL LINES

Jaroslav Roubal, Emma Anisimová and
Kateřina Prachová

Institute of Sera and Vaccines
Department of Experimental Virology
108 W. Pieck Street
101 03, Prague 10, Czechoslovakia

INTRODUCTION

The B-lymphocytes are natural target cells for Epstein-Barr virus (EBV) infection. In vivo they may be infected after clinically inapparent entry of the virus into a child or in teen-age children and young adults. Infectious mononucleosis (IM) results in 50% of cases (32,70). The infected lymphocytes are immortalized, transformed into lymphoblasts and a few cells persist in the infected individuals for life (22). They contain, as a rule, multiple copies of the viral genome (3) and express an EBV-determined DNA-binding nuclear-associated antigen (EBNA) (52,72).

A close association has been demonstrated between EBV and Burkitt lymphoma and nasopharyngeal carcinoma (for review see 20,41, and chapters in this volume by Linder, Purtilo, Wolf and Krueger). The virus may induce other types of lymphoproliferation in immunocompromised individuals (68,69). According to the hypothesis of Klein (42) the immortalization of B-cells by EBV is the first step in the process, providing these cells with a growth potential independent of external mitogenic factors. The EBNA-positive B-blasts are thought to be arrested at a certain stage of cell differentiation. The reason why they are not eliminated from the circulation, despite the action of the host's multiple protective mechanisms (for review see 43,74), is not understood. The stage of their differentiation might play a role in this failure. Continuously dividing, persisting EBNA-positive B-blasts represent preneoplastic cells that still remain under the

179

control of the host, which keeps their concentration relatively
low (42). Under conditions of antigenic stimulation (42) or
immunosuppression (68), their growth is significantly promoted.
Their enhanced proliferation is associated with an increased risk
of genetic errors, due to which, as in the case of reciprocal 8;14
translocation, a malignant clone may arise. The cytogenetic error
would thus be an ultimate step in the oncogenic process (42)
permitting the altered clone to escape the immune surveillance.

The stage of EBV-infected cells differentiation may play some
role in eliminating them from circulation, and thereby control
their proliferative potential. For studying these questions, the
use of EBV-positive B-lymphoblastoid cell lines offers definite
advantages. We review the current knowledge about the differentiation of lymphoblastoid cells, to show how cells may be modulated in vitro, and to consider the possible role of cell
differentiation in EBV-induced lymphoproliferation and EBV-induced
life-threatening diseases.

Derivation of B-Lymphoblastoid Cell Lines

EBV-positive cell lines may be isolated from the blood of
patients with infectious mononucleosis or with EBV-induced
Burkitt's lymphoma (BL), from patients with lymphoproliferative
diseases, and even from the blood of normal seropositive donors
(59). They may also be obtained after in vitro infection of
B-lymphocytes with EBV (55). Cell lines isolated from normal
donors, from patients with infectious mononucleosis, or derived in
vitro after EBV infection (lymphoblastoid cell lines, LCL) are
polyclonal and diploid for various periods of time after their
establishment (62,97), but may become "monoclonal" and aneuploid
after prolonged cultivation in vitro (9,57,59). In contrast, cell
lines derived from BL are monoclonal from the beginning and
exhibit characteristic chromosomal changes (BL-lines) (97). Each
of them represents a malignant clone proliferating in vivo.

A few EBV-negative lymphoid lines have also been derived from
lymphoproliferative malignancies. Their characteristics and
degree of differentiation usually reflect the properties of the
respective malignant clones involved in the in vivo proliferation
(59). Despite this, a certain intraclonal variation in the degree
of differentiation may occur. This has been demonstrated by Lok
et al. (49) who isolated EBV-negative cell lines BALM 3,4,5 from
the pleural effusion of a patient with poorly differentiated
diffuse lymphocytic lymphoma. Although the cells were of the same
clonal origin, as demonstrated by chromosomal and light-chain
analyses, they differed in their stage of differentiation. While
line BALM 5 was of a lymphoblastoid nature, the lines BALM 3 and
BALM 4 were plasmacytoid.

Characterization of EBV-positive Lymphoblastoid Cell Lines
(for review see ref. 59)

The overall morphology of EBV-positive cell lines is similar to that of lymphoblasts. Transmission electron microscopy shows LCL cells to possess a round or, often an irregularly shaped nucleus with finely granular chromatin and one to three prominent nucleoli. The cytoplasm is moderately extensive and contains a fairly well developed Golgi apparatus, numerous mitochondria, short cisternae of rough and smooth endoplasmic reticulum and abundant polyribosomes. Contrary to LCL lines, the ribosomes in BL lines are almost never attached to the endoplasmic reticulum and the Golgi apparatus is less prominent (59). Pleomorphism is typical of polyclonal LCL lines, but the individual lines are similar to each other. The cells of individual BL lines, due to their monoclonal origin, are morphologically homogeneous. However, their clonal origin provides individual features that distinguish them (59).

BL and LCL lines differ by a variety of other properties as well (for review see 59). Some characteristics, e.g. the glyco-protein patterns, resemble those present in small circulating lymphocytes (L-lines) or in activated B-blasts (LCL-lines). Among their various features the surface immunoglobulin receptors and immunoglobulin secretion have been studied the most extensively. These markers are closely associated with the stage of differentiation (53).

Immunoglobulins of EBV-positive Lines

LCL lines. Lymphoblastoid cell lines of non-malignant origin derived from cord lymphocytes, normal donors and infectious mononucleosis patients have been studied by Steel et al. (87). All of these lines secrete immunoglobulins. The lines obtained by EBV transformation of cord lymphocytes almost exclusively (49/50) synthesized IgM, whereas, lines from normal donors and IM patients also secreted IgG or IgA.

In the earlier studies the most frequent type of Ig receptors and type of Ig secretion detected was IgG (87,59). More recently, after improvement of the detection techniques, IgM, or IgM + IgG, or IgM + IgD have revealed to be the predominant isotypes (59). After appropriate enrichment of the minority B-cell population and after in vitro EBV transformation, even LCL expressing the less frequent Ig isotypes, like IgA (88), may be established.

The studies on immunoglobulin receptors and Ig secretion in LCL clearly demonstrate that these lines are more mature than the ones derived from BL.

BL lines. The established BL lines are arrested at an earlier stage of cell differentiation than LCL lines. A fraction of BL lines does not produce Ig. The synthesis of Ig, if present, is monoclonal and the Ig is identical with that synthesized by the tumour cells in vivo. Moreover, the Ig synthesis is almost exclusively destined to show membrane integration (59,60,62). The predominant class of Ig synthesized by BL lines is, as a rule, IgM (58,62). However, an IgG-producing line has also been described (45,62). Surface IgD in untreated BL lines has not been detected so far (93).

BL biopsy cells. Each BL line represents a malignant clone proliferating in vivo. Therefore, it is of interest to compare the surface immunoglobulin pattern of in vitro cultivated cells with that possessed by BL biopsy cells. Gunvén et al. (26) have analyzed surface immunoglobulins in 114 biopsies derived from 91 BL cases. Their results support the assumption that BL is represented by monoclonal B-cell proliferation. However, some variation in the degree of differentiation between the various BL cases has been observed: only 5% of the biopsies were surface Ig-negative, 18% were negative for mu chains and 61% for gamma chains. Delta-chain staining was absent or weakly positive in a few tumors. With regard to cell differentiation the authors concluded that the majority of the tumors expressed one predominant heavy and often one light chain. A few tumors possessed mu, gamma and one light chain and some either one heavy or one light chain or no surface Ig at all. The relatively large proportion of IgG possessing biopsy cells in comparison with the established lines was due to exogenous antibody coating the cells: in biopsies with moderate or low gamma-chain stainability both light chains were detected and it was possible to elute them at low pH. However, in many of the highly gamma-chain positive tumors studied a single light-chain staining was found, which was indicative of monoclonal gamma-chain synthesis.

Owing to the absence of delta-chain staining in BL biopsies together with a lack of delta-chain positivity in established BL cell lines (93) and owing to the low insulin binding to BL lines (4) (see below), the authors (26) concluded that the BL cells were presumably "frozen" at the stage of B cell maturation that precedes the appearance of surface IgD, which is an important marker in B cell differentiation (2,38,84,94).

Insulin Binding and Cell Differentiation

The stage of cell differentiation can be established in EBV-positive cell lines by studying insulin binding. Activated human lymphocytes express insulin receptors (47). According to

Helderman et al. (28,29,30) the insulin receptors represent a universal marker of activated lymphocytes. Åman et al. (4) have found that among 46 lines of different origin, 43 bound more insulin than normal peripheral blood lymphocytes thus resembling activated B cells. More mature cells, the EBV-positive LCL lines of normal origin or surface IgD-carrying cell lines, bound more hormone than the less differentiated BL-lines.

All IgD-carrying lines exhibit high insulin binding (4). However, the presence of surface IgD only is not sufficient for high binding of the hormone, since the majority of Ig-positive cells in peripheral blood express IgD but do not bind insulin. Moreover, a certain stage of activation that is present in the IgD-carrying cell lines is needed for the adsorption of insulin. It is likely that the expression of insulin receptors is associated with different patterns of metabolic activity of cells at different stages of development.

Spontaneously established, IM-derived cell lines bind less insulin than in vitro EBV-transformed lines derived from normal adults (4). This difference could be explained in two ways: the in vitro transformed lines may be influenced by factors involved in in vitro transformation that are not operative in vivo. Alternatively, the properties of IM lines may reflect an in vivo condition favoring selection of different cell populations, in contrast to in vitro transformation (4).

In Vitro Modulation of Differentiation Stage of BL Cell Lines

An EBV-negative cell line of BL origin, Ramos, has been used to monitor the effect of EBV infection on cell differentiation (86). This was performed by comparing some surface properties of the original cells with a series of lines converted by B95-8 or P3HR-1 strains of EBV. The authors have found the following changes. While the original Ramos cells expressed surface IgM but not IgD and had a low concentration of insulin receptors, eight of nine converted sublines expressed IgD and a variable but usually high insulin-binding capacity. These results indicate that the differentiation of the BL cell line, Ramos, is not completely "frozen" but that further differentiation can be induced by conversion with EBV. However, the viral genome per se does not seem to be sufficient to increase insulin binding, as the conversion by EBV of another EBV-negative cell line, BJAB, resulted in decreased insulin binding (4). Moreover, the EBV-converted BJAB-lines did not switch to IgD positivity.

Kishimoto et al. (40) have demonstrated that the Burkitt lymphoma cell line, Daudi, which expresses cytoplasmic and surface IgM, can be switched from IgM to IgG expression and from a membrane-bound to a secretory Ig-pattern when assisted with normal

human T cells either alone or in combination with macrophage
factors. This result supports the idea that T cells activated
against Ia-like molecules on an allogeneic B-cell line exert a
helper function switching from IgM to IgG production in Daudi
cells.

Guglielmi and Preud'homme (25) have reported that the
expression of Ig markers by the virus-nonproducer BL cell line
Raji varied during the growth of cells. The basic phenotype for
Raji cells was characterized by cytoplasmic IgM and no detectable
surface immunoglobulins. Spontaneous variation of this phenotype
was observed when the cells were cultured at low density. The
cultured cells acquired surface μ and λ chains, then also δ chains,
while they progressively lost cytoplasmic μ chains. Subsequently,
the cells lost their surface and cytoplasmic immunoglobulins and
then again displayed their basic phenotype. These different
staining patterns always proceeded in the same order. They were
not observed if the cells were cultivated at high density. It
should be recalled, however, that many others described the presence of surface IgM on Raji cells (e.g., 10,88). This discor-
dance may either be explained by differences in Raji sublines or
attributed to the conditions of cultivation. Nevertheless, these
results emphasize the necessity to strictly control conditions of
experiments monitoring cell differentiation. These authors (25)
have not found further maturation of Raji cells when cultivated
with various inducers and biologically active agents.

Induction of Differentiation in Lymphoblastoid Cell Lines by Chemical Inducers

We studied n-butyrate and 12-0-tetradecanoylphorbol-13-acetate
(TPA) induction of both virus-antigen synthesis and cell differentiation in several EBV-positive cell lines. Both drugs markedly
influence cell metabolism and interfere with cell differentiation.

Some Effects of n-butyrate and TPA on Cultured Cells

n-Butyrate is a potent inducer of virus early antigen (EA) and
viral capsid antigen (VCA) synthesis in virus producer P3HR-1
cells (51), whereas, it induces EA synthesis only in a minority of
virus-non-producer cell lines (7,51). In addition, the drug
induces erythroid differentiation in immature erythroleukemic
cells (48) and hemoglobin synthesis in human erythroleukemic
cells (5). n-Butyrate has also been shown to induce interferon in
EBV-positive lymphoblastoid Namalwa cells (56) and to affect
various morphological and biochemical properties of cultured cells
(for review see 66). This drug interferes with acetylation of
histones (76).

TPA, another inducer of EB-virus-antigen synthesis (98,99), promotes two-step carcinogenesis in mouse skin (14) and is a powerful modulator of the cell membrane by increasing fluidity (95) and interfering with the cytoskeleton (75,83). It is blastogenic for mouse and human lymphocytes (1) and induces abnormal chromatid exchanges (39). TPA is capable either of inhibiting or of inducing differentiation of both normal and malignant animal and human cells in vitro (for review see 17,96). In the mouse, TPA inhibits the spontaneous differentiation of Friend erythroleukemia cells (54,79), but it stimulates terminal cell differentiation in some myeloid leukemia cell lines (50). In man, TPA induces terminal cell differentiation in the promyelocytic-leukemia cell line HL 60 (36,80) and in some other myeloid leukemia lines (50). It also induces phenotypic and functional maturation of human histiocytic lymphoma cells (U-937) toward macrophages (61). In certain animal models in vitro the drug may inhibit differentiation or even cause dedifferentiation of normal and malignant cells (17,96). TPA regulates gene expression at both transcriptional and translational levels and complements differentiation-related changes in gene expression that have been induced by other compounds (35).

The Effects on n-Butyrate and TPA on EBV-transformed Cells Lines

We studied the effects of n-butyrate at 3mM concentration on five lymphoblastoid cell lines: 4 EBV-positive cell lines, including the virus producer P3HR-1 (34) and 3 virus-non-producer cell lines, Raji (67), NC 37 (18) and Ramos-HR-1-K (46) were employed. We also used the EBV-negative cell line Ramos (44). While P3HR-1 and Raji cells have been derived from EBV-positive African BL, the Ramos cell line has been isolated from an EBV-

Table 1. Induction of EBV-Antigens in Lymphoblastoid Cell Lines with 3mM n-Butyrate

Cells	EBV status	Per cent of IF-positive cells	
		EA	VCA
P3HR-1	producer	40-60	20-30
Raji	nonproducer	1-2	0
NC 37	nonproducer	1-2	0
Ramos	negative	–	–
Ramos-HR-1-K	nonproducer	0.5-1	0

Table 2. The Differentiation Response of Lymphoblastoid
Cell Lines to the Action of n-Butyrate

Cell Line	Differentiation	Remark	Stage of dif-ferentiation	Relative amount of different-iated cells (%)
P3HR-1	no	Virus-particle formation, virus-induced morpholo-gical changes	-	-
Raji	yes		plasmablasts plasma cells	60 20
NC 37	yes		plasmablasts or earlier stages	10-15
Ramos	no	toxicity	-	-
Ramos-HR-1-K	no	toxicity	-	-

negative case of American BL. The NC 37 cells have been reported
to be derived from the blood of a normal seropositive donor (18),
but there are some doubts about their identity (George Klein,
personal communication). Virus-antigen synthesis was detected by
the indirect immunofluorescence technique (31) and morphological
differentiation was determined by transmission electron microscopy
(TEM). Specimens for TEM observations were prepared as described
elsewhere (8).

The data on antigen induction and the morphological observations are summarized in Tables 1 and 2, respectively. The
following findings have been made. In virus producer P3HR-1
cells, n-butyrate induced not only the effective synthesis of EA
and VCA (7,51) but also the formation of virus particles, which
were mostly immature (7). The ongoing productive virus cycle was
associated with the development of virus-specific cellular
alterations; however, the overall cell morphology remained within
the range typical for lymphoblasts (7) (Figure 1).

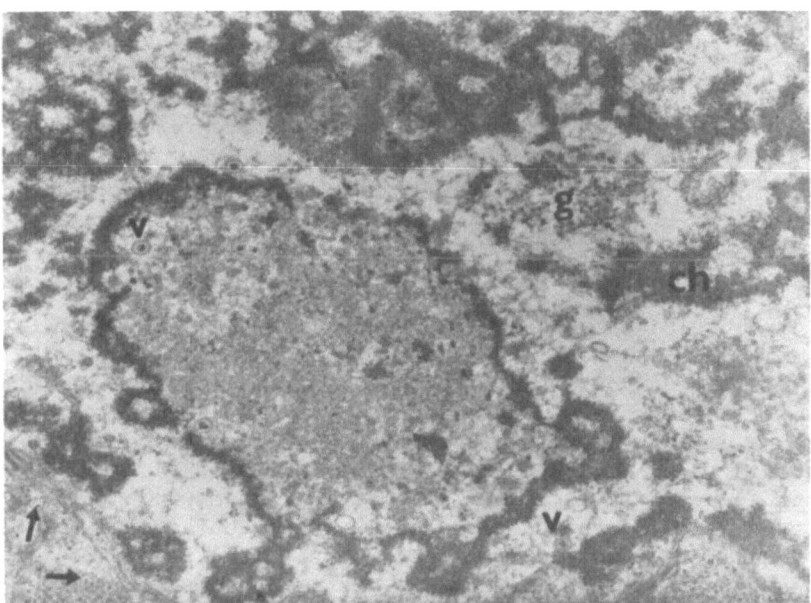

Fig. 1. Electron micrograph of a thin section through the nucleus
         of virus producer P3HR-1 cell. The nucleoplasm exhibits
         characteristic EBV-induced cytopathic changes: margina-
         tion of chromatin /ch/, reduplication of nuclear membrane
         /arrows/ and the accumulation of dense granules /g/.
         Typical immature EBV particles /V/ can be seen
         in nuclear substance. Magnification 40,500 x /Ref. 7/.

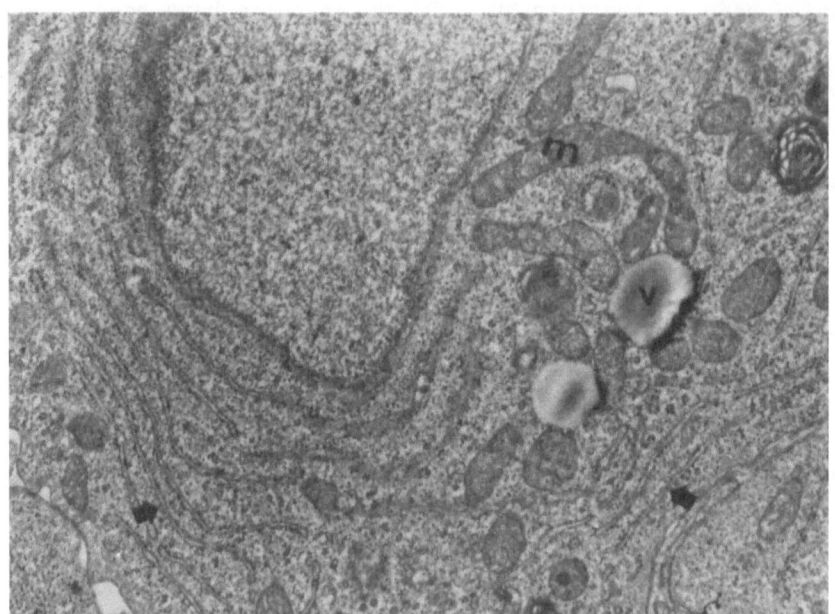

Fig. 2.   Fragment of Raji cell, 48 hrs post addition of n-
          butyrate, with features of plasmablast. The cell con-
          tains extensive regular stacks of rough cisternae of the
          endoplasmic reticulum /arrows/, well developed
          mitochondria /m/ and lipid vacuoles /v/. A portion of
          the nucleus is visible in the upper right-hand corner.
          Magnification 18,000 x /Ref. 7/.

     The response of Raji cells to this drug was different (7).
Here, n-butyrate only induced EA synthesis in a low proportion of
cells (1-2%). However, clear signs of differentiation toward
plasma cells were observed. Fourty-eight and 72 hrs after adding
the drug, a relatively large amount of rough endoplasmic reticulum
was found, mainly localized as ring-like structures around the
nucleus; as a consequence, mitochondria were pressed into zones
free of endoplasmic reticulum. The number of mitochondria
increased, lipid vacuoles appeared in the cytoplasm and the nuclei
were localized either centrally or eccentrically. These cells
representing about 80% of the cell population were classified as
plasmablasts according to criteria of Nilsson (58) (Figure 2). By
72 hrs after induction about 20% of cells were typical plasma
cells (Figure 3a, b). No signs of immunoglobulin secretion were
seen. Correspondingly, no immunoglobulins were found in the
culture fluid by radial immunodiffusing of ELISA techniques after
3 and 5 days of treatment with the drug (Roubal et al., manuscript
in preparation). The sensitivity of butyrate-treated Raji cells
to P3HR-1 virus superinfection was reduced in comparison with

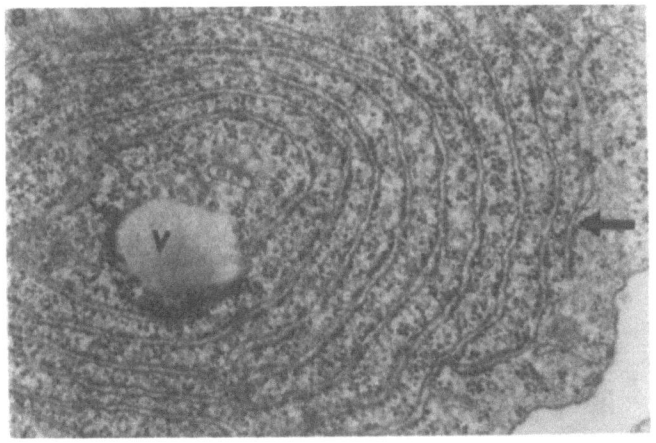

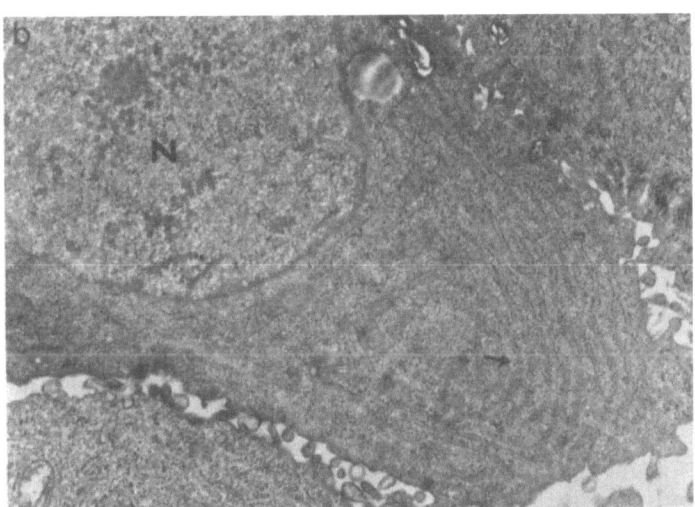

Fig. 3. a) Fragment of Raji cell 72 hrs post addition of n-
         butyrate possessing the markers of typical plasma cell.
         The enormous accumulation of rough endoplasmic reticulum,
         with parallel arrangement of its compartments, can be
         seen /arrows/. In the center a lipid vacuole /v/ is
         visible. Magnification 40,500X (ref. 7). 3b) Fragment
         of Raji cell 72 hrs post addition of n-butyrate
         possessing the markers of typical plasma cell. Cell
         contains characteristic, eccentrically located nucleus
         /N/ and large accumulation of rough endoplasmic reticulum
         /arrows/. Magnification 18,000X. (From: Anisimova, E.
         et al. Effect of n-butyrate on Epstein-Barr virus-
         carrying lymphoma lines. J. gen. Virol., 58:163, 1982.

control cultures (Roubal et al., manuscript in preparation). As
plasma cells do not express EBV receptors (58), the decrease
observed might have been the direct consequence of the loss of EBV
receptors during plasma-cell maturation. Alternatively, a
modified intracellular condition in differentiated cells might
have been unfavorable for virus-genome expression.

In NC 37 cells, n-butyrate also induced a low-level synthesis
of EA only and cell differentiation (6). However, the latter
change was not pronounced so strongly as in Raji cells. On day 3
and 5 after the addition of the drug only about 10-15% of cells
differentiated morphologically towards plasmablasts or even
earlier stages of differentiation (Table 2). No cells of typical
plasma cell morphology were observed in treated NC 37.

The n-butyrate was strongly toxic for the Ramos cell line and
its subline Ramos Hr-1-K. Only cells exhibiting degenerative
changes were observed by TEM (Anisimová, Prachová, Roubal;
unpublished results). Reasons for the toxicity of the drug for
the Ramos cell line and its derivative are unclear. Despite the
conversion of Ramos cells by EBV, they shift to a more differentiated shape (86). However, no differences between converted and
original lines in the response to n-butyrate were noted. This
prompted us to investigate the induction of virus antigens and
cell differentiation in two EBV-positive, virus-non-producer cell
lines, Raji and NC 37 by TPA (Table 3). While TPA is a potent
inducer of productive virus cycle in producer lines (98,99), it
only induces a low level of EA in non-producers (12) (Table 3).
In our tests, TPA was used either alone at a concentration of 20
ng/ml, or in a combination with 3 mM n-butyrate. This combination
was the most effective in inducing virus EA synthesis (37,64). In
Table 3, 30-50% and 10-20% of the cell population contained EA in
Raji and NC 37 cells, respectively.

TEM investigations revealed that TPA only induced early stages
of differentiation in about 7-10% of Raji cells. The morphological changes detected can be described as follows (6) (Figure 4).
Cytoplasm of the differentiated cells contained abundant
endoplasmic reticulum. The sacs of endoplasmic reticulum were
flat with frequent ribosomes attached to their surfaces in treated
cells.

The effect of the mixture of the two inducers on Raji cells
was surprisingly similar to that induced by TPA alone. However,
a larger proportion of cell population (15%) exhibited the characteristic morphological changes.

Raji cells treated with TPA or TPA plus butyrate 1.5-2.0% and
20-30% of the cells, respectively, exhibited cellular alterations
resembling some of the virus-specific changes found in the virus-

Table 3. The Effects of TPA and TPA + Butyrate on Raji and NC 37 Cells

Cells	Treatment	Percent of IF positive cells		Stages of differentiation reached	Relative amount of differentiated cells (%)	Relative amount of non-differentiated cells with virus-specific changes (%)
		EA	VCA			
Raji	TPA	1-2	0	initial stages	7-10	1.0-2.0[1]
	TPA+butyrate	20-50	0	initial stages	15	20-30[1]
NC 37	TPA	1-2	0	plasmablasts or earlier stages	10-15	0
	TPA+butyrate	10-20	0	plasmablasts or earlier stages	10-15	0

[1] only tubular structures detected
[2] Tubular structures plus additional changes detected

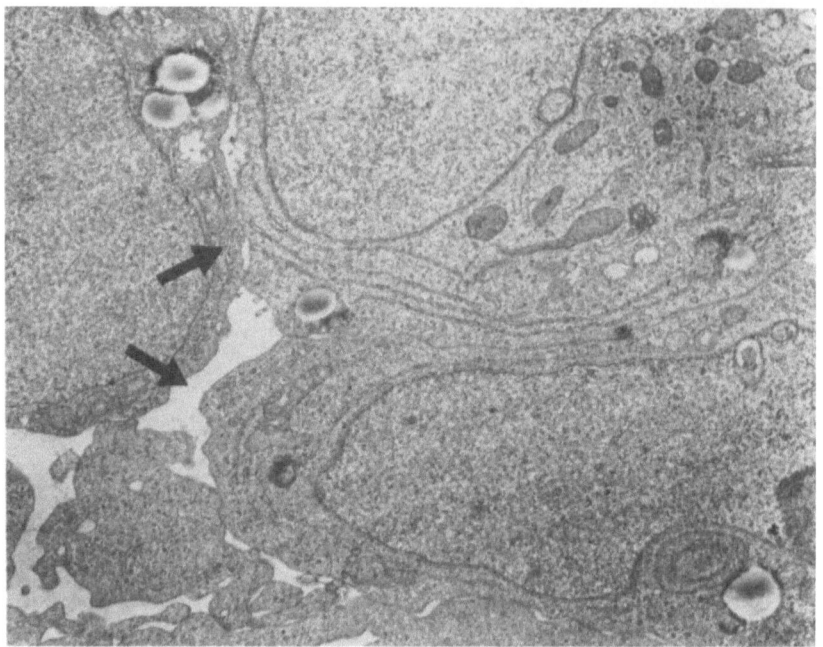

Fig. 4.   Raji cells 72 hrs post addition of TPA. Two cells
          /arrows/ at the early stage of differentiation are shown.
          The cytoplasm contains increased amount of rough
          endoplasmic reticulum. Magnification 12,200X.

producer cell line P3HR-1 (7). The cells exhibiting these alterations were undifferentiated lymphoblasts (Figure 5). In Raji
cells treated with TPA alone, hollow tubular structures appeared
in the cytoplasm (Figure 5b). When the mixture of both inducers
was used the alterations were more pronounced (Figure 5a).
Besides these structures small dense granules in the nuclei
appeared either individually or in aggregates. Reduplication of
the nuclear membrane was frequently observed; sometimes the
reduplicated regions were invaginated inside the nucleus. Margin-
ation of the chromatin, a typical alteration associated with the
productive virus cycle, was never observed. In the cytoplasm of
some cells altered mitochondria were encountered. However, the
alterations described were not always fully expressed.

     NC 37 cells cultivated in the presence of TPA or in the mix-
ture of both inducers had a strong tendency to adhere to the
plastic (6). TEM demonstrated that 72 and 120 hrs after addition
of the inducers 10-15% of cells were differentiated (Table 3).
The differentiation stopped at the plasmablast or even at earlier
stages of differentiation (Figure 6). A significantly larger
content of endoplasmic reticulum was seen in 10-15% of treated

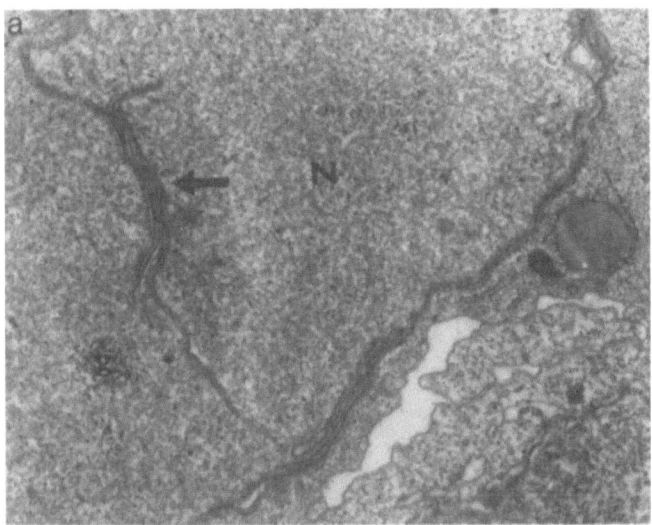

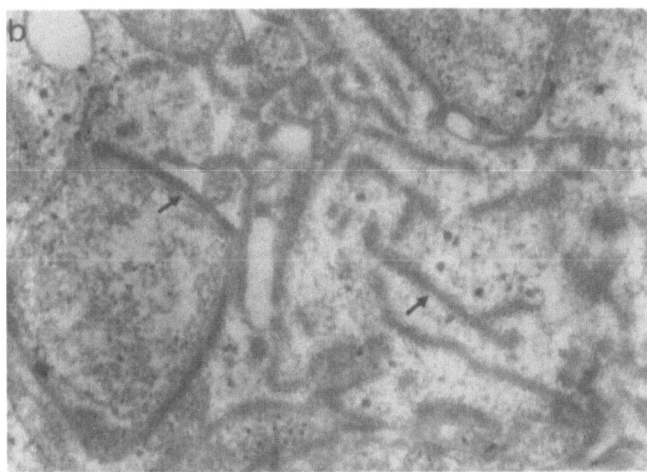

Fig. 5   a) Virus-specific-like changes in Raji cell morphology
after 72 hr treatment with TPA and n-butyrate. A thin
section throughout the nucleus /N/ is shown. A marked
reduplication of nuclear membrane with the invagination
of reduplicated region inside the nucleus, and the accumulation of dense granules /g/ are visible.
Magnification 18,000X.   b) Virus-specific-like changes in
Raji cell morphology after 72 hr treatment with TPA and
n-butyrate. A fragment of the cytoplasm containing
hollow tubular structures /arrows/ is shown.
Magnification 55,000X.

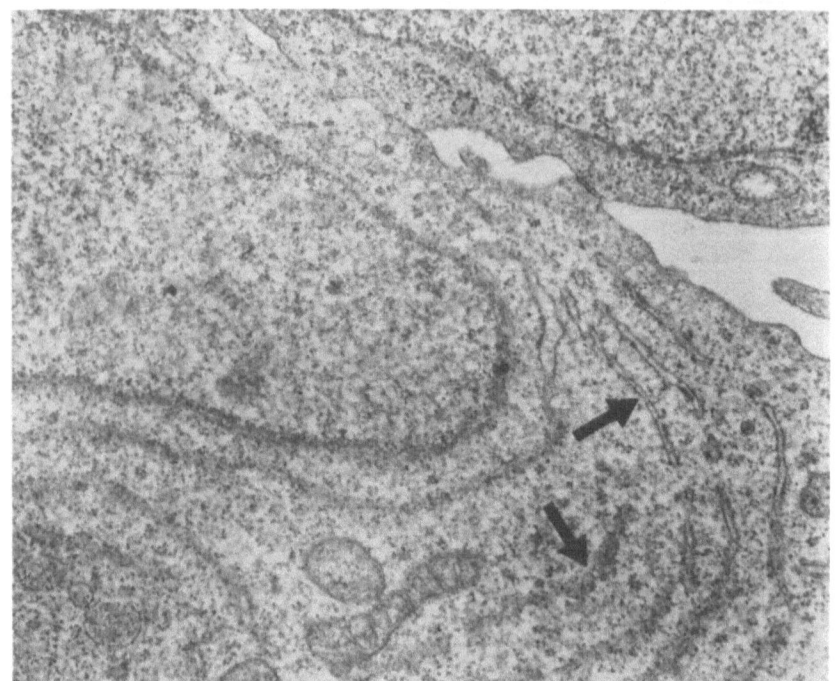

Fig. 6.   Portion of NC 37 cell differentiating towards plasmablast, 72 hrs post addition of TPA. The increased amount
of rough endoplasmic reticulum /arrows/ was detected.
Magnification 29,000X.

cells. Cisternae of endoplasmic reticulum were flat and increased
numbers of ribosomes appeared on their membranes. Frequently two
or three cisternae were found in close proximity with ribosomes
mainly localized on their outer membranes. Ribosomes prevailed
over polyribosomes.

The remaining treated NC 37 cells were lymphoblasts. However,
their shape had become irregular and frequent protrusions and
loops were detected at cell surfaces (Figure 7a, b). The protrusions, containing filamentous structures in their cytoplasm, were
sometimes very long. The loops consisted of thin strips of
cytoplasm that also possessed fine fibrils similar to those in
protrusions.

TEM of adhering NC 37 cells revealed altered lymphoblasts with
only 1-2% of cells being differentiated. In the case of NC 37,
unlike Raji cells, no cellular alterations resembling virus-
specific changes were observed in treated cultures. Reasons for
this difference are now discussed.

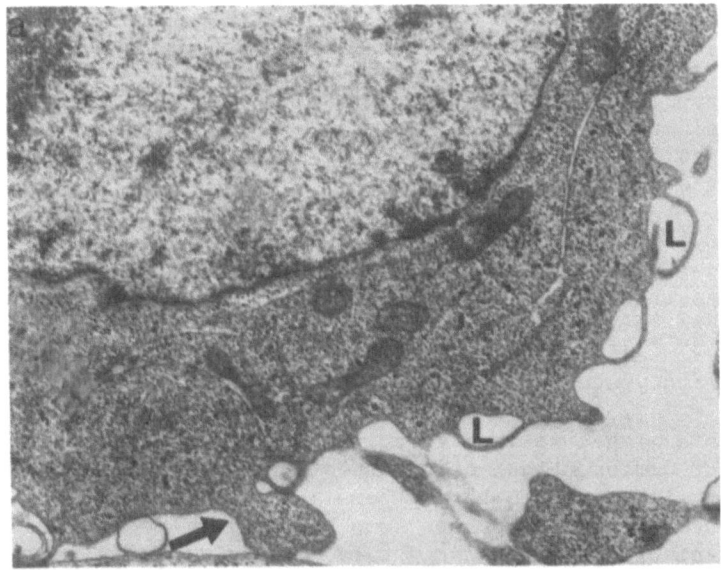

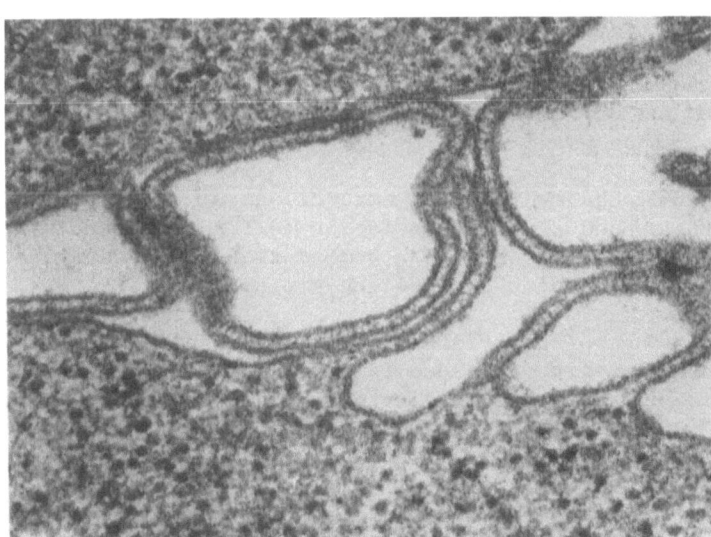

Fig. 7. a) Fragment of nondifferentiating NC 37 cell 72 hrs post
         addition of TPA. The shape of the cell is irregular with
         frequent protrusions /arrow/ and loops /L/ at the sur-
         face. Magnification 16,200X. b) Fragment of nondif-
         ferentiated NC 37 cell 72 hrs post addition of TPA. A
         larger magnification /66,000/ of the loops shown in
         Figure 7a.

Discussion of the Studies on Virus Inducer-driven Cell
Differentiation

Cell-line-dependent differentiation response. The experiments
described above indicate that the stage of differentiation at
which EBV-positive lymphoma and lymphoblastoid cells were arrested
can be influenced in vitro by the inducers employed. However, the
differentiation response is apparently dependent on both the cell
line and the inducer used.

In NC 37 cells, n-butyrate-driven differentiation was
detected in a smaller fraction of cells and reached a less activated stage than in Raji. While all three ways of induction
investigated in this study led to similar responses in NC 37
cells, there was a marked difference in the responses of Raji
cells to n-butyrate and to TPA.

At this stage, it is difficult to determine the reason for
the various differentiation responses in Raji and NC 37 lines.
The NC 37 cells, despite having been isolated from a normal donor,
were recently shown to possess some BL markers (George Klein,
personal communication) and might be similar or identical to Raji
cells (81). However, differences in the induction of the R and D
components (33) of EBV EA and in the readiness of host-cell repair
between these two lines have been reported (85,90). The various
differentiation responses also distinguish these two cell lines.
Various stages of differentiation or genetic diversification between Raji and NC 37 cells are probably involved in their differentiation responses.

Various mouse myeloid leukemia clones also differ in their
ability to respond by differentiation to TPA treatment (50). Some
of the clones respond only to a combination of TPA and the
macrophage-and-granulocyte-inducing protein.

The absence of a differentiation response in butyrate-treated
P3HR-1 cells may either be due to some cell-line-dependent properties or may be related to the cytopathogenicity of the activated
virus. This and the possible dependence between cell differentiation and virus-antigen expression will be discussed.

Inducer-dependence of differentiation response. As shown,
Raji cells differed in their ability to differentiate after the
addition of n-butyrate or TPA. Surprisingly, the mixture of both
inducers had a similar effect as TPA alone. TPA could interfere
with the terminal differentiation induced in these cells by n-
butyrate. Others report conflicting information regarding
differentiation induced by TPA: TPA can induce terminal differentiation in some systems (36,50,61,80), while in others it
interferes with it (54,79) or even causes dedifferentiation

(17,96). Only a mixture of both inducers was significantly
effective in inducing EA synthesis in Raji (37,64) (Table 3) and
NC 37 cells (Table 3).

While TPA did not induce plasma cells in Raji and NC 37 cells,
TPA driven terminal differentiation occurred in chronic lymphocytic leukemia (CLL) biopsy cells (91,92). About 90% of the CLL
cell population was involved. One to two days after addition of
the drug progression to lymphoblastoid cells occurred. On day 3
and 4 plasmacytoid cells predominated and TEM also revealed
maturation towards plasma cells. Under the influence of TPA, a
time-dependent increase in the proportion of cells containing
intracytoplasmic Ig was detected. This cytoplasmic Ig was of the
same phenotype as that detected at the cell surface of fresh,
non-induced CLL cells. A parallel decrease in cell-surface
immunoglobulin density and DNA synthesis in CLL cells was observed. Those CLL cells that had expressed surface delta chains
lost them during differentiation (91). A positive TPA response
was observed in CLL biopsies from a large proportion of patients
(82%). The patients with clinically active malignancy and/or a
large tumor-cell mass showed the greatest response to TPA, whereas
non-respondents had inactive CLL (91). In agreement with our
results, CLL cells that had differentiated to plasma cells did not
secrete immunoglobulin.

Morphological alterations not associated with cell differentiation. In Raji cells that had been cultivated in the presence
of TPA with or without n-butyrate, some cells resembling those
virus-specific changes expressed in cells that had entered a
productive virus cycle. These changes occurred in undifferentiated cells, the morphology of which remained of the lymphoblastoid type. Surprisingly, similar changes were absent from NC
37 cells that had been treated in the same manner.

Previously, we have suggested that the induction of some
virus-specific changes in cellular morphology might be associated
with the synthesis of EA rather than VCA (7). While the results
with Raji may be in line with this presumption, those with NC 37
cells seem to contradict it. However, similarly as after induction of NC 37 cells with IUDr (85), all three ways of induction
used in this study led to a significantly lower induction of the
methanol-resistant component of EA (Table 4). Therefore, some
methanol-resistant component present in induced Raji, but absent
from treated NC 37 cells, might be responsible for the appearance
of the changes (6).

As shown, the shape and cell-surface morphology were significantly changed even in undifferentiated NC 37 cells that had been
exposed to TPA. These changes might be responsible for the
tendency of treated NC 37 cells to adhere to plastic. TPA also

Table 4.   Induction of Early Antigen (EA) in Raji and NC 37
            Cell Lines by Chemical Agents

Induction used:	Percentage of EA positive cells			
	Raji		NC 37	
	Acetone fixed	Methanol fixed	Acetone fixed	Methanol fixed
Iododeoxyuridine	2.0	2.1	1.0	0
Butyrate	1.7	1.9	1.6	0
TPA	1.2	1.1	1.4	0
Butyrate plus TPA	29.4	19.1	10.1	1.7

alters the morphology of the cell membrane in Daudi BL-line (65).
After overnight treatment of Daudi with TPA, surface villi develop
and an increase in the number of osmophilic lipid bodies, disar-
rangement of mitochondria, and an increase in the number of free
ribosomes are seen.

Possible Relationship between Cell Differentiation and Virus-Antigen Expression

The question remains open whether there is any relationship
between virus genome expression and cell differentiation while
n-butyrate induced no morphological differentiation, but did
induce EBV-antigen synthesis and virus-particle formation in
producer P3HR-1 cells (7), it could induce differentiation not
associated with effective virus-antigen synthesis in non-producer
Raji (7) and NC 37 (6) cells.

This difference may either be due to an independence between
cell differentiation and virus genome expression, or to cytopathogenicity of the activated P3HR-1 virus that turns off the
macromolecular synthesis of the host (23,63,89). The latter
alternative might block differentiation. Correspondingly, the
virus-specific changes detected in TPA-treated Raji cells were
only found in those cells that did not exhibit differentiation.
This might reflect cell death when the synthesis of EA is present
(23). Alternatively, P3HR-1 cells might be a clone at a different
stage of differentiation than Raji or NC 37 cells. n-Butyrate

would then inhibit the cellular mechanisms(s) that control the
expression and replication of the EBV genome (82) leading to a
switch-on of the virus growth cycle. In latently infected cells
the expression of the virus genome is under the controls exerted
by the virus and/or the host cell. The changes in cell differentiation could modify both of these.

If virus-genome expression and cell differentiation are
associated phenomena, the following predictions could be made: 1)
for induction of virus antigens only a small shift but not
terminal differentiation is needed. 2) Cell lines not producing
virus antigens spontaneously should have an additional control
mechanism absent from the virus producers, since the combined
action of both of the inducers was needed to induce EA synthesis
efficiently.

An association between virus genome expression and cell
differentiation cannot be ruled out. In any case, the question of
dependence is very tempting since the various virus inducers,
which differ greatly in their chemical structure, have one common
denominator - they influence cell differentiation (cited from 11).

In vivo Differentiation of EBNA-Positive Cells

EBV-genome-containing cells that express EBNA have also been
found to differentiate in vivo. Robinson et al. (77,78) have
demonstrated plasmacytic differentiation in a patient with fatal
infectious mononucleosis (77) and in uncomplicated infectious
mononucleosis (78) both by morphological characterization and by
demonstrating cytoplasmic immunoglobulins. Within the first week
after the onset of symptoms of IM 70-80% of circulating EBNA-
positive cells differentiated towards plasma cells as demonstrated
by the presence of cytoplasmic immunoglobulins. IgA and IgG were
the most frequent and IgM the least frequent immunoglobulin
isotypes detected in EBNA-positive cells. While during the acute
phase of the disease about 5.5-20% of T-cell-depleted blood
lymphocytes were EBNA positive, in the 2nd or 3rd week of illness
their number sharply decreased to 0.4-1.4%. Concurrently, the
relative fraction of EBNA-positive cells containing cytoplasmic
immunoglobulins also diminished, suggesting either that the
differentiation of infected cells had changed during the disease
or that nondifferentiated EBNA-positive cells had a survival
advantage (78). This point might be of crucial importance for
understanding the life-long persistence of EBNA-positive cells in
seropositive individuals. The host's immunoregulatory mechanisms
plays an active role both in inducing the differentiation response
during the acute phase of illness and in the disappearance of
differentiated EBNA-positive cells during later periods. The
persisting cells would then be relatively resistant against the
factors eliminating them from the body. The in vitro cytotoxic

activity of natural killer cells against target cells depends on
the stage of differentiation (24,65). The sensitivity of Raji and
Daudi cells to NK cytotoxicity was increased when they had been
cultured for 24 hours in the presence of TPA. Evidently, this
increase did not depend on the presence of virus antigens in
target cells. In contrast, untreated cells did not provide good
targets (13).

A more detailed analysis of the differentiation stage of
EBNA-positive cells that may be found in BL, at various stages of
IM and in normal individuals may reveal why these cells are
arrested at a certain stage of differentiation, and how the shift
in differentiation may regulate their proliferation and influence
the action of immune mechanisms.

EBV may play an important role in inducing lymphoproliferation
in immunocompromised patients (68). Thus, opportunistic, polyclonal lymphomas may develop (69). Occasionally, the uncontrolled
or poorly controlled polyclonal lymphoproliferation can switch on
to monoclonal malignancy (69). In immunoblastic sarcoma, which
is often a polyclonal proliferation of B-cells, various degrees of
plasma-cell differentiation occur (71). Also in renal-transplant
recipients who developed lymphoproliferative diseases and in whom
EBNA-positive cells are detected (27), a varying degree of
plasma-cell differentiation, has been observed (21). The degree
of cell differentiation in immunodeficient individuals that have
developed EBV-related lymphoproliferative disease, particularly in
those in transition to monoclonal malignant lymphoma from chronic
lymphoproliferative illness, ought to be evaluated in fresh biopsy
samples.

To determine the degree of differentiation, the cells in
biopsy specimens and the resulting cell lines should be characterized. However, one should realize that the differentiation
stage of cultured cells need not necessarily reflect that present
in vivo, since the cultured cells are out of the complex influence
of the host's "milieu." Also, a possible two-step derivation of
cell lines (15,16,19,73) might prevent a direct comparison of in
vivo and in vitro characters. However, a more detailed analysis
of B-cell differentiation and plasma cell maturation is needed,
e.g. by means of monoclonal antibodies. An in vitro modulation of
the differentiation stage of EBV-positive lymphoma and lymphoblastoid cell lines by various inducers may serve as a model to
further understand events in vivo.

SUMMARY AND CONCLUSIONS

The stage of differentiation of EBV-positive lymphoma cell
lines may be modulated in vitro by n-butyrate, TPA, T-cell helper

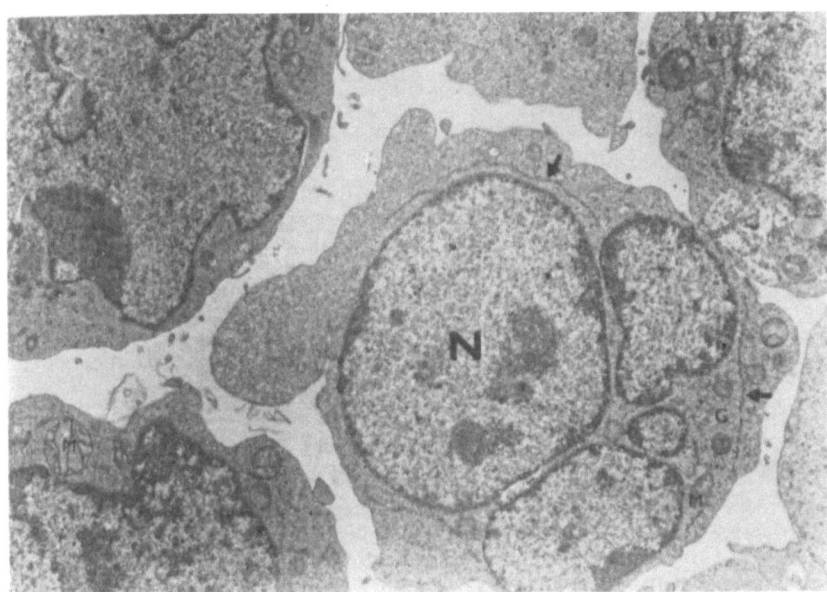

Fig. 8.   Electron micrograph of untreated Raji cells. Typical
          features of lymphoblasts may be detected: large irregular
          nucleus /N/, cytoplasm containing few mitochondria /M/,
          the Golgi apparatus /G/ and weakly-developed rough
          endoplasmic reticulum /arrows/. Magnification 8,400X.

factors, and possibly by other agents. However, apparent cell-
line dependent and inducer-dependent variations in the differentiation responses were observed. The in vitro modulation of cell
differentiation may be a useful model for studying B-cell differentiation and plasma-cell maturation in more detail, e.g. with the
use of monoclonal antibodies and cytogenetic analysis using
banding techniques (97). This may elucidate the mechanisms
operative in arrest in differentiation and potential modulations.
More detailed investigations on cell differentiation may contribute to a better understanding of the persistence of EBV immortalized cells in seropositive individuals, the processes that keep
the virus in latency, and the mechanisms involved in immune
defense against EBV-transformed cells.

REFERENCES

1.   Abb, J., Bayliss, C.J. and Deinhardt, F. Lymphocyte activa-
        tion by the tumor promoting agent 12-0-tetradecanoyl-
        phorbol-13-acetate (TPA). J. Immunol., 122:1639, 1979.
2.   Abney, E.R., Cooper, M.D., Kearney, J.F., Lafton, A.R. and
        Parkhouse, R.M.E. Sequential expression of immunoglobu-

lin on developing mouse B-lymphocytes: a systematic survey that suggests a model for the generation of
immunoglobulin isotype diversity. J. Immunol.,
120:2041, 1978.

3. Adams, A. The state of the virus genome in transformed cells
    and its relationship to host cell DNA. In: M.A. Epstein
    and B.G Achong (eds.), The Epstein-Barr virus. pp.
    125-184. New York: Springer-Verlag, 1979.

4. Åman, P., Lundin, G., Hall, K., and Klein, G. Insulin
    receptors on human lymphoblastoid lines of B-cell origin.
    Cell. Immunol., 65:307, 1981.

5. Andersson, L.C., Jokinen, M., and Gahmberg, C.G. Induction
    of erythroid differentiation in the human leukemia cell
    line K 562. Nature, London, 278:364, 1975

6. Anisimová, E., Prachová, K., and Roubal, J. Effects of n-
    butyrate and phorbol ester (TPA) on Epstein-Barr virus
    antigen induction and cell differentiation. Manuscript
    in preparation.

7. Anisimová, E., Saemundsen, A.K., Roubal, J., Vonka, V., and
    Klein, G. Effect of n-butyrate on Epstein-Barr virus-
    carrying lymphoma lines. J. gen. Virol., 58:163, 1982.

8. Anisimová, E., Tučková, E., Vonka, V., and Závadová, H.
    Ultra-structural changes induced by influenza viruses in
    permissive and non-permissive cells. Virology, 77:330,
    1977.

9. Béchêt, J.M., Fialkow, P.J., Nilsson, K., Klein, G. and
    Singh, S. Immunoglobulin synthesis and glukoso-6-
    phosphate dehydrogenase as cell markers in human
    lymphoblastoid cell lines. Exp. Cell Res., 89:275,
    1974.

10. Ben-Bassat, H., Polliack, A., Mitrani-Rosenbaum, S.,
    Reichert, F., Froimovici, M., and Goldblum, N. A com-
    parative study of human cell lines derived from patients
    with lymphoma, leukemia and infectious mononucleosis.
    Cancer, 40:1481, 1977.

11. Ben-Sasson, S.A., and Klein, G. Activation of the
    Epstein-Barr virus genome by 5-aza-cytidine in latently
    infected human lymphoid lines. Int. J. Cancer, 28:131,
    1981.

12. Bister, K., Yamamoto, N. and zur Hausen, H. Differential
    inducibility of Epstein-Barr virus in cloned, non-
    producer Raji cells. Int. J. Cancer, 23:818, 1979.

13. Blazer, B., Patarroyo, M., Klein, E., and Klein, G.
    Increased sensitivity of human lymphoid lines to natural
    killer cells after induction of the Epstein-Barr viral
    cycle by superinfection or sodium butyrate. J. Exp.
    Med., 151:614, 1980.

14. Boutwell, R.K. Function and mechanism of promoters of car-
    cinogenesis. CRC Critical Revs. Toxicol., 2:419, 1974.

15. Crawford, D.H., Rickinson, A.B., Finerty, S., and Epstein,
     M.A. Epstein-Barr (EB) virus genome-containing EB
     nuclear antigen-negative B-lymphocyte populations in
     blood in acute infectious mononucleosis. J. Gen.
     Virol., 38:449, 1978.

16. Dalens, M., Zech, L., and Klein, G. Origin of lymphoid
     lines established from mixed cultures of cord-blood
     lymphocytes and explants from infectious mononucleosis,
     Burkitt's lymphoma and healthy donors. Int. J. Cancer,
     16:1008, 1975.

17. Diamond, L., O'Brien, T.G., and Rovera, G. Tumor promoters:
     effects on proliferation and differentiation of cells in
     cultures. Life Sciences, 23:1979, 1978.

18. Durr, F.E., Monroe, J.H., Schmitter, R., Traul, K.A., and
     Hirshaut, Y. Studies on the infectivity and cytopathol-
     ogy of Epstein-Barr virus in human lymphoid cells. Int.
     J. Cancer, 6:436, 1970.

19. Epstein, M.A. and Achong, B.G. Various forms of
     Epstein-Barr virus infection in man: established facts
     and a general concept. Lancet, i:836, 1973.

20. Epstein, M.A. and Achong, B.G. The relationship of the
     virus to Burkitt's lymphoma. In: M.A. Epstein and B.G.
     Achong (eds.), The Epstein-Barr Virus. pp. 321-338.
     New York: Springer-Verlag, 1979.

21. Frizzera, G., Hanto, D.W., Gajl-Peczalska, K.J., Rosai,
     J., McKenna, R.W., Sibley, R.K., Holahan, K.P., and
     Lindquist, L.L. Polymoprhic diffuse B-cell hyperplasias
     and lymphomas in renal transplant recipients. Cancer
     Res., 41:4262, 1981.

22. Gergely, L., Czeglédy, J., Váczi, L., Szkalka, A., and
     Berényi, E. Cells containing Epstein-Barr nuclear anti-
     gen (EBNA) in peripheral blood. Acta Microbiol. Acad.
     Sci. Hung., 26:41, 1979.

23. Gergely, L., Klein, G., and Ernberg, I. Host cell macromo-
     lecular synthesis in cells containing EBV-induced early
     antigens, studied by continued immunofluorescence and
     radioautography. Virology, 45:22, 1971.

24. Gidlund, M., Örn, A., Pattengale, P.K., Jansson, M., Wigzell,
     H., and Nilsson, K. Natural killer cells kill tumor
     cells at a given stage of differentiation. Nature,
     292:848, 1981.

25. Guglielmi, P. and Preud'Homme, J.L. Immunoglobulin
     expression in human lymphoblastoid cell lines with early
     B-cell features. Scand. J. Immunol., 13:303, 1981.

26. Gunvén, P., Klein, G., Klein, E., Norin, T. and Singh, S.
     Surface immunoglobulins in Burkitt's lymphoma biopsy
     cells from 91 patients. Int. J. Cancer, 25:711, 1980.

27. Hanto, D.W., Frizzera, G., Purtilo, D.T., Sakamoto, K.,
     Sullivan, J.L., Saemundsen, A.K., Klein, G., Simmons,
     R.L., and Najarian, J.S. Clinical spectrum of

lymphoproliferative disorders in renal transplant recipients and evidence for the role of Epstein-Barr virus.
Cancer Res., 41:4253, 1981.

28.   Helderman, J.H., Reynolds, T.C. and Strom, T.B. The insulin
      receptors as a universal marker of activated lymphocytes.
      Eur. J. Immunol., 8:589, 1978.

29.   Helderman, J.H. and Strom, T.B. Emergence of insulin recep-
      tors upon alloimmune T cells in the rat. J. Clin.
      Invest., 59:338, 1977.

30.   Helderman, J.H. and Strom, T.B. Specific insulin binding
      site on T and B lymphocytes as a marker of cell activa-
      tion. Nature (London), 274:62, 1978.

31.   Henle, G. and Henle, W. Immunofluorescence in cells derived
      from Burkitt's lymphoma. J. Bacteriol., 91:1248, 1966.

32.   Henle, G., and Henle, W. The virus as an etiologic agent of
      infectious mononucleosis. In: M.A. Epstein and B.G.
      Achong (eds.), The Epstein-Barr Virus. pp. 297-320.
      New York: Springer-Verlag, 1979.

33.   Henle, G., Henle, W., and Klein, G. Demonstration of two
      distinct components in the early antigen complex of
      Epstein-Barr virus infected cells. Int. J. Cancer,
      8:272, 1971.

34.   Hinuma, Y. and Grace, J.T. Cloning of immunoglobulin pro-
      ducing human leukemia and lymphoma cells in long-term
      culture. Proc. Soc. Exp. Biol. Med., 124:107, 1967.

35.   Hoffman-Liebermann, B., Liebermann, D., and Sachs, L.
      Regulation of gene expression by tumor promoters. III.
      Complementation of the developmental program in myeloid
      leukemic cells by regulating m-RNA production and m-RNA
      translation. Int. J. Cancer, 28:615, 1981.

36.   Huberman, E. and Callaham, M.F. Induction of terminal dif-
      ferentiation in human promyelocytic leukemia cells by
      tumor-promoting agents. Proc. Natl. Acad. Sci. USA,
      76:1293, 1979.

37.   Ito, Y., Kawanishi, M., Harayama, T., and Takabayashi, S.
      Combined effect of the extracts from Croton tiglium,
      Euphorbia lathyris or Euphorbia tirucalli and n-butyrate
      on Epstein-Barr virus expression in human lymphoblastoid
      P3HR-1 and Raji cells. Cancer Letters, 12:175, 1981.

38.   Kettman, J.R., Cambier, J.C., Uhr, J.W., Ligler, F., and
      Vitetta, E.S. The role of receptor IgM and IgD in deter-
      mining, triggering and induction of tolerance in murine
      B-cells. In: G. Moller (ed.), Immunological Reviews.
      Vol. 43, pp. 69-95. Muntsgaard, Copenhagen, 1979.

39.   Kinsella, A.R. and Radman, R. Tumor promoter induces sister
      chromatid exchanges: relevance to the mechanism of car-
      cinogenesis. Proc. Natl. Acad. Sci. USA, 75:6149, 1978.

40.   Kishimoto, K., Hirano, T., Kuritani, T., Yamamura, Y.,
      Ralph, P., and Good, R.A. Induction of IgG production
      in human B lymphoblastoid cell lines with normal human T
      cells. Nature (London), 271:756, 1978.

41. Klein, G. The relationship of the virus to nasopharyngeal carcinoma. In: M.A. Epstein and B.G. Achong (eds.), The Epstein-Barr Virus. pp. 339-415. New York: Springer-Verlag, 1979.

42. Klein, G. Immune and non-immune control of neoplastic development: contrasting effects of host and tumor evolution. Cancer, 45:2486, 1980.

43. Klein, E., Ernberg, I., Masucci, M.G., Szigeti, R., Wu, Y.T., Masucci, G., and Svedmyr, E. T-cell response to B-cells and Epstein-Barr virus antigens in infectious mononucleosis. Cancer Res., 41:4210, 1981.

44. Klein, G., Giovanella, B., Westman, A., Stehlin, J.G., and Mumford, D. An EBV-genome negative cell line established from an American Burkitt lymphoma; receptor characteristics, EBV-infectability and permanent conversion into EBV-positive sublines by in vitro infection. Intervirology, 5:319, 1975.

45. Klein, G., Nilsson, K., and Yefenof, E. An established Burkitt's lymphoma line with cell membrane IgG. Clin. Immunol. Immunopathol., 3:575, 1975.

46. Klein, G., Zeuthen, J., Terasaki, P., Billing, R., Honig, R., Jondal, M., Westman, A., and Clements, G. Inducibility of the Epstein-Barr virus (EBV) cycle and surface marker properties of EBV negative lymphoma lines and their in vitro EBV-converted sublines. Int. J. Cancer, 18:639, 1976.

47. Krug, U., Krug, F., and Cuatrecasas, P. Emergence of insulin receptors on human lymphocytes during in vitro transformation. Proc. Natl. Acad. Sci. USA, 69:2604, 1972.

48. Leder, A. and Leder, P. Butyric acid, a potent inducer of erythroid differentiation in cultured erythroleukemic cells. Cell, 5:319, 1975.

49. Lok, M.S., Koshiba, H., Hant, T., Abe, S., Minowada, I., and Sandberg, A.A. Establishment and characterization of human B-lymphocytic lymphoma cell lines (BALM-3, -4 and -5). Intraclonal variations in the B-cell differentiation stage. Int. J. Cancer, 24:572, 1979.

50. Lotem, J. and Sachs, L. Regulation of normal differentiation in mouse and human myeloid leukemic cells by phorbol esters and the mechanisms of tumor promotion. Proc. Natl. Acad. Sci. USA, 76:5158, 1979.

51. Luka, J., Kallin, B., and Klein, G. Induction of the Epstein-Barr virus (EBV) cycle in latently infected cells by n-butyrate. Virology, 94:228, 1979.

52. Luka, J., Siegert, W., and Klein, G. Solubilization of the Epstein-Barr virus determined nuclear antigen and its characterization as a DNA-binding protein. J. Virol., 22:1, 1977.

53. Marchalonis, J.J. and Cone, R.E. Biochemical and biological characteristics of lymphocyte surface immunoglobulin. Transplant. Revs., 14:3, 1978.

54. Miao, R.M., Fieldsteel, A.H., and Fodge, D.W. Opposing
     effects of tumour promoters on erythroid differentiation.
     Nature (London), 274:271, 1978.
55. Miller, G. Human lymphoblastoid cell lines and Epstein-Barr
     virus: a review of their interrelationship and their
     relevance to the etiology of leukoproliferative states
     in man. Yale J. Biol. Med., 43:358, 1971.
56. Morser, J., Meager, A., and Colman, A. Enhancement of
     interferon m-RNA levels in butyric acid treated Namalwa
     cells. Febs. Letters, 112:203, 1980.
57. Nilsson, K. High frequency establishment of human
     immunoglobulin-producing lymphoblastoid lines from nor-
     mal and malignant lymphoblastoid tissue and peripheral
     blood. Int. J. Cancer, 8:432, 1971.
58. Nilsson, K. Established human lymphoid cell lines as a
     model for B lymphocyte differentiation. In: B. Serrou
     and C. Ronsenfeld (eds.), Human Lymphocyte
     Differentiation: Its Application to Cancer. pp.
     307-317. Amsterdam: Elsevier/North-Holland Biomed.
     Press, 1978.
59. Nilsson, K. The nature of lymphoid cell lines and their
     relationship to the virus. In: M.A. Epstein and B.G.
     Achong (eds.), The Epstein-Barr Virus. pp. 225-281.
     New York: Springer-Verlag, 1979.
60. Nilsson, K., Andersson, L.C., Gahmberg, C.G. and Wigzell, H.
     Surface glycoprotein patterns of normal and malignant
     human lymphoid cells. II. B-cells, B-blasts and
     Epstein-Barr virus (EBV) positive and negative B-
     lymphoid lines. Int. J. Cancer, 20:708, 1977.
61. Nilsson, K., Forsbeck, K., Gidlund, M., Sundström, C.,
     Töterman, T., Sällström, J. and Wenge, P. Surface
     characteristics of the U-937 human histiocytic lymphoma
     line. Specific changes during inducible morphologic and
     functional differentiation in vitro. In:
62. Nilsson, K. and Pontén, J. Classification and biological
     nature of established human hematopoietic cell lines.
     Int. J. Cancer, 15:321, 1975.
63. Nonoyama, M. and Pagano, J.S. Replication of viral deoxy-
     ribonucleic acid and breakdown of cellular deoxyribo-
     nucleic acid in Epstein-Barr virus infection. J.
     Virol., 9:714, 1972.
64. Ooka, T. and Calender, A. Effects of arabinofuranosylthy-
     mine on Epstein-Barr virus replication. Virology,
     104:219, 1980.
65. Patarroyo, M., Biberfeld, D., Klein, E., and Klein, G.
     12-0-tetradecanoylphorbol-13-acetate (TPA) treatment
     elevates the natural killer (NK) sensitivity of certain
     human lymphoid lines. Cell. Immunol., 63:237, 1981.
66. Prasad, K.N. and Sinha, P.K. Effects of sodium butyrate on
     mammalian cells in culture: a review. In vitro, 12:125,
     1976.

67. Pulvertaft, R.J.V. A study of malignant tumors in Nigeria
     by short term tissue cultures. J. Clin. Pathol.,
     18:261, 1965.
68. Purtilo, D.T. Epstein-Barr-virus-induced oncogenesis in
     immune deficient individuals. Lancet, 1:300, 1980.
69. Purtilo, D.T. Malignant lymphoproliferative diseases
     induced by Epstein-Barr virus in immunodeficient
     patients, including X-linked, cytogenetic, and familial
     syndromes. Cancer Genet. Cytogenet., 4:251, 1981.
70. Purtilo, D.T. and Sakamoto, K. Reactivation of Epstein-Barr
     virus in pregnant women, social factors, and immune com-
     petence as determinants of lymphoproliferative diseases.
     A hypothesis. Medical Hypothesis, 8:401, 1982.
71. Reece, E.R., Gartner, J.G., Seemayer, T.A., Joncas, J.H., and
     Pagano, J.S. Epstein-Barr virus in malignant lymphopro-
     liferative disorder of B-cells occurring after thymic
     epithelial transplantation for combined immunodeficiency.
     Cancer Res., 41:4243, 1981.
72. Reedman, B.M. and Klein, G. Cellular localization of an
     Epstein-Barr virus (EBV)-associated complement-fixing
     antigen in producer and non-producer lymphoblastoid cell
     lines. Int. J. Cancer, 11:499, 1973.
73. Rickinson, A.B., Jarvis, J.E., Crawford, D.H., and Epstein,
     M.A. Observations on the type of infection by Epstein-
     Barr virus in peripheral lymphoid cells of patients with
     infectious mononucleosis. Int. J. Cancer, 14:704, 1974.
74. Rickinson, A.B., Moss, D.J., Wallace, L.E., Rowe, M., Misko,
     I.S., Epstein, M.A., and Pope, J.H. Long-term T-cell
     mediated immunity to Epstein-Barr virus. Cancer Res.,
     41:4216, 1981.
75. Rifkin, D.B., Crowe, R.M., and Pollack, R. Tumor promoters
     induce changes in the chick embryo fibroblast cytoskele-
     ton. Cell, 18:361, 1979.
76. Riggs, M.G., Whittaker, R.G., Neumann, J.R., and Ingram, J.M.
     n-Butyrate causes histone modification in HeLa and
     Friend erythroleukemia cells. Nature (London), 268:462,
     1977.
77. Robinson, J.E., Brown, N., Andiman, W., Halliday, K.,
     Francke, U., Robert, M., Andersson-Anvret, M.,
     Horshmann, D., and Miller, G. Diffuse polyclonal B cell
     lymphoma during primary infection with Epstein-Barr
     virus. N. Engl. J. Med., 302:1293, 1980.
78. Robinson, J.E., Smith, D., and Niederman, J. Plasmacytic
     differentiation of circulating Epstein-Barr virus-
     infected B lymphocytes during acute infectious mono-
     nucleosis. J. exp. Med., 153:235, 1981.
79. Rovera, G., O'Brien, T.G., and Diamond, L. Tumor promoters
     inhibit spontaneous differentiaton of Friend erythro-
     leukemic cells in culture. Proc. Natl. Acad. Sci. USA,
     74:2894, 1977.

80. Rovera, G., Santoli, D., and Damsky, C. Human promyelocytic
     leukemia cells in culture differentiate into macrophage-
     like cells when treated with phorbol diester. Proc.
     Natl. Acad. Sci. USA, 76:2779, 1979.
81. Rymo, L., Lindahl, T., Povey, S., and Klein G. Analysis of
     restriction endonuclease fragments of intracellular
     Epstein-Barr virus DNA and isoenzymes indicate a common
     origin of the Raji, NC 37 and F265 human lymphoid cell
     lines. Virology, 115:115, 1981.
82. Saemundsen, A.K., Kallin, B., and Klein, G. Effect of n-
     butyrate on cellular and viral DNA synthesis in cells
     latently infected with Epstein-Barr virus. Virology,
     107:557, 1980.
83. Seif, R. Factors which disorganize microtubules or micro-
     filaments increase the frequency of cell transformation
     by polyoma virus. J. Virol., 36:421, 1980.
84. Seligman, M., Preud'Homme, J.L., and Brouet, J.C. Human
     lymphoproliferative disease as models of lymphocyte dif-
     ferentiaton. In: B. Serrou and C. Rosenfeld (eds.),
     Human Lymphocyte Differentiation. Its Application to
     Cancer. pp. 133-140. Amsterdam: Elsevier/North Holland
     Biomed. Press, 1978.
85. Simonová, I., Závadová, H., and Vonka, V. Differential
     expression of D and R components of Epstein-Barr virus
     early antigen after superinfection and after induction
     with 5-iododeoxyuridine. Acta Virol., 21:184, 1977.
86. Spira, G., Åman, P., Koide, N., Lundin, G., Klein, G., and
     Hall, K. Cell surface immunoglobulin and insulin recep-
     tor expression in an EBV-negative lymphoma cell line and
     its EBV-converted sublines. J. Immunol., 126:122, 1981.
87. Steel, C.M., Philipson, J., Arthur, E., Gardiner, S.E.,
     Newton, M.S., and McIntosh, R.V. Possibility of EB
     virus preferentially transforming a subpopulation of
     human B-lymphocytes. Nature (London), 270:729, 1977.
88. Steinitz, M., and Klein, G. EBV-transformation of surface
     IgA-positive human lymphocytes. J. Immunol., 125:194,
     1980.
89. Steinitz, M., Bakacz, T., and Klein, G. Interaction of the
     B95-8 and P3HR-1 substrains of Epstein-Barr virus (EBV)
     with peripheral human lymphocytes. Int. J. Cancer,
     22:251, 1978.
90. Suchánkova, A. and Vonka, V. UV-inactivation of Epstein-
     Barr virus: differences in early antigen expression in
     two different non-productive cell lines and influence of
     caffeine. Acta Virol., 22:383, 1978.
91. Tötterman, T.H., Nilsson, K., Claesson, L., Simonsson, B.,
     and Åman, P. Differentiation of chronic lymphocytic
     leukemia cells in vitro. I. Phorbol ester-induced
     changes in the synthesis of immunoglobulins and HLA-DR.
     Human Lymphocyte Differentiation, 1:13, 1981.

92. Totterman, T.H., Nilsson, K., and Sundström, C. Phorbol-
    ester-induced differentiation of chronic lymphocytic
    leukemia cells. Nature (London), 288:176, 1980.

93. Van Boxel, J.A. and Buell, D.N. IgD on cell membranes of
    human lymphoid cell lines with multiple immunoglobulin
    classes. Nature (London), 251:443, 1974.

94. Vitetta, E.S. and Uhr, J.W. Immunoglobulin-receptors
    revisited. Science, 189:964, 1975.

95. Weinstein, I.B., Lee, L.S., Fisher, P.B., Mutson, A. and
    Yamasaki, H. Action of phorbol esters in cell culture:
    mimicry of transformation, altered differentiation, and
    effects on cell membranes. J. Supramolec. Struct.,
    12:195, 1979.

96. Weinstein, I.B. and Wigler, M. Cell culture studies provide
    new information on tumor promoters. Nature (London),
    270:659, 1977.

97. Zech. K., Haglund, W., Nilsson, K., and Klein, G.
    Characteristic chromosomal abnormalities in biopsies and
    lymphoid cell lines from patients with Burkitt and
    non-Burkitt lymphomas. Int. J. Cancer, 17:47, 1976.

98. zur Hausen, H., Bornkamm, G.W., Schmidt, R., and Hecker, E.
    Tumor initiators and promoters in the induction of
    Epstein-Barr virus. Proc. Natl. Acad. Sci. USA,
    76:782-785, 1979.

99. zur Hausen, H., O'Neill, F.J., Freese, U.K., and Hecker, E.
    Persisting oncogenic herpesvirus induced by the tumour
    promoter TPA. Nature (London), 272:373, 1978.

EPSTEIN-BARR VIRUS IN NEW HOST CELLS

David J. Volsky

Department of Pathology & Laboratory Medicine
University of Nebraska Medical Center
Omaha, Nebraska

INTRODUCTION

Study of Epstein-Barr virus (EBV) is troubled by a number of vexing paradoxes. EBV was discovered 20 years ago (6,7). The biological roles and the molecular mechanisms of action of EBV remains a puzzle.

The first problem arise because EBV is ubiquitous and there is no identifiable permissive host cell system. This causative agent of infectious mononucleosis (IM) infects 70-100% of individuals in all societies (53). It can be easily recovered from the saliva and throat washings of IM patients, suggesting a route for its spread. IM patients have elevated titers of antibodies against products of the EBV reproductive cycle, i.e., the early (EA), viral capsid (VCA) and viral membrane (MA) antigens (36,53). Yet, no human primary target cell expressing EA, VCA and MA, and supporting EBV replication in vivo, has been discovered (29).

The second paradox is the strong immune response to EBV-infection vs. the viral role in oncogenesis. IM is an acute and self-limiting lymphoproliferative disease. Tight immuno-logical control subdues EBV infection (29,36,53). Only in rare cases of immunological breakdown do the "silent" infections by EBV lead to malignant B-cell proliferation. For example, children with inherited immune deficiency are at high risk of EBV-induced lymphomagenesis (40,41) as are immune suppressed transplant recipients (38), underscoring the role of immunological defense against EBV. On the other hand, in at least two malignancies, Burkitt's lymphoma (BL) and nasopharyngeal carcinoma (NPC), EBV is more than an innocent passenger affecting the tumor cells post factum (7,19,29). Cells taken from patients with BL and NPC tumors in endemic areas contain multiple copies of EBV genome and express the EBV-determined nuclear antigen, EBNA (7,19,29). As reviewed by Johnson in this monograph, inoculation of EBV into some New World monkeys may lead to lymphoproliferation and lymphoma (31). Paradoxically, however, BL and NPC patients have elevated titers to EBV-specific antigens and their cell-mediated immune effector mechanism seems to be intact as measured by various assays (7,19,29). How do the BL and NPC cells achieve autonomy from the immune system that is so efficient in eliminating EBV-infected IM lymphocytes?

A third and perhaps most difficult question stems from restriction of virus target cells by viral receptors. Owing to the presence of specific receptors on B cells, the virus is exclusively B-lymphotropic (17,29,67). How does EBV enter human epithelial cells lacking receptors for the virus? How does the virus genome present in NPC cells relate to the origin of this disease?

In summary, EBV is a unique member of the human Herpesvirus family. Ubiquitous but lacking a detectable permissive cell in humans, lymphotropic but present in epithelial cells, strongly immunogenic but associated with several malignancies - EBV is the "enfant terrible" of tumor virology. However complex and unresolved these paradoxes, EBV remains a prominent candidate for being a human tumor virus. Experiments being done in my laboratory seek to resolve some of these enigmas and limits of understanding EB viral oncogenesis.

Three limitations make the research on EBV technically and conceptually difficult. 1) Unlike other herpesviruses, EBV is highly restricted with regards to host organism and target cells (17,29,67). It cannot infect fibroblasts or epithelial cells in vitro. B-lymphocytes of humans and some other primates seemed to have been, till recently, the only target cells infectable in vitro by EBV. Within the B-lymphocytes lineage, EBV cannot infect stem cells or plasma cells. Infection is precisely restricted to B-cells possessing surface immunoglobulin and complement (C3d) receptors. IgM-secreting cells are the most susceptible targets for the virus (2,29,67). The host cell restriction of EBV precludes studying the interaction of the virus with cells which, unlike B lymphocytes, may not have mechanisms for restricting the EBV life cycle, 2) no fully permissive host cell allowing genetic recombination between viruses and production of mutants is available (7,19,29). Exposure of B-lymphocytes to EBV results in cell transformation ("immortalization") into lymphoblastoid cell lines (LCL) without evidence of advancement through the viral reproductive pathway. Only after prolonged cultivation in vitro, a few cells (1-5%) fail to control the viral

life cycle, allowing reproduction of the virus (7,19,29), 3)
finally, no convenient and inexpensive animal (i.e., murine) in
vivo model system for studying EBV-induced oncogenesis and related
immune responses has been found.

Numerous attempts to broaden the EBV host cell range beyond
primate B lymphocytes were unsuccessful (9,17,61). Although not
comprehensive, these studies indicated B lymphocytes from human
and certain primates may be the only susceptible target cells for
the virus (9,17,28,60). The EBV system has provided a paradigm of
an extraordinary target cell restriction and specialization.
Klein has postulated an evolutionary adaptation of the virus to
the C3d receptor on B-cells (67). This adaptation allows viral
latency and viral survival in B lymphocyte (67).

Bioengineering techniques are opening a new era of transferring genetic information between cells. Transfer of whole
genomes, DNA fragments or purified genes is now being done. Using
these techniques since 1980, we and others have broken through the
host cell restriction of EBV, permitting study of the interaction
between EBV, or EBV-DNA fragments, and cells usually devoid of
viral receptors. Since these cells are not ordinarily infectable
by the virus in vitro, we define them here as novel host cells.
Our laboratory is now capable of evaluating the host cell restriction of viral expression, finding permissive target cells, and
developing murine models for studying in vivo responses to
EBV-infected cells.

Techniques for Introducing Viral and Cellular Genetic Information
into Non-Susceptible Cells

Transfer of whole genomes or genome fragments between living
eukaryotic cells can be accomplished by direct microinjection
using microneedles, vesicle-cell-fusion, DNA transfection and
infection by viruses following implantation of viral receptors
onto receptor-negative cells.

Microneedles have been applied for microinjection of different molecules, including macromolecules and DNA, by Graessman
et al. and Stacey and Allfrey in 1977 (10,23,50). The material
can be injected into the cytoplasm or nucleus of living cells. The
number of injected molecules is high, can be estimated, and the
recipient cell can be observed. Disadvantages include the low
number of cells that can be injected and the necessity to use
large cells for injection. Therefore, the technique is limited
mainly to large monolayer cells and oocytes. Nevertheless,
microinjection was first used to transfer EBV genome into the
receptor-negative unnatural host cells. In 1980 Graessman and
colleagues demonstrated that EBV genes can be expressed, following
microinjection of viral DNA, in human diploid fibroblasts, African

green monkey kidney cells and rat fibroblasts (11). The expression of EBV-DNA was limited; only gene products of the early
antigen (EA) complex were detected (11). Perhaps the limited
expression was due to DNA denaturation during the purification
process, DNA shearing during the microinjection or intracellular
restriction in the unnatural host cells.

DNA transfection utilizes phagocytosis in the presence of
calcium phosphate (12). This technique is used most frequently
for introducing DNA and DNA fragments into various cells.
However, low DNA uptake by a low number of the recipient cells
(usually $10^{-6} - 10^{-5}$) is a serious limitation of this method.
Inclusion of transforming or thymidine kinase is needed to select
the successfully transfected cells. DNA recombination techniques
permit construction of recombinant plasmids in which a gene(s) of
interest is coupled to a TK gene (37,64). Transfection of such
plasmids into target TK^-cells grown in a selective (T^+) medium
will result in a selective survival of cells containing the TK and
the gene of interest. This approach has been recently used for
introducing a putative EBV-nuclear antigen (EBNA)-expressing
gene(s) into the LTK^-mouse cells (52). The selected LTK^+ mouse
cells expressed a nuclear neoantigen related to human EBNA (52).

Fusion-mediated DNA transfer technique employs membranous
vehicles for transfer (25). DNA is trapped within a membrane
vesicle and then fused with the recipient cells. Two kinds of
vesicles are presently used for DNA transfer by this technique:
artificial phospholipid vesicles (liposomes) and reconstituted
viral envelopes. Liposomes have been studied for years as simple
models for assessing the structure and function of biological
membranes and as drug carriers in vivo (reviewed in 13 and 35).
Recently, liposomes have been successfully used to introduce polio
virus genome into receptor-negative cells (65). However, since
most of the liposomes are phagocytosed and thus do not actually
fuse with eukaryotic cells, they do not serve as an efficient
vehicle. Their target cell range obviously does not include non-
phagocytosing cells, such as lymphocytes.

Reconstituted viral envelopes offer high fusion efficiency
and specific target cell recognition (25). Similar to intact
viruses, these vesicles attach preferentially to cells containing
specific receptors, fuse with cellular membranes and thus empty
their contents into the cytoplasm (25). Also resulting is the
implantation of the viral envelope components into the recipient
cell plasma membrane. The virus we use for DNA transfer is the
fusogenic Sendai virus (SV)(34). Sendai virus envelope contains
only two glycoproteins, the fusion protein F which is required for
the virus-cell fusion and the hemagglutinin protein HN which is
required for the viral recognition of the target cell (reviewed in
23 and 25). SV envelopes are prepared by solubilizing with

detergents and isolating from other viral components by ultra-
centrifugation (15,60). Removal of the detergent results in a
spontaneous formation of reconstituted membranes resembling the
original intact envelopes both structurally and functionally
(15,60). The reconstituted Sendai virus envelopes are therefore
capable of fusing with target cell membranes (15,25,60). Recently
we demonstrated that reconstitution of Sendai virus envelopes in
the presence of whole EBV particles or purified EBV DNA results in
their entrapping inside the reconstituted vesicles (ref. 47 and
unpublished results). The vesicles were used for delivering EBV or
EBV-DNA into the receptor-negative cells. This resulted in partial or full expression of EBV-related functions (47).

Reconstituted Sendai virus envelopes can also be used for
transplantation of membrane receptors between living cells
(25,39,55,58). In principle, reconstitution of Sendai virus envelopes in the presence of exogenous membrane proteins results in
the formation of hybrid vesicles. Fusion of the vesicles with
target cells incorporates the exogenous protein into the target
cell membrane (25,39,55,57). We had postulated that EBV receptors
transplanted onto receptor-negative cells would convert them into
new, though temporary, viral susceptible host cells. Since EBV
receptors are incompletely characterized (5), we adopted this
technique to implantation of fragments of purified membranes from
EBV receptor-positive cells (47,48,59,61). To prepare reconstituted hybrid vesicles, SV envelope proteins were reconstituted
with the EBV receptor-rich membrane fragments from Burkitt's
lymphoma line Raji (61). The hybrid Sendai virus-Raji membrane
vesicles (SRec-EBV) were used to transplant functional EBV receptors on practically any EBV receptor-negative cell (61). The
cells were then used as temporary receptor-positive targets for
EBV (47,48,59,61). To date, we have demonstrated expression of
EBV-DNA in more than 25 different target cells from different host
organisms (47,48,59,61 c.f. also Table 1). Among the techniques
summarized here, receptor-implantation is by far the most efficient way to introduce EBV into the virus-nonsusceptible cells.

EBV in Novel Host Cells

Table 1 lists novel, not normally infectable by EBV, host
cells from five species and summarizes the information related to
EBV-DNA expression in the bioengineered cells. It seems that the
genetic information of EBV can be expressed in virtually any cell
type from different hosts once the responsible genes are
appropriately introduced into the receptor-negative cells. The EBV
has been introduced into cells of man, mouse, rat, guinea pig, and
hamster. Unnatural target cells may be as different as mouse
B and human T lymphocytes, fibroblasts, epithelial cells and tumor
cells of a myeloid, lymphoid, erythroid, and epithelial origin.

Table 1. Expression of Epstein-Barr Virus Genes in Different Types after EBV Receptor-Implantation or Microinjection/Transfection of Viral DNA

Host	Natural unmanipulated/EBV-infectable host cell	EBV receptor-implanted EBV infected host cell	EBV-DNA-microinjected/transfected host cell	Expression of EBV-related functions			Ref.
				EBNA	Transformation	EA/VCA or virus production	
Man	Normal B lymphocyte			+	+	-	(17,32,67)
	Normal squamous epithelial cell??			-	-	-	(19,53)
		Normal B lymphocyte	Normal B lymphocyte	+	?	-	(47)
		Preleukemia B lymphocyte		+	+	-	(54,57)
				+	+	+	(56,57)
		B-cell lymphoma (P3HR-1,etc.)		+		+	(61)
		Normal T lymphocyte		-	-	+	*
		T-cell leukemia (Molt-4, 1301)		+		+ or -	(49,61)
			T-cell leukemia (Molt-4,1301)	+		+ or -	(47)
			Placental fibroblasts	?	?	+	(30)
			Embryonic fibroblasts (WI-38)	-	-	+	(11)
		Myeloma (Simpson,U-698)		+		+ or -	*
		Erythroleukemia (K562)		+		+ or -	*
		Normal nasopharyngeal epithelial cells		+	?	-	(48)

Species		Cell type				Reference
Mouse	None	Normal thymic epithelium	+	?	-	(46)
		Lung carcinoma epithelial cells (MDA-231)	+	?	-	*
		Squamous cell carcinoma(CCL-30)	-		+	(51)
		NPC cells (CNE)	-		+	(51)
		Normal B lymphocytes	+ or -	-	+	(59,61)
		Normal T lymphocytes	+ or -	-	+	(59,61)
		B-cell lymphoma (ABT6C,TL⁻)	+		+ or -	*
		T-cell leukemia (YAC-1) LTK⁻	+		+ or -	(52)
		Myeloma (P3NS-1)	+		+ or -	(61)
		Plasmocytoma (P-815)	+		+ or -	*
		Fibroblasts (3T3)	+ or -	?	-	*
		Splenocytes	+ or -	?	+	(61)(47)
Rat	None	Splenocytes	+/-	-	+	*
		Fibroblasts	-	-	+	(11)
Guinea pig	None	Splenocytes	+/-	-	+	*
Hamster	None	Splenocytes	+/-	-	+	*

* cells were EBV receptor-implanted and EBV-infected in this laboratory as described previously (17,37). EBV-determined antigens were detected by anticomplement (EBNA) and direct (EA, VCA) immunofluorescence (45) two days after infection. + or - : expression (+) or lack of expression (-) of an antigen depending on the target cell or viral substrain used (see text). +/-: low antigen expression.

The unusual host cell restriction of EBV to human B lymphocytes in vitro is determined primarily at the plasma membrane
level, due to the presence of specific EBV receptors. None of the
cells shown in Table 1 could be infected in vitro with EBV by
exposing the cells to the virus. However, viral antigens were
fully expressed after the viral genetic information was introduced
into the cells by bioengineering, i.e., after bypassing the plasma
membrane barrier (Table 1). We thus postulate that the biological
(in vivo) range of EBV may not be limited by the specificity and
exclusive presence of EBV receptors on human B lymphocytes. Many
foreign particles, including viruses, enter cells by phagocytosis
- a fairly nonspecific process (3). Many chemicals present in our
environment, such as the tumor promoters of the phorbol ester
family, modulate cell membranes, affecting the specificity and
activity of surface receptors (4). EBV may thus interact in vivo,
under certain conditions, with cells which are found in vitro to
be receptor-negative and resistant to the virus penetration.
Finally, ubiquitous influenza and herpes simplex viruses are known
to induce cell-cell fusion (16,44). Infection by these viruses
may promote fusion between EBV-harboring B lymphocytes and any
cell with which the lymphocyte gets in close contact.

Two lines of evidence suggest that EBV is not solely
restricted to B lymphocytes in vivo. One is the well known association of the virus with nasopharyngeal carcinoma (NPC) and
epithelial cells (reviewed by Krueger in this volume). Patients
with NPC have elevated antibodies to EBNA, EA and VCA
(19,29,36,52). Undifferentiated NPC cells express EBNA and
contain multiple copies of the EBV genome (19). Given these
empirical findings, epithelial cells must be infectable by EBV in
vivo. However, attempts to infect fresh epithelial cells by
intact virus in vitro have been unsuccessful (9,48). As with
other non-human B lymphocytic cells (Table 1), failure to infect
appears to be a result of the epithelial cell membrane block
against EBV penetration in vitro. Transfection of purified
EBV-DNA into epithelial cell lines has allowed limited expression
of viral antigens (51). Implantation of functional EBV receptors
onto epithelial cells from the carcinoma cell line MDA has
permitted EBV infection and expression of EBV-nuclear antigen,
EBNA (Table 1). Recently, we have investigated whether normal
human epithelial cells have EBV receptors (48). We established
primary cultures of epithelial cells from human nasopharynx, using
adenoids and tonsils removed from children. In accordance to
previous reports, also these cells could not be infected by EBV.
Using fluorescein-labeled EBV (FITC-EBV) and an Ortho cytofluorograph we demonstrated that the epithelial cells do not have
EBV receptors. However, following EBV-receptor implantation, the
cells bound FITC-EBV. Two to five days after exposure to transforming B-95-8 substrain of EBV, 1-5% of the receptor-implanted
cells expressed EBNA. EA and VCA were not detected in the

virus-infected cultures (48). Thus, normal human epithelial cells
from nasopharynx are susceptible to EBV infection when the
membrane barrier resulting from the lack of EBV receptors is
overcome by implanting receptors onto the cells. How EBV normally
penetrates into epithelial cells of nasopharynx in vivo remains
undetermined. One way to accomplish that may be by fusion of the
epithelium with EBV-infected lymphocytes. Bayliss and Wolf
suggested that cell fusion could be mediated by fusogenic proteins
present in the EBV-producer cells (1). Wolf summarizes this
hypothesis elsewhere in this volume.

The occurrence of EBV reproductive cycle in vivo is another
indication that the virus is not restricted to B lymphocytes in
all in vivo situations. IM, Burkitt's lymphoma and NPC patients
all have elevated titers of antibodies against proteins of the
EBV-lytic pathway, EA and VCA (19,36,53). Virus is shed in saliva
of these patients. Moreover, healthy persons retain anti-VCA
antibodies throughout life (19,36,53), indicating that EBV is
constantly reproduced somewhere in the individuals. And yet,
human B lymphocytes are not capable of supporting EBV lytic pathway in vitro and in vivo. Infection results in an early
expression of EBNA, followed by cell immortalization into
lymphoblastoid cell lines (LCL) which are without any detectable
lytic cycle (7,29). Peripheral lymphocytes of IM and BL patients
express EBNA but not EA and VCA (7,29). Also, BL cells
express EBNA only (7). Moreover, cells taken from the NPC tumors
stain only for EBNA but not EA or VCA (19,29). Normal epithelial
cells infected by EBV, following receptor-implantation, exclusively express EBNA (48). It thus seems likely that also nasopharyngeal epithelial cells are not capable of supporting EBV
reproduction. Where is the virus reproduced in vivo? EBV, as
for every virus, must have a permissive host cell for reproduction. It is apparent that such a permissive host cell has not
yet been detected. An early postulate was that EBV may be
reproduced in parotid gland ductal cells (32, see also Wolf in
this volume). Unfortunately, this was not followed by more
detailed studies. A systematic search of human tissues for
permissive EBV host cells is ongoing in several laboratories.

The latency imposed on EBV by a mature human B lymphocyte is
probably a result of the particular molecular controls characteristic for the differentiation stage of the lymphocyte. This
strict control of the EBV life cycle can be partially reduced by
chemicals (18,66), superinfection with EBV (43) or culturing cells
at high density or low temperatures. Until recently, these were
the only ways to study events during the EBV life cycle.

New hosts (Table 1) allow study of the life cycle of EBV in
cells from various tissues and species at different stages of
differentiation. Once inside the receptor-negative cell, EBV-DNA

is submitted to molecular controls of a given host cell. The
latter is probably related to the origin and the stage of differentiation of a host cell. As evident from the data in Table 1,
the range of cellular responses to the challenge of EBV-DNA is
between induction of EBNA cell transformation (nasopharyngeal
epithelial cells, preleukemia lymphocytes, mouse 3T3 cells) and a
full lytic cycle with low or no EBNA induction and without
causing cell transformation (mouse lymphocytes, human embryonic
fibroblasts, squamous cell carcinoma, etc.).

     Analysis of the interaction between EBV and bioengineered
cells sheds new light on the mechanisms controlling EBV-DNA
expression and the sequence of viral translational products during
the cycle. Previously, synthesis of EBNA was regarded as the
first step in the expression of EBV-DNA, in transforming and lytic
pathways of the virus in cells (8,29). T antigen, for instance,
is the first product of Simian virus-40 (SV-40) life cycle in the
productive and nonproductive infections (14). In contrast to
SV-40 or polyoma viruses, however, investigators of EBV did not
have a primary permissive system for EBV to test the above
hypothesis. Studies on the mechanisms of virus cycle were limited
to the established EBV-transformed cell lines in which the lytic
cycle can be induced by chemicals or by EBV-superinfection
(18,43,66). Consequently, only late events of the lytic pathway
(from induction of EA to viral particles release) have been partially evaluated (18,43,66). The early events, in particular, the
mechanism of the molecular "switch" between B-cell transformation
and lytic pathways could not be studied. These experimental
limits can be eleviated using our receptor transplantation technique. Analysis of the molecular events during the primary EBV
lytic cycle in permissive human T and mouse lymphocytes (Table 1,
Refs. 49,59,61) suggests that EBNA synthesis may not be required
during the EBV-lytic cycle that follows primary infection by the
virus. In EBV-infected mouse lymphocytes EBNA is expressed in
only 0.1-1.0% of the infected cells two days after infection, compared to 8-10% of EA/VCA-positive cells (59,61). Moreover, in
EBV-infected human T lymphocytes, EBNA could not be detected at
all, while the EA and VCA antigens were synthesized by a significant proportion of cells (Table 1). Also other new EBV hosts,
such as human T cell-derived Molt-4 and 1301 cells, myeloma cells,
or mouse T-cell leukemia YAC-1 cells expressed EBNA antigens in
fewer cells than EA and VCA (Table 1, Refs. 49,59,61). In certain
cells, such as placental fibroblasts, mouse lymphocytes or Molt-4,
infectious viral particles were recovered following the primary
lytic cycle (30,49,59).

     The results of these studies suggest that two different,
mutually exclusive pathways of EBV expression may occur:

TRANSFORMATION PATHWAY

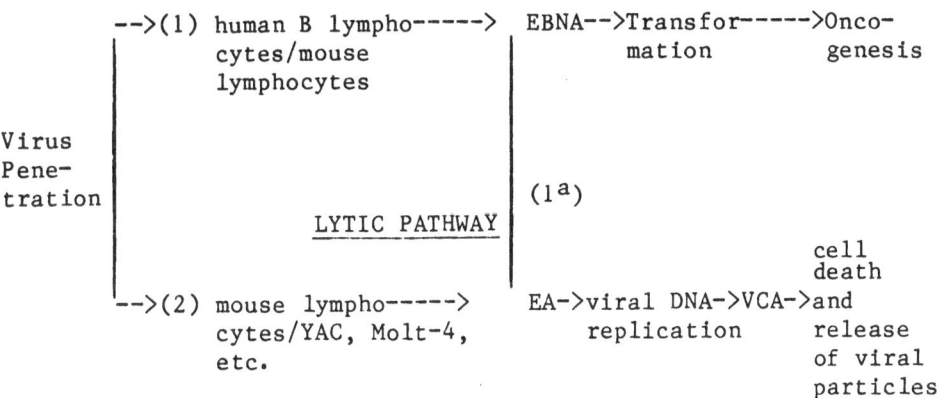

Illustrated above are: 1) the EBNA-positive transformation pathway
in human B lymphocytes, in certain mouse lymphocytes and other new
host cells which express EBNA; 1[a]) the EBNA-positive lytic pathway
after superinfection or chemical induction of EBV-positive cell
lines; 2) the lytic pathway in primarily infected cells (mouse
lymphocytes, mouse lymphoma YAC, human T-cells derived lymphoma
Molt-4, placenta fibroblasts, embryonic fibroblasts, etc. cf. Table
1) which may not require EBNA synthesis.

   EBNA is the major EBV-related protein that is characteristic
for virally-induced cell proliferation (transformation) (Ref.7,29)
and is diminished or lacking during the primary lytic cycle in the
new host cells. It is tempting to postulate that synthesis of
EBNA or association of an EBNA precursor with a cellular protein,
could block the viral reproductive cycle thereby initiating
latency. Concomitantly, the cell undergoes transformation. The
novel EBV-permissive host cell systems, such as mouse lymphocytes,
may be useful to evaluate this hypothesis. According to a recent
report, the EBV transformation-related component may consist of a
virally-coded 48K polypeptide ("true EBNA") forming a complex with
a cell-coded 53K polypeptide (26). Supposedly, the complex is
more stable than either of its components separately, which may
explain the absence or very low levels of 53K component in normal
cells (26). In the well-defined SV-40 system, a complex
comprising of the virus-coded T antigen in association with a
host protein, 53K, has been described by several laboratories
(26,27). The difference between SV-40 and EBV systems is the
transforming proteins. Synthesis of the T antigen is a prereq-
uisite for SV-40 DNA replication (14), however, EBV may replicate
without EBNA synthesis (59).

   EBNA or a related compound may regulate the EBV-cycle and
transformation by the virus. This hypothesis is testable

modifying the EBV-mouse lymphocyte interaction. The question is
asked whether the predominantly lytic system can be pushed to
cellular transformation. For instance, increasing the amount of
intracellular 53K proteins, by exposure to chemicals or microinjection, prior to or concomitantly with EBV infection, may
stabilize EBNA in mouse lymphocytes and immortalize cells.

In Vivo Studies in Mice

    Success in EBV-infection of mouse lymphocytes in vitro
(59,61) prompted us to ask the question whether we could develop
an in vivo murine model for studying EBV-host interaction. We
assumed that inoculation of syngeneic, in vitro EBV-infected mouse
lymphocytes, expressing EBNA, EA and VCA into a mouse would

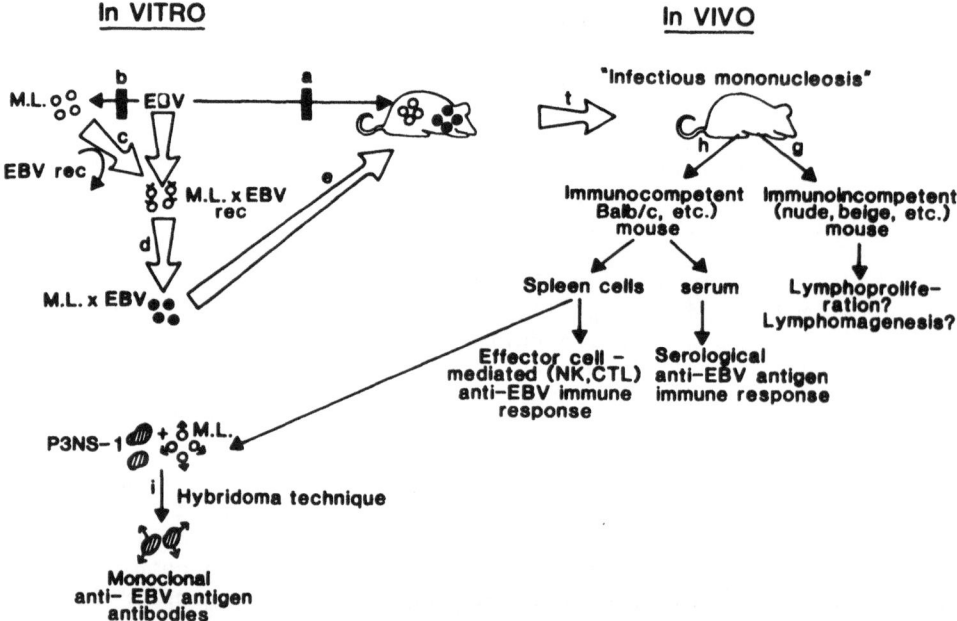

Fig. 1. In vivo murine system for studies on EBV. Mouse lympho-
          cytes (M.L.) cannot be infected by EBV in vivo (1) or in
          vitro (6). Only following functional EBV receptors (EBV
          rec) implantation into their membranes (c), the cells can
          be infected by the virus (d). Repetitive inoculations of
          EBV-infected mouse lymphocytes into syngeneic mice (e)
          promotes IM-liked disease (f). Serological and effector
          cell-mediated immune responses of the animal (h) and
          potential lymphoproliferation (g) can now be studied. An
          important benefit of the system is the possibility of
          producing monoclonal antibodies to EBNA, EA, and VCA (i).

possibly create an infectious mononucleosis (IM)-like disease. We
anticipated both humoral and effector cell-mediated immune
responses against the EBV antigen-harboring cells. In mice with
impaired immune responses, we could expect proliferation of the
EBNA-expressing mouse lymphocytes and perhaps, EBV-related mouse
lymphomas.

Figure 1 illustrates our experimental system. Mouse cells
cannot be infected by inoculating EBV into mice and other non-
primates (Step a). Neither can mouse lymphocytes (61) be infected
by EBV in vitro (Step b). Only following implantation of EBV
receptors (Step c) can mouse lymphocyte be infected by the virus
(Step d). When infected mouse lymphocytes are inoculated into
syngeneic mice (Step e), the animal is confronted with cells of
its own genetic constitution, but also viral antigens. As noted
earlier, this situation can be considered analogous to IM in
humans (Step f).   Serological and effector cell mediated immune
responses of the animal (Step h) and, potential proliferation of
pre-tumor cells can be studied (Step g). Importantly, production
of monoclonal antibodies against EBV-related antigens is now being
achieved. Previous attempts to produce monoclonal antibodies to
EBV antigens used immunization of mice with EBV-infected human
cells, causing strong xenogeneic immune response against human
proteins. Such proteins are more abundant than the EBV-related
antigens. Thus, selection of specific anti-EBV antigen producing
cells became extremely difficult. Consequently only monospecific
antibodies against membrane antigen of EBV (MA) have been selected
till now (33,43). In contrast, mice can now be immunized with
syngeneic cells in which the only immunogeneic proteins are
products of EBV-life cycle, significantly increasing chances to
obtain monoclonal anti-EBNA, EA, and VCA antibodies (Step i).
Preliminary use of the in vivo mouse model have been recently
reported (62,63) and are briefly described below.

Humoral Responses

In a typical experiment, Balb/c mouse lymphocytes are isolated and EBV-infected (59,61). On the second or third day post
infection, when the expression of EBV-determined antigens peak as
determined by immunofluorescence, the cells are washed and
inoculated intraperitoneally into syngeneic mice. The inoculation
is repeated thrice in biweekly intervals. The mice are
sacrificed 3-4 days after the last injection, their spleens
removed, and blood collected. The serum is tested for antibodies
by indirect immunofluoresence for EA, VCA, and anticomplement immunofluorescence for EBNA, using a panel of cells expressing these
antigens. We can detect antibodies against all three antigens,
EBNA, EA and VCA, in titers from 1:20 to 1:40 for anti-EBNA, and
to 1:160 for anti-EA and anti-VCA. The sera had also a virus-
neutralizing activity suggesting anti-membrane antibody (MA).

Effector Cell-Mediated Immune Response

Inoculation of mice with EBV-infected syngeneic lymphocytes provoked significant cell-mediated immune responses. For example, increased natural killer (NK) cell activity in the range of 20-30% above the control levels was found against human, mouse, and marmoset target cells. The increased NK activity probably was induced by the inoculated EBV-infected lymphocytes. In contrast, receptor-implanted but EBV-noninfected lymphocytes or EBV alone did not evoke similar increase in the NK activity. While the increased NK activity could be detected 5 days post inoculation no cytotoxic T lymphocyte (CTL) activity became evident at that time. Following consecutive inoculations of syngeneic lymphocytes, however, the CTL increased probably reflecting generation of memory T cells. CTL was measured by interacting spleen cells from inoculated Balb/c mouse against a panel of control, mock-infected or EBV-infected lymphocytes. Up to 40% of EBV-infected mouse lymphocytes were lysed by the effector cells at an E/T ratio of 100:1. Receptor-implanted cells alone or untreated lymphocytes were not lysed at all.

Monoclonal EBNA Antibodies to EBNA

Attempts to produce monoclonal anti-EBNA antibodies by immunizing mice with EBNA-positive Raji or BJAB cells have not succeeded by others because xenogeneic immunization induces strong immune response against human proteins. EBNA is probably the least abundant of all non-structural EBV-antigens, as reflected by the necessity to use a "triple-sandwich" anti-complement immunofluorescence assay (45) for its detection. EBNA is also a weak antigen, as reflected by the failure of immunization of mice with partially purified antigen preparations to stimulate significant antibody respone (J. Luka, personal communication).

Our preliminary results (see above) demonstrated that syngeneic EBV-infected mouse lymphocytes invoke strong anti-EBV antigen immune response when inoculated into syngeneic Balb/c mice (62,63). Antibody to EBNA in the mouse serum was 1:20-1:40. This is high, considering the relatively low number of EBNA-positive mouse lymphocytes (up to 1%, versus 10% of EA and VCA, see ref. 59). However, EBV-related proteins are the only immunogens presented to the syngeneic mouse. Recently, we have selected monoclonal anti-EBNA antibodies using our system and the hybridoma technique of Koehler (22). Clones which produce anti-EBNA, anti-EA or anti-VCA antibodies have been selected. It seems that monospecific anti-EBV-antigen antibodies can be produced in this system with relative ease. This approach may be applicable to life-threatening agents, such as hepatitis B and cytomegaloviruses.

In summary, our preliminary data indicate that mice mimic some of the EBV-related immune responses of humans during infectious mononucleosis. This mouse model system offers experimental opportunities inaccessible in humans. For instance, use of inbred, genetically defined strains permits evaluation of the role of histocompatibility antigens in the immune responses to EBV-infected cells. Experiments can be designed to test the effect of immune suppressors and stimulators, chemical carcinogens and environmental tumor promoters on the animal response to EBV-infected cells. Mouse experimental systems will complement marmoset models, in which marked immune deficiency resembling X-linked lymphoproliferative syndrome (XLP) in humans is observed (see articles by Johnson and Purtilo in this volume).

SUMMARY AND CONCLUSIONS

Restriction of EBV to human B lymphocytes was attributed in the past to a special relationship between the viral genetic information and intracellular control mechanisms in the differentiated B cell. Results of our studies show that the cellular restriction of EBV is primarily determined at the plasma membrane level. The presence or absence of specific viral receptors on differentiated human and certain other primate B lymphocytes determine infectability of cells. This barrier can be bypassed by employing DNA-microinjection and transfection, or transplantation of EBV receptors. EBV-DNA can thereby enter non-natural cells of various types and origins, resulting in viral infection. Transplantation of EBV receptors followed by the application of an intact virus is the most efficient of the techniques. About 10% of new target cells can be infected following receptor implantation, a similar proportion to human B lymphocytes or receptor-positive lymphoblastoid cell lines. This technique permits biochemical and molecular studies on the EBV-life cycle in new host cells. In contrast, transfection of EBV-DNA results in the expression of EBV-related functions in only one of 10^3 or 10^4 cells.

Briefly, cardinal features of the interaction of EBV with new host cells include:

1) The exclusively cell-transforming mode of interaction of the B95-8 substrain of EBV with cells human B lymphocytes is not the rule with new host cells. Depending on the host cell type, both viral substrains can induce either mostly EBNA (with little or no EA and VCA) or enter the viral lytic cycle (with little EBNA induction much expression of EA and VCA, and without causing cell transformation).

2) Obtaining EBV-transformed cell lines of non-human B cell
   origin either through "conversion" of the existing tumor
   cells to 100% EBV-positivity, or by the direct
   EBV-transformation of normal cells, is feasible.

3) Permissive (lytic) EBV systems in primarily infected cells,
   such as human T and mouse lymphocytes, have been
   established. This paves the way for molecular studies on
   the EBV-life cycle and for production of new EBV mutants.

4) Development of a murine in vivo model for studying the
   action of EBV, the influence of environmental co-factors;
   and the host immune responses which subdue the virus-
   infected cells, is in progress.

5) Infection of murine cells has facilitated the production of
   monoclonal anti-EBNA antibodies.

   EBV has been labeled by George Klein an "enfant terrible" of
human virology. As with any difficult child, novel approaches
were required to understand the motives and mechanisms of the
biological action of this enigmatic virus. New ways of studying
the EBV as reviewed above, hold promise to increase our knowledge
about this tumorigenic virus and the oncogenesis process in
general.

ACKNOWLEDGMENTS

   The author would like to thank Drs. G. Klein, I.M. Shapiro,
D.T. Purtilo, D.R. Johnson and F. Sinangil for their cooperation
and constant encouragement during the various stages of this
work. Technical assistance of C. Kuszynski, B. Volsky, L.
Pertile and M. Hedenskog are also gratefully acknowledged.
Help of Mrs. S. Blum in typing this manuscript is greatly
appreciated. This work was supported in part by the PHS
Grant #1R01 CA33386 awarded by the National Cancer Institute,
the R. Estrin Goldberg Memorial Grant for Cancer Research and
by the Nebraska Department of Health Grant LB506.

REFERENCES

1.   Bayliss, G.J. and Wolf, H. Epstein-Barr virus-induced cell
         fusion. Nature, 287:164, 1980.
2.   Bird, A.G. and Britton, S. A live human B-cell activator
         operating in isolation of other cellular influences.
         Scand. J. Immunol., 9:507, 1979.
3.   Dales, S. Early events in cell-animal virus interactions.
         Bacteriological Reviews, 37:103, 1973.

4. Dion, L. D., De Luca, L.M., and Colburn, N.H. Phorbol ester-
    induced anchorage independence and its antagonism by
    retinoic acid correlates with altered expression of spe-
    cific glycoproteins. Carcinogenesis, 2(10):951, 1981.

5. Epstein, M.A. and Achong, B.G. Introduction: discovery and
    general biology of the virus. In: M. A. Epstein and B.
    G. Achong (eds.), The Epstein-Barr Virus. pp. 1-4.
    Berlin, New York: Springer-Verlag, 1979.

6. Epstein, M.A. and Achong, B.G. Morphology of the virus and
    of virus induced cytopathologic changes. In: M.A.
    Epstein and B.G. Achong (eds.), The Epstein-Barr Virus.
    pp. 23-33. Berlin, New York: Springer-Verlag, 1979.

7. Epstein, M.A. and Achong, B.G. The relationship of the
    virus to Burkitt's lymphoma. In: M.A. Epstein and B.G.
    Achong (eds.), The Epstein-Barr Virus. pp. 321-329.
    Berlin, New York: Springer-Verlag, 1979.

8. Ernberg, I., Masucci, G., and Klein, G. Persistence of
    Epstein-Barr virus nuclear antigens (EBNA) in cells
    entering the EB viral cycle. Int. J. Cancer,
    17:197, 1976.

9. Glaser, R., Lang, C.Max, Lee, K.J., Schuller, D.E., Jacobs,
    D., and McQuattie, C. Attempt to infect nonmalignant
    nasopharyngeal epithelial cells from humans and squirrel
    monkeys with Epstein-Barr virus. J. Natl. Cancer Inst.,
    5:1085, 1980.

10. Graessmann, A., Graessmann, M., and Mueller, C. Regulatory
    function of Simian virus 40 DNA replication for late
    viral gene expression. Proc. Natl. Acad. Sci. USA,
    74:4831, 1977.

11. Graessman, A., Wolf, H., and Bornkamm, G.W. Expression of
    Epstein-Barr virus genes in different cell types after
    microinjection of viral DNA. Proc. Natl. Acad. Sci.
    USA, 77:433, 1980.

12. Graham, F. L. and Van Der Eb, A.J. A new technique for the
    assay of infectivity of human adenovirus 5 DNA.
    Virology, 52:456, 1973.

13. Gregoriadis, G. Tailoring liposome structure. Nature,
    283:814, 1980.

14. Hoggan, M.D., Bowe, W.P., Black, P.M., and Hubner, R.J.
    Production of tumor specific antigens by oncogenic
    viruses during acute cytolytic infections. Proc. Natl.
    Acad. Sci. USA, 53:12, 1965.

15. Hosaka, Y. and Shimizu, K. Artificial assembly of envelope
    particles of HVJ (Sendai virus). I. Assembly of hemo-
    lytic and fusion factors from envelopes solubilized with
    Nonidet P-40. Virology, 49:627, 1972.

16. Huang, R.T.C., Wahn, K., Klenk, D.H., and Rott, R. Fusion
    between cell membrane and liposomes containing the
    glycoproteins of influenza virus. Virology,
    104:294, 1980.

17.   Jondal, M. and Klein, G.   Surface markers on human B and T
         lymphocytes. II. Presence of Epstein-Barr virus recep-
         tors on B lymphocytes. J. Exp. Med., 138:1365, 1973.
18.   Kallin, B., Luka, J., and Klein, G.   Immunochemical charac-
         terization of Epstein-Barr virus-associated early and
         late antigens in n-Butyrate-treated P3HR-1 cells. J.
         Virol., 32:710, 1979.
19.   Klein, G.   The relationship of the virus to nasopharyngeal
         carcinoma. In: M.A. Epstein and B.G. Achong (eds.),
         The Epstein-Barr Virus. pp. 339-350. Berlin, New York:
         Springer-Verlag, 1979.
20.   Klein, G., Gergely, L., and Goldstein, G.   Two-color immu-
         nofluorescence studies on EBV-determined antigens. Clin.
         Exp. Immunol., 8:593, 1971.
21.   Klein, G., Giovanella, B., Westman, A., Steblin, J.S., and
         Mumford, D. An EBV-genome negative cell line established
         from American Burkitt lymphoma: receptor characteristics,
         EBV infectivity and permanent conversion into EBV posi-
         tive sublines by in vitro infection. Intervirol.,
         5:319, 1976.
22.   Koehler, G. and Milstein, C.   Continuous cultures of fused
         cells secreting antibody of predefined specificity.
         Nature (London), 256:495, 1975.
23.   Kulka, R.G. and Loyter, A.   The use of fusion methods for
         the microinjection of animal cells. In: F. Bronner and
         A. Kleinzeller (eds.), Current Topics in Membranes and
         Transport. Vol. 12, pp. 365-430. New York: Academic
         Press, 1979.
24.   Linzer, D. and Levine, J.J.   Characterization of a 54 K
         Dalton cellular SV-40 tumor antigen present in SV-40
         transformed cells and uninfected embryonal carcinoma
         cells. Cell, 17:43, 1979.
25.   Loyter, A. and Volsky, D.J.   The use of reconstituted
         Sendai virus envelopes as carriers for the introduction
         of biological materials into animal cells. In: G. Poste
         and J.A. Nicholson (eds.), Cell Surface Review. In
         press, 1982.
26.   Luka, J., Jornvall, H., and Klein, G.   Purification and
         biochemical characterization of the Epstein-Barr virus-
         determined nuclear antigen and an associated protein
         with a 53,000-Dalton subunit. J. Virol., 35:592, 1980.
27.   McCormick, F., Clark, R., Harlow, E., and Tjian, R.   SV-40 T
         antigen binds specifically to a cellular/53 K protein in
         vitro. Nature, 292:63, 1981.
28.   Menzes, Y., Sergneuron, J.M., Petel, P., Bourkas, A., and
         Lenoir, G. Presence of Epstein-Barr virus receptors but
         absence of virus penetration, in cells of an Epstein-Barr
         virus genome-negative human lymphoblastoid T line
         (Molt-4). J. Virol., 22:816, 1977

29. Miller, G. Biology of Epstein-Barr virus. In: G. Klein (ed.), Viral Oncology. pp. 713-734. New York: Raven Press, 1980.

30. Miller, G., Grogan,E., Heston, L., Robinson, J., and Smith, D. Epstein-Barr viral DNA: infectivity for human placental cells. Science, 212:457, 1981.

31. Miller, G., Shope, T., Coope, D., Waters, L., Pagano, J., Bornkamm, G.W., and Henle, W. Lymphoma in cotton-topped marmosets after inoculation with Epstein-Barr virus: tumor incidence, histologic spectrum, antibody responses, demonstration of viral DNA, and characterization of viruses. J. Exp. Med., 145:948, 1977.

32. Morgan, D.G., Miller, G., Niederman, J.C., Smith, H.W., and Dowably, J.M. Site of Epstein-Barr virus replication in the oropharynx. Lancet, i:1154, 1979.

33. Mueller-Lantzsch, N., George-Fries, B., Herbst, H., Zur Hausen, H. and Braun, D.G. Epstein-Barr virus strain - and group-specific antigenic determinants detected by monoclonal antibodies. Int. J. Cancer, 28:321, 1981.

34. Okada, Y., Koseki, J., Kim, J., Maeda, Y., Hashimoto, T., Kanno, Y., and Matsui Y. Modification of cell membranes with viral envelopes during fusion of cells with HVJ (Sendai virus). Exp. Cell Res., 93:368,

35. Papahadjopoulos, D., Fraley, R., Heath, T.D., and Straubinger, R.M. Liposomes: recent advances in methodology for introducing macromolecules into eukaryotic cells. Techniques in Cellular Physiology, P114:1, 1981.

36. Pearson, G.R. Epstein-Barr virus: immunology. In: G. Klein (ed.), Viral Oncology. pp. 739-767. New York: Raven Press, 1980.

37. Pellicer, A., Wagner, E.R., Kareh, A., Dewey, M.J., Reuser, A.J., Silverstein, S., Axel, R., and Mintz, B. Introduction of a viral thymidine kinase gene and the human B-globin gene into developmentally multipotential mouse teratocarcinoma cells. Proc. Natl. Acad. Sci. USA, 77(4):2098, 1980.

38. Penn, J. Host origin of lymphomas in organ transplant recipients. Transplantation, 27:214, 1979.

39. Prujansky-Jakobovits, A., Volsky, D.J., Loyter, A., and Sharon, N. Alteration of lymphocyte surface properties by insertion of foreign functional plasma membrane components. Proc. Natl. Acad. Sci. USA, 77:7247, 1980.

40. Purtilo, D.T. Epstein-Barr-virus-induced oncogenesis in immune-deficient individuals. Lancet, i:300, 1980.

41. Purtilo, D.T. Immune deficiency predisposing to Epstein-Barr virus-induced lymphoproliferative diseases: the X-linked lymphoproliferative syndrome as a model. Adv. Cancer Res., 34:279, 1981.

42. Qualtiere, L.F., Chase, R., Broman, B., and Pearson, G.R. Identification of Epstein-Barr virus strain differences

with monoclonal antibody to a member glycoprotein.
Proc. Natl. Acad. Sci. USA, 79:616, 1982.

43.   Qualtiere, L.F. and Pearson, G.R. Radioimmune precipitation
       study comparing the Epstein-Barr virus membrane antigens
       expressed on P3HR-1 virus-superinfected Raji cells to
       those expressed on cells in a B-95 virus transformed
       producer culture activated with Tumor-Promoting agent
       (TPA). Virol., 102:360, 1980.

44.   Read, G.S. Person, S., and Keller, P.M. Genetic studies of
       cell fusion induced by herpes simples virus type 1. J.
       Virology, 35:105, 1980.

45.   Reedman, B.M. and Klein, G. Cellular localization of an
       Epstein-Barr virus (EBV) associated complement-fixing
       antigen in producer and non-producer lymphoblastoid cell
       lines. Int. J. Cancer, 11:499, 1973.

46.   Seshi, B., Volsky, B., Anderson, R., Purtilo, D.T., and
       Volsky, D.J. Infection of normal human thymic epithe-
       lial cells by Epstein-Barr virus (EBV) following implan-
       tation of EBV receptors. Thymus, in press.

47.   Shapiro, I.M., Klein, G., and Volsky, D.J. Epstein-Barr
       virus coreconstituted with Sendai virus envelopes infects
       Epstein-Barr virus receptor-negative cells. Biochem.
       Biophys. Acta, 676:19, 1981.

48.   Shapiro, I.M. and Volsky, D.J. Infection of human
       nasopharyngeal epithelial cells by Epstein-Barr virus
       (EBV) following EBV receptor-transplantation. Science,
       in press.

49.   Shapiro, I.M., Volsky, D.J., Saemundsen, A., Anisimova, E.,
       and Klein, G. Infection of the human T cell-derived
       leukemia line Molt-4 by Epstein-Barr virus (EBV): induc-
       tion of EBV determined antigens and virus production.
       Virol., 120:171, 1982.

50.   Stacey, D.W. and Allfrey, V.G. Evidence of autophagy of
       microinjected proteins in HeLa cells. J. Cell Biol.,
       75:870, 1977.

51.   Stoerker, J., Parris, D., Yajima, Y., and Glaser, R.
       Pleiotropic expression of Epstein-Barr virus DNA in
       human epithelial cells. Proc. Natl. Acad. Sci. USA,
       78(9):5852, 1981.

52.   Summers, W.P., Grogan, E.Z. Shedd, D., Robert, M., Liu,
       Chun-Ren, and Miller, G. Stable expression in mouse
       cells of nuclear neoantigen after transfer of a
       3.4-megadalton cloned fragment of Epstein-Barr virus
       DNA. Proc. Natl. Acad. Sci. USA, 79:5688, 1982.

53.   de-The, G. The role of Epstein-Barr virus in human
       diseases: infectious mononucleosis, Burkitt's lymphoma
       and nasopharyngeal carcinoma. In: G. Klein (ed.), Viral
       Oncology. pp. 769-798. New York: Raven Press, 1980.

54.   Tsukuda, K., Volsky, D.J., Shapiro. I.M., and Klein, G.
       Changed patterns of human B-lymphocyte activation by

Epstein-Barr virus (EBV), following EBV-receptor implantation prior to infection. Eur. J. Immunol., 12:87,
1982.

55. Volsky, D.J. Ahrlund-Richter, L., Dalianis, T., and Klein,
     G. Implantation of mouse histocompatibility antigens
     into membranes of cultured tumor cells. Eur. J.
     Immunol., 11:341, 1981.

56. Volsky, D.J. and Anderson, R. Preleukemia patients have a
     consistent lymphocyte defect as reflected by the defi-
     ciency in Epstein-Barr virus receptors. Submitted for
     publication.

57. Volsky, D.J., Anderson, R., and Kuszynski, C. Establishment
     of permanent cultures from Epstein-Barr virus (EBV)-
     nonsusceptible human lymphocytes. In: J.W. Parker and
     R.C. O'Brien (eds.), 15th International Leukocyte
     Culture Conference. John Wiley & Sons, Inc., in press,
     1983.

58. Volsky, D.J., Cabantchik, Z.I., Beigel, M., and Loyter, A.
     Implantation of human erythrocyte anion channel into
     plasma membrane of friend erythroleukemic cells. Proc.
     Natl. Acad. Sci. USA, 76:5440, 1979.

59. Volsky, D.J., Klein, G., Volsky, B., and Shapiro, I.M.
     Production of infectious Epstein-Barr virus in mouse
     lymphocytes. Nature, 293:399, 1981.

60. Volsky, D.J. and Loyter, A. An efficient method for
     reassembly of fusogeneic Sendai virus envelopes after
     solubilization of intact virions with Triton X-100.
     FEBS Lett., 92:190, 1978.

61. Volsky, D.J., Shapiro, I.M., and Klein, G. Transfer of
     Epstein-Barr virus receptors to receptor-negative cells
     permits virus penetration and antigen expression.
     Proc. Natl. Acad. Sci. USA., 77:5453, 1980.

62. Volsky, D.J., Shapiro, I.M., and Kuszynski, C. A murine
     model system for studying the molecular mechanism of
     Epstein-Barr virus (EBV)-mediated cell transformation
     and carcinogenesis. Fed. Proc., 41:688, 1982.

63. Volsky, B. and Volsky, D.J. Anti-Epstein-Barr virus (EBV)
     immune response in mice inoculated with autologous
     EBV-infected lymphocytes. The Sixth Cold Spring Harbor
     Meeting on Herpesviruses. pp. 83. New York: Cold
     Spring Harbor Lab, 1982.

64. Wigler, M., Sweet, R., Sim, G.K., Wold, B., Pellicer, A.,
     Lacy, E., Maniatis, T., Silverstein, S., and Axel, R.
     Transformation of mammalian cells with genes from pro-
     caryotes and eucaryotes. Cell, 16:777, 1979.

65. Wilson, T., Paphadjopoulos, D., and Taber, R. The introduc-
     tion of poliovirus RNA into cells via lipid vesicles
     (Liposomes). Cell, 17:77, 1979.

66. Yamato, N., Mueller-Lantsch, N., and zur Hausen, H. Effect
     of actinomycin D and cycloheximide on Epstein-Barr virus

early antigen induction of lymphoblastoid cells. J.
Gen. Virol., 51:255, 1980.

67.   Zeuthen, J. and Klein, G.   B-cell and Epstein-Barr Virus
(EBV) associated functions in human cells and hybrids.
In: J.E. Celis, A. Graessman, and A. Loyter (eds.),
Transfer of Cell Constituents into Eukaryotic Cells.
NATO Advanced Study. Series A, pp. 235-262. New York:
Raven Press, 1980.

BIOLOGY OF EPSTEIN-BARR VIRUS

Hans Wolf

Max von Pettenkofer Institute of Hygiene and
Microbiology, University of Munich
Munich, West Germany

INTRODUCTION

Epstein-Barr virus (EBV) has been linked to infectious mono-nucleosis and to the neoplasias, nasopharyngeal carcinoma and Burkitt's lymphoma. The initial evidence of an etiologic rela-tionship was mainly derived from seroepidemiological studies (for review see ref. 1) and confirmed by nucleic acid hybridization with biopsy materials (for review see ref. 2). The work of many laboratories contributed data which does not seem to fit into a unifying concept. This paper briefly summarizes some apparently conflicting results; from these data a hypothetical model for the biology of EBV is developed.

Antibodies directed to viral capsid antigen (VCA) are present in almost the entire adult population. Although 20-30 percent of the population excrete EBV in the saliva, antibodies to EBV early antigen (EA) are usually absent. On the other hand, early anti-gens are major proteins produced during the replication of EBV and potent antigens as judged from immunoprecipitation experiments (3). How can EBV be produced in the body without causing the development of antibodies against certain antigens? EBV genome containing lymphoblastoid cell lines can be established from any individual who has recovered from an EBV infection or by infecting umbilical cord lymphocytes with EBV. Why don't the EBV genome-carrying cells proliferate in normal individuals? To date EBV receptors (in the human system of nonmalignant cells) have only been demonstrated on B lymphocytes (4,5,6), EBV genomes have been demonstrated in the epithelial cells of nasopharyngeal carcinoma (7,8,9). How does EBV manage to enter these cells? Why are EBV related malignancies geographically clustered although the virus

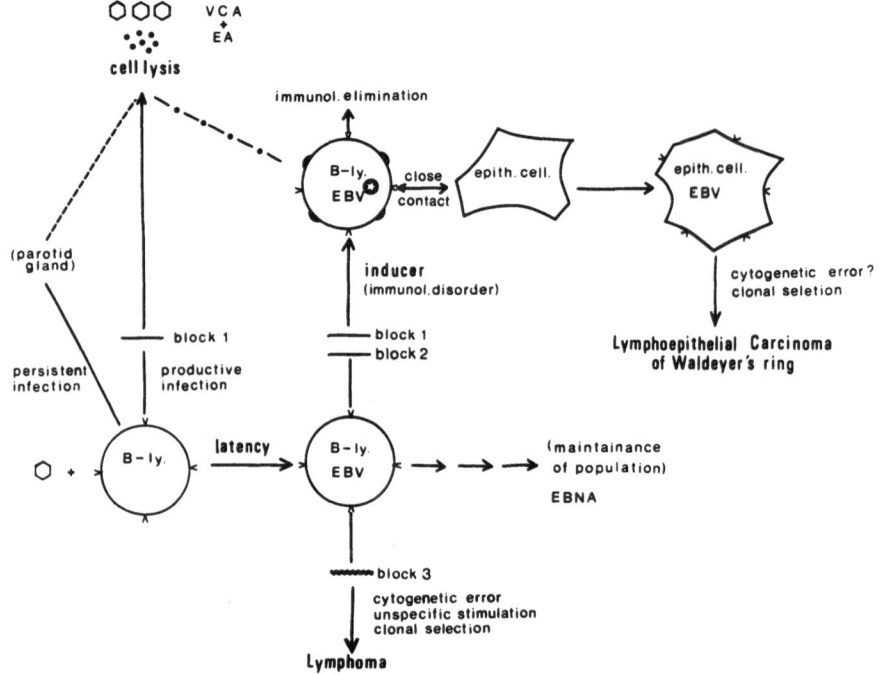

Fig. 1. Hypothesis regarding relationships and mechanisms
         involved in EBV-induced diseases. EBV is introduced into
         epithelial cells owing to close contact and subsequent
         fusion of these cells which allows virus to enter the
         epithelial cell. This gives rise to nasopharyngeal
         carcinoma after a cytogenetic error occurs in the infec-
         ted cell. Latent virus is thought to reside in parotid.
         Immunodeficiency permits infected B cells to proliferate.
         The final step in evolution of a lymphoma maybe a cyto-
         genetic error.

is ubiquitous and individual strain differences could not be
linked to the type of malignancy (10)?

     What follows is a short description of some effects of EBV in
certain model situations. From the observed properties a hypothetical scheme is derived.

Normal EBV Interaction with Host

     a) Primary infection: development of antibodies to VCA, EA
        and EBNA

     EBV enters its natural target cells (B-lymphocytes) upon pri-
mary contact (see figure). Due to the absence of block 1

(cellular response to infection), peripheral B-lymphocytes (in small numbers) enter into a lytic cycle. There is a block within the target cell which leads to a low level of EBV production. A similar block in virus genome free cells found for H. saimiri can be overcome by chemicals like phorbol esters (11). In this case production of EBV in primarily infected B-lymphocytes leads to shedding of virus containing VCA and other viral proteins (EA - early antigen) into the bloodstream and induces the production of antibodies directed to these antigens. Within a few weeks block 1 appears and virus is no longer synthesized in peripheral B-lymphocytes. This means that antigen is no longer available and antibody titers decline (VCA - viral capsid antigen) or disappear (EA). A number (ca. 0.01%) of B-lymphocytes contain EBV genomes and EBNA. These cells are subject to natural turnover and upon lysis liberate EB nuclear-associated antigen (EBNA); therefore antibody forms and persist lifelong.

b) Convalescence: maintenance of antibodies to VCA but not to EA

In seropositive individuals EBV is produced in the parotid gland (12,13,16). Upon lysis, the virus-producing cells in the vicinity of the salivary duct shed EA together with viral particles into the salivary duct. The proteins comprising the EA and VCA antigen complexes are not available to the blood stream and thus do not stimulate the production of antibodies. EA and viral particles (containing VCA) are shed in saliva and digested. Certain B lymphocytes have receptors for EBV particles containing VCA but not EA; some of the VCA is reabsorbed out of the saliva by the lymphocytes in the oropharynx and presented to the immune system as antigen. This may explain the lifelong persistence of antibodies to VCA but not to EA (13).

Special Atypical Conditions

a) Nonspecific secondary antibody titer increases to VCA and EA

Under certain circumstances block 2 (see figure) is reduced. This immunosuppression may be caused by other diseases like Hodgkin's disease and organ transplantation with its associated immune suppression. As a consequence some EBV genome carrying B-lymphocytes from the periphery may enter a lytic cycle, produce EA and VCA, and release it into the blood stream. This causes a secondary increase of antibodies to EA and VCA.

b) Development of nasopharyngeal carcinoma

Certain chemicals, including many methylation inhibitors like TPA, IUdR and cycloleucine, partially overcome block 1. This

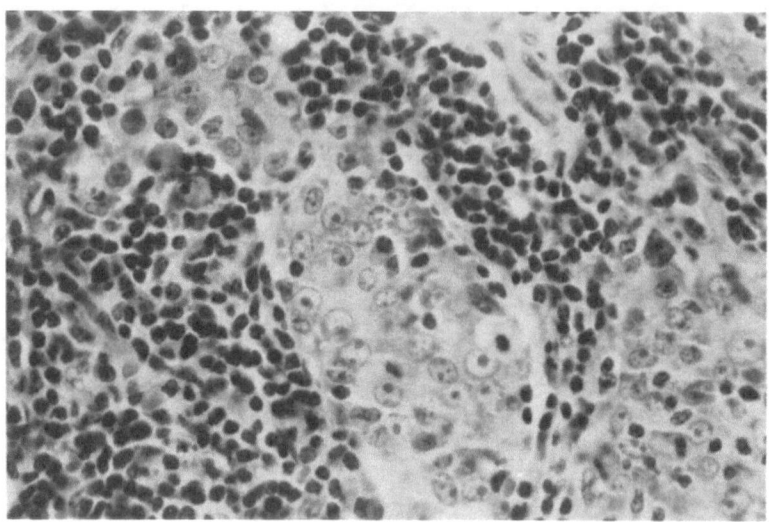

Fig. 2. Photomicrograph of undifferentiated nasopharyngeal carcinoma infiltrated by lymphoid cells. Hematoxylin and
eosin X450.

leads to an (partial?) activation of EBV in carrier lymphocytes.
Lymphocytes which express early EBV genes have the potential to
fuse to EBV receptor negative cells if they are in close contact
(14,15). If EBV-inducing chemicals in the environment are present
for many years, the likelihood of fusion of B cells with epithelial
cells is increased. A close proximity of lymphocyte and epithelial cells occurs particularly in the Waldeyer ring of the oropharynx (17). The photomicrograph displayed below of a nasopharyngeal carcinoma shows the close proximity of lymphoid cells with
the malignant epithelium. In the normal nasopharynx B cells are
located within and beneath the mucosa. Elsewhere in this book
Volsky demonstrates how EBV receptors can be transplanted to
epithelial cells by fusogenic virus. In addition, chemicals or
drugs may specifically reach the lymphocytes in the oropharynx but
not in their active form at other sites of the body. This seems
even more likely if they are administered as ingredients of folk
medication for sore throat as it may occur in the high risk areas
for NPC in China (18). As a consequence it is more likely under
these influences that EBV containing epithelial cells evolve and
that a clone grows out and forms a lymphoepithelial (nasopharyngeal) carcinoma preferentially (20). The lytic expression (block
1) of EBV in epithelial cells may be more suppressed according to
model experiments (20,21). Therefore fusion of a lymphocyte (with
already partially activated EBV genome) and an epithelial cell may
not lead to the death of the fusion product.

The presence of low levels of EBV antigens producing cells in oropharyngeal tissue which is enriched with IgA producing lymphocytes may specifically stimulate the production of IgA specific for EBV-related antigens. These antibodies in turn have a negative influence on antibody-dependent cytotoxicity (ADCC), thus their presence in high concentrations may favor further outgrowth of tumor cells. In this book Krueger describes in detail immune responses to EBV in patients with NPC.

c) Development of Burkitt's lymphoma (monoclonal malignancy)

The very strong block 3 (see figure) may, under rare circumstances, be ineffective and allow the clonal selection of a cell which differs in its antigenic makeup. Environmental mutagens (22) and nonspecific "mitogens" (malaria) (23) which facilitate clonal selection through proliferation may favor this even. Specific cytogenetic aberrations in the selected clones (24) may correlate with the altered antigenic makeup of these cells. A different view of the steps involved in the development of Burkitt's lymphoma has been published by Klein (25).

d) Development of polyclonal B Cell proliferation

Specific genetic constellations X-linked lymphoproliferative syndrome (XLP) or acquired conditions (immune suppresssed transplant recipients) determine a reduced efficiency of block 3 (cellular response to proliferating cells). Therefore the selective pressure on peripheral B-lymphocytes (which already have a potential for unlimited growth by virtue of the resident EBV genomes) may be weaker. Under less stringent selective pressure more cells may proliferate in vivo and lead to a polyclonal lymphoma (25,27). Nonspecific growth stimuli such as the graft may favor initial proliferation and facilitate the selection of cell clones. A specific cytogenetic error (25) may occur under therapy may induce a change from polyclonality to monoclonality. Harada, Purtilo and Hanto describe this conversion to monoclonality elsewhere in this book.

e) Relation to T-cell leukemia

As a side efffect of primary EBV infection, the initial proliferation of B-lymphocytes due to the early absence of block 3 (competent T-cells) apparently leads to a proliferation of T-lymphocytes. This may be caused by growth factors. This polyclonal activation of T-lymphocytes may occasionally activate T-cells with malignant growth potential and lead to a T-cell leukemia following infectious mononucleosis. Conditions c, d and e may convert from polyclonality to monoclonal malignancy when a specific cytogenetic error supervenes.

SUMMARY AND CONCLUSIONS

Several postulates of the hypothesis seem to be supported by experimental data. EBV particles have been isolated from Stensen's duct of the parotid (28). Moreover, EBV DNA containing cells, which most likely are the origin of EBV found in the saliva of normal adults, have been identified in the salivary gland (15,29). EBV-induced cell fusion (14), the activation of latent EBV genes in the lymphoblastoid cells by a number of drugs (30) which may be introduced by environmental factors (17), has been found to be sufficient to enable these cells to fuse to EBV receptor negative cells (15). The probability of fusion events should be dependent on the supply of lymphoid cells with activated early EBV genes at a site where they are in close contact to epithelial cells. An indicator for the presence of EBV activation would be elevated antibody levels of EBV related antigens.

A study contrasting areas with low and high incidence of NPC, performed in China, showed significant differences in their antibody profiles (31). In both areas EBV infections occur at a young age (1 year). This makes possible a role of early infection and the availability of certain young cells as fusion partners (32) less likely. In low NPC incidence areas, the antibody levels normalize after a few months post infection. In contrast, the antibody levels remain high for many months or years in high NPC incidence areas. This probably reflects a continuous activation of otherwise latent EBV in lymphoid cells of the peripheral blood. Fusion may be incomplete and allow transmission of EBV or lymphoid cells producing EBV with (33) karyotypes available from NPC biopsies (34) and the demonstration of EBV receptors on NPC tumor cells, but not on healthy epithelial cells of the same area (35), may point to a more complete fusion.

Noteworthy is the finding that monoclonal lymphoma (Burkitt's lymphoma, BL) lack certain cell markers as compared to lymphoblastoid cells from healthy individuals (36). Similarily, human T-cell leukemia virus (HTLV) transformed T-lymphoid cells may change their HLA markers during proliferation (37).

Although the observations described seem to support the outlined hypothesis, the conclusion must be treated with caution. A final proof or disproof may be very difficult. One way of solving this problem may be the search for lymphoid cell markers on NPC derived cells and the establishment of animal models. Elsewhere in the volume, Volsky described how Sendai virus can be used as an agent for transferring EBV receptors to epithelial cells.

REFERENCES

1. Henle, W. and Henle, G. Seroepidemiology of the virus.
    In: M.A. Epstein and B.G. Achong (eds.), The Epstein-Barr
    Virus. pp. 62-78. New York: Springer, 1979.
2. Wolf, H. The biology of Epstein-Barr virus (EBV) in rela-
    tion to NPC. In: Proceedings of UICC Workshop on
    Nasopharyngeal Carcinoma, in print, 1982.
3. Bayliss, C.G. and Wolf, H. The regulated expression of
    Epstein-Barr virus. III. Proteins specific by EBV
    during the lytic cycle. J. Virol., 56:105, 1981.
4. Jondal, M. and Klein, G. Surface markers on human B and T
    lymphocytes. II. Presence of Epstein-Barr virus recep-
    tors on B lymphocytes. J. Exp. Med., 138:1365, 1973.
5. Glaser, R., Lang, C.M., Lee, K.J., Schuller, D.E., Jacobs,
    D., and McQuattie, C. Attempt to infect nonmalignant
    nasopharyngeal epithelial cells from humans and squirrel
    monkeys with Epstein-Barr virus. J. Natl. Cancer Inst.,
    64:1085, 1980.
6. Wolf, H. and zur Hausen, H. unpublished.
7. Wolf, H., zur Hausen, H., and Becker, V. EB viral genomes in
    epithelial nasopharyngeal carcinoma cells. Nature New
    Biol., 244:245, 1973.
8. Desgranges, C., Wolf, H., de Thé, G., Shanmugaratnam, K.,
    Cammoun, N., Ellouz, R., Klein, G., Lennert, K., Munoz,
    N., and zur Hausen, H. Nasopharyngeal carcinoma. X.
    Presence of Epstein-Barr genomes in separated epithelial
    cells of tumors in patients from Singapore, Tunisia and
    Kenya. Int. J. Cancer, 16:7, 1975.
9. Klein, G., Giovanella, B.C., Lindahl, T., Fialkov, P.J.,
    Singh, S., and Stehlin, J. Direct evidence for the pre-
    sence of Epstein-Barr virus DNA and nuclear antigen in
    malignant epithelial cells from patients with poorly
    differentiated carcinoma of the nasopharynx. Proc.
    Natl. Acad. Sci. USA, 71:4737, 1974.
10. Bornkamm, G.W., Delius, H., Zimber, U., Hudewentz, J., and
    Epstein, M.A. Comparison of Epstein-Barr virus strains
    of different origin by analysis of the viral DNAs. J.
    Virol., 35:603, 1980.
11. Modrow, S. and Wolf, H. Characterization of Herpesvirus
    saimiri and Herpesvirus ateles induced proteins. J. Gen.
    Virol., in press.
12. Wilmes, E. and Wolf, H. Der Nachweis von Epstein-Barr-
    virus-genomen in der Orhspeicheldruse. Laryngol-Rhinol.,
    60:7, 1981.
13. Wolf, H., Wilmes, E., and Bayliss, G.J. Epstein-Barr virus:
    its site of persistence and its role in the development
    of carcinomas. In: Neth et al. (eds.), Modern Trends
    in Human Leukemia IV. pp. 191-196. Heidelberg, Berlin:
    Springer, 1981.

14.   Bayliss, G.J. and Wolf, H.   Epstein-Barr virus-induced cell
      fusion.   Nature, 287:164, 1980.
15.   Bayliss, C.J. and Wolf, H.   An Epstein-Barr virus early
      protein induces cell fusion.   Proc. Natl. Acad. Sci.
      USA, 78:7162, 1981.
16.   Wolf, H., Bayliss, G.J., and Wilmes, E.   Biological prop-
      erties of Epstein-Barr virus.   In: E. Grundmann, G.R.F.
      Krueger, and D.V. Ablashi (eds.), Nasopharyngeal
      Carcinoma.   Vol. 5, pp. 101-109. Gustav Fischer Verlag -
      Stuttgart, 1981.
17.   Döhnert, C.   Ober lymphoepitheliale guschwulste Erkenntnisse
      anhand der Gewekultur und vergleichender klinischer,
      morphologischer under virologischer untersuchungen.   In:
      Sitzungsbericht der Heidelberger Akademie der
      Wissenschaften.   Vol 3, pp. 96-168. Berlin:Springer,
      1977.
18.   Hirayama, T. and Ito, Y.   A new view of the etiology of
      nasopharyngeal carcinoma.   Preventive Medicine, 10:614,
      1981.
19.   Wilmes, E., Wolf, H., Deinhardt, F. and Naumann, H.H. EBV
      serology in NPC and related malignancies.   In: E.
      Grundman, G.R.F. Krueger, and D.V. Ablashi (eds.),
      Cancer Campaign.   Nasopharyngeal Carcinoma.   Vol. 5, pp.
      145-150.   Gustav Fischer Verlag - Stuttgart, 1981.
20.   Glaser, R., Zimmermann, J., St. Jeor, S., and Rapp, F.
      Demonstration of a cellular inhibitor of Epstein-Barr
      and cytomegalovirus synthesis.   Virology, 64:289, 1975.
21.   Graessmann, A., Wolf, H., and Bornkamm, G.W.   Expression of
      Epstein-Barr virus genes in different cell types after
      microinjection of viral DNA.   Proc. Natl. Acad. Sci. USA,
      77:433, 1980.
22.   Birnboim, H.C.   DNA strand breakage in human leukocytes
      exposed to a tumour promoter, phorbol myristate acetate.
      Science, 215:1247, 1982.
23.   Burkitt, D.P.   Etiology of Burkitt's lymphoma - an alter-
      native hypothesis to a vectored virus.   J. Natl. Cancer
      Inst., 42:19, 1969.
24.   Manolova, Y., Manolov, G., Keiler, J., Levan, A., and Klein,
      G.   Pseudo-Burkitt lymphoma marker 14 in lymphoblastoid
      cell lines.   Hereditas, 90:5, 1979.
25.   Klein, G.   Lymphoma development in mice and humans:
      diversity of initiation is followed by convergent
      cytogenetic evolution.   Proc. Natl. Acad. Sci. USA,
      76:1221, 1979.
26.   Purtilo, D.T.   Epstein-Barr-virus-induced oncogenesis in
      immune-deficient individuals.   Lancet, 1:300, 1980.
27.   Purtilo, D.T.   Immune deficiency predisposing to
      Epstein-Barr virus-induced lymphoproliferative diseases:
      the X-linked lymphoproliferative syndrome as a model.
      In: G. Klein and S. Weinhouse (eds.), Advances in Cancer

Research. Vol. 34, pp. 279-312. New York: Academic
Press, 1980.

28. Morgan, D.G., Miller, G., Niedermann, J.C., Smith, H.W., and
     Dowaliby, J.M. Site of Epstein-Barr virus replication
     in the oropharynx. Lancet, ii:1154, 1979.

29. Wolfe, H., Haus, M., and Wilmes, E. Submitted.

30. zur Hausen, H., Bornkamm, G.W., Schmidt, R., and Hecker, E.
     Tumor initiators and promoters in the induction of
     Epstein-Barr virus. Proc. Natl. Acad. Sci. USA, 76:782,
     1979.

31. Institute of Virology, Beijing. A study on the serum level
     of complement fixing antibody to EB virus in groups of
     individuals of Guangdong province and Beijing. Chinese
     J. Otorhinolaryngol., 13:23, 1978.

32. Jaenisch, R. Retroviruses and embryogenesis: microinjection
     of Moloney leukemia virus into midgestation mouse
     embryos. Cell, 19:181, 1980.

33. Seigneurin, J.-M., Vuillaume, M., Lenoir, G., and de Thé, G.
     Replication of Epstein-Barr virus: ultrastructural and
     immunofluorescent studies of P3HR1-superinfected Raji
     cells. J. Virol., 24:836, 1977.

34. Finerty, S., Jarvis, J.E., Epstein, M.A., Tramper, P.A.,
     Ball, G., and Giovanella, B.C. Cytogenetics of
     malignant epithelial cells and lymphoblastoid cell lines
     from nasopharyngeal carcinoma. Br. J. Cancer, 37:231,
     1978.

35. Glaser, R., de The, G., Lenoir, G., and Ho, J.H. Superinfec-
     tion of epithelial nasopharyngeal carcinoma cells with
     Epstein-Barr virus. Proc. Natl. Acad. Sci. USA, 73:960,
     1976.

36. Kintner, C.H. and Sugden, B. Identification of antigenic
     determinants unique to the surfaces of cells transformed
     by Epstein-Barr virus. Nature, 294:458, 1981.

37. Reitz, M.S., Jr., Popovic, M., Kalyanaraman, V.S.,
     Robert-Guroff, M., Broder, S., Mann, D., and Gallo, R.C.
     Human T-cell leukemia-lymphoma virus (HTLV): presence
     in a T-cell subset from infected patients. In: R. Neth,
     R. Gallo, T. Graf, K. Mannweiler, and K. Winkler (eds.),
     Modern Trends in Human Leukemia. Vol. IV. Berlin:
     Springer-Verlag, in press.

HERPESVIRUS-INDUCED LYMPHOPROLIFERATIVE DISEASES

IN NON-HUMAN PRIMATES

Donald R. Johnson

Department of Pathology & Laboratory Medicine
University of Nebraska Medical Center
Omaha, Nebraska 68105

INTRODUCTION

Non-human primate experimental models for Herpes virus-induced lymphoproliferative diseases.

The association of Herpesviruses and lymphoid cells is found in many species, including man. Examples include Marek's disease in chickens, Herpesvirus saimiri (HVS) in squirrel monkeys, Herpesvirus ateles (HVA) in spider monkeys, Herpesvirus papio (HVP) in baboons, and Epstein-Barr virus (EBV) in man. Under normal circumstances, these viruses are kept under control by multiple immunological surveillance systems. They do not induce disease except in rare instances of immunosuppression which are influenced by environmental co-factors or due to genetically determined immunodeficiency states (31). Under these circumstances of immunodeficiency, oncogenic effects of lymphotropic Herpesviruses are found. The search for an experimental model system for studying both the oncogenic potential and the mechanisms of tumor formation by the lymphotropic Herpesviruses was facilitated by the finding that certain species of New World primates were susceptible to virus-induced lymphoproliferative diseases. Of the species of primates tested as potential models for viral carcinogenesis, the marmoset (Saguinus species) has proven to be most susceptible to a broad range of viruses (69). For example, the marmoset is susceptible to EBV as are immune deficient men.

In this chapter three primate associated lymphotropic Herpesviruses and their induction of fatal lymphoproliferative diseases in cotton-topped tamarins are discussed and compared.

243

These findings may elucidate the oncogenic potential of lymphotropic Herpesviruses and information may be gained regarding
the relevance of immunosurveillance systems against certain viruses inducing neoplasms in man.

Simian Lymphotropic Herpesviruses

A. Herpesvirus saimiri (HVS) and Herpesvirus ateles (HVA)

1. Natural hosts

HVS was originally isolated from kidney cell cultures of
a squirrel monkey (Saimiri sciureus). It is carried in the
circulating T lymphocytes of the natural host (5,8,41,43,66).
On removal of lymphoid cells from squirrel monkeys, and
culture with a permissive monolayer cells, the virus is recovered. HVS is present in most squirrel monkeys but does not
induce an overt disease in the natural host, even when the
monkeys are treated with immunosuppressive agents (39). Klein
and associates have defined an HVS early antigen (EA) complex
and Pearson et al. have described late antigens (LA) and
membrane antigens on infected cells which are similar to viral
envelope antigens (29,50,51).

HVA was first isolated in 1970 from primary kidney
cultures of healthy spider monkeys (Ateles geoffroyi) (44).
As with HVS, the target cells for HVA are lymphoid cells under
natural conditions (9). HVA can also infect fibroblastic or
epithelial cell cultures in vitro leading to cytopathic
effects typical of herpesvirus (5,9). HVA and HVS share
cross-reacting viral antigens; including a virus-associated
nuclear antigen (HATNA) which is detected by an acid-fixed
nuclear-binding technique. Detection of HATNA has been found
to be related to the number of viral genome equivalents/cell
(5,9,26,29). HVA transforms marmoset monkey lymphocytes in
vitro leading to permanent T cell lines (12). Recently, HVS
have transformed marmoset T lymphocytes in vitro which had
been preconditioned with T cell growth factor (TCGF) (IL-2)
(13).

2. Experimental infection

Both HVA and HVS are highly oncogenic when inoculated
into New World primates which are closely related to their
natural host. They consistently induce a fatal lymphoproliferative disease in cotton-topped marmosets (Saguinus
oedipus), white-lipped marmosets (Saguinus fuscicollis, S.
nigricollis), and common marmosets (Callithrix jacchus)
(5,8,16,33-35,41,67-69). The infected marmosets succumb to a
rapidly progressing neoplasm. The cotton-topped marmoset

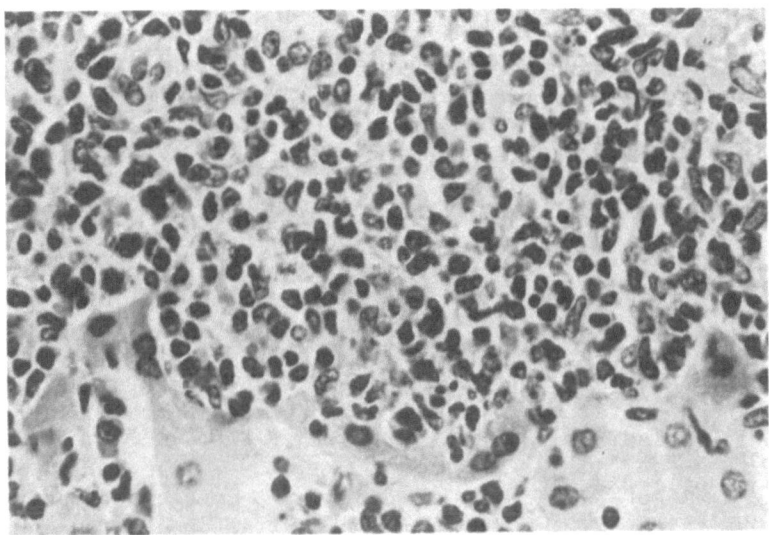

Fig. 1.   Photomicrograph of liver from cotton-topped marmoset
          infected with Herpes saimiri virus. A large sheet of
          twisted, irregular shaped T cells are seen infiltrating
          the sinuses. This is in contrast to the more uniform
          round nuclei of EBV-induced B cell proliferation (see
          figure 2). Hematoxylin and eosin X460.

shows lymphadenopathy and splenomegaly ten days to two weeks
post-inoculation. Time of death usually occurs at four to
seven weeks and depends on the dose of infecting virus. The
white-lipped marmosets have a less severe and a wider variability of disease after HVA or HVS inoculation. Both viruses
can induce a lymphoma which is universally fatal. The common
marmosets are not consistently susceptible to HVS induction of
lymphoma but they are completely sensitive to HVA.

The pathological features of the HVS and HVA-induced
lymphoproliferative diseases have been extensively described
(5,22,23,69). The major clinical features and pathological
findings after HVS and HVA injection include generalized
lymphadenopathy, hepatosplemomegaly, and leukocytosis; usually
more severe with HVS infection. Peripheral blood shows high
percentages of atypical prolymphocytes and lymphoblasts.
Necropsy reveals cellular infiltrates distributed widely
throughout lymphoid organs, liver, kidneys, and other tissues.
Dense infiltrates of lymphoreticular cells replace the normal
cytoarchitecture (Fig. 1). The experimentally induced
neoplasia due to HVS or HVA has been classified as diffuse

lymphoma of the poorly differentiated lymphocytic type
(22,23,69). HVS induced tumors are polyclonal in origin as
determined by chromosome analysis of cell lines from tumors of
hematopoietic-chimeric marmosets which contain both XX and XY
cells (38). HVS and HVA derived tumor cell lines can be
cultured in vitro as suspension cultures and they express T-
lymphocyte surface markers (5,9,12,69). Adsorption assays for
HVS and HVA reveal that T cells, thymocytes, and T cell lines
are specific targets for infection by these viruses (24,25).
The tumor cells do not express viral antigens in vivo.
However, after a short term in culture in vitro; HVS- and
HVA-carrying tumor cells express EA and LA and produce small
amounts of infectious virus (5). Tumor cells or the infected
organs of HVS or HVA infected marmosets contain significant
amounts of viral DNA which can be detected by molecular
hybridization and reassociation kinetics (16).

Marmosets infected with HVS or HVA develop antibodies to
both viral antigens, LA and EA, and virus neutralizing antibodies (29,50,51). These antibodies appear two to three weeks
post infection. Titers increase until the animals die. In
vitro cellular immune responses to HVS and HVA infected cells
have been described (1).

In summary, HVA and HVS are T lymphotropic herpesviruses
of South American non-human primates and have the ability to
transform (immortalize) lymphoid cells. The virus-carrying
potentially neoplastic cells are kept under strict immunosurveillance in the natural host, but these viruses can induce a
rapidly proliferating lymphoid malignancy when inoculated into
a closely related animal. Presumably these animals have inadequate immune responses to these viruses.

B. Epstein-Barr virus

1. Disease in man

Epstein-Barr virus or EBV is a ubiquitous virus that
infects the majority of humans around the world. EBV is the
causative agent of infectious mononucleosis (IM), a self-
limited lymphoproliferative disease of man (21). Moreover,
life-threatening EBV-carrying lymphoproliferative diseases
have been identified in immunosuppressed allograft recipients
and individuals with genetically-determined immunodeficiencies
whose immune defenses to EBV are defective (52). Most of
these diseases are polyclonal. In contrast, true neoplasms
associated with EBV, Burkitt's lymphoma and nasopharyngeal
carcinoma, are monoclonal proliferations of EBV-carrying cells
(30). In these cases, EBV may initiate by immortalizing the
target cell, but additional cellular (presumably genetic)

changes may be responsible for the emergence of the monoclonal neoplastic clone (32).

EBV in vitro has the capacity to transform normal B lymphocytes of man and certain non-human primates into continuous lymphoblastoid cell cultures (LCL) (20). The LCL established in vitro and cell lines established from infectious mononucleosis from normal seropositive donors carry the EBV genome, express an EBV specific nuclear antigen (EBNA), are polyclonal and diploid, fail to grow in the subcutaneous space in nude mice and have low cloning efficiency in agarose. In contrast, EBV-carrying Burkitt lymphoma cell lines are monoclonal, not diploid, have a specific 8;14 chromosome translocation, have the ability to grow as malignant tumors subcutaneously in nude mice, and have high cloning efficiency in agarose (14,15,37,48,70). EBV is postulated to initiate immortalization; but due to the continuous stimulation by an environmental co-factor (i.e., holoendemic malaria for Burkitt's lymphoma), chances for a cytogenetic change increase (i.e., 8;14). This specific, reciprocal translocation is thought to endow the cell with the ability to escape regulatory mechanisms and hence an autonomous neoplastic clone emerges. Cells carrying 8;14 translocation have been found to have proliferative advantage over cells without chromosomal abnormalities (18).

Recently, multiple EBV-genome and EBNA positive cells have been found within the lymphoproliferative lesions of fatal or chronic infectious mononucleosis and X-linked lymphoproliferative syndrome (XLP) and in "lymphomas" of renal transplant recipients, and one lymphoma in an ataxia telangiectasia patient (4,19,53,56-58). The exact localization and distribution of the EBV genomes, clonality, and the cytogenetic status of the proliferating lymphoid cells in these lesions, remains to be more fully characterized. Fragmentary evidence now available suggests that the majority of EBV-provoked diseases in the immunodeficient patients are polyclonal and diploid. If so, they would in all likelihood, be due to a failure of multiple immune defense mechanisms exhibited by some of these patients rather than changes at the target cellular level (40,59,60,63).

2. Experimental infection

To study the oncogenic potential of EBV and the mechanisms of oncogenesis, New World non-human primates have been used as experimental models. Cotton-topped marmosets (Saguinus oedipus), owl monkeys (Aotus species), common marmosets (Callithrix jacchus), white-lipped marmosets (Saguinus fusciocollis), and squirrel monkeys (Saimiri species) are susceptible to EBV-induced disease (7,10,28,36,61,64,65). The cotton-topped marmoset (CTM) is particularly vulnerable to EBV-induced lymphoproliferative disease. Studies with EBV and CTM have revealed anti-EBV antibodies are not found in monkeys in their natural state. EBV also can infect marmoset B lymphocytes <u>in vitro</u>. Cell-free EBV, cell-associated virus, and autologous transformed cells can induce fatal lymphoproliferative diseases in approximately one-third of inoculated animals (11,17,45,46). The histopathology has been described as similar to Burkitt's lymphoma or immunoblastic sarcoma (46). The other two-thirds of the inoculated marmosets develop inapparent infection and silent seroconversion or illness including severe lymphoid hyperplasia. The antibody response of inoculated marmosets to EBV induced antigens is often delayed and of low titer. No antibodies develop to the EBV determined nuclear antigen (EBNA) (6,46). This lack of anti-EBNA production is comparable to that seen in children with T cell defects (59).

EBV-induced lymphoproliferative disease in the cotton-topped marmoset has been considered a model of Burkitt's lymphoma in man; but the question remains whether the previously described malignant lymphoma of marmosets is a true lymphoma (i.e., a counterpart of Burkitt's lymphoma), or rather an example of a fatal infectious mononucleosis as occurring in an immunodeficient person with X-linked lymphoproliferative syndrome or in a renal transplant patient. Infection of marmoset monkeys with EBV leads to peripheral lymphadenopathy (inguinal, axillary, cervical, mandibular) first detected around three weeks after inoculation. It usually progresses to pronounced lymphadenopathy (6,28,46). At four to six weeks post-infection, approximately one-third of the animals with prominent lymphadenopathy show inactivity, weakness, anorexia, and die. Peripheral lymph nodes in the survivors decrease in size after approximately six weeks. They return to normal by eight to ten weeks post-infection. During the time of persistent lymphadenopathy, total leukocyte counts increase and the percentage of lymphocytes ranges from 30 to 85%. Atypical circulating lymphocytes are not usually detected. But with abatement of peripheral lymphadenopathy, hematologic values return to normal.

Animals that die of lymphoproliferative disease manifest peripheral and visceral lymphadenopathy, hepatosplenomegaly, enlarged tonsils and thymuses, and focal ulcerative colitis or ileitis. Mesocenteric, paraaortic and pelvic lymphadenopathy is also pronounced. Spleens are enlarged four to six times above normal in size, are friable and necrotic.

Microscopically, the disseminated lymphoproliferative lesions
are comparable to cases of fatal infectious mononucleosis
(52).

Lesions in lymph nodes, spleens, tonsils, and thymus are
characterized by extensive proliferation and/or massive necrosis. The degree of lymphoproliferation in lymph nodes is
variable from node to node, and from area to area in the same
node. Lesions range from mild follicular hyperplasia to focal
and nodular proliferation to diffuse replacement of the normal
cytoarchitecture. The nodular and diffuse proliferative
lesions are composed primarily of immunoblasts and to a lesser
extent, cells with plasmacytoid appearance; mitotic features
are numerous. The extent of necrosis varies from no necrosis
to small focal areas to diffuse necrosis of the entire node.
In the spleen, severe infiltration of lymphoid cells causing
markedly splenic enlargement is readily apparent, nearly all
lymphoid cells are necrotic. Only scattered periarterial
cuffs and small islands of subcapsular proliferating
lymphoblasts remain viable. The tonsils and thymuses are
replaced by dense immunoblastic infiltrates associated with

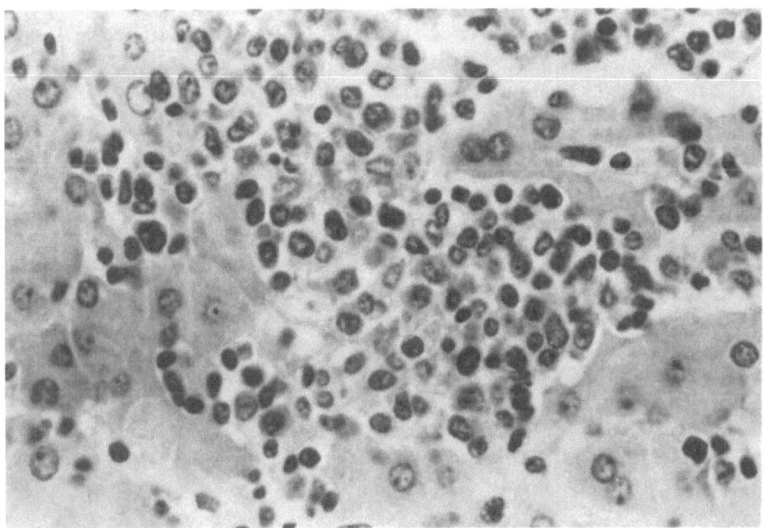

Fig. 2. Photomicrograph of liver from cotton-topped marmoset.
The animal was infected with EBV and a lymphopro-
liferative disease ensued. Note the heterogeneous popu-
lation of lymphocytes infiltrating and expanding sinuses.
Plasmacytoid features are seen. Hematoxylin and eosin
X460.

marked necrosis. Skeletal muscle underlining the tonsils is
invaded by lymphoid cells and bone marrow is hypercellular due
to immunoblastic infiltrates.

Visceral organs show extensive lymphoproliferation.
Hepatic lesions are characterized by extensive periportal and
sinusoidal infiltration of immunoblastic and plasmacytoid
cells (Fig. 2). Sites of focal ulceration in the ileum and
the colon are grossly apparent. They contain immunoblastic
infiltrates and necrosis is found. Immunoblastic infiltrates
are present in perivascular and interstitial tissues of kidney
cortices. They surround bronchi, bronchioles, and pulmonary
vessels and invade the cortex and medulla of adrenal glands.

Although the fatal lymphoproliferative disease observed
in EBV inoculated cotton-topped marmosets is superficially
similar to Burkitt's lymphoma, careful morphological examination of these tumors has revealed that they more closely
resemble fatal infectious mononucleosis in man. The proliferating cells are usually very heterogenous including many
immunoblasts and plasmacytoid cells (Fig. 2).

EBV induced tumor cells removed from animals have the
properties of B lymphocytes, express EBNA and a small percentage of these cells express EA and VCA after culture in vitro
(Table 1). These cultured tumor cells express chiefly IgM on
their surface, but a small percentage express IgG and IgD, and
both kappa and lambda staining cells. Recent studies have

Table 1. Properties of EBV-induced Marmoset Tumor Cells

1) Morphology	Lymphoblastoid, B cells
2) EBV antigen expression[1]	EBNA
	EA
	VCA
3) Surface immunoglobulin	IgM
	IgG
	IgD
4) Immunoglobulin production[2]	IgM
	IgG
5) Colony formation in agarose	Low
6) Tumorigenicity	No tumors induced in nude mice
7) Karyotype	Normal diploid

[1]EBNA = Epstein-Barr virus nuclear antigen, EA = Early antigen,
VCA = Viral capsid antigen.
[2]Immunoglobulin production in supernate of tumor cell culture.

shown that the tumor cells also can secrete IgM, IgG, and both kappa and lambda light chains into the culture medium (28). These tumor cells, when tested for ability to form colonies in agarose, show a very low cloning efficiency, comparable to in vitro established marmoset and human cell lines. They do not show the high cloning efficiency of Burkitt lymphoma cells (49). These "tumors" appear to be polyclonal lymphoproliferations as judged by the presence of immunoglobulin heavy and light chains which can be detected by both surface staining and immunoglobulin secretion in vitro. Deinhardt et al. have previously reported that cell lines established from EBV induced lymphomas in marmosets were also multiclonal by cytoplasmic immunoglobulin studies (6).

There is, however, one reported EBV induced lymphoma in marmosets which may have been monoclonal: a marker chromosome was observed in three cell lines derived from the tumor (54).

The EBV lymphoid cell lines established from marmoset tumors express surface IgD, a differentiation marker not found on Burkitt's lymphoma cells, but associated with EBV conversion as cells enter the terminal phase of cellular differentiation (62). Moreover, EBV induced marmoset tumor cells inoculated subcutaneously into nude mice showed no tumor development in these immune deficient animals (28). Thus EBV-induced lymphomas in cotton-topped marmosets are more similar to fatal infectious mononucleosis and the EBV-associated proliferations in renal transplant and XLP patients than to Burkitt's lymphoma.

The role of a specific chromosomal change in EBV induced lymphomas in lymphomagenesis can be evaluated in the marmoset experimental model. Burkitt's lymphoma derived cell lines have a reciprocal 8;14 translocation (37). Since this marker is regularly present in the monoclonal Burkitt's lymphoma, no matter whether it is EBV-carrying or EBV-negative, whereas it is equally regularly absent from EBV-transformed lymphoblastoid cell lines of normal origin, it is important and perhaps decisive in Burkitt lymphomagenesis. Previous karyotyping of EBV established LCL from cotton-topped marmosets has shown it to be relatively easy to detect major rearrangements such as deletions and translocations. Newly established lines have normal diploid chromosomes (27). Recent studies of karyotypic analysis of marmoset cell lines derived from EBV-induced lymphomas reveal no consistent deletions or translocations, indicative of the specific rearrangement similar to Burkitt's lymphoma or other lymphomas (28).

Humoral immunity to EBV is defective in marmosets. Animals inoculated with EBV develop low titer (1:20-1:40)

antibodies to VCA between six – eight weeks post-inoculation.
Antibodies to EA are also found at similar times in EBV inoculated marmosets (1:5-1:10) (28,46). Some marmosets develop
lymphoma before anti-EBV antibodies are detected. Marmosets
infected with EBV rarely develop antibody to EBNA. Animals
tested up to eighteen weeks post-infection have no antibodies
to EBNA. This poor response to EBNA is similar to what has
been reported in cases of fatal infectious mononucleosis and
the X-linked lymphoproliferative syndrome. Both may reflect
natural killer cell (NK) or T-cell defects in responding to
virus infected cells (2,3,40,55).

Also defective cell mediated immune responses of cotton-
topped marmosets to EBV transformed lymphoblastoid cell lines
have been demonstrated. Responses are markedly deficient when
compared to man (1). An example, presented in Table 2, shows
that man can react with a very powerful lymphocyte proliferation response to autologous, allogeneic, or xenogeneic cells
infected with EBV. In contrast, the cotton-topped marmoset
has very low reactivity to EBV infected autologous or allogeneic cells. The NK cell response to EBV infected cells
has also been evaluated. The NK cell may be relevant in
eliminating potential EBV tumor cells (3). As shown in Table
3, five species of marmosets were tested in an NK-cell cytotoxicity assay against two non-EBV-carrying tumor cell lines
and two EBV Burkitt lymphoma cell lines. At least in the in
vitro assay, the cotton-topped and common marmoset are deficient in killing EBV tumor cells when they are compared to
other species of marmosets or man.

The cotton-topped and common marmoset are the most
vulnerable species to EBV-induced disease. EBV-induced

Table 2. Proliferative Responses of Marmoset Lymphocytes
          to EBV-lymphoblastoid Cell Lines

Effector Cells	Stimulator Cells			
	Autologous	EBV Autologous	EBV Allogeneic	EBV Xenogeneic
Marmosets[1]	$1.05+0.04$[3]	$2.81+0.85(2.7)$	$3.70+0.58$	$11.00+4.4$
Human[2]	2.2 ∓ 0.1	$16.55 \mp 3.15(7.5)$	13.8 ∓ 5.45	35.8 ∓ 6.9

[1] 8 cotton-topped marmosets tested 3-5 times
[2] EBV-positive adults tested 3-5 times
[3] ^{3}H-Thymidine incorporation $\pm$ S.E., mean CPM X 10^3

Table 3. Comparison of Natural Killer Cell-mediated Cytotoxicity of Five Marmoset Subspecies against 4 Human Tumor Cell Lines

| Source of Natural Killer Cells | T A R G E T   C E L L S | | | |
	MOLT-4	K562	DAUDI(EBV+)	RAJI(EBV+)
1 Saguinus oedipus (Cotton-top)	25*	24	6	2
2 Saguinus fuscicollis (White-lip)	31	25	21	10
3 Saguinus mystax (White moustached)	68	99	60	56
4 Saguinus labiatus (Red bellied)	59	73	40	35
5 Callithrix jacchus (Common)	13	9	2	0
6 Human peripheral blood	71	87	43	11

*% cytotoxicity at 20:1 effector: target ratio, mean of 4 animals in each group tested two times.
MOLT-4 = Acute lymphocytic leukemia
K562 = Chronic myelocytic leukemia
Daudi = Burkitt lymphoma
Raji = Burkitt lymphoma

disease has been reported in only one white-lipped marmoset (64). Perhaps, cotton-topped marmosets have never developed the genetic apparatus required to mount a vigorous immune response (Ir) against this life-threatening lymphotropic virus. EBV evolved in man after the continents of Africa and South America had separated approximately 50 million years ago. The New World monkeys evolved after EBV arose from a Herpesvirus on the African continent. Thus cotton-topped marmosets have not been exposed to EBV during evolution and they probably have not developed immune response genes to cope with this virus. The marmoset is a very reclusive animal and thus in its natural habitat does not come into contact with man.

In man, a powerful autologous stimulation reaction occurs when normal peripheral lymphocytes are confronted with

EBV-carrying B-cell lines. Perhaps this reaction reflects the
selective preadaptation of humans to this virus or merely
reflects the way normal lymphocytes (mainly T-cells) react
toward autologous B-cells. Potentially, oncogenic viruses
that have ubiquitous occurrence in the natural host species
may select the host through fixation of appropriate Ir genes,
for efficient recognition of viral induced membrane antigens.
Hence rejection of most or all tumor cell precursors created
by the viral transformation occurs. Given that the autologous
lymphocyte stimulation reaction occurring in the EBV system is
as strong or stronger than the strongest mixed lymphocyte
culture reaction across major histocompatibility barriers, it
is conceivable that this reaction is a valid expression of
immune surveillance. Cotton-topped marmosets do have diminished autologous stimulation reactions and NK reactivity to
EBV-infected cells when compared to man. This diminished
response may explain their vulnerability to EBV induced
diseases (1). This immunologic deficiency expressed by marmosets to Herpesvirus transformed cell lines may also be
related to their hematopoietic chimerism (47).

SUMMARY AND CONCLUSIONS

     The lymphotropic Herpesviruses are important models of lym-
phomagenesis because they demonstrate lymphoproliferative diseases
in their natural hosts as well as in certain experimental hosts.
The answers to basic questions concerning the immunological
control mechanisms which have evolved and have been fixed by
selection to prevent the development of potential neoplastic cells
are now being approached. Patients under immunosuppression or
with genetic immunodeficiencies and certain experimental non-human
primate models can provide further information to explain this
complicated process. Study of the immunopathology of cotton-
topped marmosets inoculated with HVA and HVS, T-lymphotropic
herpesvirus of New World primates; and EBV and EBV-related, B
lymphotropic herpesviruses of man and the Old World primates can
help answer these clinical and basic questions. HVA and HVS in
marmosets induces a fatal lymphoproliferative disease, different
from a true neoplasia because of the multiclonal origin of the
tumor cells. As such, it may be considered a "T-cell malignant
mononucleosis." EBV, in most instances, can induce a lymphoproliferation relatively similar to a fatal infectious mononucleosis of transplant or X-linked lymphoproliferative syndrome
patients. The marmosets (particularly the cotton-topped marmoset)
are deficient in many of the multiple effectors which control
virus-carrying proliferating cell lines. Experiments need to be
done to dissect this phenomena. The similarity of these diseases
in marmosets and EBV infections in man indicate that these animals
may be a powerful model for studying the immunopathology of virus

induced lymphoproliferative diseases of humans. In addition, the uses of immunotherapy or vaccines for treating or preventing illness can be studied.

ACKNOWLEDGEMENTS

The author gratefully acknowledges the excellent assistance of Mrs. Elisabeth Levan, Mrs. Barbara Ehlin-Hendrickson, Ms. Kerstin Falk, and Dr. James Ogden. Professors Karl Lennert, George Klein, Göran Levan, Lauren Wolfe, and Dr. David Purtilo were generous in evaluating the tumor tissue and in consultation. I also wish to thank Dr. Werner Henle for EBV-antibody titrations. These studies were supported by funds provided by: The Swedish Cancer Society, Cancer International Research Cooperative (Cancirco) and NIH Grant CA 23561.

Donald R. Johnson was the recipient of a post-doctoral fellowship from the Cancer Research Institute, Inc.

We thank the Board of Health, City of Chicago, for housing the experimental animals.

REFERENCES

1. Abb, J., Abb, H., and Deinhardt, F. Cell-mediated immune response of marmosets to Herpesvirus associated antigens in vitro. Cancer Immunol. Immunother., 9:219, 1980.
2. Bar, R.S., Deler, C.J., Clausen, K.P., Hurtubise, P., Henle, W., and Hewetson, J.F. Fatal infectious mononucleosis in a family. N. Engl. J. Med., 290:363, 1974.
3. Blazar, B., Patarroyo, M., Klein, E., and Klein, G. Increased sensitivity of human lymphoid lines to natural killer cells after induction of the Epstein-Barr viral cycle by superinfection or sodium butyrate. J. Exp. Med., 151:614, 1980.
4. Britton, S., Andersson-Anvret, M., Gergely, P., Henle, W., Jondal, M., Klein, G., Sandstedt, B., and Svedmyr, E. Epstein-Barr virus immunity and tissue distribution in a fatal case of infectious mononucleosis. N. Engl. J. Med., 288:89, 1978.
5. Deinhardt, F.W., Falk, L.A., and Wolfe, L.G. Simian Herpesvirus and neoplasia. In: G. Klein and S. Weinhouse (eds.), Advances in Cancer Research. Vol. 19, pp. 167-205. New York: Academic Press, 1974.
6. Deinhardt, F., Falk, L., Wolfe, L.G., Paciga, J., and Johnson, D.R. Response of marmosets to experimental infection with Epstein-Barr virus. In: G. DeThe, M.A. Epstein and H. zur Hausen (eds.), Oncogenesis and

Herpesvirus II. Vol. 11, pp. 161-168. IARC Scientific
Publications, 1975.

7.   Epstein, M.A., Hunt, R.D., and Rabin, H. Pilot experiments
     with EB virus in owl monkeys (Aotus trivirgatus). I.
     Reticuloproliferative disease in an inoculated animal.
     Int. J. Cancer, 12:309, 1973.

8.   Falk, L.A., Wolfe, L.G., and Deinhardt, F. Isolations of
     Herpesvirus saimiri from blood of squirrel monkeys
     (Saimiri sciureus). J. Natl. Cancer Inst.,
     48:1499, 1972.

9.   Falk, L.A., Nigida, S.M., Deinhardt, F., Wolfe, L.G.,
     Cooper, R.W., and Hernandez-Camacho, J.I. Herpesvirus
     ateles: properties of an oncogenic Herpesvirus isolated
     from circulating lymphocytes of spider monkeys (Ateles
     sp.). Int. J. Cancer, 14:473, 1974.

10. Falk, L., Deinhardt, F., Wolfe, L., Johnson, D., Hilgers,
     J., and DeThe, G. Epstein-Barr virus. Experimental
     infection of Callithrix jacchus marmosets. Int. J.
     Cancer, 13:785, 1976.

11. Falk, L., Wolfe, L., Deinhardt, F., Paciga, J., Dombros, L.,
     Klein, G., Henle, W., .and Henle, G. Epstein-Barr virus:
     transformation of nonhuman primate lymphocytes in vitro.
     Int. J. Cancer, 13:363, 1974.

12. Falk, L., Johnson, D., and Deinhardt, F. Transformation of
     marmoset lymphocytes in vitro with Herpesvirus ateles.
     Int. J. Cancer, 21:652, 1978.

13. Falk, L. Personal communication.

14. Fialkow, P.J. Human tumors studied with genetic markers.
     Birth Defects, 12:123, 1976.

15. Fialkow, P.J., Klein, G., Gartler, S.M., and Clifford, P.
     Clonal origin for individual Burkitt tumours. Lancet,
     1:384, 1970.

16. Fleckenstein, B., Bornkamm, G.W., and Werner, F.J. The role
     of Herpesvirus saimiri genomes in oncogenic transfor-
     mation of primate cells. In: Comparative Leukemia
     Research 1975. Biblthca haemat. No. 43, pp. 308-312.
     Karger, Basel, 1976.

17. Frank, A., Andiman, W.A., and Miller, G. Epstein-Barr virus
     and nonhuman primates: natural and experimental infec-
     tion. Adv. Cancer Res., 23:171, 1976.

18. Fukuhara, S. and Rowley, J.D. Chromosome 14 translocations
     in non-Burkitt lymphomas. Int. J. Cancer, 22:14, 1978.

19. Hanto, D.W., Frizzera, G., Purtilo, D.T., Sakamoto, K.,
     Sullivan, J.L., Saemundsen, A.K., Klein, G., Simmons,
     R.L., and Najarian, J.S. A clinical spectrum of
     lymphoproliferative disorders in renal transplant reci-
     pients and evidence for the role of the Epstein-Barr
     virus. Cancer Res., 41:4253, 1981.

20. Henle, W., Diehl, V., Hohn, G., zurHausen, H., and Henle, G.
     Herpes-type virus and chromosome marker in normal leuko-

cytes after growth with irradiated Burkitt cells.
Science, 157:1064, 1967.

21. Henle, G., Henle, W., and Diehl, V. Relations of Burkitt's
tumor-associated herpes-type virus to infectious mononucleosis. Proc. Natl. Acad. Sci., 59:94, 1968.

22. Hunt, R.D., Melendez, L.V., Garcia, F.G., and Trum, B.F.
Pathologic features of Herpesvirus ateles lymphoma in
cotton-topped marmosets (Saguinus oedipus). J. Natl.
Cancer Inst., 49:1631, 1972.

23. Hunt, R.D., Melendez, L.V., King, N.W., Gilmore, C.E.,
Daniel, M.D., Williamson, M.E., and Jones, T.C.
Morphology of a diseases with features of malignant
lymphoma in marmosets and owl monkeys inoculated with
Herpesvirus saimiri. J. Natl. Cancer Inst., 44:447,
1970.

24. Johnson, D.R., Klein, G., and Falk, L. Interaction of
Herpesvirus ateles and Herpesvirus saimiri with primate
lymphocytes. I. Selective adsorption of virus by
lymphoid cells. Intervirology, 31:21, 1980.

25. Johnson, D.R., Ernberg, I., and Klein, G. Interaction of
Herpesvirus ateles with marmoset lymphocytes. II.
Identification of target cell population and stimulation
of DNA synthesis after infection in vitro.
Intervirology, 14:202, 1980.

26. Johnson, D.R., Ohno, S., Kaschka-Dierich, C., Fleckenstein,
B., and Klein, G. Relationship between Herpesvirus
ateles-associated nuclear antigen (HATNA) and the number
of virus genome equivalents in HVA-carrying lymphoid
lines. J. Gen. Virol., 52:221, 1981.

27. Johnson, D., Levan, G., Klein, G., Nigida, S., and Wolfe, L.
Chromosomes and cell surface markers of marmoset lymphocytes and Epstein-Barr virus-transformed marmoset cell
lines. Cancer Genetics and Cytogenetics, 8:101, 1980.

28. Johnson, D.R., Wolfe, L.G., Levan, G., Klein, G., Ernberg,
I., and Aman, P. Epstein-Barr virus induced lymphoproliferative disease in cotton-topped marmosets. In press.

29. Klein, G., Pearson, G., Rabson, A., Ablashi, D.V., Falk, L.,
Wolfe, L., Deinhardt, F., and Rabin, H. Antibody reactions to Herpesvirus saimiri (HVS)-induced early and late
antigens (EA and LA) in HVS-infected squirrel, marmoset
and owl monkeys. Int. J. Cancer, 12:270, 1973.

30. Klein, G. The Epstein-Barr virus and neoplasia. N. Engl. J.
Med., 293:1353, 1975.

31. Klein, G. and Klein, E. Immune surveillance against virus-
induced tumors and non-rejectability of spontaneous
tumors: contrasting consequences of host versus tumor
evolution. Proc. Natl. Acad. Sci., 74:2121, 1977.

32. Klein, G. Lymphoma development in mice and humans: diversity
of initiation is followed by convergent cytogenetic
evolution. Proc. Natl. Acad. Sci., 76:2442, 1979.

33.   Laufs, R. and Fleckenstein, B.   Susceptibility to Herpesvirus
      saimiri and antibody development in Old and New World
      monkeys. Med. Microbiol. Immunol., 158:227, 1973.
34.   Laufs, R. and Melendez, L.V.   Oncogenicity of Herpesvirus
      ateles in monkeys. J. Natl. Cancer Inst., 51:599, 1973.
35.   Laufs, R., Steinke, H., Steinke, G., and Petzold, D. Latent
      infection and malignant lymphoma in marmosets (Callithrix
      jacchus) after infections with two oncogenic herpes-
      viruses from primates. J. Natl. Cancer Inst.,
      53:195, 1974.
36.   Leibold, W., Huldt, G., Flanagan, T.G., Anderson, M., Dalens,
      M., Wright, D.H., Voller, A., and Klein, G.
      Tumorigenicity of Epstein-Barr virus (EBV) transformed
      lymphoid line cells in autologous squirrel monkeys. Int.
      J. Cancer, 17:533, 1976.
37.   Manolov, G. and Manolova, Y. Marker band in one chromosome
      14 from Burkitt lymphomas. Nature, 234:33, 1972.
38.   Marczynska, B., Falk, L., Wolfe, L., and Deinhardt, F.
      Transplantation and cytogenetic studies of Herpesvirus
      saimiri-induced disease in marmoset monkeys. J. Natl.
      Cancer Inst., 50:331, 1973.
39.   Martin, L.N. and Allen, W.P. Response to primary infection
      with Herpesvirus saimiri in immunosuppressed juvenile and
      newborn squirrel monkeys. Infect. Immun., 12:528, 1975.
40.   Masucci, M.G., Szigeti, R., Ernberg, I., Bjorkholm, M.,
      Mellstedt, H., Henle, G., Henle, W., Pearson, G.,
      Masucci, G., Svedmyr, E., Johansson, B., and Klein, G.
      Cell-mediated immune reactions in three patients with
      malignant lymphoproliferative diseases in remission and
      abnormally high Epstein-Barr virus antibody titers.
      Cancer Res., 41:4292, 1981.
41.   Melendez, L.V., Daniel, M.D., Hunt, R.D., and Garcia, F.G.
      An apparently new herpesvirus from primary kidney
      cultures of the squirrel monkey (Saimiri sciureus). Lab.
      Anim. Care, 18:374, 1968.
42.   Melendez, L.V., Daniel, M.D., Garcia, F.G., Fraser, C.E.O.,
      Hunt, R.D., and King, N.W. Herpesvirus saimiri. I.
      Further characterization studies of a new virus form from
      the squirrel monkey. Lab. Anim. Care, 19:372, 1969.
43.   Melendez, L.V., Hunt, R.D., Daniel, M.D., Garcia, F.G., and
      Fraser, C.E.O. Herpes saimiri. II. An experimentally-
      induced malignant lymphoma in primates. Lab. Anim. Care,
      19:378, 1969.
44.   Melendez, L.V., Hunt, R.D., King, N.W., Barahona, H.H.,
      Daniel, M.D., Fraser, C.E.O., and Garcia, F.G.
      Herpesvirus ateles, a new lymphoma virus of monkeys.
      Nature New Biol., 235:182, 1972.
45.   Miller, G., Shope, T., Lisco, H., Stitt, D., and Lipman, M.
      Epstein-Barr virus: transformation, cytopathic changes

and viral antigens in squirrel monkey and marmoset leukocytes. Proc. Natl. Acad. Sci. USA, 69:383, 1972.

46. Miller, G., Shope, T., Coope, D., Waters, L., Pagano, J.,
     Bornkamm, G.W., and Henle, W. Lymphoma in cotton-topped
     marmosets after inoculation with Epstein-Barr virus:
     tumor incidence, histologic spectrum, antibody responses,
     demonstration of viral DNA, and characterization of
     viruses. J. Exp. Med., 145:948, 1977.

47. Nickerson, D., and Gergozian, N. Functional capabilities of
     marmoset T and B lymphocytes in primary in vitro antibody
     formation. Cell. Immunol., 57:408, 1981.

48. Nilsson, K., Giovanella, B., Stehling, J.S., and Klein, G.
     Tumorigenicity in human hematopoietic cell lines in athymic
     nude mice. Int. J. Cancer, 19:337, 1977.

49. Nilsson, K. The nature of lymphoid cell lines and their
     relationship to the virus. In: M.A. Epstein and B.G.
     Achong (eds.), The Epstein-Barr Virus. pp. 225-281.
     Berlin: Springer-Verlag, 1979.

50. Pearson, G., Ablashi, D., Orr, T., Rabin, H., and Armstrong,
     G. Intracellular and membrane immunofluorescence
     investigations on cells infected with Herpesvirus
     saimiri. J. Natl. Cancer Inst., 49:1417, 1972.

51. Pearson, G.R., Orr, T., Rabin, H., Cicmanec, J., Ablashi,
     D., and Armstrong, G. Antibody patterns to Herpesvirus
     saimiri-induced antigens in owl monkeys. J. Natl. Cancer
     Inst., 51:1939, 1973.

52. Purtilo, D.T. Immune deficiency predisposing to Epstein-Barr
     virus-induced lymphoproliferative syndrome as a model.
     In: G. Klein and S. Weinhouse (eds.), Advances in Cancer
     Research. Vol. 34, pp. 279-312. New York: Academic
     Press, 1981.

53. Purtilo, D.T., Sakamoto, K., Saemundsen, A.K., Sullivan,
     J.L., Synnerholm, A-C., Anvret, M., Pritchard, J.,
     Sloper, C., Sieff, C., Pincott, J., Pachman, L., Rich,
     K., Cruzi, F., Cornet, J-A., Collins, R., Barnes, N.,
     Knight, J., Sandstedt, B., and Klein, G. Documentation
     of Epstein-Barr virus infection in immunodeficient patients
     with life-threatening lymphoproliferative diseases by
     clinical, virological, and immunopathological studies.
     Cancer Res., 41:4226, 1981.

54. Rabin, H., Neubauer, R., Hopkins, R., and Levy, B.
     Characterization of lymphoid cell lines established from
     multiple Epstein-Barr virus (EBV-induced lymphomas) in a
     cotton-topped marmoset. Int. J. Cancer, 20:44, 1977.

55. Rickinson, A.B., Moss, D.J., Wallace, L.E., Rowe, M., Misko,
     I.S., Epstein, M.A., and Pope, J.H. Long-term T-cell-
     mediated immunity to Epstein-Barr virus. Cancer Res.,
     41:4216, 1981.

56. Robinson, J.E., Brown, N., Andiman, W., Halliday, K.,
     Francke, U., Robert, M., Andersson-Anvret, M., Horstmann,

D., and Miller, B. Diffuse polyclonal B cell lymphoma during primary infections with Epstein-Barr virus. N. Engl. J. Med., 302:1293, 1980.

57. Saemundsen, A.K., Berkel, A.I., Henle, W., Henle, G., Anvret, M., Sanal, Z., Ersoy, F., Caglar, M., and Klein, G. Epstein-Barr virus-carrying lymphoma in a patient with ataxia telangiectasia. Brit. Med. J., 282:425, 1981.

58. Saemundsen, A.K., Purtilo, D.T., Sakamoto, K., Sullivan, J.L., Synnerholm, A-C., Hanto, D., Simmons, R., Anvret, M., Collins, R., and Klein, G. Documentation of Epstein-Barr virus infection in immunodeficient patients with life-threatening lymphoproliferative diseases by Epstein-Barr virus complementary RNA/DNA and viral DNA/DNA hybridization. Cancer Res., 41:4237, 1981.

59. Sakamoto, K., Freed, H., and Purtilo, D.T. Antibody responses to Epstein-Barr virus in families with the X-linked lymphoproliferative syndrome. J. Immunol., 125:921, 1980.

60. Seeley, J.K., Sakamoto, K., Ip, S., Hansen, P., and Purtilo, D.T. Abnormal subsets in the X-linked lymphoproliferative syndrome. J. Immunol., 127:2618, 1981.

61. Shope, T., Dechairo, D., and Miller, G. Malignant lymphoma in cotton-topped marmosets after inoculation with Epstein-Barr virus. Proc. Natl. Acad. Sci. USA, 70:2487, 1973.

62. Spira, G., Aman, P., Koide, N., Lundin, G., Klein, G., and Hall, K. Cell-surface immunoglobulin and insulin receptor expression in an EBV-negative lymphoma cell line and its EBV-converted sublines. J. Immunol., 126:122, 1981.

63. Sullivan, J.L., Byron, K., Brewster, F., and Purtilo, D.T. Deficient natural killer cell activity in the X-linked lymphoproliferative syndrome. Science, 210:543, 1980.

64. Sundar, S.K., Levine, P.H., Ablashi, D.V., Leiseca, S.A., Armstrong, G.R., Cicmanec, J.L., Parker, G.A., and Nonoyama, M. Epstein-Barr virus-induced malignant lymphoma in a white-lipped marmoset. Int. J. Cancer, 27:107, 1981.

65. Werner, J., Wolf, H., Apodaca, J., and zurHausen, H. Lymphoproliferative disease in a cotton-topped marmoset after inoculation with infectious mononucleosis-derived Epstein-Barr virus. Int. J. Cancer, 15:1000, 1975.

66. Wright, J., Falk, L.A., Collins, D., and Deinhardt, F. Mononuclear cell fraction carrying Herpesvirus saimiri in persistently-infected squirrel monkeys. J. Natl. Cancer Inst., 57:959, 1976.

67. Wright, J., Falk, L.A., Wolfe, L.G., Ogden, J., and Deinhardt, F. Susceptibility of common marmosets (Callithrix jacchus) to oncogenic and attenuated strains of Herpesvirus saimiri. J. Natl. Cancer Inst., 59:1475, 1977.

68. Wolfe, L.G., Falk, L.A., and Deinhardt, F. Oncogenicity of
     Herpesvirus saimiri in marmoset monkeys. J. Natl. Cancer
     Inst., 47:1145, 1971.

69. Wolfe, L.G., and Deinhardt, F. Overview of viral oncology
     studies in Saguinus and Callithrix species. Prim. Med.,
     10:96, 1978.

70. Zech, L., Haglund, U., Nilsson, K., and Klein, G.
     Characteristic chromosomal abnormalities in biopsies and
     lymphoid cell lines from patients with Burkitt and
     non-Burkitt lymphomas. Int. J. Cancer, 17:47, 1976.

RELATIONSHIP OF IMMUNE DEFICIENCY AND ONCOGENIC VIRUSES TO MALIGNANT B CELL LYMPHOMAS: MOUSE AND MAN

Paul K. Pattengale

Departments of Pathology and Microbiology
USC School of Medicine, 2025 Zonal Avenue
Los Angeles, CA 90033

INTRODUCTION

With the exception of the dualtropic murine leukemia virus (MuLV)-induced polymorphic B cell lymphoma in young C57BL/6 mice, and the Epstein-Barr virus (EBV)-induced polymorphic B cell lymphoma in immunodeficient patients, it is apparent that the vast majority of spontaneously occurring B cell lymphomas in immuno-deficient mice and men are not causally linked to overt inducing agents (e.g., oncogenic viruses) (Table 1). For this reason, the comparative features of dualtropic MuLV-induced and EBV-induced B cell diseases are discussed, as well as the association of B cell lymphomas with congenital and acquired immunodeficiencies.

Congenital Immunodeficiency and B Cell Lymphomas: Mouse versus Man

Congenital athymic (nude) mice do not show a significant increase in the overall incidence of cancer (i.e., both carcinomas and sarcomas) (26,27); however, spontaneously occurring B cell lymphomas are significantly increased in nu/nu NIH(S) homo-zygotes, as compared to age matched nu/+ heterozygotes (16). As seen in Table 2, 42.5% of nu/nu homozygotes had B cell lymphomas occurring at a mean age of 17 months versus 8.9% at a median age of 26 months in nu/+ heterozygous NIH(S) mice. Virtually all of the B cell morphologic subtypes of mouse lymphomas and related leukemias were represented in the nu/nu homozygotes (17,18) (see Table 3). These included B cell lymphomas of small lymphocytes [16%] (Figure 1), follicular center cells (FCC) [61%] (Figure 2), immunoblasts [16%] (Figure 3), and plasma cells [7%] (Figure 4). Using the Dunn classification for murine lymphoreticular neoplasms

Table 1. Correlation of Inducing Stimuli and Immunodeficiency with the Development of B Cell Lymphomas in Various Strains of Mice as Compared to Man

Type of Inducing Stimuli	Host	Pre and/or co-existing immune deficiency	Type of B cell lymphoma	Comments	References
Dualtropic Murine Leukemia Virus (MuLV)	C57BL/6 mice	None known	Polymorphic B cell immunoblastic lymphoma	Polyclonal B cell lesion is induced with high efficiency and short latency in young mice	23
Unknown (environmental, retrovirus?)	nu/nu (NIH[S]) mice	Athymic (ie., nude)	Small lymphocytic, follicular center cell (FCC), immunoblastic, and plasma cell lymphomas	Occur spontaneously at a mean age of 17 months	16
Unknown	me/+ (C57BL/6) mice	Decreased number and activity of B cells	B cell derived follicular center cell (FCC) lymphomas	Occur spontaneously at approximately 1 year	19
Unknown	BALB/c mice	Age	Follicular center cell (FCC), lymphoblastic and immunoblastic B cell lymphomas	Monoclonal B cell lesions occur spontaneously at a mean age of 2 years	22
Epstein-Barr virus (EBV)	Man	X-linked lymphoproliferative syndrome (XLP), iatrogenic immunosuppression (ie., transplant recipients)	Polymorphic B cell lymphomas (ie, primarily immunoblastic)	B cell lesions are most commonly EBV-containing and polyclonal	5,24
Unknown	Man	Age	Primarily B cell-derived follicular center cell (FCC) lymphomas	Monoclonal B cell lesions occur spontaneously in the later decades of life	10-12

Table 2. Spontaneous B Cell Lymphomas Occurring in NIH(S)-Nude Mice

	Total Mice	Age at Death from Lymphoma (mos.) Range	Mean	Number of B Cell Lymphomas	%Total Incidence of B Cell Lymphoma
nu/nu	73	7-32	17	31[a]	42.5%
nu/+	45	21-34	26	4[b]	8.9%

[a]19/31 (61%) were lymphomas of follicular center cell (FCC) type, 5/31 (16%) were lymphomas of small B lymphocytes, 5/31 (16%) were lymphomas of B immunoblasts, and 2/31 (7%) were lymphomas of plasma cells.

[b]2/4 (50%) were lymphomas of small B lymphocytes, 1/4 (25%) was a lymphoma of B immunoblasts, and 1/4 (25%) was a lymphoma of FCC cells.

Table 3.   Immunomorphologic Classification of Murine Lymphoma and
           Related Leukemias as Proposed by Pattengale and Taylor
           (1981)[a]

Morphologic[b] (Lymphoid Cell Morphology)	Immunologic Type[c] B Cell	T Cell	Non-B Non-T Cell
Follicle Center Cell[d]	+	0	0
Small Cell Type	+.	0	0
Large Cell Type	+	0	0
Large & Small (mixed) Cell Type	+	0	0
Plasma Cell	+	0	0
Immunoblast	+	(+)	(+)
Small Lymphocyte	+	(+)	(+)
Lymphoblast	+[e]	+	+

[a]The proposed classification refers only to lymphoid cell,
lymphocyte-derived neoplasms and therefore excludes those
derived from the monocyte/macrophage/ histiocyte series (i.e.,
true histiocytic lymphoma). It is also stressed that the
diagnosis of lymphoma/leukemia is based <u>primarily</u> on morphologic
criteria and is then <u>subsequently</u> combined with immunologically-
based parameters.

[b]The morphologic cell types listed are those which have been
observed and documented to date. If analogous to man, one would
expect to observe additional cell types such as the cerebriform
lymphocyte (i.e., Sezary-Mycosis Fungoides T cell) and the
plasmacytoid B lymphocyte (i.e., Waldenstroms macroglobulinemia),
as well as others.

[c]A B cell is defined as having <u>easily</u> detectable surface and/or
cytoplasmic immunoglobulin; a T cell is defined as having <u>easily</u>
detectable surface Thy 1 (i.e., theta antigen); a non-B non-T
cell is defined as lacking <u>both</u> easily detectable Thy 1 and surface and/or cytoplasmic immunoglobulin. + = already observed
and documented; (+) = not yet observed but expected; 0 = not
observed or expected.

[d]Follicular center cell (FCC) lymphomas with a marked lymph node
follicular pattern analogous to those appearing in man have not
yet been well documented. FCC lymphomas can also contain equally
prominent mixtures of both large and small FCC cell types (i.e.,
FCC lymphoma, large and small cell type).

[e]Lymphoblastic lymphoma of B cells is considered by some to be a
follicle center cell (FCC) lymphoma (9), and by others to be a
separate category (8).

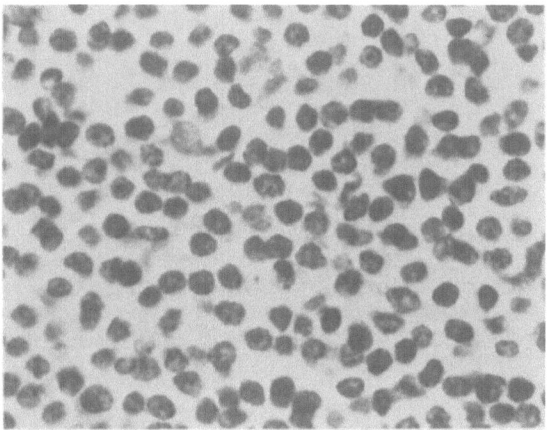

Fig. 1.   Lymphoma of small lymphocytes (i.e., small lymphocytic
          lymphoma). Note the small, non-cohesive, and round to
          slightly irregular lymphoid cells with scant cytoplasm
          and mature, condensed chromatin. H&E; lymph node, nu/nu
          NIH(S) mouse, 16 months X1000.

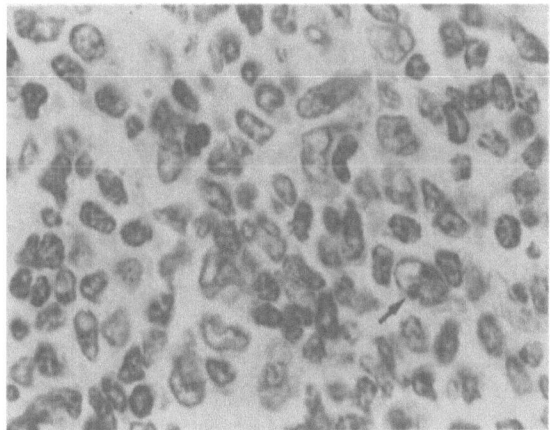

Fig. 2   Lymphoma of small and large follicle center cells (i.e.,
          FCC lymphoma, small and large, mixed, FCC type). Note
          the equal predominance of small as well as large (cleaved
          [irregular shaped] and noncleaved) follicle center cells.
          Often, large noncleaved follicle center cells have two
          prominent nucleoli which are juxtaposed to the nuclear
          membrane (see arrow). This process also stained positive
          for cytoplasmic, monoclonal IgM-lambda using specific
          immunoperoxidase staining. H&E; spleen, NFS/N mouse, 17
          months X1000.

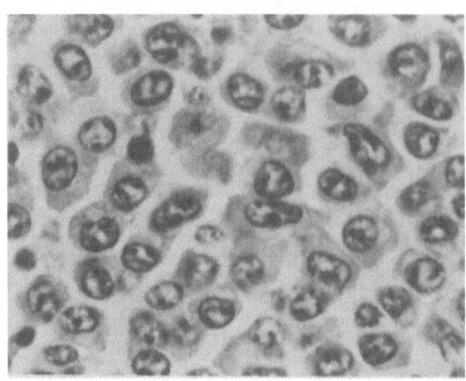

Fig. 3   Lymphoma of B immunoblasts (i.e., immunoblastic lymphoma,
          B cell type). Note the monomorphous population of non-
          cohesive, large lymphoid cells with round to oval, ve-
          sicular nuclei with prominent and distinct nucleoli. In
          addition, the nuclei are eccentric and occasionally have
          clumped, peripherally marginated, clockface-like chroma-
          tin (i.e., plasmacytoid features). Also note the moder-
          ately (i.e., amphophilic) dense cytoplasm. H&E; spleen,
          Balb/c mouse, 17 months X1000.

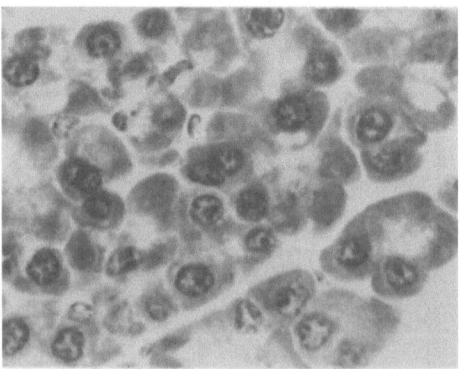

Fig. 4.   Lymphoma of plasma cells (i.e., plasma cell lymphoma).
          Note the monomorphous population of intermediate to
          large plasma cells with dense, amphophilic cytoplasm and
          eccentric nuclei with clockfaced chromatin. Also note
          the presence of occasional prominent nucleoli. This
          process stains positive for cytoplasmic, monoclonal
          IgG_1-kappa using specific immunoperoxidase staining.
          H&E; bowel mesentery, young adult Balb/c mouse carrying
          the ascites plasmacytoma MOPC 300 X1000.

(2,3), the lymphomas would be designated as lymphocytic, reticulum cell, or plasma cell neoplasms. The comparative features of the Dunn versus the Pattengale-Taylor classification for mouse lymphoma and related leukemias are illustrated in Table 4. This nu/nu NIH(S) athymic model of spontaneous B cell lymphoma is useful in exploring mechanisms of B cell lymphoma development, especially as related to the absence of post-thymic regulatory T cells. The role of environmental antigens and retroviruses in this model are also unknown, and essentially unexplored.

Preliminary information indicates the me/+ (i.e., viable motheaten heterozygote) C57BL/6 mouse, which has a congenital decrease in the number and activity of splenic B lymphocytes (28), experiences a high incidence of spontaneous B cell-derived follicular center cell (FCC) lymphomas as compared to normal C57BL/6 mice of the same age (19). Possibly follicular center B cells in the C57BL/6-me/+ mouse, although significantly decreased in numbers and activity, are more susceptible to neoplastic transformation. Although not as well documented as the nu/nu NIH(S) model, the C57BL/6-me/+ model has congenital immunodeficiencies of either T or B cells associated with the high incidence of spontaneous B cell lymphoma.

Strains of mice with congenital immunodeficiencies of natural killer (NK) cells frequently have lymphoproliferative disorders. The beige mouse (i.e., C57BL/6-bg/bg), with a NK deficiency (25), frequently develops lymphoproliferative disorders (25). Careful morphologic documentation has been lacking. In contrast, the SJL/J mouse, also having decreased NK activity from birth (25), has been documented to develop a high incidence of (i.e., >90%) spontaneous reticulum cell sarcomas, type B (i.e., RCS[B] of Dunn) at approximately one year of age (5). However, the evaluation of this presumably B cell derived lesion by immunomorphologic classifications (17,18) has been exceedingly difficult. This difficulty arises because lymphoproliferative disorder in the SJL/J mouse is heterogeneous (i.e., mixtures of lymphoblasts, follicle center cells, B immunoblasts, plasma cells, histiocytes, and macrophages). One possible unifying hypothesis considers that the neoplastic event occurs in a B cell progenitor (i.e., prepreB or pre B) capable of full differentiation (i.e., through the entire B cell morphologic spectrum) to immunoglobulin-secreting plasma cells. Oncogenic viruses have not been readily demonstrated in these strains. Furthermore, a selective natural killer (NK) cell deficiency (i.e., only involving NK cells) in these strains is unlikely, since other immunodeficiencies exist.

When evaluating and comparing the relationship of human congenital immunodeficiencies to B cell lymphomas, the situation becomes somewhat difficult, since the described lymphomas have been characterized using the earlier Rappaport classification.

Table 4.   Comparison of the Proposed Classifications
for Murine Lymphoma and Related Leukemias[a]

Dunn 1954   Pattengale-Taylor 1981

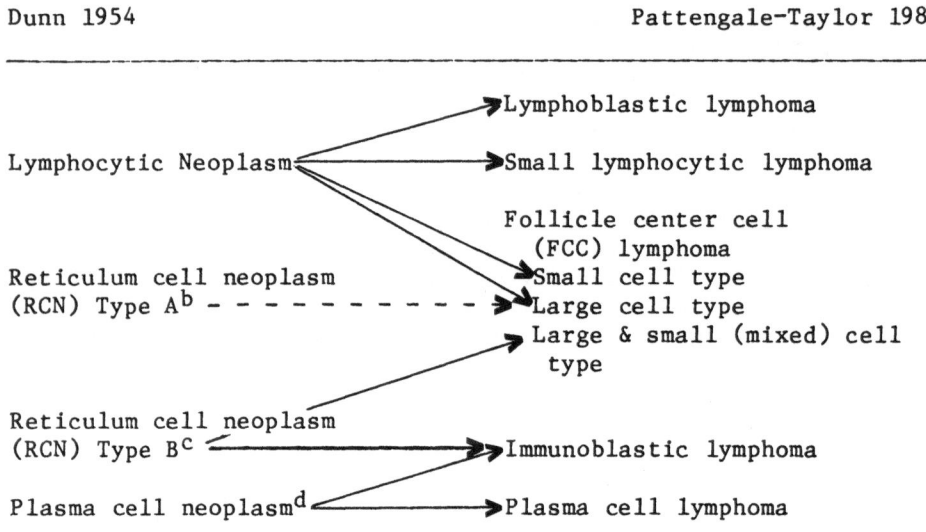

Lymphocytic Neoplasm

Lymphoblastic lymphoma

Small lymphocytic lymphoma

Follicle center cell
(FCC) lymphoma
Small cell type
Large cell type
Large & small (mixed) cell
type

Reticulum cell neoplasm
(RCN) Type A[b]

Reticulum cell neoplasm
(RCN) Type B[c]

Immunoblastic lymphoma

Plasma cell neoplasm[d]

Plasma cell lymphoma

[a]As proposed by Dunn, lymphocytic neoplasms can be localized
(i.e., lymphoma) or generalized (i.e., leukemia) involving the
peripheral blood and bone marrow compartments. By comparison
and direct analogy, lymphomas of lymphoblasts, small lymphocytes, and follicle center cells can manifest with secondary
leukemia phases (i.e., lymphoma/leukemias). RCN, Type C is considered by Dunn to be nonneoplastic and nonlymphoid in origin.
[b]The majority of RCN, Type A as proposed by Dunn is considered to
be derived from true histiocytic cells (i.e., true nonlymphoid,
phagocytic histiocytes) and rarely can present as a monocytic
leukemia. The dotted line stresses the fact that a minority of
RCN, Type A represent large FCC cell lymphomas.
[c]Although RCN, Type B is now considered not to be representative
of Hodgkin's disease, it can include both prelymphomatous, non-
neoplastic lymphoproliferations as well as true lymphoid cell
lymphomas (i.e., large FCC and immunoblastic cell types). A
lymphoma is defined as a lymphoid cell neoplasm (i.e., an autonomous monoclonal new growth, presumably derived from one cell).
In contrast, a prelymphoma is defined as a conditioned, atypical
lymphoid cell hyperplasia derived from more than one cell (i.e.,
nonmonoclonal, oligo- or polyclonal derivation), and which has a
propensity to progress to a true lymphoid cell neoplasm with
time.
[d]As stated by Dunn, a proportion of plasma cell neoplasms were
formed by typical well-differentiated plasma cells, while others
were formed of a cell type resembling a reticulum cell (i.e., a B
immunoblast with plasmacytoid features).

For example, histiocytic lymphomas have been described in
Wiskott-Aldrich syndrome, ataxia telangiectasia, agammaglobulinemia, hypogammaglobulinemias, DeGeorge's syndrome, Chediak-
Higashi, etc. (31). Whether or not these lymphomas are B cell
derived is unknown. Immunomorphologic classifications of mouse
(17,18) and human lymphomas are based on the concept that the
immune system is divided into T and B cell types. Neoplastic
conversion occurs within morphologically distinct T and B cell
subtypes (8,9). Continuing immunomorphologic studies of lymphoma
(i.e., Lukes-Collins [9] and Kiel classifications [8]) will likely
better document B cell subtypes of lymphoma in congenitally
immunodeficient patients. Discussed later in this chapter is the
relationship of EBV to the development of B cell lymphomas in
immunodeficient patients (i.e., X-linked lymphoproliferative
syndrome - XLP and immunosuppressed transplant recipients). Some
of the histiocytic lymphomas previously described in congenitally
immunodeficient patients (i.e., non-XLP) may possibly be B cell
derived and EBV-related. Merino elsewhere describes patients with
Chediak-Higashi disease (i.e., and other congenital immunodeficiencies) which exhibit B cell lymphoproliferations, presum-ably
related to EBV.

Acquired Immunodeficiency and B Cell Lymphomas: Mouse Versus Man

Here I discuss relationships of acquired immunodeficiencies
to the development of B cell lymphomas. Graft versus host disease
(GVHD) produces immunodeficiencies in F_1 hybrid mice injected with
semiallogeneic parental cells. For example, (C57BL/6 x
DBA/2)F_1 hybrids injected intravenously with parental C57BL/6
spleen cells undergo GVHD associated with the depression of T and
B cell and NK cell activity (20). Many of these mice develop B
cell lymphomas at approximately 18-24 months of age (1,21).
Knowledge regarding oncogenic retroviruses (i.e., in this
multistep, long latency model of GVHD) and the development of
malignant B cell lymphoma is lacking at the present time.

Since aging is considered by many to be an aid acquired immunodeficiency, it is noteworthy that some inbred strains of aged
mice frequently exhibit spontaneous B cell lymphomas (18).
Pattengale and Frith (22), using the recently proposed immunomorphologic classification (Table 3), determined that 54 out of 61
(i.e., 89%) lymphomas, spontaneously occurring in female BALB/c
mice at the age of 20 months and older (mean age 24 months), were
B cell-derived. Cytoplasmic immunoglobulin (CIg) was demonstrated
in 43 of 54 (i.e., 80%) of these B cell lymphomas using immunoperoxidase techniques. The most predominant B cell morphologic
subtypes were B cell lymphomas of follicular center cells (i.e.,
FCC lymphoma).

In contrast to murine GVH systems, GVH reactions produced in HLA-identical, allogeneic, immunosuppressed bone marrow transplant recipients are not associated with a significant increase in B cell malignant lymphomas (30) (although an occasional case has been reported [6]). This apparent discrepancy may relate to the that the murine GVH system is semiallogeneic (i.e., H-2 mismatched for parental donor cells) and does not involve immunosuppression of the F_1 recipient. On the other hand, aging in humans (i.e., as in murine populations) is associated with a significant increase of spontaneous B cell lymphomas. As for the BALB/c mouse (22), there is a direct analogy between mouse and man using immuno-morphologic criteria and similarities in age-related frequency of B cell lymphomas. For example, in the recent BALB/c study by Pattengale and Frith (22), the majority of lymphomas (i.e., 77%) occurred in old female mice (i.e., >20 months of age) and were B cell derived. The most common B cell types was a lymphoma

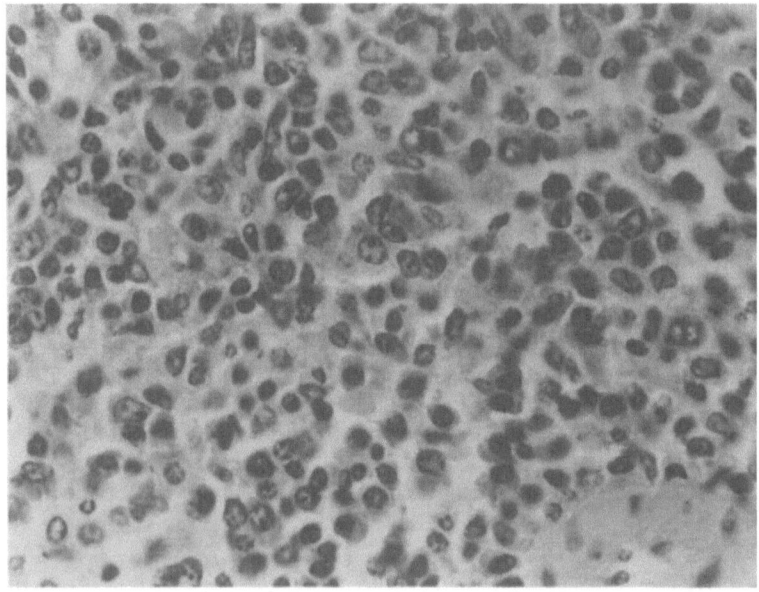

Fig. 5.   Polymorphic B cell immunoblastic lymphoma in a C57BL/6
          mouse. Note the presence of immunoblasts admixed with a
          prominent component of plasmacytoid cells. Although
          staining polyclonally for intracytoplasmic immunoglobulin
          (Ig), this B cell process was widespread and clinically
          aggressive as evidenced by sarcomatous destructive
          lesions in visceral organs. H&E; kidney, young adult
          C57BL/6 mouse injected with dualtropic-MuLV 10 weeks pre-
          viously X450.

derived from follicular center cells [i.e., FCC lymphomas (60% of cases)]. These findings were comparable to recent large studies of human adult non-Hodgkin's lymphomas (10-12). Among 790 cases (12) 585 (i.e., 74%) were B cell-derived when combined morphologic and immunologic criteria were used. Similarly, the majority (i.e., 389/585 = 66%) of these B cell-derived, adult non-Hodgkin's lymphomas were judged to be of follicular center cell (FCC) origin (i.e., 389/790 = total incidence of 49%). These age-associated monoclonally-derived B cell lymphomas in mouse and man are not overtly related to oncogenic viruses.

Of recent interest and relevance to acquired immunodeficiencies in humans is the recently described gay-related immunodeficiency syndrome (GRID) or acquired immunodeficiency syndrome (AIDS) (4,7,13,29). Elsewhere in this volume, Abrams discusses this syndrome. This syndrome is manifested by acute bouts of illness with severe acquired immunodeficiencies involving T lymphocytes and NK cells, and usually a concomitant infection with cytomegalo-virus (CMV). An alarming number of these patients develop rapidly disseminating Kaposi's sarcoma (i.e., which contains CMV DNA). B cell lymphoproliferative disorders also occur in the GRID syndrome (14). The relationship of the Epstein-Barr virus (EBV) to the B cell processes observed in GRID patients is being investigated in several laboratories. The association of EBV to AIDS will be considered in the next section (see below).

Comparative Features of Dualtropic Retrovirus and Epstein-Barr Virus Induced B Cell Lymphoproliferative Disease in Mouse and Man

As summarized in Table 5, noteworthy differences prevail between MuLV (i.e., RNA virus)-induced and EBV (i.e., DNA virus)-induced B cell lymphoproliferative diseases. However, the polymorphic, polyclonal, normal diploid, immunoblastic B cell lymphomas are strikingly similar (23). They both (i.e., mouse [Figure 5] and man [Figure 6]) show a predominance of plasmacytoid immunoblasts (i.e., eccentric nucleus with prominent amphophilic cytoplasm) associated with plasmacytoid lymphocytes and plasma cells. This polymorphic appearance (i.e., many forms of B lymphoid cells) is also associated with polyclonality as measured by isotype analysis for heavy chain and light chain isotypes. In the dualtropic MuLV-induced murine lesion, the proliferating polyclonally-derived B cells are normal diploid on karyotype analysis, and are not transplantable to nonimmunosuppressed syngeneic recipients. EBV-related (i.e., and containing) polymorphic lymphomatous B cells, by analogy would also likely be normal diploid, and unable to be transplanted subcutaneously in nude mice (i.e., in contrast to the EBV-associated Burkitt's lymphoma, which transplants subcutaneously). Polyclonally EBV-infected and transformed B cells in vitro (i.e., B lympho-blastoid cell lines [BLCL]) transplant to the immunologically

Table 5. Similarities and Dissimilarities of Dualtropic MuLV-Induced B Cell Disease in the C57BL/6 Mouse Versus EBV-Induced B Cell Disease in Man

	MuLV-Induced Disease	EBV-Induced Disease
1. Virus Properties	RNA-containing Type C retrovirus with dualtropic host range (i.e., infects mouse and non-mouse cells)	DNA containing enveloped herpesvirus
2. Natural Host	Cloned dualtropic MuLV produces B cell disease only after inoculation of susceptible mouse strain (i.e., disease is not naturally occurring in C57BL/6 mice)	EBV is ubiquitous in the human population and is etiologically related to naturally-occurring human B cell disease (e.g., infectious mononucleosis [IM])
3. Type of B cell lymphoproliferative disease	Polymorphic, polyclonal immuno-blastic B cell lymphoma is inducible with high efficiency and short latency after intra-peritoneal (i.p.) inoculation of virus into healthy mice	IM is usually self-limited. Association of EBV with monoclonal-derived B cell derived Burkitt's lymphoma is at present circumstantial. EBV is etiologicaly related, however to the development of polymorphic, polyclonal B cell lymphomas in immunodeficient individuals
4. Temporal association of polymorphic B cell lymphoma with prior immunodeficiency state	None known	Temporal association with pre-existing congenital (i.e., XLP) or iatrogenic (i.e., transplant-related) immunodeficiency

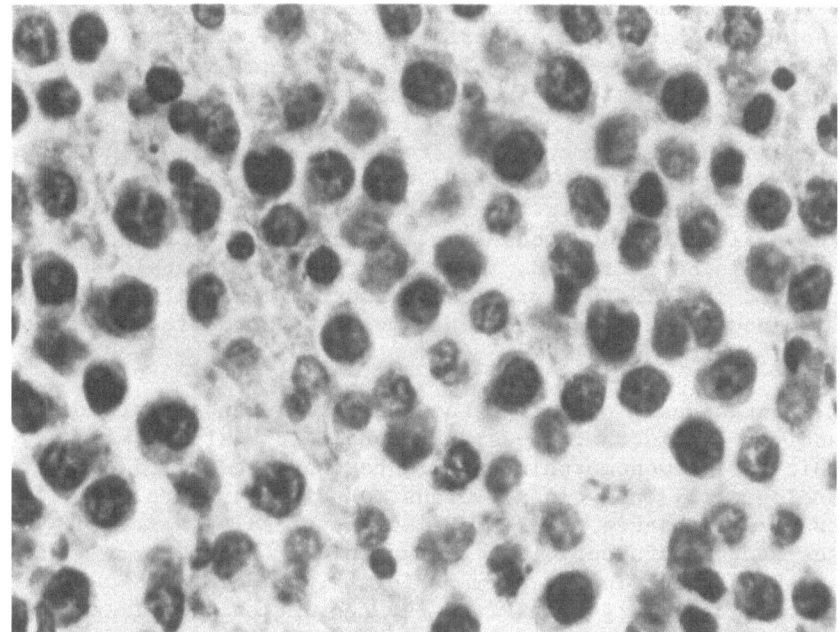

Fig. 6. Polymorphic B cell immunoblastic lymphoma of the central
nervous system in a young man with XLP who had chronic
infectious mononucleosis. Although morphologically
diagnosed as an immunoblastic lymphoma (i.e., sarcoma) of
B cells, it was polyclonal with respect to Ig isotypes
(i.e., IgA, IgG, IgM) but predominance of
IgM-kappa-containing cells were found. Note the large
cells and small plasmacytoid cell component. H&E;
central nervous system X850.

privileged nude mouse brain. By direct analogy, one would predict
that the polymorphic lymphomatous B cells obtained from immunodeficient patients would grow in the nude mouse brain.

The occurrence of a viral-induced, polymorphic, polyclonal B
cell (immunoblastic) malignant lymphoma is conceptually troublesome. Traditionally, a malignant lymphoma is defined as a
lymphoid cell neoplasm which is derived monoclonally (i.e., from
one cell) and which is truly autonomous in growth characteristics.
Although clinically and pathologically <u>malignant</u>, the polymorphic
B cell proliferation (as described above) departs from the traditional definitions of neoplasia by being polyclonal and unable to
be transplanted (i.e., conditioned or nonautonomous). Furthermore,
it is often diploid (i.e., in contrast to the characteristic nonrandom aneuploidy often observed in true malignancy). An opera-
tional definition of the polymorphic B cell lymphomas as

opportunistic and prelymphomatous (i.e., a conditioned atypical B lymphoid cell hyperplasia, derived from more than one cell [i.e., nonmonoclonal, olig- or polyclonal derivation] and having a propensity to progress to a true lymphoid cell neoplasm) is proposed.

Although this progression from normal diploid, conditioned polyclonality (e.g., polymorphic) to (nonrandom) aneuploid, autonomous monoclonality (e.g., monomorphic) has never been observed in the dualtropic MuLV mouse system, occasional instances of this occurring in EBV-infected, immunodeficient individuals have been documented (5,24) This progression might be causally related to the immunodeficiency state, since young C57BL/6 mice are immunologically quite normal.

Spontaneously occurring human B cell immunoblastic lymphomas, in addition to further in-depth morphologic evaluation (i.e., polymorphic versus monomorphic) should be continued to be evaluated immunologically (polyclonal versus monoclonal), virologically (presence or absence of EBV) and karyotypically (normal diploid versus nonrandom aneuploid). The clinical treatment of a virally (i.e., EBV) conditioned, normal diploid, polyclonal B cell lesion is theoretically different from the conventional anti-neoplastic therapy used to treat monoclonal B cell lesions (i.e., anti-viral strategies versus chemotherapeutic and/or radiotherapeutic strategies). Accurate diagnoses are therefore mandatory for making the appropriate choices of clinical treatment.

SUMMARY AND CONCLUSIONS

In summary, the ubiquitous herpesvirus, EBV, under the appropriate circumstances of immunodeficiency (i.e., congenital and/or acquired) can condition the in vivo growth of polyclonally-derived B lymphocytes. Although the B cell lymphoproliferation is polymorphic and polyclonal, the disease is often clinically and pathologically malignant, killing the patient. An analogous model system in the C57BL/6 mouse is described, which is inducible with dualtropic murine leukemia virus (MuLV). It too, results in a polyclonal, polymorphic immunoblastic lymphoma of B cells.

The relationship of B cell lymphomas to congenital and acquired immunodeficiency in the mouse was discussed. Thus far direct evidence for oncogenic retroviruses is lacking. The increased frequency of malignant B cell lymphomas in a variety of mice with pre- and/or co-existing immunodeficiencies (i.e., nude, motheaten, GVH-induced F_1 hybrids, and aged BALB/c) is somewhat analogous to human B cell lymphomas developing in parallel with congenital or acquired immunodeficiencies. The lymphomas occurring in these patients are difficult to evaluate since they were classified according to the earlier Rappaport classification. Finally, I emphasize that spontaneous B cell lymphomas (i.e., primarily follicular center cells [FCC] lymphomas) arising in aging BALB/c mice (i.e., presumed acquired immunodeficiency) are immunomorphologically similar to spontaneous B cell lymphomas (i.e., primarily FCC lymphomas) of the non-Hodgkin's type arising in older, adult human populations.

REFERENCES

1.   Armstrong, M.Y.K., Schwartz, R.S., and Beldotti, L. Neoplastic sequelae of allogeneic disease. III. Histological events following transplantation of allogeneic spleen cells. Transplantation, 6:1380, 1967.
2.   Dunn, T.B. Normal and pathologic anatomy of the reticular tissue in laboratory mice, with a classification and discussion of neoplasms. J. Natl. Cancer Inst., 14:1281, 1954.
3.   Dunn, T.B. and Deringer, M.K. Reticulum cell neoplasm, Type B, or the "Hodgkin's-like lesion" of the mouse. J. Natl. Cancer Inst., 40:771-820, 1968.
4.   Durack, D.T. Opportunistic infections and Kaposi's sarcoma in homosexual men. N. Engl. J. Med., 305:1465, 1981.
5.   Frizzera, G., Hanto, D.W., Gajl-Peczalska, K.J., Rosai, J., McKenna, R.W., Sibley, R.K., Holahan, K.P. and Lindquist, L.L. Polymorphic diffuse B-cell hyperplasias and lymphomas in renal transplant recipients. Cancer Res., 41:4262, 1981.
6.   Gossett, T., Gale, R., Flushman, H., Austin, G.E., Sparkes, R., and Taylor, C.R. Immunoblastic sarcoma in donor cells after bone marrow transplantation. N. Engl. J. Med., 300:904, 1979.
7.   Gottlieb, M.S., Schroff, R., Schanker, H.M., Weisman, J.D, Fan, P.T., Wolf, R.A., and Saxon, A. Pneumocystis carinii pneumonia and mucosal candidiasis in previously healthy homosexual men. N. Engl. J. Med., 305:1425, 1981.
8.   Lennert, K., Stein, H., and Kaiserling, E. Cytological and functional criteria for the classification of malignant lymphomata. Br. J. Cancer, 31(Suppl. 2):1, 1975.
9.   Lukes, R.J. and Collins, R.D. New approaches to the classification of the lymphomata. Br. J. Cancer, 31(Suppl. 2):1, 1975.
10. Lukes, R.J., Taylor, C.R., Parker, J.W., Lincoln, T.L., Pattengale, P.K., and Tindle, B.H. A morphologic and immunologic surface marker study of 299 cases of non-Hodgkin's lymphomas and related leukemias. Am. J. Pathol., 90:461, 1978.

11.   Lukes, R.J., Parker, J.W., Taylor, C.R., Tindle, B.H.,
      Cramer, A.D., and Lincoln, T.L. Immunologic approach to
      non-Hodgkin's lymphoma and related leukemias. An analy-
      sis of the results of multiparameter studies of 425
      cases. Sem. Hematol., 15:322, 1978.
12.   Lukes, R.J., Taylor, C.R., and Parker, J.W. Immunologic
      surface marker studies in the histopathological diagno-
      sis of non-Hodgkin's lymphomas based on multiparameter
      studies of 790 cases. In: S.A. Rosenberg and H.S.
      Kaplan (eds.), Advances in Malignant Lymphoma:
      Etiology, Immunology, Pathology, and Treatment. Vol. 3.
      Bristol-Myers Symposia, New York: Academic Press, in
      press.
13.   Masur, H., Michelis, M.A., Greene, J.B., Onorato, I.,
      Vandestouwe, R.A., Holzman, R.S., Wormser, G., Brettman,
      L., Lange, M., Murray, H.W., and Cunningham-Rundles, S.
      An outbreak of community-acquires Pneumocystis carinii
      pneumonia. Initial manifestation of cellular immune
      dysfunction. N. Engl. J. Med., 305:1431, 1981.
14.   Meyer, P. Personal communication.
15.   Murphy, E.D. SJL/J, a new inbred strain of mouse with a
      high, early incidence of reticulum cell neoplasms. Proc.
      Am. Assoc. Cancer Res., 4:46, 1963.
16.   Parker, J.W., Joyce, J., and Pattengale, P. Spontaneous
      neoplasms in aged athymic (nude) mice. In: Proceedings
      of the Third International Workshop on Nude Mice. pp.
      347-358. New York: Gustav-Fischer, 1982.
17.   Pattengale, P.K. and Taylor, C.R. Immunomorphologic classi-
      fication of murine lymphomas and related leukemias. In:
      Proceedings of the Rodent Lymphoma Workshop, Marsh 4-5,
      pp. 72-79. Available from the National Center for
      Toxicological Research, Jefferson, Arkansas, 1981.
18.   Pattengale, P.K. and Taylor, C.R. Experimental models of
      lymphoproliferative disease: the mouse as a model for
      human non-Hodgkin's lymphomas and related leukemias.
      Am. J. Pathol. (in press).
19.   Pattengale, P.K. and Schultz, L.D. - unpublished com-
      munications.
20.   Pattengale, P.K., Ramstedt, U., Gidlund, M., Orn, A.,
      Axberg, and Wigzell, H. Natural killer (NK) activity in
      (C57BL/6xDBA/2)F_1 hybrids undergoing acute and chronic
      graft-versus-host (GVHD) disease. Eur. J. Immunol.
      (in press).
21.   Pattengale, P.K. - unpublished observations.
22.   Pattengale, P.K. and Frith, C.H. Immunomorphologic classi-
      fication of spontaneous lymphoid cell neoplasms
      occurring in female BALB/c mice. J. Natl. Cancer
      Inst., 70:169, 1983.
23.   Pattengale, P.K., Taylor, C.R., Twomey, P., Hill, S.,
      Jonasson, J., Beardlsey, T., and Haas, M.

Immunopathology of B cell lymphomas induced in C57BL/6 mice by dualtropic murine leukemia virus (MuLV). Am. J. Pathol., 107:362, 1982.

24. Pattengale, P.K., Taylor, C.R., Panke, T., Tatter, D., McCormick, R.A., Rawlinson, D.G. and Davis, R.L. Selective immunodeficiency and malignant lymphoma of the central nervous system. Possible relationship to the Epstein-Barr virus. Acta Neuropathol. (Berl.), 48:165, 1979.

25. Roder, J.C., Karre, K., and Kiessling, R. Natural killer cells. Prog. Allergy (Basel), 28:66, 1981.

26. Rygaard, J. and Povlsen, C.O. The mouse mutant nude does not develop spontaneous tumors. Acta Pathol. Microbiol. Scand. (B), 82:99, 1974.

27. Rygaard, J. and Povlsen, C.O. The nude mouse vs. the hypothesis of immunological surveillance. Transplant. Rev., 28:43, 1976.

28. Shultz, L.D. and Green, M.C. Motheaten, an immunodeficient mutant of the mouse. II. Depressed immune competence and elevated serum immunoglobulin. J. Immunol., 116:936, 1976.

29. Siegal, F.P., Lopez, C., Hammer, G.S., Brown, A.E., Kornfeld, S.J., Gold, J., Hassett, J., Hirschman, S.Z., Cunningham-Rundles, C., Adelsberg, B.R., Parham, D.M., Siegal, M., Cunningham-Rundles, S., and Armstrong, D. Severe acquired immunodeficiency in male homosexuals, manifested by chronic perianal ulcerative herpes simplex lesions. N. Engl. J. Med., 305:1439, 1981.

30. Storb, R. Personal communication.

31. Waldman, T.A., Strober, W., and Blaese, R.M. Symposium on the relationship of immunodeficiency to cancer. Ann. Int. Med., 77:605, 1972.

ALLOGRAFT TRANSPLANT CANCER REGISTRY

Israel Penn

Department of Surgery
University of Cincinnati Medical Center
Veterans Administration Medical Center
3200 Vine Street
Cincinnati, Ohio 45220

INTRODUCTION

Advances in our understanding of cancer derive from the recent discovery that immune deficiency is associated with an increased frequency of malignancies, particularly lymphomas. This increase has been observed both in naturally occurring diseases (23,47) and in conditions produced by iatrogenic depression of immunity (76-86). A prime example is the immunosuppressed state induced in organ transplant recipients. In 1968, we first drew attention to an increased incidence of neoplasms in this group of patients (76). Since then, we have maintained an informal allograft transplant cancer registry. Physicians from many countries have generously contributed their data. The cases reported up to September 1982 are summarized here.

Incidence of Malignancies

The Cincinnati (formerly Denver) Transplant Tumor Registry (CTTR) has information on 1592 types of neoplasia that arose in 1497 organ transplant recipients. Of these, 1463 patients received kidney, 29 heart, 2 hepatic and 3 bone marrow transplants. Analysis of data on 11,857 patients reported by 17 major renal transplant centers in Europe, Australia, and the United States reveals an incidence of cancer arising de novo after transplantation ranging from 1% to 16% (average 4%) in series of patients ranging from 470 to 1131 individuals.

In a series of 182 cardiac transplant recipients who underwent 199 transplantations the incidence was 10% (113). Elsewhere in this monograph Bieber discusses this in detail. The small numbers of liver or bone marrow transplant recipients in this series may reflect the short survival of patients undergoing these procedures. Additional information regarding this group is provided in chapters by Neudorf and Meuwissen and associates. An important factor in the case of the bone marrow recipients may be the very different immunosuppressive regimen used as opposed to renal, hepatic, or cardiac allograft recipients. Immunosuppression is given more or less continuously over many months or years whereas bone marrow recipients are given a short burst of intensive immunosuppression immediately before transplantation followed by an approximately 100 day course of immunosuppression designed to prevent or treat graft versus host disease (GVHD). Thereafter, no further immunosuppression is usually given except in patients with protracted GVHD.

The marked variations in the prevalence of cancer among renal transplant recipients may reflect significant differences in the intensity of immunosuppressive therapy administered at different centers. A more likely explanation is that some centers report all malignancies, no matter how trivial, whereas others report only florid types. The true incidence of malignancies is greater than the average figure of 4%: many centers include individuals treated in the early years of transplantation when patient survival was often short; also recipients with short lengths of follow-up are included. The importance of these factors is brought out by the study of Sheil et al. (99). Of 683 patients, 109 (16%) developed cancer (80% of which were skin neoplasms). However, if only the 459 patients who survived for at least six months are considered the incidence is 24%.

The frequency of cancer does increase with the length of follow-up after transplantation. Of 418 renal transplant patients who survived at least one year 26% had tumors; at 10 years 14 of 30 survivors (47%) were so afflicted (99). Similarly, the actuarial risk of developing cancer in 124 cardiac transplant recipients, was $2.7 \pm 1.9\%$ at one year and $25.6 \pm 11.0\%$ at 5 years (53). These statistics mandate following transplant patients indefinitely.

Age of Patients

The average age of the transplant recipients was 39.9 years (range 7 months to 70 years). Those with lymphomas were slightly younger (38.8 years) than recipients with nonlymphomatous tumors (40.1 years). Overall, 49% of the recipients were under 40 years of age, a relatively young group compared with the age of cancer patients in the general population.

Sex of Patients

Sixty-seven percent of patients were male and 33% female. These figures were similar in recipients with lymphomas and nonlymphomatous tumors. The data merely reflects the 2:1 ratio of male to female patients who undergo renal transplantation.

Time of Appearance of Tumors

The tumors appeared an average of 51 (range 1-204) months after transplantation. Lymphomas tended to appear earlier (average 29 months) than other malignancies (average 57 months). Overall, the neoplasms appeared relatively soon after transplantation as compared with other oncogenic stimuli in man which usually take 15 to 20 years or more before they produce their effects (85).

Previous Tumors in Recipients

Controversial is whether or not there is an increased incidence of cancer in patients receiving chronic dialysis therapy (85). This problem needs to be resolved as it may bear on the frequency of tumors in patients after transplantation. Of the tumors reported to the CTTR, 4.6% appeared within 4 months after transplantation. Either these neoplasms had very rapid induction times or some of them were present, but not clinically manifest, at the time of transplantation.

Nineteen patients had malignancies treated before transplantation. The cancers that appeared after this procedure bore no known relationship to the previous neoplasms in 14 recipients. However, in 5 there was a morphological or etiological connection between the two types of cancer. One patient with basal cell skin cancers before transplantation developed a cutaneous malignant melanoma after transplantation. A second recipient, who had been successfully treated for multiple myeloma, developed a pulmonary immunoblastoma. A third patient who had a gastric lymphosarcoma treated with radiotherapy 17 years previously developed an adenocarcinoma of the stomach that appeared after transplantation. Two recipients with Hodgkin's disease and myeloma respectively developed Kaposi's sarcoma after transplantation. Kaposi's sarcoma is often associated with other malignancies (9).

Malignancies in the Donors

Cancer cells may be transmitted with the allograft from a donor with cancer. They may survive and become clinically manifest in the immunosuppressed recipients. Thus it is necessary to examine for dissemination of cancer from the donors. In the present series nine donors had malignancies. Six had primary tumors

of the central nervous system, one had a carcinoma of the
bronchus, one had a cylindroma of salivary gland origin, and one
had been treated for carcinoma of the colon within 5 years of
transplantation. The neoplasms that developed in the recipients
bore no known relationship to the cancers in their respective
donors.

Types of Malignancy

The tumors recorded in the CTTR up till September 1982 are
listed in Table 1. Non-lymphomatous tumors occurred in 1201 recipients, lymphomas in 279 and both types in 17. More than one
variety of cancer was present in 95 patients so that 1592 types of
malignancy were encountered. The tumors most frequently seen in
the general population including carcinomas of the lung, prostate,
colon and rectum, female breast, and invasive carcinoma of the
uterine cervix were not increased in frequency in transplant recipients. However, certain neoplasms were remarkably common in

Table 1. De Novo Cancers in Organ Allograft Recipients

Type of Tumor	No. of Patients
Cancers of the skin and lips	604
(excluding 34 patients with carcinoma of the vulva, perineum, penis or scrotum)	
Solid lymphomas	291
Carcinomas of uterus	114
Cervix (103)	
Body (11)	
Carcinomas of the lung	75
Carcinomas of colon and rectum	59
Leukemias	42
Carcinomas of breast	47
Metastatic carcinomas	40
(primary site unknown)	
Carcinomas of the head and neck (exluding thyroid, para-thyroid, and eye)	38
Carcinomas of the kidney	35
Host kidney (31)	
Allograft kidney (4)	
Carcinomas of thyroid	25
Carcinomas of liver and bile ducts	23
Carcinomas of urinary bladder	24
Cancers of stomach (2 carcinoid tumors)	20
Ovarian cancers	20
Testicular carcinomas	19
Soft tissue sarcomas	22
Cancers of the pancreas	16
Carcinomas of prostate gland	12
Brain Neoplasms	10
Miscellaneous tumors	56
	TOTAL 1592

[a]There were 1497 patients of whom 95 had more than one type of tumor

these patients. In two epidemiologic studies non-Hodgkin's
lymphomas were increased 28 fold and 49 fold, respectively over
that observed in the age matched population (40,49). Skin cancers
were common. They were in part determined by the amount of exposure to sun (82). In regions with relatively little sun, the
incidence was increased four to seven fold. With high actinic
exposure the frequency rose almost 21 fold above the already high
prevalence observed in the general population of those areas.
Almost all the increase was in squamous cell carcinoma. Possibly
some increase occurred in malignant melanoma (82). A special type
of skin cancer, involving the vulva and perineum, was also a
surprisingly common finding (Table 1). Many afflicted patients
were young, an unusual finding in that tumors in these locations
generally occur in older people in the general population. A few
patients gave a history of herpes genitalis or condyloma acuminatum. Perusal of the Table indicates a remarkably high incidence
of Kaposi's sarcoma. It comprises only 0.6% of all cancers in the
general population of the United States but makes up 3.5% in
transplant patients. If we omit non-melanoma skin cancers and
in-situ carcinomas of the cervix which are excluded from most
cancer statistics, the frequency becomes 5%. In-situ carcinomas
of the cervix of the uterus showed a 14 fold increase over that
seen in the age-matched population.

Lymphomas

    The focus of this book is lymphomas and thus detailed
discussion is provided (Table 2). In transplant patients these
neoplasms show several unusual features when compared with their
pattern in the general population. Lymphomas make up 3% to 4% of
all tumors in communities at large. In contrast, they comprised
291 of 1592 tumors (18%) in transplant patients. If we exclude
non-melanoma skin cancers and in-situ carcinomas of the uterine
cervix the corrected frequency was 26%. I have included Kaposi's
sarcoma among the lymphomas as some pathologists believe that they
belong in this category of neoplasms. However, as the cell of
origin of Kaposi's sarcoma is still a matter of controversy (109),
its inclusion among the lymphomas may not be justified.
Endothelial cell origin of Kaposi's is likely. See the chapter by
Sonnabend on Kaposi's sarcoma in male homosexuals. If we exclude
the 55 cases of Kaposi's sarcoma from the above statistics, the
frequency of lymphomas is 19%. This figure still reflects the
disproportionately high prevalence of lymphomas among transplant
patients. (Kaposi's sarcoma will be discussed in a later section
of this report.)

    Classification of the lymphomas remains problematic. There
are about 50 histological classifications of lymphoma (108).
Ideally we would classify all the tumors according to the cell of
origin such as T cell, B cell, null cell, etc. Unfortunately,

only a small number of tumors listed in Table 2 have been studied
by immunological techniques. To date all 25 cases studied immunologically were of B cell origin. To my knowledge no lymphoma of T
cell origin has been described in organ transplant recipients.

We are left with a hodge-podge of terms for the tumors.
Taylor (108) has emphasized that different morphological expressions of lymphoma, which formerly were classified as distinct and
separate diseases, are not absolutely distinct one from another,
they frequently merge. In addition to the problem of classifying
lymphomas, pathologists have great difficulty in distinguishing
certain "immunoproliferations" from true "lymphomas" (18). The
problem is compounded in transplant patients whose lymphoid
tissues are exposed to a number of foreign antigens, including
those of the allograft, heterologous anti-lymphocyte globulin, a
broad spectrum of infectious agents, and a variety of medications.
The lesions may appear to be malignant on morphological grounds,
but immunoperoxidase and other cell marker techniques reveal the
"lymphomas" are polyclonal (34). Hanto describes this later in
this section of the book. These may represent a proliferative
phase of poorly differentiated lymphoid cells midway in development between an EBV-induced polyclonal lymphoproliferative process
and a monoclonal lymphoma. A transition from the polyclonal
infiltrates to monoclonal tumors has been postulated. These
findings have therapeutic implications. The polyclonal lymphoproliferations should not be treated with chemotherapeutic agents.
Instead immunosuppression should be reduced and antiviral agents
such as Acyclovir® or interferon should be administered.

Table 2. Solid Lymphomas in Organ Transplant Recipients

Reticulum cell sarcomas[a]	146[b]
Kaposi's sarcomas	55[b]
Unclassified lymphomas	34
B cell lymphomas	25
Lymphosarcomas	10
Hodgkin's disease	9
Plasma cell lymphomas	6
Lymphoreticular malignancies	4
Burkitt's lymphoma	1
Histiocytic medullary reticulosis	1
TOTAL	291

[a]Also classified as "histiocytic lymphoma,"
 "microglioma," "immunoblastic sarcoma,"
 "reticulosarcoma," and "large cell lymphomas."
[b]One patient had Kaposi's sarcoma and a reticulum
 cell sarcoma.

Several other lymphoproliferative disorders must be distinguished from lymphomas in transplant patients, including immunoblastoid lymphadenopathy (61), lymphomatoid granulomatosis (33), lymphoid hyperplasia induced by antilymphocyte or anti-thymocyte globulin therapy (24), and toxoplasmosis (46). In addition, diphenylhydantoin (dilantin), used in seizure disorders, in dialysis, and renal transplant patients, may cause pseudo-lymphomas and even lymphomas (17).

Unusually uncommon is Hodgkin's disease (HD). Only 9 cases of HD occurred among 236 patients (4%) with lymphomas whereas in the general population it comprises 34% of all lymphomas and is the most common subtype of lymphoma in any age group (78,83-85). In three recipients HD was localized involving a regional lymph node area in 2 patients and the liver in one. The other 6 recipients had widespread disease most commonly involving multiple lymph node areas. In all, 7 of the 9 patients (78%) had lymph node involvement. HD is also underrepresented as a malignancy in children with primary immune deficiency.

Of the patients with non-Hodgkin's lymphomas 6 had plasmacytomas. In 3 the tumor was localized to the small bowel, the large bowel, and the brain, respectively. The other 3 patients had widespread disease.

The remaining 221 patients with non-Hodgkin's lymphomas had a variety of tumors. Reticulum cell sarcomas predominated. In

Table 3. Non-Hodgkin's Lymphomas Involving Brain
or Spinal Cord[a]

Organs Involved	No. of Patients
Brain only	67[b]
Brain and multiple organs	13[b]
Brain and lungs	2
Spinal cord only	1
CNS (site not specified)	2
Brain and lymph nodes	1
Brain, spinal cord and lymph nodes	1
Brain and renal allograft	1
TOTAL	88

[a]Excludes 1 patient with involvement of the pituitary gland, 2 with meningeal involvement and 1 with involvement of the retina and optic nerve.
[b]Excludes one patient in each category with multiple myeloma.

several series in the general population extranodal involvement
occurred in from 24% to 48% of cases (21,91). In contrast, among
these 221 patients extranodal involvement occurred in 173 (78%).
Of those with nodal involvement 45 patients had widespread
involvement of the liver, lungs, spleen, bone marrow, small bowel,
colon, and brain. Only 3 patients had nodal lesions isolated to a
single area. Extranodal localization to a single organ or
occurred in 124 patients (56%). Of these recipients 71 (57%) had
lymphoma localized in the central nervous system (CNS). Overall
88 of the 221 patients (40%) had CNS involvement (Table 3).
Patients with meningeal involvement were not included in these
statistics. Almost always the brain was affected. Frequently,
the brain tumors had multicentric distribution. The remarkably
high frequency of involvement of the brain contrasts with a 1%
incidence of cerebral involvement by non-Hodgkin's lymphoma in a
series of 1039 patients in the general population (meningeal
involvement occurred in 3.7%) (38).

Possibly the brain involvement is due to poor immunological
reactions so that lymphoma cells, that arise in the brain itself
or are carried there from other regions, grow readily in this
privileged site (78,85). Clues to the mechanisms which allow
EBV-associated lymphoproliferative disorders to invade the CNS
come from studies in nude mice (28A). Subcutaneous injection of
aneuploid Burkitt lymphoma cells results in tumor formation,
whereas injection of diploid polyclonal lymphoblastoid cell lines
are rejected, presumably by natural killer cells. In contrast,
both cell lines will grow as tumors if injected into the CNS. The
physician should consider a lymphoma of the CNS whenever a
transplant patient develops neurological symptoms. Thorough
evaluation is necessary, i.e., examination of the cerebrospinal
fluid, computerized axial tomography, electroencephalography,
radionuclide brain scan, and cerebral angiography. These tests
assist in excluding more common causes of neurological symptoms

Table 4. Leukemias in Organ Transplant Recipients

Myeloid leukemia	2
Acute myeloblastic leukemia	11
Chronic myeloid leukemia	11
Erythroleukemia	6
Monocytic leukemia	1
Acute monoblastic leukemia	3
Acute myelomonoblastic leukemia	2
Acute leukemia (undifferentiated)	3
Acute lymphoblastic leukemia	2
Chronic lymphocyte leukemia	1

including hypertensive encephalopathy, meningitis, brain abscess or intracranial hemorrhage.

Another striking feature in the 221 patients was the frequency of lymphomatous involvement of the allograft. It occurred in 30 renal transplant recipients, 1 cardiac allograft patient and 1 hepatic transplant recipient. In at least 4 patients the tumor presented in the soft tissues at the sites of injection of antilymphocyte globulin (11,16,113).

As lymphomas are common in transplant patients one might expect that leukemias would also be frequent. However, only 3 of 42 leukemias could definitely be identified as lymphocytic (Table 4). The majority of leukemias arose from granulocytes, or less frequently, from monocytes.

Owing to the inevitable transplantation of substantial numbers of donor lymphocytes with an allograft, the question arise whether the lymphomas arises from donor or host origin. Most lymphomas arise from host lymphocytes in transplantation studies in animals (28). Studies of sex chromatin or of HLA specificities on donor and recipient lymphocytes and lymphoma cells in one liver and 5 renal transplant recipients showed that all arose from host cells, while in a bone marrow transplant patient the tumor was of donor origin (29,80).

Sixteen of 30 tumors (53%) that occurred in 29 cardiac allograft recipients were lymphomas. Bieber describes this in great detail in the next chapter. Several observations deserve discussion. An increased incidence of lymphoma was found in young patients with idiopathic cardiomyopathy and in those who required retransplantation (6). However, these variables did not correlate when evaluated by multivariate analysis (113). Firstly, patients who present with idiopathic cardiomyopathy are younger than those with atherosclerotic coronary artery disease. Certain investigators think that the observed relationship between preexisting cardiac disorders and the lymphoma may reflect the patient's age rather than the pretransplant diagnosis (113). However, in two epidemiologic studies in renal transplant recipients, no consistent variations in risk of developing lymphoma according to age at transplantation could be found (40,49).

Secondly, there is no support for the theory that patients with idiopathic cardiomyopathy are more prone to lymphoma than the general cardiac transplant population (113). Thirdly, the degree of immunosuppression is related to the development of lymphoma. Patients undergoing multiple cardiac allografts have a significantly increased risk (113). In the overall CTTR series, 15% of patients who developed lymphomas had undergone two or more transplantations, whereas for the patients with nonlymphomatous

tumors – it was 10%. In two epidemiologic studies in renal
transplant recipients, no difference in the risk of developing
lymphoma was found between patients who underwent multiple as
opposed to single transplants (49), but a significant relationship
was found in the other study (41).

Radiotherapy or combination chemotherapy or both have greatly
improved the prognosis of patients in the general population
suffering from Hodgkin's disease and non-Hodgkin's lymphoma. In
contrast, lymphomas in transplant patients have poor prognoses.
Only 18% of patients in the present series are currently alive.
Admittedly, not all the deaths were from lymphoma. The dismal
outlook for these patients was borne out by a study showing that
mortality of renal transplant recipients with lymphomas was
increased 48 fold over that seen in the general population (48).

Kaposi's Sarcoma

Transplant patients with Kaposi's sarcoma (KS) were generally
young averaging 41 years (range 25-59 years). [Abrams and
Sonnabend describe this cancer in male homosexuals elsewhere in
this monograph.] Their tumors appeared from 3 to 101 months after
transplantation (average 16 months). In the general population KS
occurs mainly in young black males in tropical Africa and in
whites of Eastern European Jewish or North Italian ancestry
(109). In transplant patients the 55 cases occurred in 10
patients of Jewish background (including 9 Israelis), 8 blacks, 4
Arabs, 4 Italians, 3 Greeks, 3 Brazilians, and 19 of various
ancestries, mostly of West European origin.

Thirty-seven patients (67%) with KS had involvement of the
skin, oropharyngolaryngeal mucosa, or both. Visceral involvement,
particularly of the gastrointestinal tract or respiratory system,
occurred in 18 recipients (33%). Eight of the 37 patients (22%)
with nonvisceral lesions had complete or partial remissions
following cessation or reduction of immunosuppressive therapy.
Although spontaneous remissions of Kaposi's sarcoma do occur
occasionally, the high frequency of remissions suggests that the
changes in treatment or immunity played a significant role.
Twenty-six of 37 patients (70%) with nonvisceral involvement and 4
of 18 with visceral KS (22%) are currently alive. The deaths in
patients with visceral lesions were usually caused by their KS,
while in patients with non-visceral involvement death came from
other causes. The behavior of Kaposi's sarcoma in transplantation
patients is more benign than that seen in immunodeficient homosexual men (102). These patients have a high incidence of KS,
lymphadenopathy, fever and weight loss, features attesting to the
often generalized nature of their disease. There is a high
mortality rate in these men.

One should suspect Kaposi's sarcoma whenever a transplant recipient develops reddish blue macules or plaques in the skin or oropharyngeal mucosa, or "granulomas" that fail to heal (78,81-85). If the diagnosis is confirmed a thorough evaluation is necessary to exclude visceral involvement.

Skin and Lip Cancers

The most common tumors reported to the CTTR were carcinomas of the skin and lips (38% of the neoplasms). Their frequency increases with the length of follow-up after transplantation (63,82,98). In recipients from Australia, the overall frequency of skin cancer was 5%. The prevalence was 8% in survivors of at least one year after transplantation and it was 17% in survivors of four years or longer (63). In addition, 28% of the four-year survivors had premalignant keratoses.

The pathologic types reported to the CTTR are shown in Table 5. Features distinguishing these skin neoplasms from those seen in the general population included reversal of ratio of the basal cell to squamous cell carcinomas (63,82,98). Another difference is the youth of the transplant patients (i.e., 30 years younger than the community at large) (82). In addition, multiple cutaneous malignancies occurred in 263 of 604 transplant recipients (44%), an incidence in this worldwide collection of patients comparable to that seen only in areas of high sunshine exposure.

Most skin cancers were of low-grade malignancy and were readily controlled with conventional therapy. Lymph node metastases occurred in 40 patients, 33 of whom had squamous cell

Table 5. Carcinomas of the Skin and Lips

Type of Tumor	No. of Patients
Squamous cell carcinomas	317
Basal cell carcinomas	171
Squamous and basal cell carcinomas	81
Malignant melanoma	24[a]
Unclassified	8
Malignant sweat gland carcinoma	2[b]
Intracystic sebaceous gland carcinoma	1
TOTAL	604

[a]Five patients also had a squamous cell carcinoma, and another had multiple basal cell carcinomas.
[b]One patient also had a basal cell carcinoma; another also had basal and squamous cell carcinomas.

carcinomas and 7 with malignant melanomas. Of the squamous cell
carcinomas that involved lymph nodes, 25 involved the skin only, 4
the lips, and 4 with skin and lip involvement. However, in three
patients with skin and lip involvement, the clinical picture
suggested that the metastases probably arose from the skin
lesions. Metastatic skin cancer caused the deaths of 35 patients,
23 with squamous cell carcinomas and 12 of 24 with malignant
melanomas. Of the fatalities caused by squamous cell carcinomas,
17 were caused by lesions arising in the skin, 3 by lesions from
the lips, and 3 from lesions involving the lips and skin, but the
skin lesions apparently were responsible for the lethal metastases. These findings are in keeping with a more than ten fold
increased mortality from squamous cell carcinoma of the skin in
Australian renal transplant recipients (48).

Etiology of the Tumors

Probably a complex interplay of multiple factors is required
even in the development of a single type of tumor. We shall consider the roles played by disturbances of immunity; oncogenic
viruses; oncogenic effects of immunosuppressive agents; possible
co-oncogenic properties of these compounds; other potentially
oncogenic treatments; and variations in individual susceptibility
to neoplasia (77,78,85).

DISTURBANCES OF IMMUNITY

There are several ways by which deficient immune reactions may
aid the development of neoplasms.

Immune Surveillance

According to the immune surveillance hypothesis (7,9,110) a
major function of immunity is to control cancer. During daily
wear and tear millions of cells require replacement. Occasional
cells undergo mutations, some of which have malignant potential.
According to the hypothesis, the immune system recognizes aberrant
cells and destroys them. Only when a rare tumor cell escapes surveillance does a cancer become evident. Immune surveillance is
not involved in the induction of cancers but only in the control
of clinically unrecognized in-situ tumors (43).

T lymphocytes are regarded as playing a key role in immune
surveillance. However, these cells alone cannot account for the
control of incipient neoplasms. Recent data suggests that natural
killer (NK) cells, macrophages, and possibly polymorphonuclear
leukocytes play important roles in surveillance (37,106). Supporting this view are studies in beige mice which have a selective and
marked defect in NK activity. They have a high frequency of

lymphomas (93).   Patients with the Chediak-Higashi syndrome have
similar immune defects (94).   Their lymphoproliferative diseases
are described by Merino in this volume and elsewhere (15).   The
frequent occurrences of lymphomas in organ transplant recipients
may also be related to severely depressed NK activity (59).

The immune surveillance concept has stirred controversy
(43,55,69,78,85,96,106).   One criticism leveled at the hypothesis
is that if it is correct, we should observe an increase of all
cancers, not only certain tumors.   However, perhaps if organ
transplant recipients lived long enough they would develop tumors
which usually have a long latent period of 15 or 20 years or more,
such as carcinomas of the breast, bronchus, prostate and colon in
similar proportions to those seen in the general population (43).
However, many patients die at an earlier stage from intercurrent
infections and lymphomas.

Critics of the immune surveillance hypothesis also argue that
if the theory is correct we should observe cancers in immunologically privileged sites, i.e., the anterior ocular chamber, the
hamster's cheek pouch, and possibly the brain (69,105).   These
criticisms can be refuted.   Malignancies are unlikely to arise in
the anterior chamber of the eye since it contains very few mitotic
cells (43).   In addition, lymphomas frequently occur in the brains
of organ transplant recipients as described above.   Presently it
is unwise to dismiss the surveillance hypothesis as being invalid.

Immune Stimulation

When mixtures of immune lymphocytes and malignant cells were
injected into irradiated animals accelerated neoplastic growth was
observed when low lymphocyte-to-tumor ratios were used.   However,
with higher ratios inhibition of growth was found.   These findings
form the basis of the immune stimulation theory (89) which
suggests a weak immune reaction, rather than inhibiting tumor
growth, stimulates it.   The effects of immunological reactions on
their target tissues may be considered biphasic: stimulation of
cell division and growth occurs at one level, and inhibition of
growth and destruction of cells at another.   This theory is difficult to prove and it does not account for the disproportionally
high frequency of certain tumors.

Chronic Antigenic Stimulation

Repeated or continuous antigenic stimulation in several
experimental models has resulted in malignant lymphomas
(2,5,28,44,66,107,111).   Chronic stimulation of lymphoid tissues
may lead to hyperplasia and eventually neoplasia.   This sequence
of events is analogous to experiments producing neoplasms in
hyperstimulated target organs after disrupting endocrine feedback

mechanisms (22). The frequent occurrence of lymphomas, particularly reticulum cell sarcomas, in organ transplant recipients
may be related to the prolonged presence of an allograft having
foreign histocompatibility antigens, or to antigenic stimulation
from infectious agents. Lukes and Collins (60) have shown that
reticulum cell sarcomas have the morphology of antigen-stimulated
lymphocytes and hence call them "immunoblastic sarcomas."

Chronic antigenic stimulation may also cause lymphomas by
activating endogenous C-type oncornaviruses. Hirsh et al. (39)
have shown that rejection of skin grafts placed in Balb/c(H-2^d)
mice from A/J (H-2^a) or DBA/2(h-2^d) donors activated viruses,
which when injected in NIH-Swiss mice induced thymic lymphomas.

One model for producing lymphomas through chronic antigenic
stimulation involves the establishment of chronic GVHD in adult
F_1 hybrid mice (28). Chronic GVHD may also activate C-type
viruses and continued viral replication in blastogenic lymphoid
tissue may progress to neoplastic proliferation (39). Similar
mechanisms may explain the development of lymphomas in organ
transplant recipients. Donor lymphocytes or lymphoid tissues are
invariably transplanted with the kidney, liver or heart and may
possibly cause GVHD. However, if GVHD causes post transplant
lymphomas in man, it is curious that these neoplasms occur
frequently after renal or cardiac transplantation in which GVHD is
virtually unknown. In contrast, only rarely lymphomas are
observed after bone marrow transplantation (29), which is frequently complicated by GVHD, but in which long term survival has
been accomplished (100). Chapters by Neudorf and Meuwissen discuss
this aspect in greater detail elsewhere in this book. It seems
possible that when large numbers of survivors are followed for
prolonged periods, more lymphomas will be observed.

A hypothesis that may explain the frequent occurrence of
Kaposi's sarcoma in transplant patients implicates a chronic immunological reaction between antigenically altered lymphoid cells
and normal lymphocytes (112). In the course of this local GVHD an
angiogenesis factor is liberated and intense proliferation of
mesenchymal and endothelial cells occurs. During this process an
oncogenic virus is either transferred to or induced in the cells
responsive to the angiogenesis factor and induces their malignant
transformation.

Impaired Immunoregulation

Since cellular and humoral feedback mechanisms are important
in controlling the extent of immune reactions (85) defective
control may permit unrestrained proliferation of lymphoid cells
ultimately leading to the development of lymphomas. This may
account for the unusually high incidence of lymphomas in organ

transplant recipients. One postulate is that thymic suppressor function, which normally restricts lymphoid proliferation, is impaired thus permitting unregulated growth and lymphomagenesis (25). Furthermore, once loss of regulation occurs, the defensive capabilities of the immune system are disrupted and other, nonlymphoid, malignancies may appear.

Another theory is based on observations that immunological reactions may activate latent oncogenic viruses (2,39,96). Continuous antigenic stimulation of partially immunodeficient mice may cause the development of lymphoreticular neoplasms (2,56). As many patients described in this study also are only partially immunodeficient, it is postulated that defective antibody production fails to control lymphocyte proliferation and leads to derepression of the virogene and the activation of oncogenic viruses in an environment that favors their replication. Viruses shed from lymphoblasts infect cells in the microenvironment of the immunologic reaction causing their malignant transformation (96).

Loss of Reactivity to Tumor Antigens in Transplant Patients

The following data form the basis of a theory proposed by F.H. Bach (3). Some renal transplant recipients become specifically non-responsive to certain alloantigens present on the graft when tested in the mixed lymphocyte culture test (4). In addition, the use of pooled allogeneic normal cells to produce allo-sensitization of normal lymphocytes from a patient with leukemia leads to the development of cytotoxic T lymphocytes that are capable of lysing the patient's own leukemia cells (117,118). This observation suggests that alloantigens are actually cross-reactive with tumor-associated antigens or that cancer cells actually express certain alloantigens of the species other than those carried by normal cells of the patient. The hypothesis is that alloantigens on the graft are cross-reactive with or directly expressed on certain neoplastic cells that arise in the patient and since the renal allograft recipient has lost immunological reactivity to alloantigens, there is a concomitant loss of reactivity to the tumor (3).

Immunosuppression from Blood Transfusions

Experiments in rats have revealed that blood transfusions cause nonspecific immunosuppression. Animals transfused before inoculation of cancer cells have accelerated tumor growth when compared with controls (20). As pretransplant blood transfusions have a beneficial effect on the outcome of cadaveric renal transplants in man, the question arises whether the nonspecific immunosuppression produced by transfusions may increase the risk of cancer. Examination of the Transplant Tumor Registry data did

not show any increased incidence of tumors in transfused patients
as compared with nontransfused controls (74).

The other subjects that may relate disturbances of immunity
with the development of cancer are the spontaneous regression of
lymphomas and the effects of interferons.

Spontaneous Regression of Lymphomas

De novo lymphomas or Kaposi's sarcomas in several transplant
patients have undergone partial or complete regression, usually
after reduction or cessation of immunosuppressive therapy
(24,34,81,85). We may postulate that as the patient's immune
systems recovered from their suppressed state they not only
destroyed the malignancies but also prevented further proliferation of oncogenic viruses. However, we must bear in mind that
there are other possible explanations for the spontaneous remission of lymphomas (54). Hanto discusses this further in this
volume.

Interferons

The interferons have profound biological effects including
interference with replication of oncogenic viruses, and inhibition
of growth of cancer cells (30). The latter response may result
from their direct effects on malignant cells, or from their
actions on the immune system, or from neutralization of some of
the deleterious effects of tumor-secreted substances (30). The
immune system and the interferon system are closely linked (14).
Fiala discusses these relationships in this book. Several
immunosuppressive agents limit both antibody secretion and
interferon production in parallel. These include x-irradiation,
corticosteroids, cyclophosphamide, antilymphocyte serum, actino-
mycin, and 6-mercaptopurine (the active metabolite of azathioprine) (14,77). Use of these agents may contribute to the
development of neoplasms through reduced interferon production.
Against this theory are findings that cyclophosphamide, azathioprine and 6-mercaptopurine do not affect interferon responses
or the protective effects of interferon inducers (34).

ONCOGENIC VIRUSES

The short induction time of many of the malignancies, especially the lymphomas in transplant recipients, is compatible with
a viral etiology. Important ways oncogenic viruses can act in
organ transplant recipients include: a) As mentioned above, an
immunological reaction, such as rejection of a transplanted organ,
may activate latent endogenous oncornaviruses (12,39) and b)

immunosuppressed patients are susceptible to a great variety of infectious agents including viruses (1,10,103,104). Frequently infections are caused by EBV, herpes simplex types 1 (HSV-1) and 2 (HSV-2), cytomegalovirus, varicella-zoster virus, and papilloma-virus (84). These viruses are thought to cause certain malignan-cies in animals and man. The role of EBV in lymphomagenesis in immunodeficient individuals is discussed elsewhere by many authors in this book. One question arises: If EBV causes lymphomas in transplant patients, why do we not see an increased incidence in these indivduals ot the other cancer in man that is believed to be EBV-related, namely nasopharyngeal carcinoma (NPC)? Immune deficient children carrying EBV-induced lymphoproliferative disorders do not develop NPC. Three chapters in this volume by Wolf, Krueger and Volsky discuss NPC.

Other herpesviruses may be oncogenic under certain conditions. Several in vitro studies show that HSV-1 and HSV-2 may cause transformation of animal and human cells in culture (70,73,90). Johnson discusses and illustrates lymphoproliferative diseases induced by herpesviruses in monkeys elsewhere in the book. Several herpesviruses have caused lymphoproliferative tumors in chickens and primates, and renal adenocarcinomas in frogs (50). Uterine cancer has been induced in mice after prolonged exposure to HSV, types 1 and 2 (114). The high incidence of skin and lip cancers in organ transplant recipients may be related to infec-tions with HSV-1 (57,116) or varicella-zoster virus (115). HSV-2 has been postulated as a cause of uterine cervical carcinoma in women (50,90). It may possibly account for the increased inci-dence of this tumor in organ transplant patients (78,87). Cytomegalovirus has been isolated from tissue cultures of Kaposi's sarcoma in the general population (26). It also may be related to the outbreak of Kaposi's sarcoma in homosexual males (102), and to the high incidence of this cancer in organ transplant recipients.

There are at least eleven different types of wart (papilloma) virus. In the general population certain types of warts of the skin undergo malignant transformation and serve as a model for the study of oncogenesis (27,62). Examples are epidermodysplasia verruciformis and the venereal wart of condyloma acuminatum (27,88). Since wart virus infections are frequent in organ transplant recipients (51,84), it is possible that they may contribute to their frequent skin, vulvar, and perineal cancers (Table 1). They may also play a role in causing uterine cervical dysplasia and carcinoma (97).

Non-oncogenic viruses may enhance the effect of known car-cinogens. Experiments in mice subjected to various non-oncogenic virus infections and treated with a chemical carcinogen caused an increased prevalence of benign and malignant tumors (101).

Sonnabend, Witkin and Purtilo note elsewhere in the monograph
that male homosexuals are apt to develop cancers similar to renal
transplant recipients - Kaposi's sarcoma, non-Hodgkin's lymphoma
or squamous cell carcinomas which could be due to cytomegalovirus,
EBV or papilloma virus, respectively.

Oncogenic and Co-oncogenic Effects of Immunosuppressive Agents

The commonly used immunosuppressive agents are azathioprine,
prednisone or methylprednisolone, ALG, and cyclosphosphamide. With
the exception of cyclophosphamide, data is insufficient concerning
their carcinogenicity. Most experimental tumors developed only
when these agents were combined with physical or chemical carcinogens, with foreign protein, with virus infections, or were
used in animals such as NZB mice, suffering from autoimmune
diseases. However, the agents apparently did not cause
"spontaneous" malignancies when administered alone (36,42,52,56,
72,77). Azathioprine may be carcinogenic in man (42) but the
agent is rarely used by itself. No direct carcinogenicity has
been attributed to prednisone or ALG in humans. Possibly these
three agents may be co-oncogens in man promoting environmental
carcinogens such as sunlight, tobacco, or radiation. The incidence of skin cancers in hairless mice repeatedly exposed to
ultraviolet light was increased by the prolonged administration of
azathioprine (52). If these results can be extrapolated to man,
they may explain the high incidence of skin cancers seen in organ
allograft recipients. Dysplasia of the uterine cervical epithelium occurs after treatment with a number of immunosuppressive
agents including azathioprine (32,45,95). This agent, with a
HSV-2 infection, may account for the high incidence of carcinoma
of the cervix in transplant patients.

Cyclosporin A has been associated with lymphomas. Widespread
lymphomas occurred in 12 of 97 primates who survived at least two
weeks after transplantation of the heart or the heart and lungs
(92). Bieber describes this in this volume. All presented in 55
animals who had received Cyclosporin A either as a single medication or in combination with other immunosuppressive agents. In
man, Cyclosporin A has been used in approximately 1400 patients.
Concern has been expressed that 13 of 15 neoplasms that developed
following its use were lymphomas (86), and that 4 of the tumors
occurred in a series of 31 cardiac transplant patients treated
with this agent (75). In addition a fifth recipient had a
disseminated lymphoproliferative disorder not meeting the criteria
for malignant lymphoma. The 13 lymphomas appeared in a remarkably
short time after transplantation (average 6 months). Only one
patient was treated exclusively with Cyclosporin A. Development
of the tumors may have been related to the intensity of the
immunosuppressive regimen used: lower doses are associated with a
decreased incidence of lymphomas (8). Hanto and others have

implicated EBV in the development of lymphomas following the use of this agent (12,13,92). He discusses evidence for EBV as the etiological agent of these lymphomas in this book.

Total lymphoid irradiation has been associated with the development of lymphomas in two renal transplant recipients. However, they had been treated with splenectomy, azathioprine, prednisone and ALG (71). In summary, the development of neoplasia cannot be blamed on a single immunosuppressive agent. More likely immunosuppression in general is responsible.

Other Potentially Oncogenic Treatments

The transplant patients may have been exposed to other potentially oncogenic treatments that may have acted independently or may have been co-oncogenic with the immunosuppressive agents. Several examples may be cited. Renal transplant recipients sometimes manifest de novo carcinomas in their own kidneys after transplantation. These may have been caused by previous phenacetin abuse. Isoniazid which is used in the prevention and treatment of tuberculosis is a potential carcinogen (67). As mentioned above diphenylhydantoin (Dilantin) may cause pseudolymphomas or true lymphomas (17,58).

Variations in Susceptibility to Cancer

Animals and patients vary in their genetic susceptibility or resistance to the various oncogenic stimuli discussed above. One variable involves the genetic factors that control the enzymatic activation of chemical carcinogens. Wide individual variation prevails in carcinogen metabolism. The ratio of metabolic activation to deactivation of carcinogens may play a role in the development of neoplasms (35,68). Another important variable, which may determine why some animals and patients develop cancers and others do not, is the regulation of the immune response by the major histocompatibility system (65). Yet another variable, that may affect an individual's susceptibility or resistance to viral infections or neoplasms is the level of interferon secretion (31).

SUMMARY AND CONCLUSIONS

Organ transplantation and its associated immunosuppression is complicated by an increased incidence of certain cancers. Some are common neoplasms in the general population (skin cancers and in-situ carcinomas of the uterine cervix) while others are uncommon (lymphomas, Kaposi's sarcomas and vulvar and perineal carcinomas). The development of disproportionate numbers of these tumors after a relatively short latent period serves as a challenge to define etiology. Firstly, to replace the current

blunderbuss assault on the immune system by a sophisticated and
specific approach ensuring immunologic unresponsiveness only to
the antigens of the allograft but leaving immunity otherwise
unscathed. Secondly, to study the tumors to discover how and what
causes them. Studies done in collaboration by groups lead by
Hanto, Purtilo and Klein have demonstrated EBV genome in
lymphoproliferative diseases in transplant patients [see Cancer
Research 42:4208-4304, 1982].

In addition, time is ripe for a combined clinico-pathological
study of the lymphomas reported to the CTTR by a group of experts
so that these tumors can be characterized by immunologic cytogenetic, histologic and virologic techniques. A better
understanding of the tumors and their etiology may provide us with
means for their prevention or cure.

ACKNOWLEDGEMENTS

The author wishes to thank his many colleagues throughout the
world who have generously contributed data concerning their
patients to the CTTR.

REFERENCES

1.   Allen, D.W. and Cole, P. Viruses and human cancer. N.
        Engl. J. Med., 286:70, 1972.
2.   Armstrong, M.Y.K., Ruddle, N.H., Lipman, M.B., and Richards,
        F.F. Tumor induction by immunologically activated murine
        leukemia virus. J. Exp. Med., 137:1163, 1973.
3.   Bach, F.H. Personal communication, 1981.
4.   Bach, M.L., Engstrom, M.A., Bach, F.H., Etheredge, E.E., and
        Najarian, J.S. Specific tolerance in human kidney
        allograft recipients. Cell. Immunol., 3:161, 1972.
5.   Balls, M. and Ruben, L.N. Lymphoid tumors in amphibia: a
        review. Prog. Exp. Tumor Res., 10:238, 1968.
6.   Bieber, C.P., Hunt, S.A., Schwinn, D.A., Jamieson, S.A.,
        Reitz, B.A., Oyer, P.E., Shumway, N.E., and Stinson, E.B.
        Complications in long-term survivors of cardiac
        transplantation. Transplant. Proc., 13:207, 1981.
7.   Burnet, F.M. Immunological surveillance in neoplasia.
        Transplant. Rev., 7:3, 1971.
8.   Calne, R.Y., Rolles, K., White, J.G., Thiru, S., Evans,
        D.B., Henderson, R., Hamilton, D.L., Boone, N.,
        McMaster, P., Gibby, O., and Williams, R. Cyclosporin-A
        in clinical organ grafting. Transplant. Proc., 13:349,
        1981.
9.   Caro, W.A. Tumors of the skin. In: S.L. Moschella, D.M.
        Pillsbury, H.J. Hurley, Jr. (eds.), Dermatology. pp.

1323-1406. Philadelphia: W.B. Saunders, Co., 1975.

10.   Coleman, D.V., Gardner, S.D., and Field, A.M. Human
       polyomavirus infection in renal allograft recipients.
       Br. Med. J., 3:371, 1973.

11.   Cotton, J.R., Sarles, H.E., Remmers, A.R. Jr., Lindley,
       J.D., Beathard, G.A., Cottom, D.L., Fish, J.C.,
       Townsend, C.M. Jr., and Ritzmann, S.E. The appearance
       of reticulum cell sarcoma at the site of antilymphocyte
       globulin injection. Transplantation, 16:154, 1973.

12.   Crawford, D.H., Thomas, J.A., Janossy, G., Sweny, P.,
       Fernando, O.N., Moorhead, J.F., and Thompson, J.H.
       Epstein-Barr virus nuclear antigen positive lymphoma
       after Cyclosporin A treatment in patients with renal
       allograft. Lancet, i:1355, 1980.

13.   Crawford, D.H., Sweny, P., Edwards, J.M.B., Janossy, G., and
       Hoffbrand A.V. Long-term T-cell mediated immunity to
       Epstein-Barr virus in renal-allograft recipients
       receiving Cyclosporin A. Lancet, i:10, 1981.

14.   Declerq, E. and Merigan, T.C. Current concept of inter-
       feron and interferon production. Ann. Rev. Med., 21:17,
       1970.

15.   Dent, P.B., Fish, L.A., White, J.G., and Good, R.A.
       Chediak-Higashi Syndrome. Observations on the nature of
       the associated malignancy. Lab Invest., 15:1634, 1966.

16.   Deodhar, S.D., Kuklinca, A.G., Vidt, D.G., Robertson, A.L.,
       and Hazard, J.B. Development of reticulum-cell sarcoma
       at the site of antilymphocyte globulin injection in a
       patient with renal transplant. N. Engl. J. Med.,
       280:1104, 1969.

17.   Editorial: Is phenytoin carcinogenic? Lancet, ii:1071,
       1971.

18.   Editorial: Looking at lymphomas. Lancet, ii:306, 1979.

19.   Ehrlich, P. Uber den jetzigen stand der Karzinomforschung.
       In: The Collected Papers of Paul Ehrlich. Vol. 2, p.
       550. London: Pergamon Press, 1957.

20.   Francis, D.M.A. and Shenton, B.K. Blood transfusion and
       tumour growth: evidence from laboratory animals.
       (Letter to the Editor). Lancet, ii:871, 1981.

21.   Freeman, C., Berg, J.W., and Cutler, S.J. Occurrence and
       prognosis of extranodal lymphomas. Cancer, 29:252,
       1972.

22.   Furth, J. Conditioned and autonomous neoplasms: a review.
       Cancer Res., 13:477, 1953.

23.   Gatti, R.A. and Good, R.A. Occurrence of malignancy in
       immunodeficiency diseases. A literature review.
       Cancer, 28:89, 1971.

24.   Geis, W.P., Iwatzuki, S., Molnar, Z., Giacchino, J.L.,
       Kerman, R.H., Ing, T.S., and Hano, J.E. Pseudolymphoma
       in renal allograft recipients. Arch. Surg., 113:461,
       1978.

25. Gershwin, M.E. and Steinberg, A.D. Loss of suppressor func-
     tion as a cause of lymphoid malignancy. Lancet,
     ii:1174, 1973.
26. Giraldo, G., Beth, E., and Hagenau, F. Herpes-type virus
     particles in tissue culture of Kaposi's sarcoma from
     different geographical regions. J. Natl. Cancer Inst.,
     49:1509, 1972.
27. Gisser, S.D. Papovavirus and squamous cell carcinoma.
     Human Pathol., 12:190, 1981.
28. Gleichmann, E., Gleichmann, H., Schwartz, R.S., Weinblatt,
     A., and Armstrong, M.Y.K. Immunologic induction of
     malignant lymphoma: identification of donor and host
     tumors in the graft-versus-host model. J. Natl. Cancer
     Inst., 54:107, 1975.
28A. Giovanella, B., Nilsson, K., Zech, L., Yim, O., Klein, G.,
     and Stehlin, J.S. Growth of diploid, Epstein-Barr
     virus-carrying human lymphoblastoid cell lines
     heterotransplanted into nude mice under immunologically
     privileged conditions. Int. J. Cancer, 24:103, 1979.
29. Gossett, T.C., Gale, R.P., Fleischman, H., Austin, G.E.,
     Sparkes, R.S., and Taylor, C.R. Immunoblastic sarcoma
     in donor cells after bone-marrow transplantation. N.
     Engl. J. Med., 300:904, 1979.
30. Gresser, I. Antitumor effects of Interferon. In: F.F.
     Becker (ed.), Cancer. A Comprehensive Treatise. Vol.
     5, pp. 521-571. New York: Plenum Press, 1977.
31. Grossberg, S.E. The interferons and their inducers:
     molecular and therapeutic considerations. N. Engl. J.
     Med., 287:13, 79, 122, 1972.
32. Gupta, P.K., Pinn, V.M., and Taft, D.D. Cervical dysplasia
     associated with azathioprine (Imuran) therapy. Acta
     Cytol., 13:373, 1969.
33. Hammar, S. and Mennemeyer, R. Lymphomatoid granulomatosis
     in a renal transplant recipient. Hum. Pathol., 7:111,
     1976.
34. Hanto, D.W., Sakamoto, K., Purtilo, D.T., Simmons, R.L., and
     Najarian, J.S. The Epstein-Barr virus in the pathogenesis
     of post-transplant lymphoproliferative disorders.
     Surgery, 90:204, 1981.
35. Harris, C.C. The carcinogenicity of anticancer drugs: a
     hazard in man. Cancer, 37:1014, 1976.
36. Hattan, D. and Cerilli, G.J. Spontaneous reticulum cell
     sarcomas developing in C3H/HeJ mice on prolonged immuno-
     suppressive therapy. Transplantation, 11:580, 1971.
37. Herberman, R.B. and Ortaldo, J.R. Natural killer cells:
     their role in defenses against disease. Science,
     214:24, 1981.
38. Herman, T.S., Hammond, N., Jones, S.E., Butler, J.J., Byrne,
     G.E. Jr., and McKelvey, E.M. Involvement of the central
     nervous system by non-Hodgkin's lymphoma. The Southwest

Oncology Group Experience. Cancer, 43:390, 1979.

39. Hirsch, M.S., Proffitt, M.R., and Black, P.H. Autoimmunity, oncornaviruses, and lymphomagenesis. Contemp. Topics Immunobiol., 6:209, 1977.

40. Hoover, R. and Fraumeni, J.F. Jr. Risk of cancer in renal transplant recipients. Lancet, ii:55, 1973.

41. Hoover, R. and Fraumeni, J.F. Jr. Cancer risks in renal transplant recipients. Cited by Kinlen, L. (ref. 49), in press.

42. IARC monographs on the evaluation of the carcinogenic risk of chemicals to humans. Some antineoplastic and immunosuppressive agents. Vol. 26, pp. 33. Lyon. World Health Organization, International Agency for Research on Cancer, 1981.

43. Ioachim, H.L. The stromal reaction of tumors: an expression of immune surveillance. J. Natl. Cancer Inst., 57:465, 1976.

44. Jerusalem, C. Relationship between malaria infection (Plasmodium berghei) and malignant lymphoma in mice. Z. Tropenmed. Parasitol., 19:94, 1968.

45. Kay, S., Frable, W.J., and Hume, D.M. Cervical dysplasia and cancer development in women on immunosuppression therapy for renal homotransplantation. Cancer, 26:1048, 1970.

46. Kayhoe, D.E., Jacobs, L., Beye, K.K., and McCullough, N.B. Acquired toxoplasmosis: observations on two parasitologically proved cases treated with pyrimethamine and triple sulfonamides. N. Engl. J. Med., 257:1247, 1957.

47. Kersey, J.H., Spector, B.D. and Good, R.A. Primary immunodeficiency diseases and cancer: the Immunodeficiency-Cancer Registry. Int. J. Cancer, 12:333, 1973.

48. Kinlen, L.J., Sheil, A.G.R., Peto, J., and Doll, R. Collaborative United Kingdom-Australian study of cancer in patients treated with immunosuppressive drugs. Br. Med. J., 2:1461, 1979.

49. Kinlen, L. Immunosuppressive therapy and cancer. Cancer Surveys, in press.

50. Klein, G. Herpes viruses and oncogenesis. Proc. Natl. Acad. Sci. USA, 69:1056, 1972.

51. Koranda, F.C., Dehmel, E.M., Kahn, G., and Penn, I. Cutaneous complications in immunosuppressed renal homograft recipients. J. Am. Med. Assoc., 229:419, 1974.

52. Koranda, F.C., Loeffler, R.T., Koranda, D.M. and Penn, I. Accelerated induction of skin cancers by ultraviolet radiation in hairless mice treated with immunosuppressive agents. Surg. Forum, 26:145, 1975.

53. Krikorian, J.G., Anderson, J.L., Bieber, C.P., Penn, I., and Stinson, E.B. Malignant neoplasms following cardiac transplantation. J. Am. Med. Assoc., 240:639, 1978.

54. Krikorian, J.G., Portlock, C.S., Cooney, P., and Rosenberg,
     S.A. Spontaneous regression of non-Hodgkin's lymphoma:
     a report of nine cases. Cancer, 46:2093, 1980.
55. Kripke, M.L. and Borsos, T. Immune surveillance revisited.
     J. Natl. Cancer Inst., 51:1393, 1974.
56. Krueger, G. The significance of immunosuppression and anti-
     genic stimulation in the development of malignant
     lymphomas. In: E. Grundmann and R. Gross (eds.), The
     Ambivalence of Cytostatic Therapy, Recent Results in
     Cancer Research. Vol. 52, pp. 88-95. Berlin:
     Springer-Verlag, 1975.
57. Kvasnicka, A. Relationship between herpes simplex and lip
     carcinoma IV. Selected cases. Neoplasma, 12:61, 1965.
58. Li, F.P., Willard, D.R., Goodman, R. and Vawter, G.
     Malignant lymphoma after diphenylhydantoin (Dilantin)
     therapy. Cancer, 36:1359, 1975.
59. Lipinski, M., Tursz, T., Kreis, H., Finale, Y., and Amiel,
     J-L. Disassociation of natural killer cell activity and
     antibody-dependent cell-mediated cytotoxicity in kidney
     allograft recipients receiving high-dose immuno-
     suppressive therapy. Transplantation, 29:214, 1980.
60. Lukes, R.J. and Collins, R.D. Immunologic characterization
     of human malignant lymphomas. Cancer, 34:1488, 1974.
61. Lukes, R.J. and Tindle, B.H. Immunoblastic lymphadenopathy:
     a hyperimmune entity resembling Hodgkin's disease. N.
     Engl. J. Med., 292:1, 1975.
62. Lutzner, M.A. Epidermodysplasia verruciformis. An autoso-
     mal recessive disease characterized by viral warts and
     skin cancer. A model for viral oncogenesis. Bull.
     Cancer, 65:169, 1978.
63. Marshall, V. Premalignant and malignant skin tumors in
     immunosuppressed patients. Transplantation, 17:272,
     1974.
64. Matas, A.J., Simmons, R.L., and Najarian, J.S. Chronic
     antigenic stimulation, herpes virus infection, and
     cancer in transplant patients. Lancet, i:1277, 1975.
65. McDevitt, H.O. Regulation of the immune response by the
     major histocompatibility system. N. Engl. J. Med.,
     303:1514, 1980.
66. Metcalf, D. Induction of reticular tumors in mice by
     repeated antigenic stimulation. Acta Unio Int. Contra
     Cancrun, 19:657, 1963.
67. Miller, C.T. Isoniazid and cancer risks (Letter to the
     Editor). J. Am. Med. Assoc., 230:1254, 1974.
68. Miller, D.G. On the nature of susceptibility to cancer.
     Cancer, 46:1307, 1980.
69. Möller, G. and Möller, E. The concept of immunological sur-
     veillance against neoplasia. Transplant. Rev., 28:3,
     1976.

70. Munyon, W., Kraiselburd, E., Davis, D., and Mann, J.
     Transfer of thymidine kinase to hymidine kinaseless L
     cells by infection with ultraviolet-irradiated Herpes
     simplex virus. J. Virol., 7:813, 1971.
71. Najarian, J.S., Sutherland, D.E.R., Ferguson, R.M., Simmons,
     R.L., Kersey, J., Mauer, S.M., Slavin, S., and Kim, T.H.
     Total lymphoid irradiation and kidney transplantation: a
     clinical experience. Transplant. Proc., 13(1):417,
     1981.
72. Nehlsen, S.L. ATS-mediated immunosuppression and tumor
     risk. Behring Institute Mitteilungen, Marburg,
     Behringwerke AG pp. 201-203, 1972.
73. O'Neill, F.J. and Miles, C.P. Chromosome changes in human
     cells induced by herpes simplex, Types 1 and 2. Nature,
     223:851, 1969.
74. Opelz, G. Transfusions and malignancy. (Letter to the
     Editor) Lancet, ii:1057, 1981.
75. Oyer, P.E., Stinson, E.B., Jamieson, S.W., Hunt, S., Reitz,
     B.A., Bieber, C.P., Schroeder, J.S., Billingham, M., and
     Shumway, N.E. One year experience with Cyclosporin A in
     clinical heart transplantation. Heart Trans., in press.
76. Penn, I., Hammond, W., Brettschneider, L., and Starzl, T.E.
     Malignant lymphomas in transplantation patients.
     Tranplant. Proc., 1:106, 1969.
77. Penn, I. Malignant tumors in organ transplant recipients.
     New York: Springer-Verlag, 1970.
78. Penn, I. Tumors arising in organ transplant recipients. In:
     G. Klein and S. Weinhouse (eds.), Advances in Cancer
     Research. Vol. 28, pp. 31-61. New York: Academic Press,
     1978.
79. Penn, I. Host origin of lymphomas in organ transplant re-
     cipients. Transplantation, 27:214, 1979.
80. Penn, I. Tumors in allograft recipients (Letter to the
     Editor). N. Engl. J. Med., 30:385, 1979.
81. Penn, I. Kaposi's sarcoma in organ transplant recipients:
     report of 20 cases. Transplantation, 27:8, 1979.
82. Penn, I. Immunosuppression and skin cancer. Clin. Plastic
     Surg., 7:361, 1980.
83. Penn, I. Malignant lymphomas in organ transplant recip-
     ients. Transplant Proc., 13:736, 1981.
84. Penn, I. The price of immunotherapy. Cur. Prob. Surg.,
     18(11):682, 1981.
85. Penn, I. The occurrence of cancer in immune deficiencies.
     Cur. Prob. Cancer, 6(10):1, 1982.
86. Penn, I. Malignancies following the use of Cyclosporin A in
     man. Cancer Surveys, in press.
87. Porreco, R., Penn, I., Droegemueller, W., Greer, B. and
     Makowski, E. Gynecologic malignancies in immuno-
     suppressed organ homograft recipients. Obstet. Gynec.,
     45:359, 1975.

88. Powell, L.C. Jr. Condyloma acuminatum: recent advances in
     development, carcinogenesis and treatment. Clin.
     Obstet. Gynecol., 21:1061, 1978.
89. Prehn, R.T. Do tumors grow because of the immune response
     of the host? Transplant. Rev., 28:34, 1976.
90. Rapp, F. Question: do herpes viruses cause cancer?
     Answer: of course they do. J. Natl. Cancer Inst.
     (Editorial), 50:825, 1973.
91. Reddy, S., Pellettiere, E., Saxena, V., and Hendrickson,
     F.R. Extranodal non-Hodgkin's lymphoma. Cancer,
     46:1925, 1980.
92. Reitz, B.A., Bieber, C.P., and Pennock, J.L. Cyclosporin A
     and lymphoma in non-human primates. In: R.Y. Calne and
     D.J.G. White (eds.), Proceedings International Symposium
     on Cyclosporin A. Elsevier North Holland Biomedical
     Press, in press.
93. Roder, J. and Duwe, A. The beige mutation in the mouse
     selectively impairs natural killer cell function.
     Nature (London), 278:451, 1979.
94. Roder, J.C., Haliotis, T., Klein, M., Korec, S., Jett, J.R.,
     Ortaldo, J., Herberman, R.B., Katz, R., and Fauci, A.S.
     A new immunodeficiency disorder in humans involving NK
     cells. Nature (London), 284:553, 1980.
95. Schramm, G. Development of severe cervical dysplasia under
     treatment with azathioprine (Imuran). Acta Cytol.,
     14:507, 1975.
96. Schwartz, R.S. Another look at immunologic surveillance.
     N. Engl. J. Med., 293:181, 1975.
97. Shah, K.H., Lewis, M.G., Jenson, A.B., Kurman, R.J., and
     Lancaster, W.D. Papillomavirus and cervical dysplasia.
     Lancet, ii:1190, 1980.
98. Sheil, A.G.R., Mahoney, J.F., Horvath, J.S., Johnson, J.R.,
     Tiller, D.J., May, J., and Stewart, J.H. Cancer and sur-
     vival after cadaveric donor renal transplantation.
     Transplant. Proc., 11:1052, 1979.
99. Sheil, A.G.R., Mahoney, J.F., Horvath, J.S., Johnson, J.R.,
     Tiller, D.J., Stewart, J.H., and May, J. Cancer
     following successful cadaveric renal transplantation.
     Tranplant. Proc., 13:733, 1981.
100. Shulman, H.M., Sullivan, K.M., Weiden, P.L., McDonald, G.B.,
     Striker, G.E., Sale, G.E., Hackman, R., Tsoi, M., Storb,
     R., and Thomas, E.D. Graft versus host syndrome in man.
     A long-term clinicopathologic study of 20 Seattle
     patients. Amer. J. Med., 69:204, 1980.
101. Southam, C.M., Tanaka, S., Arata, T., Simkovic, D., Miura,
     M., and Petropolos, S.F. Enhancement of responses to
     chemical carcinogens by nononcogenic viruses and anti-
     metabolites. Prog. Exp. Tumor. Res. (Basel), 11:194,
     1969.

102. Special report. Epidemiologic aspects of the current
      outbreak of Kaposi's sarcoma and opportunistic infec-
      tions. N. Engl. J. Med., 306:248, 1982.
103. Spencer, E.S. and Andersen, H.K. Clinically evident, non-
      terminal infections with herpes viruses and the wart
      virus in immunosuppressed renal allograft recipients.
      Br. Med. J., 3:251, 1970.
104. Stevens, D.A. Immunosuppression and virus infections.
      Transplant. Proc., 5:1259, 1973.
105. Stutman, O. Immunodepression and malignancy. Adv. Cancer
      Res., 22:261, 1975.
106. Stutman, O. Immunological surveillance. In: Origins of
      Human Cancer. pp. 729-750. Cold Spring Harbor
      Laboratory, 1977.
107. Suciu-Foca, N., Dumitrescu, V., Lazar, C. and Nachtigal, M.
      Host and tumor modifications associated with serial
      heterotransplantation of tumors through immunologically
      tolerant animals. Cancer Res., 30:1681, 1970.
108. Taylor, C.R. Classification of lymphoma. New "thinking" on
      old thoughts. Arch. Pathol. Lab. Med., 102:549, 1978.
109. Templeton, A.C. Kaposi's sarcoma. In: R. Andrade, S.L.
      Gumport, G.L. Popkin, and T.D. Rees (eds.), Cancer of
      the Skin. Biology-Diagnosis-Management. pp. 1183-1225.
      Philadelphia: W.B. Saunders Co., 1976.
110. Thomas, L. Discussion of Medawar, P.B. Reactions to homo-
      logous tissue antigens in relation to hypersensitivity.
      In: H.S. Lawrence (ed.), Cellular and Humoral Aspects of
      the Hypersensitive States. pp. 529-532. New York: Paul
      Hoeber, 1959.
111. Walford, R.L. and Hildemann, W.H. Life span and lymphoma-
      incidence of mice injected at birth with spleen cells
      across a weak histocompatibility locus. Amer. J.
      Pathol., 47:713, 1965.
112. Warner, T.F.C.S. and O'Loughlin, S. Kaposi's sarcoma: a
      byproduct of tumor rejection. Lancet, ii:687, 1975.
113. Weintraub, J. and Warnke, R.A. Lymphoma in cardia
      allograft recipients. Clinical and histological features
      and immunological phenotype. Transplantation, 33:347,
      1982.
114. Wentz, W.B., Reagan, J.W., Heggie, A.D., Fu, Y-S., and
      Anthony, D.D. Induction of uterine cancer with inac-
      tivated herpes simplex virus, 1 and 2. Cancer, 48:1783,
      1981.
115. Wyburn-Mason, R. Malignant change arising in tissues
      affected by herpes. Br. Med. J., 2:1106, 1955.
116. Wyburn-Mason, R. Malignant change following herpes simplex.
      Brit. Med. J., 2:615, 1957.
117. Zarling, J.M., Robins, H.I., Raich, P.C., Bach, F.H., and
      Bach, M.L. Generation of cytotoxic T lymphocytes to

autologous human leukemia cells by sensitization to
pooled allogeneic normal cells. Nature, 274:269, 1978.

118. Zarling, J.M. and Bach, F.H. Continuous culture of T cells
cytotoxic for autologous human leukemia cells. Nature,
280:685, 1979.

LYMPHOMA IN CARDIAC TRANSPLANT RECIPIENTS ASSOCIATED WITH

CYCLOSPORIN A, PREDNISONE AND ANTI-THYMOCYTE GLOBULIN (ATG)

Charles P. Bieber, Richard L. Heberling, S.W. Jamieson, Phillip E. Oyer, Michael Cleary, Roger Warnke, Ari Saemundsen, George Klein, Werner Henle, and E.B. Stinson

Departments of Cardiovascular Surgery and Pathology
Stanford University Medical Center
Stanford, California 94305
The Southwest Foundation for Research
San Antonio, Texas 78284
The Institute for Tumor Biology
Karolinska Institute
Stockholm 60 Sweden
and the Joseph Stokes, Jr. Research Institute
Children's Hospital
Philadelphia, PA

INTRODUCTION

Cardiac transplantation has been used since 1968 to restore cardiac function in selected patients with otherwise unmanageable heart disease. In these recipients successful outcome of the procedure has been highly dependent upon effective management of allograft rejection using immunosuppressive agents. Prior to 1980 these agents included Azathioprine, corticosteroids and anti-thymocyte globulin - ATG (conventional therapy). In 1980 cyclosporin A, a fungal product whose therapeutic effect appears to result from its ability to block allograft directed T cell cytotoxic responses while leaving intact T cell suppressor responses, was substituted for azathioprine in the conventional therapy regimen (cyclosporin A therapy) (1,2). Although outcome of transplantation has been favorably effected in patients treated with cyclosporin A (79% one year survival vs. 63% in conventionally treated recipients) morbidity due to lymphoma has increased.

Among the initial 200 cardiac recipients given conventional therapy, 10 lymphomas were recorded. Lymphoma occurred most com-

monly in young recipients with idiopathic cardiomyopathy (3,4).
The most common presenting site was the brain (5) followed by the
lungs (2), ATG injection site (2), and liver (1). Two of these
recipients responded favorably to whole brain irradiation and were
free of disease three and five years following treatment; a third
recipient with involvement of brain had systemic involvement at
time of diagnosis and died shortly thereafter. The remaining two
brain lesions were occult and were detected at autopsy following
death from unrelated causes. Neither of the recipients presenting
with lung disease had recurrence following surgical resection and
local irradiation. The remaining three recipients with lymphoma
died from systemic disease. Histologic sections were all
interpreted as diffuse large cell lymphomas and negative for Ig
markers (5). The biology of these lymphomas was unclear. The
absence of Ig markers prevented confirmation of B cell lymphoma,
however, the histology was comparable to the B cell lymphoma
reported by other investigators (6). Epstein-Barr virus (EBV)
genomes were detected by nucleic acid hybridization studies in two
tumors, consistent with B cell origin (7). Whether they were true
neoplasias or perhaps EBV infection in a severe immunodeficient
host is uncertain. Irrespective of the "true" nature of the
biology, however, it was apparent that these tumors were clinically malignant; a rapid growth and spread was observed.

Additional observations have been made in the 39 most recent
cardiac recipients who had received cyclosporin A. Five lymphomas
have developed in these 39 recipients. In this report we provide
histologic, biologic, and clinical features associated with the
occurrence of lymphoma in these recent recipients. Also similar
findings in cyclosporin A treated monkey allograft recipients who
also develop lymphoma are discussed.

MATERIAL AND METHODS

Thirty-nine cardiac recipients were transplanted at Stanford
University Medical Center between December 1980 and June 1982.
All patients received cyclosporin A at 17 mg/Kg/day initially.
This was reduced over a two week period to maintain a serum level
of 150-250 ng/ml. In addition, all received prednisone 1
mg/Kg/day initially but then tapered to a maintenance dose of .2
mg/Kg/day. Twenty-six recipients initially received anti-
thymocyte globulin made in rabbits at 3 mg/Kg/day for a total of
three doses. Rejection episodes were treated by augmentating corticosteroids and in 13 instances reinstitution of ATG. Thirty-one
of the 39 recipients received ATG for prophylaxis and/or treatment
of rejection.

Serological Studies

Pre and posttranplant serum samples were studied for antibody titers to EBV viral capsid antigen (VCA), diffuse (D) and restricted (R), early antigen (EA) and nuclear-associated antigen (EBNA) (8). These studies were provided by Dr. Werner Henle, Philadelphia Children's Hospital, Philadelphia, Pennsylvania.

Tissue Typing

HLA determination of tumor cells teased from affected lymph nodes were typed in the laboratory of Dr. Rose Payne. Suspensions of teased cells were examined by light microscopy to assure cytologic conformation to the lymphoma.

Histology

Histologic examination of routine and frozen tissue sections was performed by Dr. Roger Warnke. Studies of cell surface markers were by methods previously described (5).

Nucleic Acid Hybridization Studies

Frozen aliquots of tumor tissue from 3 recipients and 2 non human primates were submitted to Ari Saemundsen in Dr. George Klein's laboratory for EBV genome assay of isolated DNA by nucleic acid hybridization techniques (7,9). Hybridization studies were also performed by Dr. Cleary in the Stanford laboratories.

Non Human Primates

Previous studies documented a 44% incidence of lymphoma in cynomolgus (Macaca fasicularis) cardiac allograft recipients immunosuppressed at least two months by cyclosporin A (10). A cynomolgus B cell line containing Herpes virus (CHV) was established from explants of lymphoma (11). The virus has properties similar to EBV in that human sera positive for EB-VCA and EA antibodies were shown by immunofluorescence techniques to react with the cynomolgus B cell line. The cynomolgus monkeys seronegative for antibodies to CHV were given 2×10^{8} cells containing CHV. Cells were radiated with 2000 rads to prevent proliferation and injected subcutaneously into the right thigh of each animal. Prior to inoculation each monkey received three daily 3 mg/Kg doses of ATG. Concomitant with virus injection the animals were given cyclosporin A 6 mg/Kg/day intramuscularly in the left thigh. The animals were examined daily for tumors. Serology was performed by Dr. Richard Heberling, Southwest Foundation for Research and Education, San Antonio, Texas.

Table 1. Clinical Features of Cardiac Recipients Receiving Cyclosporin A/
Prednisone/ATG Who Developed Lymphoma

Table 1. Clinical Features of Cardiac Recipients Receiving Cyclosporin A/
Prednisone/ATG Who Developed Lymphoma

Patient	Age/Sex	Presenting disease	HLA Type donors	Recipient	Tumor	Histology	Onset (mos)	Stage	VCA	EB Serology R	D	EBNA
205	39M	CAD	A1,2B8,37	ND	ND	DLCL	4	IV	320/160	160/20	-/-	80/20
208	39M	RHD	A2,32,B7,61	A3,31B35	ND	DLCL	6	IV	320/2560	-/40	-/-	160/80
214	40M	CAD	A3,24B27,63	A3,26B7	ND	DLCL	5	IV	1240/1280	20/20	-/-	10/-
225	46M	CAD	A29,33,B13,35	A2,B5,18	A2,B5,18	DLCL	3	I	320/5120	10/320	-/-	80/40
234	32M	CAD	A2,28B8,62	A1,25B8	A1,25B8	DLCL	3	III	-/640[5]	-/10	-/-	2/-

1. CAD - coronary artery disease; RHD rheumatic heart disease
2. DLCL - diffuse large cell lymphoma
3. Incidental finding at autopsy - death due to complications of ruptured splenic artery aneurysm
4. Reciprocals of serum titer measured preop and at time of tumor diagnosis
    (ie., 320/160 VCA of 1/320 preop and 1/160 at diagnosis; a - indicates no reactivity at 1/10 dilution)
5. IgM anti-VCA -/40.

Table 2. Lymphoma in Cardiac Recipients at Risk Three Months or Greater Following Transplantation

Treatment Group	Period	Recipients (No)	1 yr. survival (%)	Cumulative yrs. at risk	Lymphomas (No)	%Incidence yr. at risk
I. Corticosteroids Azathioprine Equine ATG	1968–1973	38	47	151.7	2	1.3%
II. Corticosteroids Azathioprine Rabbit ATG	1973–1980	108	63	343.8	8	2.3%
III. Corticosteroids Rabbit ATG cyclosporin A	1980–1981	31	79	26.5	5	18.9%
IV. Corticosteroids cyclosporin A	1982–	8	---	2.5	0	0

RESULTS

Clinical Studies

Five lymphomas developed in 31 recipients treated with a combination of cyclosporin A, prednisone, and ATG. These 31 recipients had a cumulative risk of 26.5 years yielding a lymphoma incidence/year at risk of 18.9%. This figure was in contrast to the previous figure of 2% per year at risk for recipients treated with prednisone, azathioprine and ATG (3). In contrast to previous experience, lymphoma occurred in older age recipients and in recipients presenting with arteriosclerosis (Tables 1 and 2). Incidence of lymphoma did not relate to cyclosporin dose, mean serum levels of cyclosporin recorded, ATG dose or number of ATG courses. Lymphoproliferative disorders have not occurred in eight patients treated with cyclosporin and prednisone alone, however, cumulative survival is presently only 2.5 years and the longest at risk period is 6 months.

All five lymphomas were diffuse large cell lymphomas of the immunoblastic type (Figure 1). Tumors were examined for Ig

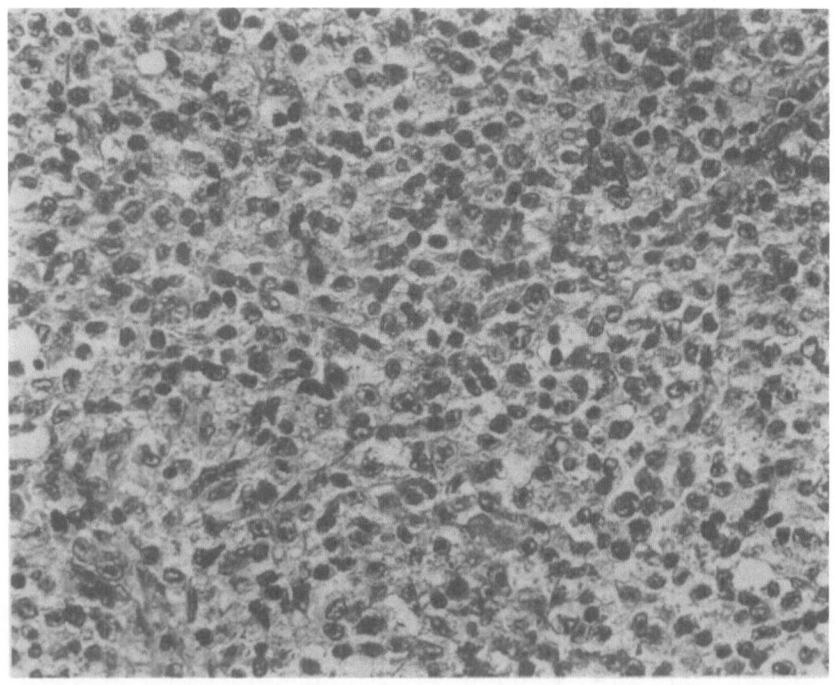

Fig. 1.   Inguinal lymph node with diffuse large cell lymphoma from patient 214.

markers in four instances. Three were negative. A fourth (pt. 234) had a more complicated pattern of staining. Tissue from an involved lymph node was predominantly negative for Ig but areas of Ig staining were noted. Ig staining revealed both kappa and lambda markers. Lambda markers, however, were most evident. In a splenic tumor nodule a larger proportion of cells were Ig positive, although most remained Ig negative. However, lambda positive cells were in the vast majority. In addition, all patients' tumors were stained with monoclonal antibodies to HLA-DR and four T cell antigens (Leu1, 2a, 3a, and 4). All were positive for HLA-DR and all negative for T cell antigens. In two instances viable tumor cells were obtained for HLA typing. In both instances tumor cells clearly possessed the HLA A and B haplotype of the cardiac recipient (Table 2).

Antibody titers to EBV-VCA, EA-R, D, and EBNA antigens were determined in 26 recipients. Twenty-four had antibody to VCA in preoperative sera. Eleven had antibody to EA, mostly R and 23 had anti-EBNA. At one month posttransplant, all 26 had antibodies to VCA and an additional 6 (17 total) antibodies to EA and 25 had antibodies to EBNA. Antibody determinations were made in 20 recipients at the end of 5 months. All remained VCA seropositive, however, two developed EA antibodies.

Antibodies to VCA and EA were present either preoperatively or at time of tumor diagnosis in all recipients who developed lymphoma (Table 3). The presence of elevated EA titers were evidence of EBV reactivation or recent infection.

Table 3. EBV Serology in Cardiac Recipients Receiving Cyclosporin A, Corticosteroids, and ATG

Serologic status	Pretransplant (patients)	1-5 Mos. Posttransplant (patients)
Seronegative (VCA-D-R-EBNA-)	2	0
Latent (VCA+D-R-EBNA+)	16	9
Active (VCA+,D+,R+,EBNA+)	8	17*

*Lymphoma only occurred in patients with evidence of reactivated infection.

In four instances, frozen tumor tissue was available for EB-DNA hybridization studies. All had cRNA/DNA filter hybridization results of >6 genome copies per cell.

Experimental studies in two monkeys inoculated with CHV are preliminary. In one, right groin adenopathy, proximal to the virus inoculation site, became apparent one week following injection. By two weeks this adenopathy had resolved and the monkey remained asymptomatic. However, at four months adenopathy recurred in the right groin. It rapidly grew to the size of a golf ball and the animal died in 2 days. Necropsy revealed a diffuse large cell lymphoma of the immunoblastic type limited to the right inguinal and lower para-aortic lymph nodes (Figure 2). The remaining monkey has no evidence of disease. In both seronegative animals, antibody titers to CHV increased to 1/80 at two weeks following inoculation. At the time of lymphoma diagnosis, the

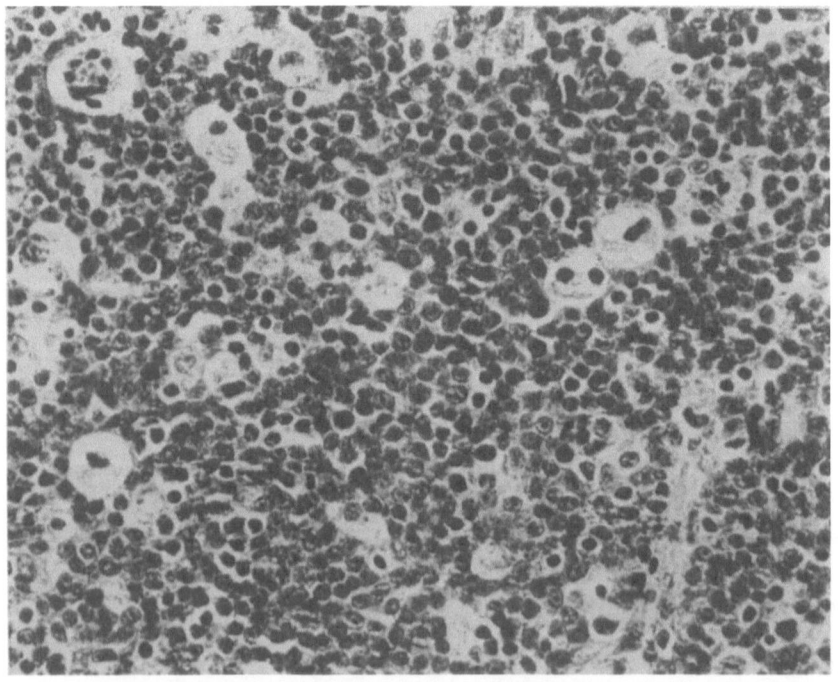

Fig. 2. Right inguinal large cell lymphoma in monkey administered cynomolgus herpes virus in the right thigh. Animal pretreated with ATG and maintained on cyclosporin A. Numerous histiocytes within immunoblastic lesion result in a resemblance of this tumor to African Burkitt's lymphoma.

titer in the monkey was 1/160 (or greater) and in the non
afflicted animal, it was 1/80. DNA hybridization studies for
human EB DNA were negative. Previous studies of monkey lymphomas
have not revealed the presence of human EB genome equivalents.

DISCUSSION

These studies demonstrate that a moderate to high incidence of
lymphoma can be anticipated in organ graft recipients treated with
cyclosporin A in combination with prednisone and ATG. Our
findings are comparable to other clinical transplant programs who
have also reported an increased incidence of lymphoproliferative
diseases when cyclosporin A was used (12,13). Clearly an increase
in the incidence of lymphoma relative to rates observed in
conventionally treated cardiac recipients and to rates reported
from other transplant centers is found when cyclosporin A is used.
A major difference in immunosuppressive protocol used at Stanford
relative to other centers using cyclosporin A has been our
inclusion of the use of ATG for prevention or treatment of
rejection. Cyclosporin A and ATG synergistically enhance the
immunodeficiency predisposing to lymphoproliferative diseases.
Cardiac recipients treated with combined immunosuppression exhibit
a reduction in the incidence of rejection but unfortunately, this
appears to result in an increase occurrence of lymphomas.

The results of our studies strongly implicate EB virus in the
pathogenesis of the lymphoproliferative diseases. Recent reactivation of EB was detected in all patients developing lymphoma.
Furthermore, lymphoma only developed in patients who demonstrated
evidence of EB reactivation. Hybridization studies demonstrated
the presence of EB genomes in all four instances where tissue
was available for examination.

EBV reactivation in recipient B cells under conditions of
immunosuppression may ultimately lead to unchecked outgrowth of
primitive B cell clones. B cell outgrowth can be achieved in
vitro by exploiting cyclosporin A's ability to inhibit T cell
cytotoxicity for autologous EB virus infected B cells (14,15).
Thus it seems reasonable to assume that treatment with cyclosporin
A and ATG facilitates reactivation and outgrowth of latent or
newly EBV infected cells. The resulting immunosuppression allows
a clinical spectrum ranging from infectious mononucleosis to
lymphoma to emerge.

Lymphoma developing among conventionally treated cardiac
recipients have previously been reported to be diffuse large cell
lymphomas which lack T or B cell markers (5). Lymphomas developing among the cyclosporin/prednisone/ATG treated patients have a
similar histology. The absence of Ig surface markers on most

tumors could have resulted from either loss of Ig expression or
failure of complete differentiation of immunoblasts. Evidence for
polyclonality such as described by Frizzera and co-workers is
suggested by surface Ig studies on tissue taken from recipient 234
(15). The preponderance of tumor cells with lambda markers in the
splenic site may represent one line of tumor cells while the cells
without Ig markers and those with kappa markers represent others.
Another measure of clonality would be to detect chromosomal alterations. To date this has not been accomplished.

The degree of immunosuppression resulting from combination
cyclosporin/prednisone/ATG is difficult to assess because the in
vitro assays are insensitive. Following ATG therapy, patients are
relatively devoid of circulating T cells for a period of one to
three weeks. Thus it is impossible to perform in vitro assays.
In contrast, recipients administered cyclosporin/prednisone
without ATG have no decrease in T cell numbers, mitogen stimulation indices or natural killer cell activity from that observed in
normal controls (16). Unfortunately, the frequency and severity
of rejection is also high in these latter patients. Whether the
degree of immunosuppression needed to assure continuous cardiac
function can ever be achieved, without a risk of lymphoma, may
depend on whether the disease can be defined sufficiently so that
effective countermeasures for its prevention or cure be taken. To
this end the strong association of disease with EB virus both by
serology and direct assay of tumor for EB viral genomes becomes
important. Participation of the EB virus in the pathogenesis of
disease offers the possibility that either anti-viral therapy such
as has been proposed by Hanto and associates or vaccination
against appropriate EB viral antigens such as suggested by
Epstein might effectively control disease (17,18). A possible
model for developing such therapy is described in this report.
Lymphoma developing in immunosuppressed monkeys administered CHV
share virtually all the histologic, biologic and clinical characteristics of lymphoma in immunosuppressed patients. Monkey tumors
are generally immunoblastic by histologic criteria, grow in an
explosive fashion, disseminate widely, and are associated with a
herpesvirus similar to EBV. Additional primate studies are in
progress to establish if there is indeed a necessity for CHV virus
in lymphoma development. Once established the immunologic deficit
requirements for development of these clinically malignant disorders could perhaps be defined.

ACKNOWLEDGEMENTS

     This work was supported in part by grants from the National
Heart and Lung Institute, HL13108.

REFERENCES

1. Oyer, P.E., Stinson, E.B., Jamieson, S.W., Hunt, S.A.,
    Billingham, M., Scott, W., Bieber, C.P, Reitz, B.A., and
    Humway, N.E. Cyclosporin A in cardiac allografting: a
    preliminary experience. Transpl. Proc., in press.
2. Hess, A.D. and Tutschka, P.J. Effect of Cyclosporin A on
    human lymphocyte responses in vitro. J. Immunol.,
    124:2601, 1980.
3. Bieber, C.P., Hunt, S.A., Schwinn, D.A., Jamieson, S.W.,
    Reitz, B.A., Oyer, P.E., Shumway, N.E., and Stinson, E.B.
    Complications in long-term survivors of cardiac
    transplantation. Transpl. Proc., 13:207, 1981.
4. Pennock, J.L., Oyer, P.E., Reitz, B.A., Jamieson, S.W.,
    Bieber, C.P., Wallwork, J., Stinson, E.B., and Shumway,
    N.E. Cardiac transplantation in prospective for the
    future. J. Thorac. and Cardio. Surg., 83:168, 1982.
5. Weintraub, J. and Warnke, R.A. Lymphoma in cardiac
    allotransplant recipients. Clinical and histologic
    features in immunologic phenotype. Transplant., 33:347,
    1982.
6. Frizzera, G., Hanto, D., Kazmiera, J., Gajl-Peczalska, J.,
    Rosai, J., McKenna, R.W., Sibley, R.K., Holahan, K.P.,
    and Lindquist, L.L. Polymorphic diffuse B cell
    hyperplasias and lymphomas in renal transplant reci-
    pients. Cancer Res., 41:4262, 1981.
7. Saemundsen, A.K., Klein, G., Cleary, M., and Warnke, R.
    EBV-carrying lymphoma in cardiac transplant recipients.
    Lancet, ii:158, 1982.
8. Henle, W., Henle, G., Zajac, B., Pearson, G., Waubke, R.,
    and Scriba, M. Differential reactivity of human sera
    with EBV-induced "early antigens." Science, 169:188,
    1970.
9. Saemundsen, A.K., Purtilo, D.T., Sakamoto, K., Sullivan,
    J.L., Synnerholm, A.C., Hanto, D.W., Simmons, R.L.,
    Anvret, M., Collins, R., and Klein, G. Documentation of
    EB virus infections in immunodeficient patients with
    life-threatening lymphoproliferative diseases by EB
    virus complementary RNA/DNA and viral DNA/DNA hybridiza-
    tion. Cancer Res., 41:4237, 1981.
10. Bieber, C.P., Pennock, J.L., and Reitz, B.A. Lymphoma in
    Cyclosporin A treated non human primate allograft recip-
    ients in malignant lymphomas. In: H.S. Kaplan and S.
    Rosenberg, p. 219. New York: Academic Press, 1982.
11. Heberling, R.L., Bieber, C.P., and Kalter, S.S. Establish-
    ment of a lymphoblastoid cell line from a lymphomatous
    Cynomolgus monkey. In: D.S. Yohn and J.R. Blakeslee
    (eds.), Advances in Comparative Leukemia Research.
    pp. 385-386. Amsterdam: Elsevier Biomedical, 1982.

12.   Calne, R.Y., Rolles, K., and Thiru, S. Cyclosporin ini-
          tially as the only immunosuppressant in 34 recipients of
          cadaveric organs. Lancet, ii:1033, 1979.
13.   Crawford, D.H., Thomas, J.A., and Janossy, G. Epstein-Barr
          virus nuclear antigen positive lymphoma after
          Cyclosporin A treatment in patients with renal
          allograft. Lancet, i:1355, 1980.
14.   Crawford, D.H., Sweeny, P., Edwards, J.N., Janossy, G., and
          Hoffbrand, A.V. Long-term T cell-mediated immunity to
          EB virus in renal allograft recipients receiving
          Cyclosporin A. Lancet, i:10, 1981.
15.   Bird, A.G., McLachlan, S.M., and Britton, S. Cyclosporin A
          promotes spontaneous outgrowth in vitro in EB virus
          induced B cell lines. Nature, 289:300, 1981.
16.   Prieksaiks, J. - Personal communication.
17.   Hanto, D.W., Frizzera, G., Gajl-Peczalska, J., Purtilo, D.T.
          Klein, G., Simmons, R.L., and Najarian, J.S. The EB
          virus in the pathogenesis of posttransplant lymphoma.
          Transplant. Proc., 13:756, 1981.
18.   Epstein, M.A. Vaccine control of EB virus-associated tumors
          in the Epstein-Barr virus. In: M.A. Epstein, and B.G.
          Achong (eds.), The Epstein-Barr Virus. pp. 440-448.
          Berlin, Heidelberg, New York: Springer-Verlag, 1979.

LYMPHOPROLIFERATIVE DISEASES IN RENAL ALLOGRAFT RECIPIENTS

Douglas W. Hanto[1], Glauco Frizzera,
Kazimiera J. Gajl-Peczalska, David T.
Purtilo[2], and Richard L. Simmons

Departments of Surgery and Laboratory Medicine
Pathology, University of Minnesota Health Sciences
Center, Minneapolis, Minnesota 54555[1]
Departments of Pathology and Laboratory Medicine
Pediatrics and the Eppley Institute for Research in
Cancer and Allied Diseases, University of Nebraska
Medical Center, Omaha, Nebraska 68105[2]

INTRODUCTION

The incidence of lymphoproliferative disorders (LPD) is
increased in many groups of immune deficient patients - recipients
of organ transplants, individuals with genetically determined
immunodeficiency or autoimmune diseases, and patients following
chemotherapy or radiation therapy (20,35,36,46). Because of
their histological features and clinical aggressiveness, these
lymphoproliferations have been labelled malignant lymphomas in
renal allograft recipients.

Such malignant lymphomas make up 20% of the cancers that
develop after transplantation, the second most common after
squamous cell carcinoma of the skin and lips (40%) (35,36). Most
reports have classified a majority of these malignant lymphomas as
reticulum cell sarcoma and have emphasized several peculiar
characteristics: their incidence is 350 times that in the
age-matched general population; the central nervous system is
affected in half of the cases, and most of these are limited to
the central nervous system (CNS); many cases have a short interval
from transplantation to diagnosis (20,35,36,43). Because these
lymphoproliferative disorders occur infrequently in any one series
(incidence 1 to 2%), the systematic investigation of the clinical,
histologic, immunologic or etiologic features, has been delayed.
Many theories of causation have been invoked, including impaired

321

immune surveillance mechanisms (27), chronic antigenic stimulation
(11), reactivation of latent oncogenic herpesviruses (30), and
direct oncogenic effects of immunosuppressive drugs (35,36) but
none have been proven. One of the more attractive theories is
that reactivation of oncogenic herpes viruses, especially the
Epstein-Barr virus (EBV), is responsible. EBV, an infectious and
oncogenic virus, transforms B-lymphocytes inducing a polyclonal
proliferation in vitro (40) and in vivo (39); it causes infectious
mononucleosis in humans (17) and a fatal lymphoproliferative
disorder in cotton-topped marmosets (9,31); it has also been
linked to Burkitt's lymphoma (25), nasopharyngeal carcinoma (26),
and the lymphoproliferative disorders that occur in patients with
X-linked lymphoproliferative syndrome (XLP) (37,38) and ataxia
telangiectasia (41). In renal transplant recipients, oropharyngeal shedding of EBV occurs in 47% to 87% (4,47) compared to 17% in
normal seropositive individuals (3). In addition, significant
rises in antibodies to EBV are common after transplantation (5).
Clinical illness due to EBV, however, has not been clearly defined
in these patients (5,29).

We have now studied 12 renal allograft recipients with a
spectrum of lymphoproliferative disorders (10,12-14). These
patients have been characterized by two distinct clinical patterns
of disease: 1) an acute infectious mononucleosis-like illness
with fever, pharyngitis, and lymphadenopathy, or 2) symptoms and
signs of solid tumor masses. These lymphoproliferative disorders
can be characterized morphologically as polymorphic diffuse B-cell
hyperplasia, polymorphic diffuse B-cell lymphoma, or immunoblastic
B-cell sarcoma. On histologic grounds they can be differentiated
from infectious mononucleosis, other reactive lymphoid hyperplasias, and Burkitt's lymphoma. Immunologic cell typing and
cytogenetic studies have shown that these lymphoproliferative
disorders may be either polyclonal or monoclonal B-cell proliferations. Furthermore, there is evidence that these lymphoproliferative disorders may evolve from polyclonal to monoclonal lymphoproliferations. The Epstein-Barr virus has been implicated as the
cause of these lymphoproliferative disorders on the basis of
serologic evidence, the presence of the Epstein-Barr nuclear
antigen (EBNA), and molecular hybridization techniques which
demonstrate EBV-specific DNA sequences in tumor specimens. As a
result of these findings, the new antiviral drug, Acyclovir®
(Burroughs-Wellcome, Research Triangle Park, NC), has been used to
successfully induce remission during the polyclonal growth phase.
Acyclovir® is also effective in suppressing the oropharyngeal
shedding of EBV. Acyclovir® seems to be ineffective in the
monoclonal lymphomas.

The patients studied are 12 renal allograft recipients who
developed lymphoproliferative disorders following transplantation
at the University of Minnesota. Our 1% overall incidence of

Table 1. Clinical Characteristics of Post-Transplantation
Lymhoproliferative Disorders

Group I	Group II
Infectious Mononucleosis-like Illness (42%)	Localized Tumor Masses (58%)
(a) Young patients (<20 yrs)	Older patients (>45 yrs)
(b) Short interval from transplantation to diagnosis (mean 11 mos.)	Long interval from transplantation to diagnosis (mean 42 mos.)
(c) Symptoms of viral illness (fever, pharyngitis, lymphadenopathy)	Symptoms related to solid tumor masses (confined to CNS 28%)
(d) Widespread disease	Less widespread, primarily extranodal
(e) High mortality (80%)	High mortality (71%)
(f) Short clinical course (mean survival 3 mos.)	Longer clinical course (mean survival 9 mos.)

"post-transplantation lymphoma" is similar to that reported in
multicenter tumor registries (35,36).

Clinical Characteristics

Patients can be divided into two groups, I and II, based on
their clinical presentation (Table 1). Group I (five cases)
patients had an infectious mononucleosis-like illness with
widespread disease. In contrast, patients in group II (seven
cases) had localized tumor masses confined to the central nervous
system in only 28% of the cases; other sites such as the oropharynx, liver, intestine were more frequently involved. Within these
two groups there are several distinguishing characteristics.

Group I: These five patients were typically young (less than
20 years) and became ill soon after transplantation or antirejec-
tion therapy, i.e., during periods of maximal immunosuppression
(Table 2). Their symptoms resembled an acute viral illness

Table 2. Summary of Clinical Characteristics of Lymphoproliferative Disorders after Renal Transplantation

Patient Age/Sex	Interval from Tx (months)	#Previous rejection episodes	Symptoms/Signs	Other organ involvement at diagnosis	Outcome (time after diagnosis)	Organ Involvement[b]
Group I						
1 (19/M)	0.5	-	Fever, sore throat, generalized lymphadenopathy, malaise	—	Died (10 days)	Disseminated
2 (15/M)	3.5	+(3)	Fever, sore throat, cervical lymphadenopathy	—	Died (8 mos.)	LN, tonsil, brain
3 (15/M)	5	-	Fever, sore throat, cervical lymphadenopathy, enlarged parotid	Parotid infiltrate[a]	Died (2 weeks)	LN, parotid, TK, brain, heart, colon, thyroid, lungs
4 (13/F)	33	+(3)	Fever, malaise, creatinine liver function tests	Liver infiltrate[a]	Alive	—
5 (11/F)	12	+(2)	Fever, malaise, rash, lung nodules	Lung nodules	Died (2 mos.)	LN, liver, BM, TK, brain, heart, lungs
Group II						
6 (52/F)	13	-	Headache	—	Died (15 mos.)	Brain
7 (51/F)	50	-	Headache, confusion, blurred vision	—	Died (7 mos.)	Brain
8 (62/F)	60	-	Incidental hard palate tumor	Hard palate mass	Alive	—
9 (68/M)	96	-	Sore throat, dysphagia, exophytic tumor at base of tongue	Oropharyngeal mass	Died	LN, liver, BM, TK
10 (28/M)	33	-	Fever, hematochezia, liver scan defect	Liver masses	Died	Liver
11 (28/M)	13	-	Fever, abdominal pain, hematochezia	Small bowel mass	Died	No residual tumor
12 (47/M)	28	+(1)	Fever, malaise, lung nodules	Lung nodules	Died	TK, lung, LN

[a]The parotid and liver involvement were characterized by invasive, B cell infiltrates without tumor mass formation.
[b]Abbreviations: LN, lymph node; TK, transplanted kidney; BM, bone marrow.

including fever, pharyngitis, and lymphadenopathy. These patients typically had widespread disease which was rapidly lethal in 4 of 5 patients, mean survival, 3 months from the time of diagnosis.

The mean age at diagnosis was 15 years (range, 11 to 19 years). The mean interval from transplantation to diagnosis was 11 months (range, 2 weeks to 33 months) and was less than 1 year in four patients. Three patients had received two transplants. Two patients received total lymphoid irradiation (TLI) (4,050 and 3,250 rads) prior to a second transplant. Three patients had been treated for rejection in the preceding 6 months. Concomitant cytomegalovirus (CMV) and herpes simplex virus (HSV) infections occurred in four and two patients, respectively.

Case Histories. A 19 year-old male received a renal transplant from his mother (Figure 1). Routine immunosuppression consisted of azathioprine, prednisone, and anti-lymphocyte globulin. On the 17th post-transplant day, he complained of mild bilateral knee pain, and his temperature rose to 102° F. During the next two weeks, the patient developed generalized nontender lymphadenopathy, fever to 105° F, profound weakness, anorexia, burning sore throat, difficulty in swallowing, and deteriorating renal function. Routine bacteriologic, viral, and fungal culture results were negative. During this time the number of immuno-blasts and plasmacytoid cells on the peripheral blood smear increased from occasional to as many as 17,500 mm-3 on the 26th post-transplant day. Azathioprine was discontinued and his prednisone dosage was tapered. A supraclavicular lymph node biopsy on the 26th post-transplant day was interpreted as poly-morphic diffuse B-cell hyperplasia. Cell marker studies on this lymph node revealed a polyclonal B-cell proliferation. The patient required hemodialysis and constant sodium bicarbonate infusions secondary to progressive metabolic acidosis and hepatic failure.

On the 28th post-transplant day, cyclophosphamide, cytosine arabinoside and methylprednisolone were started, and a reduction in the lymphadenopathy was noted the following day. A trephine bone marrow biopsy demonstrated that 37% of the cells on the bone marrow smears were immunoblasts and plasmacytoid cells. Blood cultures grew alpha-streptococci. Liver function continued to deteriorate, and the patient died on the 30th post-transplant day. At autopsy, all lymph node groups and most organs (including brain, liver, gallbladder, lungs, large bowel, appendix, adrenals, transplanted kidney, testicles, skin and thymus) were involved in the lymphoproliferative process. In retrospect, it was discovered that the patient's college roommate had developed infectious mononucleosis approximately one month before the patient's transplant. His heterophil titer prior to transplant was negative, but by the 25th post-transplant day the titer was

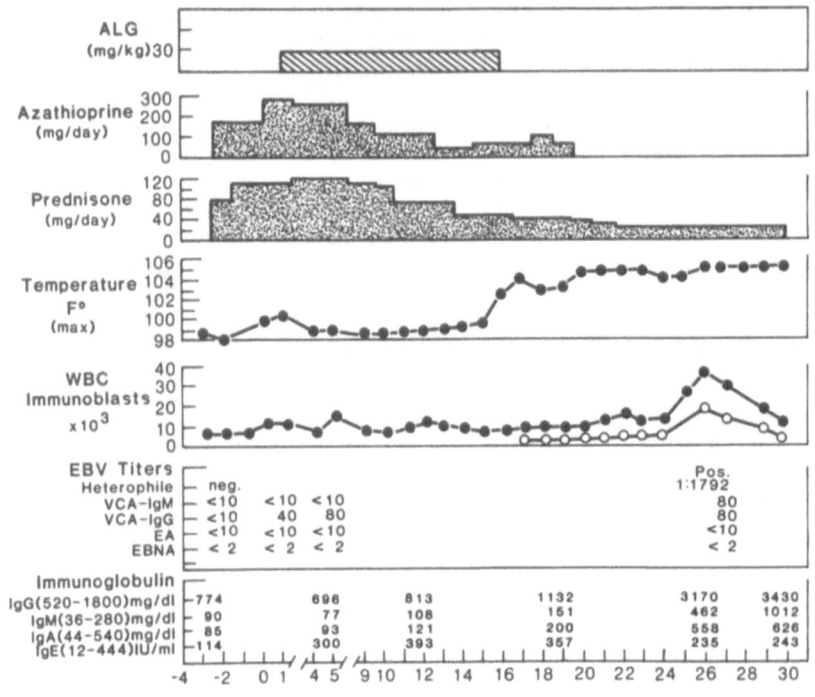

Fig. 1. A diagramatic representation of a 19-year-old recipient
(No. 1) of a renal allograft who was exposed to infectious mononucleosis one month prior to transplantation.
Widespread lymphadenopathy was followed by the appearance
of immunoblasts in the peripheral blood. EBV antibody
titers suggested a primary EBV infection and heterophil
antibodies were present in the serum. A polyclonal
increase in serum immunoglobulin was demonstrated. A
lymph node biopsy demonstrated polymorphic diffuse B cell
hyperplasia which was polyclonal. Four weeks after
transplantation, the patient died of a disease that
resembled fatal infectious mononucleosis.

positive at 1:1792 after guinea pig kidney absorption. Initial
antibody titers included anti-VCA IgG titer <1:10, IgM <1:10,
anti-EA <1:10, and anti-EBNA <1:2. The anti-VCA IgG titer rose
to 1:40 and 1:80 on the first and fifth post-transplant day. The
anti-VCA IgM titer rose to 1:80 on the 27th day. In addition, a
polyclonal increase in the quantitative serum immunoglobulins was
noted (Fig. 1). This patient, who lacked pre-existing antibodies
to EBV and was exposed to infectious mononucleosis just prior to
transplantation and immunosuppression, had a clinical course
characterized by a disseminated, rapidly progressive lympho-

proliferative process similar to cases of fatal infectious mononucleosis.

Three other patients (No. 2,3,5) had less aggressive, but ultimately fatal, lymphoproliferative processes (Table 2). Two patients (No. 2,3), both 15 years old, initially had fever, sore throat, malaise, and lymphadenopathy 3 1/2 and 5 months after transplantation, respectively. Biopsy specimens of their lymph nodes indicated polymorphic B cell lymphoma. One patient (No. 3) died two weeks after diagnosis of an intracerebral hemorrhage into a frontal lobe tumor; at autopsy the disease involved his brain, heart, parotid, colon, thyroid, and lungs. The other patient (No. 2) who is described in depth in the section titled therapy, had a polyclonal B cell proliferation which was EBNA positive and was treated on three occasions with Acyclovir®. Although the tumor initially responded to Acyclovir® therapy, it was later resistant and the patient died with widespread disease. The tumor had evolved from a polyclonal to a monoclonal B cell proliferation.

An 11-year-old girl (No. 5) developed fever, malaise, an urticarial skin rash, and bilateral nodular lung infiltrates 12 months ater transplantation and was believed to have CMV infection. She developed signs of a viral myocarditis, complete heart block, respiratory failure and seizures, and died two months after admission for a widely disseminated lymphoproliferation. At autopsy she had polymorphic B cell lymphoma involving lymph nodes, liver, bone marrow, transplanted kidney, brain, heart, and lungs.

One patient in this group is still alive (No. 4). This patient developed fever, malaise, rising creatinine levels, and elevated hepatic enzymes after treatment for three rejection episodes in the preceding eight months. The involved transplanted kidney was removed and immunosuppression discontinued; biopsy-proved lesions (polymorphic B cell lymphoma) involving the liver regressed over the subsequent two months. The patient has no evidence of disease more than five years later on hemodialysis. Review of the renal biopsy preceding her third course of therapy for rejection showed evidence of polymorphic B cell lymphoma.

Group II (seven patients): This clinical pattern appeared in older patients more than 1 year after transplantation and has a longer, yet equally lethal course (Table 1). All seven of our patients had symptoms of a solid tumor (Table 2). The mean age at the time of diagnosis was 53 years (range, 28 to 68 years); six patients were older than 45 years. The mean interval from transplantation to diagnosis was 42 months (range, 13 months to 8 years). Two patients had received a second transplant after rejecting the first. Only one patient had been treated for rejection within a year prior to diagnosis. Only one patient had concomitant CMV or HSV infections. In most cases, the initial

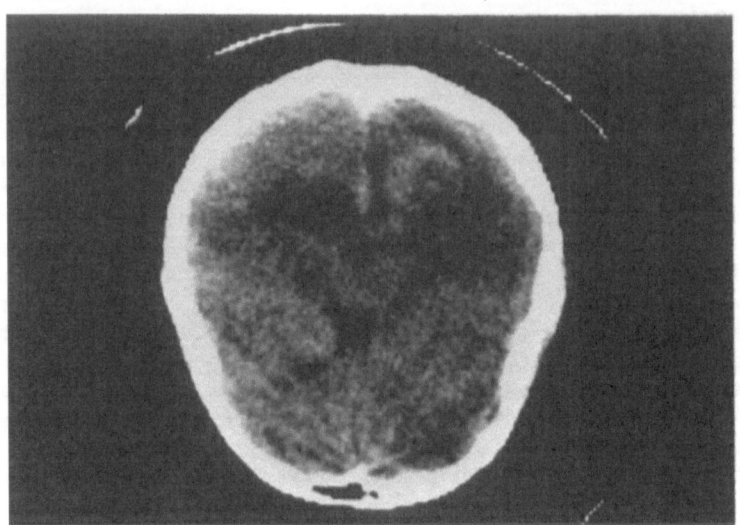

Fig. 2.   A cranial CT scan in a patient (No. 7) with headache,
          diplopia, blurred vision and polymorphic B cell lymphoma.
          A peripherally enhancing centrally lucent lesion is pres-
          ent in the right frontoparietal region.

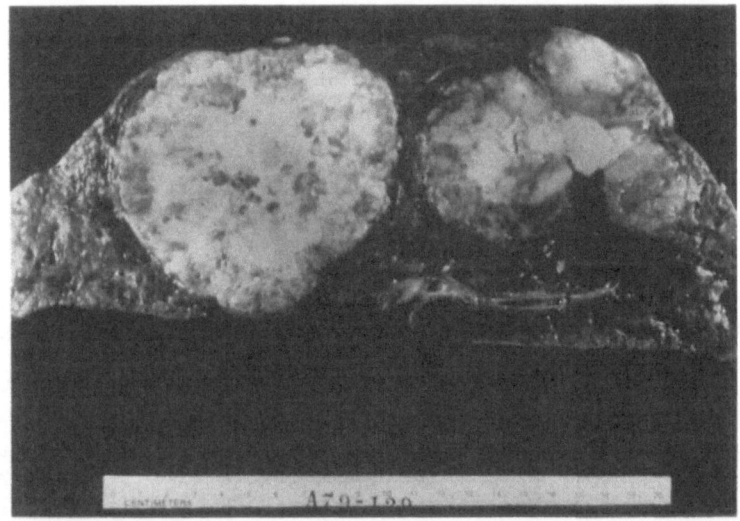

Fig. 3.   Gross features of metastatic polymorphic B cell lymphoma
          at autopsy. (Adapted from Frizzera, G. et al. Poly-
          morphic diffuse B-cell hyperplasias and lymphomas in
          renal transplant recipients. Cancer Res. 41:4262,
          1981. Courtesy of Cancer Research.)

symptoms were caused by a localized tumor mass in the brain, oropharynx, liver, or bowel (Table 2). Two patients had disease confined to the CNS (No. 6,7) in the occipital and frontal lobes, respectively. One patient (No. 6) was treated with 5,200 rads whole-brain irradiation and died 15 months later of a presumed CNS recurrence. A second patient (No. 7) (Figure 2) was treated with 4,600 rads whole-brain irradiation plus 1,000 rads to the posterior brain and died of multifocal recurrent CNS disease 7 months after diagnosis. One patient (No. 9), who had a tumor excised from the base of his tongue, developed a solitary cervical lymph node metastasis 6 months later. He died 15 months after the initial diagnosis of progressive liver involvement, in spite of chemotherapy and a reduction in immunosuppression. At autopsy massive tumor nodules were found in both hepatic lobes (Figure 3). A small bowel tumor was resected in one patient (No. 11) who died 9 months later of Pneumocystis carinii pneumonia without evidence of tumor. One patient (No. 10) with a liver mass eroding into the colon died 6 weeks after a hepatic resection with tumor involvement of the remaining lobe. Another patient (No. 12) who was

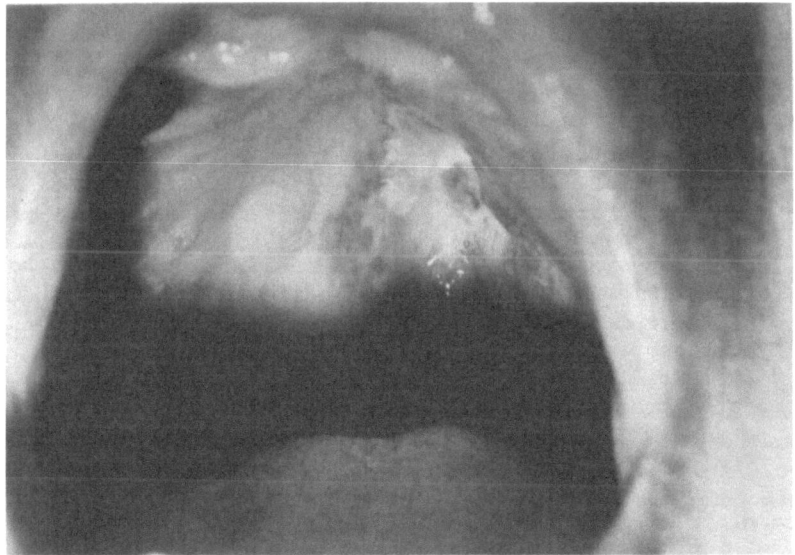

Fig. 4.   A photograph of the palate of a patient showing an ulcerated infiltrating lesion prior to biopsy. Histologically the tumor was polymorphic diffuse B-cell hyperplasia. (Adapted from Hanto, D.W. et al. Clinical spectrum of lymphoproliferative disorders in renal transplant recipients and evidence of the role of Epstein-Barr virus. Cancer Res. 41:4253, 1981. Courtesy of Cancer Research).

admitted with fever and lung nodules, developed progressive renal
and hepatic dysfunction and died 3 months after admission with
kidney, lung, and lymph node involvement. One patient (No. 8) had
a localized hard palate lesion that regressed while she was taking
a reduced dose of azathioprine (Figure 4). She subsequently
rejected her kidney, and has had no evidence of disease almost 5
years later on hemodialysis.

The clinical course in the five patients who died in Group II
was longer (mean, 9 months; range, 3 to 15 months) than in Group
I. The lymphoproliferative process usually was less widespread
than in Group I, although the sites of involvement were similar
(lymph nodes, transplanted kidney, brain, liver, oropharynx, bone
marrow, lungs, and gastrointestinal tract).

PATHOLOGY

Because the work of Frizzera et al. (10) these lymphoproliferative disorders can now be classified according to clearly
defined histologic criteria.

The lymphoid processes in these patients had morphologic
features of B cell proliferations and two classes can be
distinguished: polymorphic diffuse B cell hyperplasia (PDBH) and
polymorphic diffuse B cell lymphoma (PBL) (Table 3). Polymorphic
diffuse B cell hyperplasia is characterized by a polymorphic, diffuse, invasive B cell proliferation involving follicular center
cells (FCC) (small-cleaved and large non-cleaved) and lymphocytes
with varying degrees of plasmacytic differentiation (lympho-
plasmacytoid lymphocytes, plasma cells) and immunoblasts without
nuclear atypia (Figure 5). Polymorphic diffuse B cell lymphoma
can be distinguished from polymorphic diffuse B cell hyperplasia
primarily by the presence of large immunoblasts with marked
nuclear atypia and extensive necrosis (Fig. 5). PDBH can be
differentiated from other reactive lymphoid hyperplasias by its
diffuse pattern which replaces the normal germinal center architecture. Polymorphic B cell lymphoma can be differentiated from
the more commonly confused immunoblastic B cell sarcoma by the
presence of follicular center cells which are not present in the
latter. It is important to stress that the morphologic diagnosis
however, does not completely correlate with the clinical presentation or biologic behavior of the lymphoproliferative disorder.

Cell Marker studies: Immunologic cell typing was performed on
cell suspensions and frozen tissue sections, as previously
described (10,15). In brief, surface immunoglobulin and
cytoplasmic immunoglobulin were studied in suspensions of viable
cells and frozen tissue sections with fluorescein-conjugated
monospecific antibodies against heavy or light chains. Fc recep-

Table 3. Morphologic Characteristics of Post-Transplantation Lymphoproliferative Disorders[a]

Type of lesion	FCCs[b]	Plasmacytic differentiation	Large lymphoid cells	Atypical immunoblasts	Invasiveness	Necrosis
"Nonspecific" reactive lymphoid hyperplasia	++ (GC)	++	+/++	-	-	-
Polymorphic diffuse B cell hyperplasia (PDBH)	++ (D)	++	++/+++	-	+	-
Polymorphic diffuse B cell lymphoma (PBL)	++ (D)	+	++/+++	+/+++	+	+++
Immunoblastic B cell sarcoma	-	+	+++	+/+++	+	+

[a]Adapted from Frizzera et al. (10).
[b]FCC, follicular center cells; GC, germinal centers; D, diffuse.

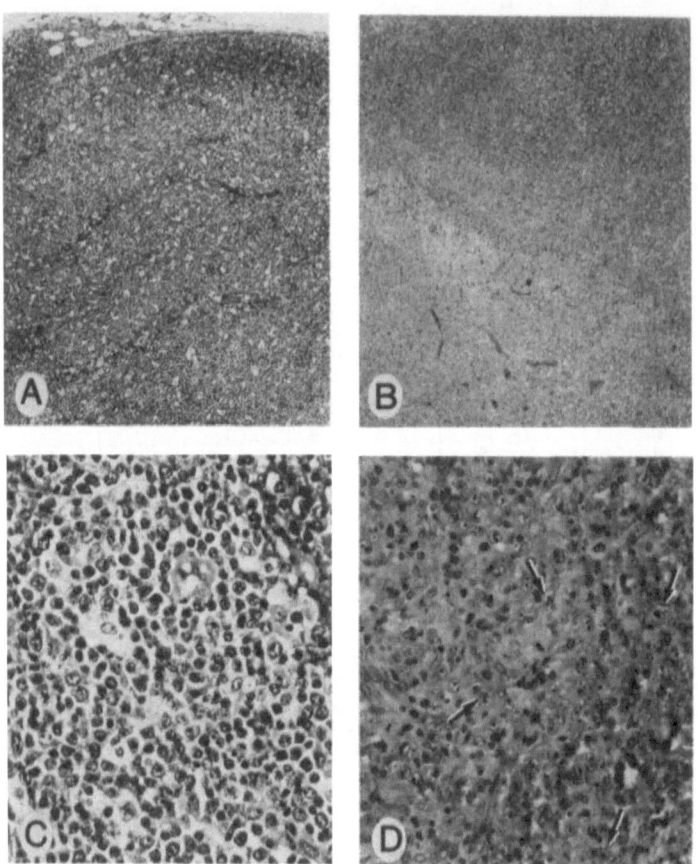

Fig. 5. Histology of post-transplantation lymphoproliferative
diseases. (a) PDBH (lymph node, patient No. 1).
Reactive, diffuse lymphoid hyperplasia with the characteristic moth-eaten appearance seen in infectious
mononucleosis. There is absence of necrosis. (Original
magnification x64). (b) PBL (liver, patient No. 9).
Half of the microscopic field shows viable tumor (top)
contrasted with extensive coagulative necrosis in the
remainder. (Original magnification x64). (c) PDBH
(lymph node, patient No. 1). This lymphoid proliferation
is characterized by the regularity of the nuclear
features of the large cells and by the abundant small
cell component with plasmacytic differentiation.
(Original magnification x400). (d) PBL (liver, patient
No. 9). This proliferation is characterized by large
cells with frequent nuclear atypia (arrows). (Original
magnification x400).

Table 4.   Cell Marker and Cytogenetic Studies in Four Patients with
Post-Transplantation Lymphoproliferative Diseases

Patient	Biopsy Site	Immunoglobulin (Surface or cytoplasmic)	Fc Receptors	Complement Receptors	Cytogenetic abnormalities
Group I					
1	Lymph node	Polyclonal	ND	ND	ND
2	Lymph node (16 weeks)	Polyclonal	+	–	ND
	Lymph node (31 weeks)	Polyclonal	+	–	ND
	Lymph node (39 weeks)	Monoclonal	+	–	ND
Group II					
8	Hard palate	Polyclonal	+	–	ND
9	Lymph node	Polyclonal	+	–	Trisomy 14

aNo satisfactory metaphases obtained for evaluation.

tors were studied with fluoresceinated aggregated human IgG, and
complement receptors were studied with bovine erythrocytes sensitized with IgM and mouse complement. Cell suspensions and
tissue sections were studied with the fluorescence microscope
equipped with Ploem epifluorescence and phase contrast, which
allows evaluation of the size of morphologic features of positive
and negative cells. The cell markers described were present on
cytologically malignant cells and could be differentiated from
those on normal cells. Binding of unsensitized sheep erythrocytes
was studied in cell suspension only.

A proportion of malignant cells from all tissues examined
(No. 1,2,8,9) demonstrated surface or cytoplasmic immunoglobulin
(or both) of the IgM, IgG, or IgA class and kappa or lambda
specificity (Table 4). Several interesting findings were made.
In one case (No. 9), chromosomal analysis of 12 metaphases from an
involved lymph node showed nine with a normal extra number 14
chromosome confirmed by G-banding. Cell markers in this case
demonstrated that a majority of cells expressed surface and
intracytoplasmic immunoglobulin of polyclonal specificity, but
there was also a smaller population of large atypical Fc and
complement receptor-positive cells negative for surface cytoplasmic immunoglobulin. These cells might have represented a
component of reactive, large follicular center cells (10) or they
might be a more undifferentiated cell population (23), and might
be the clone with the trisomy 14 (12,14). In a second patient,
who also had a polyclonal B cell proliferation by immunologic cell
typing, an extra normal number 3 chromosome was identified (Hanto,
unpublished observation). These chromosomal abnormalities may
represent examples of the cytogenetic events which result in the
transformation of these polyclonal B cell proliferations into
monoclonal tumors with enhanced autonomous malignant growth
potential (10,12-15).

Virology. Four of nine patients (No. 1,2,8,9) studied
demonstrated serologic evidence of primary (one) or reactivation
(three) EBV infection (Table 5). The other five patients showed
no such evidence. Patient #1, exposed to infectious mononucleosis
prior to transplantation, had evidence of a primary EBV infection
with a significant rise in the anti-VCA IgM and IgG titers from
<1:10 to 1:80. This patient also developed a high heterophil
antibody titer and polyclonal increase in serum immunoglobulins.
No other patient had detectable heterophil antibodies. Three
patients had serologic evidence of reactivation EBV infections
with sixfold (No. 2), tenfold (No. 9), and sixfold (No. 8) rises in
the anti-VCA IgG titers. Five patients had no diagnostic changes
in anti-VCA IgG, IgM titers, however, four patients demonstrated
persistently high anti-VCA IgG titers. No patient had diagnostic
changes in anti-EA or anti-EBNA and only six patients had detectable anti-EA or anti-EBNA at any time in their course. Only four

Table 5. EBV Serology in Patients with Post-Transplantation Lymphoproliferative Disorders[a]

Patient	Anti-VCA[b]		Anti-EA	Anti-EBNA	Interpretation
	IgG	IgM			
Group I					
1	<10	<10	<10	<2	Primary EBV infection
	80	80	<10	<2	
2	40	<2	<5	5	Reactivated EBV infection
	320	<2	<5	<2	
3	10	<2	<5	20	"Long past" EBV infection
	<5	<2	<5	<2	
4	320	<10	5	20	"Long past" EBV infection
	160	<10	<10	20	
Group II					
8	320	--	320	320	Reactivated EBV infection
	2560	--	--	--	
9	160	--	40	80	Reactivated EBV infection
	5120	--	<5	160	
10	640	2	10	40	"Long past" EBV infection
	640	2	5	40	
12	640	<10	5	<2	"Long past" EBV infection
	160	<10	5	10	

[a]VCA, viral capsid antigen; EA, early antigen; EBNA, Epstein-Barr nuclear antigen.
[b]Reciprocals of the viral antibody titer.

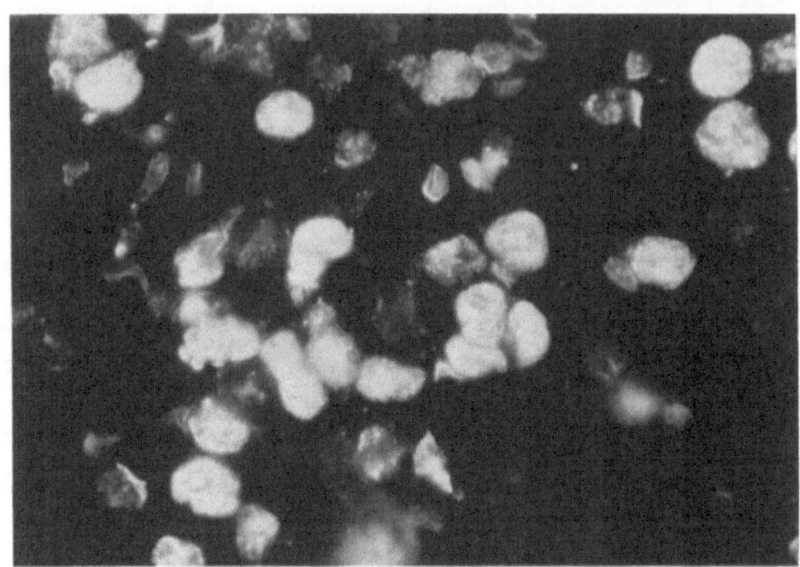

Fig. 6. Anticomplement immunofluorescence staining for the
         Epstein-Barr nuclear antigen, showing brightly staining
         positive cells on touch imprints from the lymph node.
         (Adapted from Hanto, D.W. et al. The Epstein-Barr virus
         in the pathogenesis of posttransplant lymphoproliferative
         disorders. Surgery 90:204, 1981. Courtesy of the
         C.V. Mosby Company.)

of the 12 patients were tested for evidence of oropharyngeal
shedding of EBV but all four had positive results. A touch
imprint of one tumor was stained for the presence of EBNA, and a
majority of the cells were strongly positive (Figure 6).
Utilizing EBV cRNA/DNA filter hybridization and/or vDNA/DNA
reassociation analysis, or both multiple copies of the EBV genome
were found in all eight specimens tested (Table 6).

   Therapy. Primary CNA lesions are still best treated by whole
brain irradiation, although the recurrence rate is high and survival time short in our series. Cessation of immunosuppression
and transplant nephrectomy might improve these results, but this
is speculative. Two heart transplant recipients with CNS lymphomas at Stanford University have achieved long-term survival
without recurrence after whole brain irradiation (C. Bieber,
personal communication). Localized gastrointestinal lymphomas may
be successfully excised as demonstrated in our patient (No. 11)
and in the series by Calne (2a).

Table 6. Epstein-Barr Virus Genomes in Tumor
Specimens in Post-Transplantation
Lymphoproliferative Diseases[a,b]

Patient	Biopsy Specimen	cRNA/DNA filter hybridization	cDNA/DNA Reassociation
Group I			
2	Lymph node	ND[c]	3
3	Brain	9	ND
	Parotid	9	14
	Heart	4	ND
Group II			
8	Palate	8	ND
9	Lymph node	<1	2
	Liver	13	7
10	Liver	3	5

[a]Expressed as EBV genome equivalents per cells (41).
[b]Adapted from Hanto et al. (14)
[c]ND = Not done.

More recent work suggests antiviral therapy may be worthy of
consideration in selected patients (15,16). Our results suggested
that polymorphic diffuse B cell hyperplasia and polymorphic diffuse B cell lymphoma were EBV-carrying polyclonal B cell proliferations. It was, therefore, reasonable to believe that antiviral therapy might be effective in these disorders. Acyclovir®
(9-[(2-hydroxyethoxy)-methyl]-guanine) is a new synthetic antiviral agent that has low toxicity for normal cells, but has strong
in vitro inhibitory activity against the replication of herpesviruses within the infected cells, including varicella-zoster
virus, herpes simplex virus and herpes simiae virus (B virus) (8).
Acyclovir® inhibits EBV DNA replication only in virus producing
cell lines such as P3HR-1; but it has no effect on viral DNA
replication in non-virus-producing cell lines (e.g., Raji) (6,7).
Clinical use of Acyclovir® in patients with EBV infections had not
been previously reported.

We have recently reported a patient (No. 2) who had clinical
signs and symptoms of infectious mononucleosis (fever, sore

throat, and cervical lymphadenopathy), but heterophil antibodies
and atypical lymphocytosis were absent (15). Serologic studies
were consistent with a reactivated EBV infection. Oropharyngeal
shedding of EBV was demonstrated. The lymph node biopsy was
classified as polymorphic B cell lymphoma and was a polyclonal
B cell proliferation, as defined by the presence of surface and
cytoplasmic immunoglobulin of both kappa or lambda specificity on
cytologically malignant cells. The tumor was EBNA-positive and
contained multiple copies of the viral genome. In this patient,
Acyclovir® therapy at a dose of 500 mg/M2 every eight hours effectively erradicated oropharyngeal shedding of EBV, as well as that
of herpes simplex virus, but it had no demonstrable effect on concurrent cytomegalovirus shedding. These results were consistent
with the relative susceptibility to these viruses to Acyclovir® in
vitro (6-8). EBV shedding recurred when Acyclovir® was stopped,
although herpes simplex virus shedding did not.

A dramatic resolution of fever and symptoms occurred concomitantly with Acyclovir® therapy. Furthermore, there was objective regression of the lymphoproliferative process involving lymph
nodes, tonsils, and bone marrow. We proposed that by inhibiting
the production of transforming virus, Acyclovir® effectively
interrupted the continued lytic infection of additional B lymphocytes (15). Unfortunately, treatment for an episode of rejection
two months after the initial course of Acyclovir® was associated
with recurrence of the lymphoproliferative disease one month
later, suggesting marginal immunologic control of the B-cell proliferation by host defenses. A second and then a third dramatic
clinical and objective response of the tumor to Acyclovir® provided
compelling evidence of the therapeutic efficacy during the
polyclonal-growth phase of this tumor, especially when combined
with a reduction in immunosuppressive agents.

Acyclovir® was not associated with resolution of the lymphoproliferation during the last recurrence. Aggressive tumor growth
continued in spite of Acyclovir® therapy. Simultaneously there was
a histologic change of the lesion from a polymorphic lymphoma to a
monomorphic immunoblastic proliferation. Most importantly,
although the initial lesions with polymorphic cell composition
expressed surface immunoglobulin or cytoplasmic immunoglobulin (or
both) of polyclonal specificity, the later masses were almost
entirely immunoblastic in composition, and were monoclonal B-cell
proliferations expressing only IgG kappa surface immunoglobulin or
cytoplasmic immunoglobulin, or both.

This case offers support for our previous hypotheses that
polyclonal B cell proliferation can sometimes evolve into
monoclonal tumors with enhanced potential for malignant growth,
similar to the changes that may occur in the development of
Burkitt's lymphoma (25) and in malignant lymphomas of Sjögrens

syndrome (50). As noted previously, it is likely that Acyclovir® was effective early in the disease because it interrupted the lytic cycle of EBV replication responsible for the polyclonal B-cell proliferation. By interrupting the polyclonal proliferation, Acyclovir® therapy may have unmasked the monoclonal B cell proliferation, presumably composed of latently infected (and therefore, Acyclovir® insensitive) B cells. These speculations are consistent with in vitro studies showing that Acyclovir® inhibits virus production in producer cell lines and that such lines remain latently infected as long as Acyclovir® is present. With removal of Acyclovir®, virus production resumes. It is likely that the persistence of host immunoincompetence increases the likelihood of recurrence.

We have subsequently treated an additional three patients with Acyclovir® with both polymorphic diffuse B cell hyperplasia and polymorphic B cell lymphoma, all of which were polyclonal B cell proliferations. We have successfully induced remission in all of these patients and they remain alive and well 8, 6, and 4 months after therapy (Hanto, unpublished observation). One additional patient who presented with a monoclonal B cell proliferation which contained EBV specific DNA sequences did not respond to Acyclovir® (16). This failure is consistent with our hypothesis that the monoclonal tumor is composed of latently infected and, therefore, Acyclovir®-insensitive B lymphocytes.

SUMMARY AND CONCLUSIONS

Previous reports of the lymphoproliferative disorders following renal transplantation have emphasized the high incidence of CNS involvement, the short interval between transplantation and diagnosis, and the high mortality (1,35,36,43). Matas et al. hypothesized that reactivation of latent EBV infections in the presence of the allogeneic graft (acting as a chronic antigenic stimulus) and pharmacological immunosuppression, might be responsible for the increased incidence of malignant lymphoma in transplant recipients (30). Hertel et al. demonstrated a polyclonal B-cell proliferation in nearly all cases of malignant lymphoma reviewed. They used immunoperoxidase staining of tumor biopsy specimens to determine the presence of cytoplasmic immunoglobulin (19). Some patients had serological evidence of EBV infection and a relationship between lymphoproliferative disorders and EBV in immunosuppressed patients was again proposed. Several lines of evidence in 12 patients, including clinical, pathologic, serologic, and molecular hybridization studies, now provide the strongest link to date between EBV and these abnormal lymphoproliferative disorders (10,12-14).

The 12 patients reported here demonstrate a clinical spectrum of disease, and two main groups have been identified. Young patients (<20 years) presented with symptoms of a viral illness, often with classic signs and symptoms of infectious mononucleosis, including fever, sore throat, malaise, and lymphadenopathy. The lymphoproliferative disorder occurred during high levels of immunosuppression either soon after transplantation or shortly after treatment for graft rejection. Concomitant HSV and CMV infections were common. The clinical course was that of a rapidly progressive, disseminated lymphoproliferative process with a high mortality rate (80%). The interval from diagnosis to death was short and only one patient (No. 4) in this group survived; she had been managed by transplant nephrectomy and cessation of immunosuppression.

The initial presentation and subsequent clinical course in the older patients contrasted sharply. Seven older patients (>45 years) developed their symptoms long after transplantation with localized tumor masses often confined to the CNS but more frequently involving other organ sites. There was no evidence of acute infections. Their clinical courses were that of a less widespread and more slowly progressive solid malignancy capable of widespread metastasis with a high mortality rate. Only one patient (No. 8) still survives 2.5 years after resolution of a palatal tumor and rejection of the transplanted kidney while on a reduced dose of azathioprine.

The histologic and cell marker studies provided the initial evidence for a link between EBV and these LPD. EBV infection of B lymphocytes, which have been shown to have EBV receptors on their surface (24), induces a polyclonal B cell proliferation in vitro (40) and in vivo (39). All 12 patients had abnormal lymphoproliferative processes with morphologic features of B cells. Cell marker studies (immunofluorescence and immunoperoxidase) clearly demonstrate the presence of a polyclonal B cell proliferation in all four cases in which adequate tissue was available. This is strong evidence for the proposed role of EBV as the initiator of these lymphoproliferative disorders, because EBV can induce such changes in vivo and in vitro. The polyclonal increase in serum immunoglobulins in one patient (No. 1) is also indicative of the polyclonal activation of B-cells by EBV.

The possibility of a transition from a polyclonal B-cell proliferation to a monoclonal cancer, similar to that which may occur in the development of Burkitt's lymphoma (25) and the malignant lymphomas of Sjogrens syndrome (50), is suggested by the detection of a cell population characterized by an extra marker chromosome 14 in the lymph node of one patient (No. 9), and an extra chromosome 3 in another patient (Hanto, unpublished observation). Although cell marker studies performed on this tissue demonstrated

that a majority of cells expressed surface and cytoplasmic immunoglobulin of polyclonal specificity, there was also a small
population of large atypical Fc and C' receptor-positive cells
which lacked surface and cytoplasmic immunoglobulin. These could
represent a component of reactive large follicular center cells
(10) or, as we have speculated previously, they might represent a
more undifferentiated cell population (23) and might be the clone
identified by trisomy 14. This cytogenetic change may result in
the emergence of an autonomous monoclonal tumor with enhanced
malignant growth potential. For example, human diploid
lymphoblastoid cell lines transformed by EBV will grow in the
brains of nude mice but do not survive if injected subcutaneously
(32). In contrast, aneuploid BL cell lines will grow both subcutaneously and intracerebrally in nude mice.

Although there are too few cases with documented tumor
subpopulations with cytogenetic abnormalities to be sure of this
hypothesis, the link between EBV and post-transplantation lymphoma
is much more firm. The seroepidemiological evidence is still
weak. Only four patients had serologic evidence of a primary or
reactivation EBV infection temporally related to diagnosis of the
lymphoproliferative disorder. Only one patient demonstrated an
antibody pattern consistent with a "current primary EBV
infection," as well as marked heterophil antibody response (17).
Anti-VCA IgG antibody levels were increased in three patients consistent with a reactivation EBV infection. Anti-VCA IgM was not
measured in two patients, but the presence of anti-EBNA excludes a
primary infection. Anti-EA was present in both patients and has
also been observed in patients with Hodgkin's disease and reactivation EBV infection (18). Four patients did not seroconvert to
EBV but had evidence of "long past" EBV infections characterized
by the absence of anti-VCA IgM, stable anti-VCA, and the presence
of anti-EBNA. One of these patients had a persistently high
anti-EA titer which is occasionally seen in patients with
relatively high levels of anti-VCA IgG but is unusual in transplant patients. The absence of increasing antibody to EBV may
reflect impaired humoral immunity. Sakamoto et al. (42) have
demonstrated impaired antibody responses to EBV in individuals
with the X-linked lymphoproliferative syndrome. Furthermore, it
has been noted that antibody responses to CMV infections, especially lethal infection, are variable in renal transplant
patients, and an absent or declining antibody response is regarded
as a poor prognostic sign (45).

Of greatest importance is the identification of EBV genomes
in all 5 patients studied by EBV cRNA/DNA filter hybridization and
vDNA/DNA reassociation analysis. In addition, a majority of cells
were EBNA positive on a touch imprint prepared from one specimen.
These results are essentially similar to those which have been
used to make the association between EBV and Burkitt's lymphoma,

nasopharyngeal carcinoma and the lymphoproliferative disorders seen in the X-linked lymphoproliferative syndrome and ataxia telangiectasia (26,41).

There is increasing awareness of the importance of the immune status of the host in EBV infections. Normally, resolution of infectious mononucleosis is mediated by EBV-specific cytotoxic T-lymphocytes (49), specific antibodies directed against virally determined antigens (17), and possibly augmented natural killer cell activity (48). However, fatal cases of infectious mono-nucleosis do occur and are often associated with subtle immune deficiencies (2,34,37-39). Cotton-top marmosets have impaired in vitro cellular responses, do not produce antibody to EBNA, and are susceptible to a fatal lymphoproliferative disorder induced by EBV (31). Treatment with azathioprine and prednisone increases their susceptibility. Renal transplant recipients have impaired cellu-lar and humoral immune responses, including markedly depressed natural killer cell activity (28), are susceptible to a variety of opportunistic infections, and shed EBV in the saliva (47). Herpes virus infections have been themselves associated with inverted T4-T8 ratios in peripheral blood (44). The differences in biologic behavior of the lymphoproliferative diseases seen in these 6 cases are probably best explained by differences in host responsiveness. For example, the younger patients were more immunosuppressed and developed a more disseminated lymphoproliferative disorder which had more rapid clinical courses. Furthermore, the more frequent association of prior or concomitant CMV infection in the younger patients may also reflect their lack of immunologic reactivity. On the other hand, CMV is known to be a profoundly immuno-suppressive virus (21,22) and may predispose to the development of primary or reactivation EBV infection. Prospective studies of specific immune functions in these patients are required to deter-mine the relative importance of impaired humoral and cellular immunity.

The importance of EBV and iatrogenic immunosuppression in the pathogenesis of these disorders cannot be overemphasized if we are to alter the outcome. Early diagnosis, reduction in immuno-suppression, and antiviral therapy may improve the poor prognosis at least during the polyclonal growth phase.

ACKNOWLEDGEMENTS

This research was supported by grant AM 13083 from the United States Department of Health Service.

REFERENCES

1. Anderson, J.L., Bieber, C.P., Fowles, R.E., and Stinson, E. Idiopathic cardiomyopathy, age, and suppressor-cell dysfunction as a risk determinants of lymphoma after cardiac transplantation. Lancet, ii:1174, 1978.

2. Britton, S., Anderson-Anvret, M., Gergely, P., Henle, W., Jondal, M., Klein, G., Sandstedt, B., and Svedmyr, E. Epstein-Barr-virus immunity and tissue distribution in a fatal case of infectious mononucleosis. N. Engl. J. Med., 298:89, 1978.

2a. Calne, R.Y., Roller, K., Thiru, S., McMaster, P., Craddock, G.N., Aziz, S., White, D.J.G., Evans, D.B., Dunn, D.C., Henderson, R.G., and Lewis, P. Cyclosporin A initially as the only immunosuppressant in 34 recipients of cadaveric organs: 32 kidneys, 2 pancreas, and 2 livers. Lancet, ii:1033, 1979.

3. Chang, R.S., Lewis, J.P., and Abildgaard, C.F. Prevalence of oropharyngeal excreters of leukocyte-transforming agents among a human population. N. Engl. J. Med., 289:1325, 1973.

4. Chang, R.S., Lewis, J.P., Reynolds, R.D., Sullivan, M.J., and Neuman, J. Oropharyngeal excretion of Epstein-Barr virus by patients with lymphoproliferative disorders and by recipients of renal homografts. Ann. Intern. Med., 88:34, 1978.

5. Cheeseman, S.H., Henle, W., Rubin, R.H., Tolkoff-Rubin, N.E., Cosimi, B., Cantell, K., Winkle, S., Herrin, J.T., Black, P.H., Russell, P.S., and Hirsch, M.S. Epstein-Barr virus infections in renal transplant recipients. Effects of antithymocyte globulin and interferon. Ann. Intern. Med., 93:39, 1980.

6. Colby, B.M., Shaw, J.E., Elion, G.B., and Pagano, J.S. Effect of Acyclovir [9-(2-hydroxyethoxymethyl)guanine] on Epstein-Barr virus DNA replication. J. Virol., 34:560, 1980.

7. Datta, A.K., Colby, B.M., Shaw, J.E., and Pagano, J.S. Acyclovir inhibition of Epstein-Barr virus replication. Proc. Natl. Acad. Sci., USA, 77:5163, 1980.

8. Elion, G.B., Furman, P.A., Fyfe, J.A., de Miranda, P., Beauchamp, L., and Schaeffer, H.J. Selectivity of action of an antiherpetic agent, 9-(2-hydroxyethoxymethyl) guanine. Proc. Natl. Acad. Sci., USA, 74:5716, 1977.

9. Frank, A., Andiman, W., and Miller, G. Epstein-Barr virus and nonhuman primates: natural and experimental infection. Adv. Cancer Res., 23:171, 1976.

10. Frizzera, G., Hanto, D.W., Gajl-Peczalska, K.J., Rosai, J., McKenna, R.W., Sibley, R.K., Holahan, K.P., and Lindquist, L.L. Polymorphic diffuse B-cell hyperplasias

and lymphomas in renal transplant recipients. Cancer
Res., 41:4253, 1981.

11.   Gleichmann, E., Gleichmann, H., Schwartz, R.W., Weinblatt,
      Al, and Armstrong, M.Y.K. Immunologic induction of
      malignant lymphoma: identification of donor and host
      tumors in the graft-versus-host model. J. Natl. Cancer
      Inst., 54:107, 1975.

12.   Hanto, D.W., Frizzera, G., Gajl-Peczalska, K., Purtilo,
      D.T., Klein, G., Simmons, R.L., and Najarian, J.S. The
      Epstein-Barr virus (EBV) in the pathogenesis of post-
      transplant lymphoma. Transplant. Proc., 13:756, 1981.

13.   Hanto, D.W., Sakamoto, K., Purtilo, D.T., Simmons, R.L.,
      and Najarian, J.S. The Epstein-Barr virus in the
      pathogenesis of posttransplant lymphoproliferative
      disorders. Surgery, 90:204, 1981.

14.   Hanto, D., Frizzera, G., Purtilo, D.T., Sakamoto, K.,
      Sullivan, J., Saemundsen, A.K., Klein, G., Simmons, R.L.,
      and Najarian, J.S. Clinical spectrum of lymphprolif-
      erative disorders in renal transplant recipients and
      evidence for the role of Epstein-Barr virus. Cancer
      Res., 41:4253, 1981.

15.   Hanto, D., Frizzera, G., Gajl-Peczalska, K., Sakamoto, K.,
      Purtilo, D.T., Balfour, H., Simmons, R.L., and Najarian,
      J.S. Epstein-Barr virus-induced B-cell lymphoma after
      renal transplantation. N. Engl. J. Med., 306:913, 1982.

16.   Hanto, D., Frizzera, G., Gajl-Peczalska, K.J., Simmons,
      R.L., Najarian, J.S., and Balfour, H.H., Jr. N. Engl.
      J. Med., 307:896, 1982.

17.   Henle, G. and Henle, W. The virus as the etiologic agent
      of infectious mononucleosis. In: M.S. Epstein and B.G.
      Achong (eds.), The Epstein-Barr Virus. pp. 297-320.
      New York: Springer-Verlag, 1979.

18.   Henle, W. and Henle, G. Epstein-Barr virus (EBV) in related
      serology in Hodgkin's disease. Natl. Cancer Inst.
      Monogr., 36:79, 1973.

19.   Hertel, B.F., Rosai, J., Dehner, P., and Simmons, R.L.
      Lymphoproliferative disorders in organ transplant
      recipients. Lab. Invest., 36:340, 1977

20.   Hoover, R. and Farumeni, J.F., Jr. Risk of cancer in
      renal-transplant recipients. Lancet, ii:55, 1973.

21.   Howard, R.J., Miller, J., and Najarian, J.S. Cytomegalo-
      virus-induced immune suppression. II. Cell mediated
      immunity. Clin. Exp. Immunol., 18:119, 1974.

22.   Howard, R.J. and Najarian, J.S. Cytomegalovirus-induced
      immune suppression. I. Humoral immunity. Clin. Exp.
      Immunol., 18:109, 1974.

23.   Johansson, B., Klein, E., and Haglund, S. Correlation
      between the presence of surface localized immunoglobulin
      (Ig) and the histological type of human malignant
      lymphomas. Clin. Immunol. Immunopathol., 5:119, 1976.

24. Jondal, M. and Klein, G. Surface markers on human B and T
     lymphocytes. II. Presence of Epstein-Barr virus recep-
     tors on B lymphocytes. J. Exp. Med., 138:1365, 1973.
25. Klein, G. Lymphoma development in mice and humans:
     diversity of initiation is followed by convergent cyto-
     genetic evolution. Proc. Natl. Acad. Sci., USA,
     76:2442, 1979.
26. Klein, G. The relationship of the virus to nasopharyngeal
     carcinoma. In: M.A. Epstein and B.G. Achong (eds.), The
     Epstein-Barr Virus. pp. 339-350. New York: Springer-
     Verlag, 1979.
27. Klein, G. and Klein, E. Immune surveillance against virus-
     induced tumors and nonrejectability of spontaneous
     tumors: contrasting consequences of host versus tumor
     evolution. Proc. Natl. Acad. Sci., USA, 74:2121, 1977.
28. Lipinski, M., Tursz, T., Kreis, H., Finale, Y., and Amiel,
     J.L. Dissociation of natural killer cell activity and
     antibody-dependent cell-mediated cytotoxicity in kidney
     allograft recipients receiving high-dose immuno-
     suppressive therapy. Transplantation (Baltimore),
     29:214, 1980.
29. Marker, S.C., Ascher, N.L., Kalis, J.M., Simmons, R.L.,
     Najarian, J.S., and Balfour, H.H., Jr. Epstein-Barr
     virus antibody responses and clinical illness in renal
     transplant recipients. Surgery (St. Louis), 85:433,
     1979.
30. Matas, A.J., Simmons, R.L., and Najarian, J.S. Chronic
     antigenic stimulation, herpesvirus infection, and cancer
     in transplant recipients. Lancet, i:1277, 1975.
31. Miller, G. Experimental carcinogenicity by the virus in
     vivo. In: M.A. Epstein and B.G. Achong (eds.), The
     Epstein-Barr Virus. pp. 352-372. New York: Springer-
     Verlag, 1979.
32. Nilsson, K., Giovanella, B.C., Stehlin, J.S., and Klein, G.
     Tumorigenicity of human hematopoietic cell lines in
     athymic nude mice. Int. J. Cancer, 19:337, 1977.
33. Pagano, J.S. and Shaw, J.E. Molecular probes and genome
     homology. In: M.A. Epstein and B.G. Achong (eds.), The
     Epstein-Barr Virus. pp. 109-146. New York: Springer-
     Verlag, 1979.
34. Penman, H.G. Fatal infectious mononucleosis: a critical
     review. J. Clin. Pathol., 23:765, 1971.
35. Penn, I. Malignancies associated with immunosuppressive or
     cytotoxic therapy. Surgery (St. Louis), 83:492, 1978.
36. Penn, I. The price of immunotherapy. Curr. Probl. Surg.,
     18:681, 1981.
37. Purtilo, D.T. Epstein-Barr-virus-induced oncogenesis in
     immune deficient individuals. Lancet, i:300, 1980.
38. Purtilo, D.T., Paquin, L., DeFlorio, D., Virzi, F., and
     Sakhuja, R. Immunodiagnosis and immunopathogenesis of

the X-linked recessive lymphoproliferative syndrome.
Semin. Hematol., 16:309, 1979.

39. Robinson, J.E., Brown, N., Andiman, W., Halliday, K.,
     Francke, U., Robert, M.F., Andersson-Anvret, M.,
     Horstmann, D., and Miller, G. Diffuse polyclonal B-cell
     lymphoma during primary infection with Epstein-Barr
     virus. N. Engl. J. Med., 302:1293, 1980.

40. Rosen, A., Gergely, P., Jondal, M., Klein, G., and Britton,
     S. Polyclonal Ig production after Epstein-Barr virus
     infection of human lymphocytes in vitro. Nature
     (London), 267:52, 1977.

41. Saemundsen, A.K., Purtilo, D.T., Sakamoto, K., Sullivan,
     J.L., Synnerholm, A-C., Hanto, D.W., Simmons, R.,
     Anvret, M.A., Collins, R., and Klein, G. Documentation
     of Epstein-Barr virus infection in immunodeficient
     patients with life-threatening lymphoproliferative
     diseases by Epstein-Barr virus complementary RNA/DNA
     and viral DNA/DNA hybridization. Cancer Res., 41:4237,
     1981.

42. Sakamoto, K., Freed, H.J., and Purtilo, D.T. Antibody
     Responses to Epstein-Barr virus in families with the X-
     linked lymphoproliferative syndrome. J. Immunol.,
     125:921, 1980.

43. Schneck, S.A. and Penn, I. De novo brain tumours in renal-
     transplant recipients. Lancet, 1:983, 1971.

44. Schooley, R.T., Hirsch, M.S., Calvin, R.B., Cosimi, A.B.,
     Tolkoff-Rubin, N., McCluskey, R.T., Burton, R.C.,
     Russell, P.S., Herrin, J.T., Delmonico, F.L., Giorgi,
     J.V., Henle, W., and Rubin, R.H. Association of herpes-
     virus infections with T-lymphocyte-subset alterations,
     glomerulopathy, and opportunistic infections after renal
     transplantation. N. Engl. J. Med., 308:307, 1983.

45. Simmons, R.L., Matas, A.J., Rattazzi, L.C., Balfour, H.H.,
     Howard, R.J., and Najarian, J.S. Clinical charac-
     teristics of the lethal cytomegalovirus infection
     following renal transplantation. Surgery (St. Louis),
     8:537, 1977.

46. Spector, B.D., Perry, G.S., III, and Kersey, J.H.
     Genetically determined immunodeficiency diseases (GDID)
     and malignancy: report from the Immunodeficiency-Cancer
     Registry. Clin. Immunol. Immunopathol., 11:12, 1978.

47. Strauch, B., Andrews, L., Siegel, N., and Miller, G.
     Oropharyngeal excretion of Epstein-Barr virus by renal
     transplant recipients and other patients treated with
     immunosuppressive drugs. Lancet, 1:234, 1974.

48. Sullivan, J.L., Byron, K.S., Brewster, F.E., and Purtilo,
     D.T. Deficient natural killer cell activity in the X-
     linked lymphoproliferative syndrome. Science, 210:543,
     1980.

49.   Svedmyr, E. and Jondal, M. Cytotoxic effector cells
         specific for B cell lines mononucleosis. Proc. Natl.
         Acad. Sci., USA, 72:1622, 1975.
50.   Zulman, J., Jaffe, R., and Talal, N. Evidence that the
         malignant lymphoma of Sjogrens syndrome is a monoclonal
         B-cell neoplasm. N. Engl. J. Med., 299:1215, 1978.

CHRONIC MONONUCLEOSIS

Martin Tobi*[1] and Abraham Morag[2]

[1]Department of Internal Medicine
University of Chicago
Chicago, IL 60637
*Present Address - Laboratory Immunology
NCI, NIH
Bethesda, MD 20205
[2]Division of Clinical Virology, Section of Virology
Hadassah-Hebrew University Medical School
Jerusalem, Israel

INTRODUCTION

Since its discovery in 1964 (1) and implication as the main cause of the infectious mononucleosis (IM) syndrome (2), the Epstein-Barr virus (EBV) has become a common archetype of human latent viral infections (3). This has been ascribed to its infection of B lymphocytes (4) and a resultant permanent viral carrier state (3). These genome carrying cells may give rise to continuous EBV-containing lymphoblastoid cell lines in in vitro cultures established from the peripheral blood and lymph node lymphocytes of seropositive individuals (5). With the characterization of the specific antibody responses in IM (6), their application in the elucidation of atypical cases of EBV infection became evident (7), particularly in children (8) and in 50-60% of adults where the minimal criteria for the diagnosis of IM (9) are not fulfilled (10,11). Given the high incidence of exposed individuals (80% by late adolescence), the recognized tendency of herpes viruses to reactivation (3), the persistent carrier state, and the predisposition to atypical infections, it might be expected that recurrent or prolonged atypical EBV infections would be commonly reported.

Before the knowledge of the existence of EBV and its relation to IM, such case reports (12) were unusual and often were lacking in essential data. In 1962, Bender (13) noted that cases of IM recurrence were rare and found only one case of 1,000 examined over 20 years satisfying strict hematologic and serologic criteria existing at the time. In his review, he cited only one of 12 purported cases of chronicity and recurrence of IM in a female at ages 11 and 19 and 21 reported by Kaufman (14) as being of special interest. Isaacs in 1948 described persistence of symptoms and signs of IM from 3 months to 4 years after onset of acute IM in 53/206 patients (42) 50% of these for more than one year. In general, these patients had similar features to our patients described below, 2/3 being female.

With the development of accurate techniques of diagnosis of EBV infection, case reports of atypical manifestations of EBV could be documented. One case report of a serological recurrence of IM on the basis of seropositivity prior to the illness was reported by Chang (15) purportedly confirming an earlier report (16) of three such cases. Unfortunately, a full serological profile was not performed. Further cases with such a profile in patients with persisting symptomatology after IM have been performed by Horwitz et al. (17) and Banatvala et al. (18) and this will provide a basis for later discussion. A case of a 25-year old man with a positive heterophile response with persistence of symptoms of malaise and weight loss four years after IM was reported by Askinazi et al. (19) with few other criteria for the IM syndrome and an antibody profile suggestive of a past EBV infection.

Recent reports of chronic EBV infections in patients with some form of immune deficiency constitute an important group and may provide the clue to pathogenesis of such atypical infections (20-24). Sophisticated immune studies may be required to uncover such deficiencies (23) which are generally unavailable in the general hospital or office setting.

Recently, we described a group of patients with prolonged atypical illness with serology suggestive of an EBV association without evidence for an immunodeficiency or underlying wasting disease (25). These patients are described, their physical symptoms and signs discussed in terms of past experience, and serological profile contrasted with those of known chronic EBV cases above.

Serological studies of Paul-Bunnell-Davidsohn (PBD) tests, determination of specific IgG, IgM to viral capsid antigen (VCA) of EBV, antibodies to the Diffuse (EAD) and Restricted EAR) components of the early antigen (EA) complex and Epstein-Barr nuclear antigen (EBNA) were performed as described elsewhere (26).

The indirect immunofluorescence method was used to measure antibodies to EBV and cytomegalovirus (CMV). Materials are likewise detailed (25).

The first two patients presented to the Internal Medicine Department of Hadassah University Hospital, Mt. Scopus, Jerusalem concurrently in February 1980. The first, a young female student of 25, had persistent low grade pyrexia and malaise since November 1979, when she had presented to the Students' Health Service with malaise, fever, and was found to have a mild cervical lymphadenopathy. On follow-up, a transient splenomegaly and mild weight loss of 10 lbs. was documented. In February, three months after the onset of her disease, she was found to have IgG anti-VCA 1:256, IgM anti-VCA 1:32, and anti-EAR 1:8, anti-EAD <1:8, anti-EBNA 1:40, and a diagnosis of atypical EBV infection was made. The heterophile antibody (PBD) was negative and besides a relative lymphocytosis of up to 56% of normal morphology, no criteria for the diagnosis of acute mononucleosis were fulfilled. In view of her prolonged course of illness, a serological survey was performed. Only evidence for past CMV exposure was documented. Tests for rheumatoid and antinuclear factor were negative. Liver function tests were normal. T and B cell functions including quantitative immunoglobulin estimations were normal. Past skin testing showed allergy to penicillin and housedust mites. Serial antibody testing of up to 18 months of the illness revealed an essentially unchanged profile while the malaise, low grade fever and lymphocytosis persisted.

The second patient, a young man of 19, had an acute febrile illness in February 1980 with generalized lymphadenopathy and significant hepatosplenomegaly. Heterophile testing was negative but a morphologically normal relative lymphocytosis of 50% was documented with an anti-VCA IgG titer of 1:512 and IgM anti-VCA of 1:32, and a diagnosis of atypical EBV infection was made. Unfortunately, not enough sera remained for anti-EA and anti-EBNA determinations. Exacerbations of fever continued monthly and he underwent an extensive workup to exclude a possible underlying malignancy. Investigations were unrevealing and immune testing, as in the first patient, revealed no abnormality. Liver function tests, liver biopsy, bone marrow aspiration, and culture for tuberculosis were unrewarding. Toxoplasma studies as well as autoimmune serology were negative. IgM anti-VCA titer remained elevated at 1:32 and in addition, anti-EAR titers were >1:8 throughout the follow-up period of 18 months. The patient's history is positive for severe allergy to penicillin and several analgesics.

The occurrence of two patients with evidence for prolonged EBV infection prompted a review of EBV serological results at the Division of Clinical Virology, Hebrew University Hadassah Medical

Table 1. Summary of Signs and Symptoms in Seven Patients
with Chronic Atypical Illness Associated with
Epstein-Barr Virus Infection

Signs and Symptoms	1	2	3	4	5	6	7
Fever	+	+	+	+	+	+	-
Lymphadenopathy	+	+	-	+	+	-	+
Enlarged liver	-	+	-	-	-	+	-
Enlarged spleen	+	+	-	+	+	+	-
Weight loss	+	+	+	-	+	+	-
Lymphocytosis	+	+	-	+	+	+	-
Malaise	+	+	+	+	+	+	-
Weakness	-	-	+	+	-	+	-
Anxiety state	-	-	+	-	+	-	-
Abdominal pains, nausea, etc	-	+	+	-	-	-	-
Myalgia	-	-	+	-	-	-	-
Thyroiditis	-	-	+	-	-	+	-
History of allergy	+	+	-	-	+	-	-

School which revealed five other patients with persistent IgM
anti-VCA responses in a non-declining titer for a duration of at
least six months. The physicians responsible for the follow-up of
these patients were contacted and questioned with regard to their
symptom complexes and physical signs. These are summarized in
Table 1 and serological profile in Table 2. All these patients
had chronic complaints related to low grade fever, lymphadenopathy
or malaise. A history of allergy was elicited in about half.
Only one patient, a man of 23, had had classical heterophile
positive IM fulfilling all criteria. His course of disease was
slightly different from his fellow sufferers in that he would
experience malaise, fever, lymphadenopathy, and liver function
abnormality almost every month on a recurrent rather than persistent basis. He has a persistent splenomegaly and has
thalassemia minor for which he does not receive treatment.

These patients were all followed up for the minimum of one
year with largely no change in symptoms nor serological profile.
The IgM anti-VCA showed little tendency to decline and the
anti-EAR, where positive, did likewise. Follow-up continues and a
full EBV immunocompetence study is intended.

Table 2. Serological Studies in Seven Patients with
Prolonged Atypical Illness

Patient	Date of onset	Months of Illness	EBV VCA* IgG	EBV VCA* IgM	EBV EA* R	EBV EA* D	EBNA	Cytomegalovirus IgG	Cytomegalovirus IgM	PBD* test
1	Nov. 1979	0	ND*	ND	ND	ND	ND	ND	ND	ND
		3	1:256	1:32	1:8	<1:8	1:40	1:32	<1:8	ND
		5	1:512	1:64	ND	ND	ND	1:32	<1:8	Neg
		7	1:512	1:64	1:8	<1:8	1:80	1:16	<1:8	ND
		14	1:256	1:64	1:8	<1:8	1:160	ND	ND	ND
		18	1:256	1:64	1:8	<1:8	1:80	1:16	<1:8	ND
2	Feb. 1980	1	1:512	1:32	ND	ND	ND	1:64	1:8	Neg
		4	1:128	1:16	ND	ND	ND	1:128	1:8	Neg
		6	1:128	1:16	1:8	<1:8	1:40	1:128	<1:8	ND
		13	1:128	1:16	1:8	<1:8	1:80	1:64	<1:8	ND
		14	1:256	1:32	1:16	<1:8	1:40	1:128	<1:8	ND
		18	1:128	1:32	1:8	<1:8	1:20	1:32	<1:8	ND
3	March 1980	0?	ND	ND	ND	ND	ND	ND	ND	ND
		3	1:256	1:32	<1:8	<1:8	1:80	1:32	<1:8	Neg
		5	1:256	1:32	<1:8	<1:8	1:80	ND	ND	ND
		9	1:512	1:64	1:8	<1:8	1:40	1:8	<1:8	ND
		13	1:128	1:64	<1:8	<1:8	1:160	1:32	<1:8	ND
		15	1:128	1:32	<1:8	<1:8	ND	1:16	<1:8	ND
4	Sept. 1978	0?	ND	ND	ND	ND	ND	ND	ND	++
		10	1:256	1:16	1:32	<1:8	1:160	1:128	1:32	ND
		15	1:512	1:32	1:32	<1:8	1:320	1:128	<1:8	ND
		18	1:512	1:32	ND	ND	ND	1:64	<1:8	Neg
		26	1:512	1:32	1:32	<1:8	1:160	ND	ND	ND
		29	1:256	1:32	1:32	<1:8	1:80	ND	ND	ND
5	Nov. 1979	0	ND	ND	ND	ND	ND	ND	ND	ND
		1	1:512	1:32	<1:8	<1:8	1:40	1:64	<1:8	ND
		3	1:512	1:64	<1:8	<1:8	1:40	ND	ND	Neg
		12	1:128	1:32	<1:8	<1:8	1:80	ND	ND	ND
		16	1:128	1:32	<1:8	<1:8	1:80	1:32	<1:8	ND
6	Oct. 1978	0	ND	ND	ND	ND	ND	ND	ND	ND
		4	1:512	1:64	<1:8	<1:8	1:80	1:32	<1:8	ND
		15	1:128	1:16	<1:8	<1:8	1:320	1:32	<1:8	ND
7	May 1979	1?	1:512	1:64	ND	ND	ND	ND	ND	ND
		8	1:512	1:32	1:8	<1:8	1:160	1:128	1:16	ND
		9	1:512	1:32	1:8	<1:8	1:80	1:128	1:16	ND
		17	1:128	1:32	1:8	<1:8	ND	1:64	1:8	ND
		23	1:128	1:32	1:8	<1:8	1:80	ND	ND	ND

*PBD = Paul-Bunnell-Davisohn test, VCA = viral capsid antigen; EA = early antigen; EBNA =
Epstein-Barr nuclear antigen. ND = not done.

SYMPTOMATOLOGY AND CLINICAL FINDINGS WITH REGARD TO CLASSICAL IM

Malaise, Fever and Fatigue

Eighty to 100% of patients with acute IM will have these
manifestations (27), although a corresponding proportion of the
above patients experienced this, these are non-specific features
of many chronic illnesses. The fever was always low grade never
much more than 38°C, usually more noticeable in the evening, but
unassociated with chills which occur in 40-60% or sweats (80-95%),
of acute IM cases (28). The malaise developed by midday and
patients often would have to cancel their afternoon activities and
return to bed, often to sleep until the next day. In general, the
lethargy of acute IM resolves in 2-3 weeks in 60-70% of cases, but
in the remainder may persist for many weeks (27) particularly
after severe liver involvement (8,17).

Lymphadenopathy, Splenomegaly and Pharyngitis

Most patients had a regional lymphadenopathy (27) contrasting
with the generalized lymphadenopathy of 80-100% in acute IM.
Where a biopsy was performed, a morphological diagnosis of
reactive hyperplasia was made. The sore throat seen in 80-100%
of acute IM patients was unusual amongst the above patients. The
transient splenomegaly in most cases resolved without recurrence
but at presentation corresponds to the 50-70% seen in acute IM.
No splenic tenderness was observed [(15-30%) in acute IM (28)].

Neurologic and Psychiatric Features

Anxiety or depression may not be obvious in the patient in
the stages of acute illness, however, Cadie et al. (29) on the
basis of a questionnaire and 36 home visits in 31 patients up to
one year after acute IM in a prospective study, found that half of
20 females suffered from mild depression after the illness. There
was no difference from the control premorbid state in males. In
those women with preceding anxiety states, these worsened.
Hendler (30) reviewed the literature on this subject and presented
two case reports of severe depression in a teenage boy and girl
after acute IM with objective central neurological sequelae. Two
of five females of the above patients suffered from minor psychiatric therapy and a third declined psychiatric evaluation.

Hepatomegaly, Myalgia and Abdominal Pain (27,28)

These are unusual in acute IM, ranging 10-25%, accordingly
these were unusual features in the above patients, but when
present were troublesome and represented a therapeutic problem.

Bradycardia

Thirty-five to fifty percent of acute IM patients may have
bradycardia (28). The case of putative chronic EBV infection
described by Askinazi had bradycardia 1(19). Patient 3 had a
documented episode during her illness--her thyroid function at the
time was normal and she was not taking any B-blocking agents.

Criteria for Diagnosis of Atypical Prolonged Illness Associated with EBV

Despite occasional similarities in symptoms to the above
features of acute IM, the patients did not share sufficient
features to conform to a particular syndrome. The hematologic and
serologic criteria are best discussed once the cases of chronic
EBV infection in the immunodeficient has been considered.

Table 3. Summary of Clinical and Serological Features of Patients with Chronic Infectious Mononucleosis

Patient	Clinical Features	Anti-VCA Antibodies			EBNA	Heterophile	Comment
		IgM	IgG	EA			
"A" 5 yrs. old female ill 19 mos.	Initial rash, fever, malaise At 6 months hepatosplenomegaly lymphadenopathy, leucocytosis, thrombocytopenia. At 1 yr. wt. loss, blasts in blood	1:320	1:20,000	1:10,000	1:40	Negative	Fatal EBV infection, EBNA in lymph nodes and blood Interferon secretion impaired EA, EBNA response positive (ref 20).
"B" 21 yrs. old Male ill 24 mos.	Fever, hepatomegaly after splenectomy and multiple transfusions. Initially 23% atypical	1:20 ?	1:80,000 1:640 1:320	1:20,000 1:320 1:20	1:30 ? ?	Negative	Persistent IM, impaired mitogen responses and T-cell depletion (ref 22).
H.W. 10 yrs. old Male ill 18 mos.	Relapsing fever, hepatosplenomegaly. Lymphadenopathy. 59% relative lymphocytosis 2% atypical lymphocytes	?	1:2560	1:320	1:40	Positive	Fatal IM, low mitogen response of lymphocytes. Polyclonal hypergammaglobulinemia. EBV genomes detected in liver (24).
J.W. 18 yrs. old Male recurrence in 3 years	Fatigue, headache, pharyngitis Lymphadenopathy. 70% relative lymphocytosis. 6% atypical lymphocytes.	1:40	1:80	1:20	<1:2	Positive	Recurrent IM and family history. EBV genome in lymph node (ref 24).
Sister of J.W. 21 years old Female ill 24 mos.	Clinical features not described Partial defective IgM deficiency	<1:2	1:80	1:40	1:10	?	Chronic IM and subtle immunodeficiency (ref 24).
B.N. 18 mos. old Female ill 16 mos.	Rash, hepatosplenomegaly, weight loss, lymphadenopathy, pancytopenia 38% lymphocytes on peripheral smear. No atypical cells.	?	1:1280	1:640	1:160	Negative	Chronic IM, improved after splenectomy. EBV in spleen (ref 24).
A.H. 10 yrs. old Male ill >6 mos.	Recurrent fever, pallor, malaise, hepatosplenomegaly, pancytopenia and few atypical lymphocytes.	<1:10 <1:10	1:1280 1:1280	1:320(D) 1:320(D)	1:2 1:2	Negative	Chronic IM. Impaired cellular response to EBNA positive cells (ref 24).
T.F. 9 yrs old ill 18 mos.	Fever, lymphadenopathy pharyngitis, splenomegaly, pneumonitis	1:40 1:20	1:2560 1:5120	1:640(D) 1:640	1:40 1:40	Positive	As for patient A.H. EBNA + PBL (ref 23).

Abbreviations: EBV = Epstein-Barr virus, IM = Infectious mononucleosis, VCA = Viral capsid antigen, EA = Early antigen complex, EAD = Diffuse component of EA, EBNA = Epstein-Barr nuclear antigen, PWM = Pokeweed mitogen, PBL = Peripheral blood lymphocytes.

Chronic EBV Infections in Immunodeficient Individuals

The cases to be considered are presented as primary EBV infections which were either persistent or progressed to a fatal polyclonal lymphoproliferative disease. All patients had been ill for at least four months. Some lack a continuous serological follow-up but specific studies of EBV immune mechanisms render them most important to our developing understanding of such infections. The patients most studied in this regard are those with the X-linked lymphoproliferative (XLP) syndrome described by Purtilo (24). These patients are described elsewhere in this book, but attention will be drawn briefly to their atypical, serological findings. Patients described below are summarized in Table 3.

The case of a five year old girl described by Virelizier et al. (Pt. A - Table 3) (20) was studied by specialized EBV and immunological testing during her illness. She had been reasonably well except for upper respiratory infections until onset of illness of a skin rash and transient fever. A few months thereafter fever, fatigue and anorexia were noted and five months later lymphadenopathy appeared. Hematologically, there was anemia, leucocytosis of 21,000 cells/cu. mm with 80% neutrophils, and a thrombocytopenia of 65,000/mm. A polyclonal hypergammaglobulinemia was documented and a lymph node biopsy showed reactive hyperplasia, but repeated bone marrow aspirations were not rewarded by a specific diagnosis. A year after the onset of her illness, the patient deteriorated--suffering a significant weight loss, fever, lymphadenopathy, and hepatosplenomegaly with 42% lymphocytes in the peripheral smear. Microbiological studies were negative. The PBD test was of an insignificant titer. Corticosteroid treatment resulted in some resolution of adenopathy and splenomegaly but the patient developed interstitial pneumonitis and the steroids were discontinued. EBNA negative blast cells of a B cell polyclonal origin were found in increasing numbers. The child expired despite therapy with multiple cytotoxic agents, 19 months after the onset of disease. The only immune abnormality evident was the failure of her lymphocytes to produce immune interferon. One percent of lymph node and blood lymphocytes were EBNA positive four months after anti-EBV antibodies were first detected. The cellular response to EBV antigens was intense. A follow-up of serial EBV serologies showed very high IgG anti-VCA (1:20,000 - 1:80,000 initial-terminal) IgM anti-VCA 1:320-1:20; anti-EA 10,000 - 20,000; anti-EBNA 1:40 - 1:320. These serological findings accompanied by the results of the above positive EBV tests support a diagnosis of persistent EBV infection (17,36) but the role of deficient immune interferon secretion in this disease is yet unknown.

The case of a 21 year old man (Pt. B - Table 3) splenectomized
secondary to trauma, necessitating many blood transfusions who
then developed a persistent IM with transient immunodeficient, was
described by Purtilo et al. (22). His disease began 25 days
post-operatively with high fever, leucocytosis of 50,000 with a
lymphocytosis of 61% with 23% atypical lymphomononuclear cells and
biopsy proven hepatitis. Bacterial cultures were negative, and
over more than one year IgG anti-VCA was >1:320, anti-EA 1:32
-1:20 (in declining titer) and CMV titer showing a past infection.
The heterophile antibody was negative and abnormally decreased
response to B and T cell mitogens were documented with a persistently low number of T cells by E rosette formation. In the early
stages of the disease, the patient had hypogammaglobulinemia.
Unfortunately, IgM anti-VCA levels were not given for EBV nor CMV,
and no premorbid serological testing was performed. An early and
late anti-EBNA evaluation would have been most informative. The
data is, however, highly suggestive of an EBV infection. An
analogy of the XLP syndrome was drawn on the basis of the clinical
features.

Amongst the other cases of chronic or recurrent EBV illnesses
in immunodeficient individuals, summarized in Table 3, Purtilo
described four cases, one, H.W., succumbed to his disease (24).
Two males, H.W. and J.W., ages 10 and 18, and two females, the
sister of J.W. age 21 and B.N. age 18 months. The pattern of
illness was atypical, hematologic findings described in three show
a relative lymphocytosis in the males with an insignificant
proportion of atypical lymphocytes. Heterophile responses were
positive in two. Serology showed varying IgG anti-VCA, significant anti-EA and positive anti-EBNA titers in all but J.W. where
the profile resembles one of the patterns of reactivity after EBV
exposure in the XLP syndrome (21). Other findings are summarized
in the table as are the two male cases as described by Masucci et
al. (23) as having chronic IM. One 10 year old (A.H.) and (T.F.)
a 9 year old with illness duration of six and 18 months, respectively. Both had atypical illnesses with fever, hepatomegaly, or
splenomegaly. Additional hematologic features are summarized in
Table 3. A.H. -- had negative IgM anti-VCA, anti-EAD and the low
anti-EBNA titers similar to J.W., whilst T.F. had high IgM anti-VCA
(likewise IgG anti-VCA and anti-EAD) with a normal anti-EBNA
titer. Both showed weak immune reactions to EBNA positive
material but normal responses to a plant mitogen contrasting with
the XLP syndrome.

A common clinical syndrome was absent, however, persistence of
a prolonged illness with serology supportive of EBV activity and
various different immune aberrations were found. These patients
may represent a spectrum of severity of chronic EBV infection with
the mild cases represented by our patients.

The Significance of Antibody Profiles in Chronic EBV Syndromes

The hematologic features of acute IM may be imitated by other acute viral conditions (31,32) and even in chronic states of yet undetermined etiology, lymphocytosis with a significant proportion of atypical lymphocytes has been shown to persist (33). These features are, therefore, of limited usefulness in their specificity and heavy reliance is therefore placed on specific antibody tests.

The Heterophile Antibody

Whilst 90% positivity in adult cases of acute IM is documented (6), this antibody has limited use in chronic cases. In none of the putative cases reported by Isaacs (42) was the heterophile test >1:64. All our cases were negative in this context, and in the immunodeficient patients, 4/7 had negative responses (Table 3). Depending on the method of determination, it may remain detectable in 75% up to one year after acute IM as shown in one prospective study (34). This might result in misleading diagnoses if disregarded. In the case report of prolonged persistence of this antibody in the asymptomatic patient by Askinazi (19), the EBV antibody profile was not supportive of active infection. Thus, while a persistent positive response is wholly dependent on other serological tests for the diagnosis, a negative test does not exclude the likelidhood of a chronic EBV infection.

IgM and IgG Anti-VCA Antibodies

The IgM anti-VCA test, a difficult laboratory technique, is present in 100% of acute IM (6). This antibody declines in titer and is negative in all patients by one year (7). No patients were found to be positive prior to the onset of acute disease in another (34). In the study of IgM anti-VCA in various EBV-associated disease states, Banatvala (18) described one female with prolonged lassitude and recurrent lymphadenopathy, six months after acute IM with persistence of the IgM response for that time period. Prolonged IgM responses in patients with complications of viral infections or in the immunosuppressed were highlighted. Where measured in the immunodeficient patients, it was positive in 2/3 of the cases (Table 3). False IgM anti-VCA positivity may be seen in the presence of rheumatoid factor (RF) (35), but all our patients were RF negative. Sera from a control group of patients less than a year after acute IM tested in our laboratory did not show IgM antibodies. IgM anti-VCA has been found in 50% of asymptomatic patients positive for EA antibodies and attributed to reactivation (36). The IgM response in reactivated infection with other herpesvirus infections has been documented (37). Despite the supportive evidence which exists for detectable IgM in prolonged illness or reactivation in EBV and other viral infec-

tions, convincing evidence for IgM anti-VCA as the specific marker
is lacking. The findings of persisting, non-declining serial
titers of IgM anti-VCA in symptomatic patients with no intervening
underlying illness and with persistently positive specific antibodies is supportive of an illness closely associated with EBV. The
presence of IgG anti-VCA is an indication of past infection and
when positive in a situation of prolonged illness, usually does
not confer much diagnostic information. Relatively high levels
were seen in the immunodeficient patients described. Sumaya (36)
found a positive correlation with anti-EA positivity in an asymptomatic rural population with high titers to IgG anti-VCA.
Persistent serial titers higher than the geometric mean titers of
the general population may, therefore, be an indicator of EBV
activity but they are of no definite diagnostic value in this
setting.

Anti-EA Antibodies

Antibodies to the D (approximately 70%) and only occasionally
to the R component of the EA complex are found in adults with
early acute IM (6). However, generally, the D and R components
are not differentiated in many studies. In the immunodeficient as
may be seen from Table 3, anti-EA may be extremely elevated but is
not a usual feature in the XLP syndrome (21) although anti-EA may
be present (24). Their presence is of uncertain significance in
the asymptomatic (36) but in the cases of prolonged symptomatology
after acute IM (17), R antibodies persisted for many months in
patients symptomatic for up to 39 months. Remarkably, of those
with late anti-EAR antibody responses, 3/7 had recurrent symptoms.
IgG anti-VCA and EA antibodies may be elevated in many unrelated
disorders such as ataxia telangiectasia, Hodgkin's disease,
rheumatoid arthritis, systemic lupus erythematosus, sarcoidosis
and organ transplants (41). This does not necessarily imply a
causal relationship of EBV to these conditions (17). The D and R
antibody responses in nasopharyngeal carcinoma and Burkitt's
lymphoma have been well characterized (38,39). Sumaya (36)
postulated that the presence of R antibodies was due to endogenous
reactivation of virus. In the cases summarized herein, the
demonstration of EBNA and EBV genome in blood or tissue specimens
in the presence of elevated anti-EA titers supports this view.
The XLP patients with IM lacking anti-EA, despite ongoing EBV
infections, suggests that this interpretation might not be
universally applicable. In our patients, 4/7 had continuously low
but clearly discernable titers of anti-EAR while no EAD antibody
was detected. Although the latter component's response in acute
IM where positive (70%), roughly parallels that of IgM anti-VCA
(6), data is insufficient to suggest that its persistence is of
the same significance as the IgM anti-VCA in this group of
patients. Two of four of the patients described by Horwitz et
al. (17) who had recurrent symptoms following IM were positive for

anti-EAD at recurrence while all 4 were positive for anti-EAR. Of
anti-EAD detected in the patients in Table 3, it should be borne
in mind that it may be difficult to discern low levels of anti-EAR
in the presence of dominant anti-EAD titers (17).

Anti-EBNA

This antibody arising in the late convalescent phase in 100%
of patients with IM (6) is a useful test if sera is available
early in the putative chronic EBV infection. Unfortunately, such
estimations were not possible in our patients. In the XLP
patients and two of the immunodeficient cases (Table 3), anti-EBNA
titers were absent, as is the case in ataxia telangiectasia and
Behcet's disease which suggests an immune function abnormality
(41). In Table 3, A.H. had low titer anti-EBNA and T.F. a normal
titer, yet both showed impaired or absent cell-mediated immune
responses to EBNA (23). The pathogenesis of such a response is
yet to be elucidated but the presence of low anti-EBNA titers
suggests an impaired eradication of transformed EBNA positive
cells. This may account for the chronicity (40). No clue to this
is provided by the normal anti-EBNA titers in our patients, but
specialized studies are intended to rule out the possibility of a
subtle EBV-specific immune deficiency. The high incidence of
allergy and presence of thyroiditis in two patients (Table 1) may
be clues to an altered immune state in these patients.

Elevated (2'-5')-Oligo-A Synthetase Activity

It became necessary to demonstrate a chronic infective process
of viral origin to support our serological data. Since interferon
defends against viral infection (43) it was reasoned that interferon levels (or effects thereof) should be elevated chronically
in these patients. A low molecular weight inhibitor of viral
protein synthesis, (2'-5')-oligo-Adenylate, has been postulated to
be produced through interferon's activity in inducing the
(2'-5')-oligo-A synthetase enzyme (44). By assaying this enzyme
in peripheral blood mononuclear cells, a sensitive measurement of
interferon activity can be made (45). Schattner et al. showed
increased levels of this synthetase activity in varied acute viral
infections in 41 patients varying from 100 to 1940% of the normal
mean value (46). A group of patients with other non-infective
diseases generally had far lower activities, exceptions being
collagen diseases and EBV related malignancies. Measurement of
the enyzme activity in 6/7 of our patients, including an additional 2 patients with the same criteria who have since been
included in this group, yielded values in excess of 340% of the
normal mean value (47). A group of control acute IM patients had
a mean activity of 458% which fell to 95% 3-4 weeks after the
onset of disease (Table 4). Whilst these results do not necessarily support the contention that these patients are suffering

Table 4. (2'-5') Oligo A in Infections Associated
with Epstein-Barr Virus

Patient No.	Duration of Illness in Months Prior to Enzyme Determination	(2'-5') Oligo A Synthetase [Activity (% of Normal Mean Value]
1	18(15)[a]	750
2	14(14)	700
	18(18)	700
3	15(12)	460
4	30(20)	340
5	16(16)	515
7	23(23)	340
8	16(5)	575
9	12(10)	370
Acute IM[b]	------	458
IM-Recovery[c]	3-4 weeks	95

[a]Numbers in parenthesis indicate duration in months after initial
serological finding of elevated IgM to VCA.
[b]Mean level of activity in nine patients during acute stage of
infectious mononucleosis (range: 210-700).
[c]Mean level of activity in two patients 3-4 weeks after acute
stage of infectious mononucleosis

from an ongoing EBV infection, it is reasonable to submit that in
the absence of demonstrable collagen disease or EBV related
malignancy, these patients seem to maintain a state of interferon
activity usually observed in viral infections inter alia, acute
IM. Obviously, more studies are needed before this may be
confirmed and immune aberrations in the interferon system be ruled
out.

A Diagnostic Eponym

Horwitz et al. (17) suggested that intermittent activation of
the EBV carrier state probably occurs, but it was not known if
such a reactivation could be accompanied by symptoms of either
relapse or chronic mononucleosis. He emphasized the importance of
such features as the presence of atypical lymphocytes from which
IM derives its name. Very few of the chronic cases discussed here
had the minimal criteria for the diagnosis (9) of the IM syndrome.
From this aspect, it would appear that to call this entity Chronic
IM might be a misnomer. We are unable at the present level of
knowledge to delineate the pathologic process as one of a continuous primary infection nor a continuous reactivation to allow an

accurate etiological description. The appellation of "prolonged
atypical illness associated with serological evidence of persistent EBV infection" is too cumbersome. Bender (13) in the
prediscovery days of EBV suggested that the hematologic criteria
be strictly adhered to until the cause was discovered. It is well
established that at least 80% of the general population carry
latent EBV in B lymphocytes and thus, literally have "chronic EBV
infection." A more appropriate term would be chronic EBV illness,
implying prolonged symptoms. Until the pathogeneses of these
chronic diseases are elucidated, one may do worse than adhere to
the popular term "chronic mononucleosis", a contraction of Isaacs'
term "Chronic Infectious Mononucleosis" (42).

    We would suggest that this diagnosis be based on the existence
of a clinically atypical illness for at least a year's duration
with specific serology supportive of EBV activation in the absence
of apparent manifestation of serious underlying disease with a
commitment to careful surveillance. An international registry for
this disease, as has been established for the XLP syndrome, might
aid further study.

    A condition which should be tested for chronic mononucleosis
is habitual hyperthermia of young females described in a well
known medical text (48) as follows: "The patient may have
temperatures ranging from 37.2 - 38°C regularly or intermittently
for years and also usually has a variety of complaints characteristic of psychoneurosis, such as fatigability, insomnia, bowel
distress, vague aches, and headaches. Prolonged careful study and
observation fails to reveal evidence of organic disease.... The
diagnosis of this syndrome can be made with reasonable certainty
after a suitable period of observation and study, and if the
patient can be convinced of its validity, a real service will have
been rendered."

SUMMARY AND CONCLUSIONS

    A brief historical review of chronic and recurrent IM dating
from the post-Paul-Bunnell-Davidsohn era is presented. The
symptoms and signs of recently reported groups of patients with
serological evidence for prolonged EBV infection are compared to
those of classical acute IM. Unique immunodeficient cases of
chronic or recurrent IM gleaned from the recent literature are
presented. The antibody profiles to EBV in these conditions are
discussed in relation to acute IM, the seemingly normal and
immunodeficient groups with chronic IM. The results and implications of an unique interferon activity test in the former is
presented and discussed. A convenient diagnostic eponym, the
establishment of an international registry, and other disease
entities, possibly masquerading as chronic EBV, are suggested.

ACKNOWLEDGMENTS

     Zohar Ravid, Ph.D. of the Division of Clinical Virology,
Hadassah Medical Center, Jerusalem who performed the serological
studies. Drs. Revel and Schattner who performed the (2'-5')oligo-
A synthetase assay. Drs. Chowers, Feldman-Weiss, Ben-Chitrit,
Michaeli, Shalit, Knobler, Neuman, Gamus and Herman for providng
the patients, Professor Y. Menczl for permission to publish the
Mt. Scopus patients and to Dr. Ian Munro, editor of Lancet, for
kindly allowing the reproduction of Tables from the published
originals. Ms. Linda Alcorn for secretarial assistance. This
paper is dedicated to the memory of Baruch Feldman, M.D.

REFERENCES

1.   Epstein, M.A., Achong, B.G., and Barr, Y.M. Virus particle
      in cultured lymphoblasts from Burkitt's lymphoma. Lancet,
      $\underline{i}$:702, 1964.
2.   Henle, G., Henle, W., and Diehl, V. Relation of Burkitt's
      tumour associated with herpes-type virus to infectious
      mononucleosis. Proc. Natl. Acad. Sci. USA, $\underline{59}$:94,
      1968.
3.   Epstein, M.A. and Achong, B.G. Various forms of EBV infec-
      tion in man: estalished facts and a general concept.
      Lancet, $\underline{ii}$:836, 1973.
4.   Pattengale, P.K., Smith, R.W., and Gerber, P. Selective
      transformation of B lymphocytes by EB virus. Lancet,
      $\underline{ii}$:93, 1973.
5.   Nilsson, K., Klein, G., Henle, W., and Henle, G. The
      establishment of lymphoblastoid lines from adult and
      fetal human lymphoid tissue and its dependence on EBV.
      Int. J. Cancer, $\underline{8}$:443, 1971.
6.   Henle, W., Henle, G.E., and Horwitz, C.A. Epstein-Barr
      virus-specific diagnostic tests in infectious mono-
      nucleosis. Human Path., $\underline{5}$:551, 1974.
7.   Hallee, T.J., Evans, A.S., Niederman, J.C., Brooks, C.M.,
      and Voegtly, J.H. IM at the U.S. military academy.
      Yale J. Biol. Med., $\underline{3}$:182, 1974.
8.   Karzon, D.T. Infectious mononucleosis. Adv. Pediat.,
      $\underline{22}$:231, 1976.
9.   Horwitz, C.A. Practical approach to the diagnosis of
      infectious mononucleosis. Postgraduate Med., $\underline{65}$:179,
      1979.
10.   Niederman, J.C., Evans, A.S., Subrahmanyah, L., and
      McCollum, R.W. Prevalence, incidence and persistence of
      EB virus antibody in young adults. N. Engl. J. Med.,
      $\underline{282}$:361, 1970.
11.   Joint investigation by University Health Physicians and
      P.H.L.S. Laboratories. Infectious mononucleosis and its
      relationship to EBV antibody. Br. Med. J., $\underline{4}$:643, 1971.

12.   Paterson, J.K. and Pinninger, J.L. Case of recurrent
      infectious mononucleosis. Br. Med. J., 2:476, 1955.
13.   Bender, C.E. Recurrent mononucleosis. J. Am. Med. Assoc.,
      182:954, 1962.
14.   Kaufman, R.E. Recurrences of infectious mononucleosis.
      Amer. Practit., 1:673, 1950.
15.   Chang, R.S. EBV virus-seropositive person is susceptible
      to infectious mononucleosis. N. Engl. J. Med., 292:925,
      1975.
16.   Stevens, D.A., Pry, T.W., and Manaker, R.A. Infectious
      mononucleosis -- Always a primary infection with herpes-
      type virus? J. Natl. Cancer Inst., 44:533, 1970.
17.   Horwitz, C.A., Henle, W., Henle, G. et al. Clinical
      evaluation of patients with infectious mononucleosis and
      development of antibodies to the R component of the EB
      virus-induced early antigen complex. Am. J. Med.,
      58:330, 1975.
18.   Banatvala, J.E., Best, J.M., and Wallter, D.K. EBV-specific
      IgM in infectious mononucleosis, Burkitt's lymphoma and
      nasopharyngeal carcinoma. Lancet, i:1205, 1972.
19.   Askinazi, C., Cole, F.S., and Brosch, J.L. Positive
      differential heterophil antibody tests -- persistence in
      a symptomatic patient. J. Am. Med. Assoc., 236:1492,
      1976.
20.   Virelizier, J.L., Lenoir, G., and Griscelli, C. Persistent
      EBV infection in a child with hypergammaglobulinemia and
      immunoblastic proliferation associated with a selective
      defect in immune interferon secretion. Lancet, ii:231,
      1978.
21.   Sakamoto, K., Freed, H.J., and Purtilo, D.T. Antibody
      responses to EBV in families with the X-linked lymphopro-
      liferative syndrome. J. Immunol., 125:921, 1980.
22.   Purtilo, D.T., Paquin, L.A., Sakamoto, K., Hutt, L.M., Yang,
      J.P.W., Sparling, S., Beberman, N., and McAuley, R.A.
      Persistent transfusion associated infectious mono-
      nucleosis with transient acquired immunodeficiency. Am.
      J. Med., 68:437, 1980.
23.   Masucci, M.G., Szigeti, R., Ernberg, I., Masucci, G., Klein,
      G., Chessel, J., Sieff, C., Lie, S., Glomstein, A.,
      Businco, L., Henle, W., Henle, G., Pearson, G.,
      Sakamoto, K., and Purtilo, D.T. Cellular immune defects
      to EBV-determined antigens in young males. Cancer Res.,
      41:4284, 1981.
24.   Purtilo, D.T., Sakamoto, K., Saemundsen, A.K., Sullivan,
      J.L., Synnerholm, A.C., Andersson-Anvret, M., Pritchard,
      J., Sloper, C., Sieff, C., Pincott, J., Pachman, L.,
      Rich, K., Cruzi, F., Cornet, J., Collins, R., Barnes,
      N., Knight, J., Sandstedt, B., and Klein, G.
      Documentation of EBV infection in immunodeficient
      patients with life-threatening lymphoproliferative

diseases by clinical, virological and immunopathological
studies. Cancer Res., 41:4226, 1981.

25. Tobi, M., Morag, A., Ravid, Z. et al. Prolonged atypical
    illness associated with serological evidence of persistent
    EBV infection. Lancet, 1:61, 1982.

26. Lennette, E.M. and Schmidt, N.J. (eds.) Diagnostic Proce-
    dures for Viral, Rickettsial and Chlamydial Infections.
    5th edition, pp. 441-470. Washington, D.C. American
    Public Health Association, 1979.

27. Schleupner, C.J. and Overall, J.C. Infectious mono-
    nucleosis and EBV. II. Clinical picture, diagnosis,
    management. Postgrad. Med., 65:95, 1979.

28. Finch, S.C. Infectious mononucleosis. In: R.L. Carter
    and H.G. Penman (eds.), Infectious Mononucleosis. pp.
    19-46. Oxford and Edinburgh: Blackwell Scientific
    Publications, 1969.

29. Cadie, M., Nye, F.J., and Storey, P. Anxiety and depression
    after infectious mononucleosis. Brit. J. Psychiat.,
    128:559, 1976.

30. Hendler, N. and Leary, W. Psychiatric and neurologic
    sequelae of infectious mononucleosis. Am. J. Psych.,
    135:842, 1978.

31. Evans, A.S. Epstein-Barr and infectious mononucleosis.
    N. Engl. J. Med., 286:836, 1972.

32. Evans, A.S. Infectious mononucleosis and related syndrome.
    Am. J. Med. Sci., 276:325, 1978.

33. Gordon, D.S., Jones, B.M., Browning, S.W., Spira, T.J., and
    Lawrence, D.N. Persistent polyclonal lymphocytosis of B
    lymphocytes. N. Engl. J. Med, 307:232, 1982.

34. Evans, A.S., Niderman, J.C., Cenabre, L.C., West, B., and
    Richards, N.A. A prospective evaluation of heterophile
    and EBV-specific IgM antibody tests in clinical and sub-
    clinical infectious mononucleosis: specificity and
    sensitivity of the tests and persistence of antibody.
    J. Inf. Dis., 132:546, 1975.

35. Henle, G., Lynette, E.T., Alspaugh, M.A., and Henle, W.
    Rheumatoid factor as a cause of positive reactions in
    tests for Epstein-Barr virus specific IgM antibodies.
    Clin. Exp. Immunol., 36:415, 1979.

36. Sumaya, C.V. Endogenous reactivation of Epstein-Barr
    virus infections. J. Inf. Dis., 135:374, 1977.

37. Ross, C.A.C. and McDavid, R. Specific IgM antibody in serum
    of patients with herpes-zoster infections. Br. Med. J.,
    5:522, 1972.

38. Henle, G., Henle, W., and Klein, G. Demonstration of two
    distinct components in the early antigen complex of
    Epstein-Barr virus infected cells. Int. J. Cancer,
    8:272, 1971.

39. Henle, W., Ho, H.C., Henle, G., and Kwan, H.C. Antibodies
    to EBV-related antigens in nasopharyngeal carcinoma.

Comparison of active cases with long-term survivors. J. Natl. Cancer Inst., 51:361, 1973.

40. Klein, G. and Purtilo, D.T. Summary: symposium on Epstein-Barr virus induced lymphoproliferative disease in immuno-deficient patients. Cancer Res., 41:4302, 1981.

41. Henle, W. and Henle, G. Epstein-Barr virus-specific serology in immunologically compromised individuals. Cancer Res., 41:4222, 1981.

42. Isaacs, R. Chronic infectious mononucleosis. Blood, 3:898, 1948.

43. Baron, S. and Dianzani, F. General consideration of the interferon system. Tex. Rep. Biol. Med., 35:1, 1977.

44. Baglioni, C. Interferon-induced enzymatic activities and their role in the antiviral state. Cell, 17:255, 1979.

45. Minks, M.A., Benvin, S., Maroney, P.A., and Baglioni, C. Synthesis of (2'-5')-oligo (A) in extracts of interferon-treated HeLa cells. J. Biol. Chem., 254:5058, 1979.

46. Schattner, A., Wallach, D., Merlin, G., Hahn, T., Levin, S., and Revel, M. Assay of an interferon-induced enzyme in white blood cells as a diagnostic and in viral diseases. Lancet, ii:497, 1981.

47. Morag, A., Tobi, M., Ravid, Z., Schattner, A., and Revel, M. Elevated [2'-5']-oligo A synthetase activity in patients with prolonged illness associated with serological evidence of persistent EBV infection. Lancet, i:744, 1982.

48. Harrison's Principles of Internal Medicine. 9th Edition Eds. Isselbacher, Adams, Braunwald, Petersdorf, and Wilson. 10: Chills and Fever. R.G. Petersdorf, pp. 60-67, 1980.

ADDENDUM

The authors wish to make it clear that the data regarding the IgM anti-VCA results found in our 7 cases from Jerusalem have not been confirmed in a reference laboratory. We would, therefore, caution our readers that these results should not be viewed as universally applicable at this stage. We have, however, repeated and confirmed our original results using 3 different sources of anti-human-IgM, -chain specific globulin from Miles-Yeda, Ltd.; Rehavot, Israel; Behring Institute, Frankfurt, Germany; and Tago, Inc., Burlingame, California. A recently published case of chronic mononucleosis by Edson et al. in the Journal of Immunology, 130:919, 1983, had IgM anti-VCA titers of similar duration and quantitation to our patients.

THE SYNDROME OF ACQUIRED IMMUNODEFICIENCY AMONG

A SUBSET OF HOMOSEXUAL MEN

Joseph A. Sonnabend[1],
Steven S. Witkin[2],
Ruth B. Purtilo[3], and
David T. Purtilo[3]

[1]49 West 12th Street
New York, NY 10011
[2]Department of Obstetrics and Gynecology
The New York Hospital
Cornell Medical Center
525 East 68th Street
New York, NY 10021
[3]Department of Humanities and Jurisprudence and
the Department of Pathology and Laboratory Medicine
University of Nebraska Medical Center
42nd & Dewey Avenue
Omaha, NE 68105

INTRODUCTION

The etiologic basis for recent occurrence of an acquired immunodeficiency syndrome (AIDS) among a group of homosexual men, predominantly in New York City, San Francisco and Los Angeles remains unexplained. Manifestations of the syndrome include opportunistic infections, autoimmunity, chronic lymphadenomegaly, and malignancies. The syndrome has no acceptable established diagnostic definition. The multiple diverse mainifestations are an essential feature.

A prevailing view is that a new and unique transmissible agent may be responsible for AIDS, thus linking the disease occurring in homosexual men with a similar syndrome seen among Haitians, intravenous drug users, young children, and hemophiliac patients (1). Thus we have been prompted to develop a model for establishing the genesis of the syndrome at this time. We propose that AIDS does not require the person-to-person transmission of a

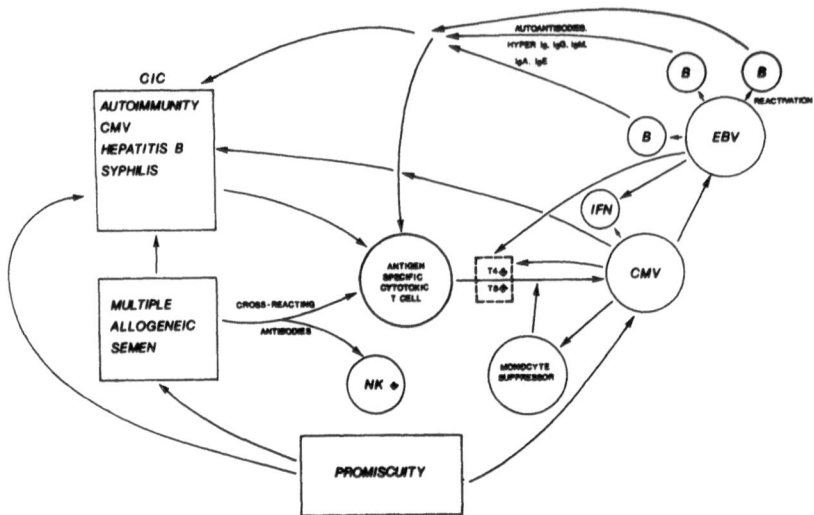

Fig. 1. Summary of multifactorial bases of acquired immune
         deficiency in a subset of homosexuals. Abbreviations:
         CMV, cytomegalovirus; CIC, circulating immune complexes;
         NK, natural killer cell; EBV, Epstein-Barr virus.

unique, previously unidentified, infectious agent. Rather than
invoke a single common infectious etiology, our model proposes
that different pathways can lead to disorders of immune regulation
and outlines the mechanisms that may lead to AIDS in homosexual
men. A parallel or similar disorder occurs in renal transplant
recipients, who experience the same diverse infections, Kaposi's
sarcoma (KS), squamous cell carcinomas and B cell lymphomas.
Elsewhere in this book Penn documents the similarities in the
types of neoplasms. As is the case with the men with AIDS, renal
transplant recipients have an acquired immunologic disorder due to
immunosuppressive therapy.

Hypothesis

     Any hypothesis regarding the genesis of AIDS must include an
explanation for the occurrence of the syndrome at the present
time. "Why now?" We suggest that the new element is an unprecedented level of sexual promiscuity that has developed among a
subgroup of homosexual men in New York, San Francisco, Los Angeles,
and some other large urban centers since the late 1960's. Homosexual patients with KS and Pneumocystis carinii pneumonia (PCP)
have reported sexual contact with an unusually large number of
different partners. This has been a consistent finding in the few
epidemiologic surveys that have been reported (2).

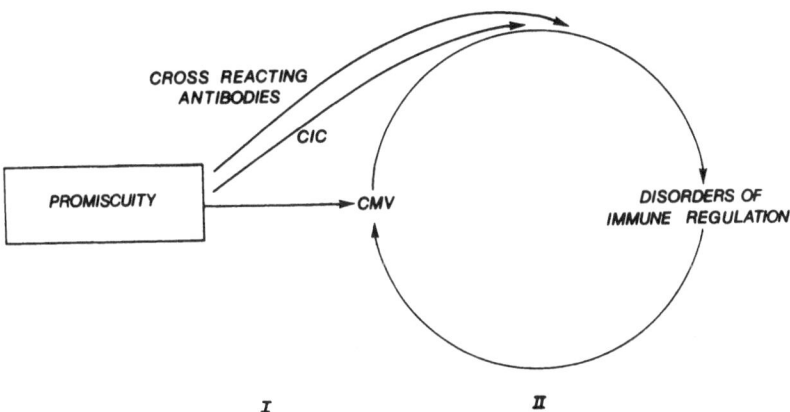

Fig. 2.   The biphasic natural history of acquired immunodeficiency
          syndrome is summarized. I. is an acquisition phase which
          is probably reversible and lasts for many months to
          years. In contrast, phase II is a progressive and
          presently not reversible. CIC, circulating immune
          complexes; CMV, cytomegalovirus.

     We suggest that two distinct stages may be recognized in the
development of the syndrome. An initial reversible stage of
acquisition is followed by a self sustaining stage of progression.
During the first stage the cumulative effects associated with promiscuity result from repeated infection with cytomegalovirus
(CMV), reactivation of Epstein-Barr virus (EBV), and immune
responses to spermatozoa. Each of these factors will be discussed
(Figure 1).

     The syndrome in males appears to be biphasic (see Figure 2).

PROBABLE ETIOLOGIC FACTORS IN AIDS

Cytomegalovirus and immunoregulatory defects

     Infection with CMV evokes several responses from the immune
system. Activation of T8 suppressor/lytic T cells accompanies a
reduction in the ratio of T4 helper T cells and thus the T4 to T8
ratio is reversed. These changes resemble those seen in acute
infections with EBV, but unlike EBV, T subset aberrations may
persist for up to a year following primary infections with CMV
(3,4). In addition, infection with CMV induces a population of
monocytes with suppressor activity (5). Autoreactive antibodies
have been associated with CMV infections, as has the appearance of
circulating immune complexes (CICs) (6,7). CMV as well as other
herpesvirus-infected cells express Fc receptors (8,9).

Noteworthy associations regarding CMV infections and sexual promiscuity include:

1. CMV is excreted in saliva, urine and semen. Viral titers are probably highest in semen (10).

2. Asymptomatic carriage of CMV in semen may persist for over a year (11).

3. CMV antibody has been detected in 94% of homosexual, and 54% of heterosexual men attending a clinic for sexually transmitted diseases. IgM isotype was detected in 57% of homosexual men compared with 4% of heterosexual men (12,13).

4. The prevalence of CMV viruria among homosexual men attending a clinic was 7-14%. The excretion rate would probably have been higher had semen been sampled (12). Highly promiscuous populations may have very high carrier rates.

5. Reinfection with CMV can occur. More than one strain of CMV can be shown to be present by comparing nucleic acid fragments from different viral isolates (14).

The frequency with which an individual will be reinfected with CMV will be a function of both the number of different sexual contacts, as well as the prevalence of CMV carriage in the population with whose members the individual interacts. In New York City, during the past 10 years, the prevalence of CMV carriage in populations of highly promiscuous men was probably at least 10%. Owing to this carriage rate exposure to CMV would therefore be repeated, and innocula may be massive. Another consequence of CMV infection could be the reactivation of other latent herpes viruses, in particular, EBV (15).

Reactivation of Epstein-Barr virus

Almost all adults carry EBV in latency in B cells. Primary infection usually occurs silently in children. EBV infects B cells which possess receptors for the virus (16) and activates B cells to immunoglobulin synthesis. EBV is thus a polyclonal activator, and can act in the absence of T cell help (17,18) (Figure 1). All 65 of the patients we have studied for EBV have been seropositive (S. Harada, J. Sonnabend and D. Purtilo - unpublished observations). Many of the men with AIDS show chronic lymphadenomegaly and evidence of polyclonal B cell activation despite the virtual absence of T helper cells in some of the patients (19). Initially lymphoid tissues are hypoplastic. About a third of B cells exposed in vitro can be infected by EBV, and about 10%

of infected cells will be activated to immunoglobulin synthesis (20). Among the mechanisms that have evolved to deal with this B cell infection are natural killer (NK) cells (21). In addition, suppressor T cells (with a surface phenotype defined by a T8 monoclonal antibody) are activated to suppress B cell activation and proliferation (21). In seropositive individuals a different type of cytotoxic T cell is rapidly activated. Unlike the suppressor/lytic T cell evoked during a primary infection, these T cells (memory T cells) from seropositive individuals are specific for EBV infected B cells (22). Harada and associates discuss the role of memory T cells in another chapter of this book. The suppressor and memory T cells also differ in the kinetics of suppression of B cell activation to immunoglobulin synthesis (22). The viral antigen specific T cell is also HLA restricted, but while T8 cytotoxic cells recognize viral antigens on the surface of the infected cell in the context of class I major histocompatibility complex (MHC) products, cytotoxic T cells with a T4 surface phenotype recognize antigens in the context of class II MHC products (23). HLA restricted antigen specific cytotoxic T cells are generated during many viral infections, including CMV infection (24).

We propose that, by virtue of their immunosuppressive effects, CMV and possibly other viruses cause recurrent EBV reactivation. Multiple herpes virus infections (15) and reactivation of EBV have been seen in other immunodeficiency disorders not directly resulting from viral infections. Administration of the immunosuppressive drug, cyclosporin A, for example, has been associated with reactivation of EBV (25,26). Among agents that induce EBV in vitro are corticosteroids (27). Often, patients with AIDS develop chronic lymphadenomegaly and other features of chronic infectious mononucleosis (28). Abrams discusses this in detail in the accompanying chapter.

The resemblance of AIDS patients to renal transplant recipients has been mentioned. Importantly, renal transplant recipients specific T cell immunity to EBV is impaired (29), and the lymphomas that they develop contain EBV genome (30). Similarly, Ziegler et al. (31) have found EBV genome in B cell lymphomas, resembling Burkitt's lymphoma, in patients with AIDS.

With successive bouts of EBV reactivation, increasing numbers of B cells would be driven to immunoglobulin synthesis and a variety of antibodies including some autoantibodies, produced. Many patients show evidence of enhanced immunoglobulin synthesis, involving IgG, IgA, IgM (32) and even IgE isotypes (Joyce Wallace, personal communication). This occurs despite diminished T helper function. The T cell-independent, polyclonal activation of B cells by EBV could explain this paradox (Figure 1).

Polyclonal activation of B cells and autoimmunity

     Many AIDS patients show evidence of autoimmunity. Documented
clinically, is a thrombocytopenia associated with anti-platelet
antibodies (33). Likely leukopenia and some unexplained rashes
frequently observed in these patients could also result, at least
in part, from autoimmune response. Antinuclear antibody (ANA) was
found in two of 37 homosexual men with AIDS at a titer of 1:100,
and two-thirds of these men had ANA titers of 1:10; 3/37 had
elevated titers to ssDNA, 4/37 exhibited rheumatoid factor, and
13/37 had circulating immune complexes by the Clq binding assay
(J. Sonnabend, unpublished observations). Cryoglobulins are
detectable in serum during the course of infectious mononucleosis
(34). Thus we predict their presence in AIDS. An unusual acid
labile form of interferon has been detected in the sera of many
homosexual AIDS patients (35). This type of interferon has been
found in systemic lupus erythematosus and other autoimmune
diseases. Its presence in AIDS is further evidence for an
autoimmune component in this disease. Possibly additional
clinical manifestations of autoimmunity will become apparent as
observations are extended.

Immune responses to semen

     Repeated exposure of men per rectum to multiple allogeneic
semens induces deleterious immune responses. Witkin and Sonnabend
studied immune responses to spermatozoa in 18 homosexual men.
Anti-sperm antibodies of IgG and IgA isotypes were found in 10 and
2 of the 18 men, respectively. Circulating immune complexes were
elevated in two-thirds of the men and sperm related antigen found
in the sera of some (36). Thus one possible factor contributing
to immunological impairment could be CICs (Figures 1 and 2)
associated with sperm related antigens. There are antigens
expressed on cells in the ejaculate including HLA antigens and
gangliosides that are shared by lymphocytes (36). For example,
spermatozoa express a ganglioside antigen, asialo GM_1, which is
also present on NK cells (38). Approximately 38% of men (13 of
21) with AIDS complicated by opportunistic infection or cancer
showed anti-asialo GM_1 antibodies whereas 0 of 19 asymptomatic
males showed this antibody in their blood. Moreover, a strong
negative correlation ($p<0.001$) was found between the presence of
anti-asialo GM_1 antibodies and the absolute number of T4 (helper)
lymphocytes (39). Many AIDS patients show diminished NK function
(32). Antibodies to asialo GM_1 would contribute to this, a
possibility we are presently investigating. Repeated exposure to
different allogeneic semens may eventually lead to the appearance
of antibodies autoreactive with T lymphocytes and NK cells (40).
Multiple anti-HLA antibodies will probably be found in promiscuous
homosexual men who have never received blood transfusions. The
diversity of the anti-HLA antibodies may in fact provide an

objective measure of promiscuity. Our preliminary studies of 20 AIDS patients reveal one-half possess lymphocytotoxic antibodies. Given the recent appearance of AIDS in homosexual men, exposure to allogeneic semen cannot in itself be responsible for the morbidity. We propose that immune responses to semen may provide a background of immune suppression not only promoting repeated CMV infections, but also exacerbating the immunologic disorders.

Circulating immune complexes in AIDS

CICs have been detected in many patients with AIDS. Our additional observations have shown a clear correlation between promiscuity and the presence of CICs: thirteen of thirteen homosexual patients with KS and six of ten promiscuous homosexual men had CICs, while these were present in only one out of eight non-promiscuous homosexual men (Witkin, Safai, Krim, and Sonnabend, unpublished observations). Undoubtedly, many different antigens form immune complexes in these men. Hepatitis B, syphilis, and CMV are among the infectious agents which are highly prevalent in these men and which can be associated with immune complexes (Figures 1 and 2). Additional contributions to the CICs may appear once autoantibodies are produced. A further contribution is from sperm related antigens, and indeed their presence in CICs in promiscuous homosexual men who have antibodies to spermatozoa has already been demonstrated (36).

Mechanisms of disease acquisition, and transition to a self-sustaining stage

We propose that the first stage of disease acquisition is a period of frequent sexual contact with different partners who carry CMV and thus repeated infection with this virus occur. These repeated infections are associated with an accumulation of effects which in aggregate eventually result in a switch to a self-sustaining, progressive condition characterized by an inability of cytotoxic lymphocytes to clear CMV and other infectious agents. The critical concept during the initial stage is that of a cumulative process involving:

a. An increasing level of CICs which may react with Fc or complement receptors on some T lymphocytes and interfere with their cytotoxic function. Herpes virus infected cells, including CMV-infected cells, express Fc receptors and thus may bind CICs and block target recognition by cytotoxic lymphocytes.

b. The appearance in increasing concentrations of antibodies that are cross reactive with cytotoxic T cells and NK cells. The specific targets may be regulatory or effector T cells. The consequence is impaired cytotoxicity. Antibodies reactive with T

lymphocytes and NK cells may result from polyclonal B cell activation, or from immunization by cross reactive antigens present in
the ejaculate.

c. A diminishing ratio of T4 helper to T8 suppressor cells.
The action of cytotoxic T lymphocytes would be susceptible to T8
suppression. CMV and EBV infections, as well as toxoplasmosis
(which is common in AIDS) have been associated with T subset
aberrations. These changes are evoked by antigens expressed on
the surface of the infected cell. Persistence of infection would
maintain these subset changes.

Table 1. Infectious and Non-infectious Diseases in the
          Acquired Immunodeficiency Syndrome[*]

Cytomegalovirus infections
Herpes simplex virus infectious (progressive and severe)
Reactivated Epstein-Barr virus infections
Herpes varicella-zoster

Tuberculosis
Atypical mycobacterial infections

Cryptococcosis
Gastrointestinal candidiasis
Coccidioidomycosis
Histoplasmosis

Cerebral and occular toxoplasmosis
Pneumocystis carinii pneumonia
Cryptosporidiosis
Strongyloidiasis

Progressive multifocal leukoencephalopathy
Autoimmune thrombocytopenia
Leukopenia
Unexplained generalized lymphadenomegaly
Nephrotic syndrome
Progressive "wasting syndrome"

Kaposi's sarcoma
Non-Hodgkin's lymphoma
Squamous cell cloacal carcinoma

---

[*]Sources: Centers for Disease Control surveillance
             data New York City Department of Health
             monthly meeting on AIDS

These three general influences, autoantibodies, CICs, and a decrease in ratio of T4:T8 subsets, conspire to inhibit an effective cytotoxic response to CMV infected cells. The relative contribution of each might vary with each patient.

Eventually the immunosuppression becomes irreversible and self-sustaining and independent of promiscuous sexual behavior. The sustained immunoregulatory disorders impair cytotoxic responses to other intracellular parasites, which are responsible for opportunistic infections.

Figure 2 summarizes the mechanism of self-perpetuation; the essential feature of this second stage is an inability to mount an effective cytotoxic immune response against CMV infected cells.

The diversity of the infectious and non-infectious manifestations that have been reported in association with this syndrome is apparent in the Table 1. The serious opportunistic infections occur predominantly in the profoundly immunocompromised patient. However, we have observed less immunocompromised patients who have recovered from some of the same infections and remained free from recurrence. These observations are consistent with our two-stage model. It is, therefore, clearly of benefit to recognize patients in the first stage of acquisition. We have recognized laboratory features that we think indicates early disease. Hence we are formulating diagnostic criteria, based on a combination of these indicators and clinical findings.

Our model offers a conceptual framework to formulate approaches to defining pathogenetic mechanisms and developing rational basis for intervention. We seek corroboration of our hypothesis. For example, one can compare CMV excretion rates among different populations distinguished by different levels of promiscuity and sexual preferences, and correlate these rates with the prevalence of AIDS. Perhaps the behavioral and cultural aspects that appear to be associated with the genesis of AIDS are the most troublesome; they are also critical, because they suggest an explanation for the occurrence of the syndrome at a particular time and location. Here too, it should be possible to document whether significant changes in patterns of sexual behavior have occurred in New York City during recent years. We have embarked on such a study.

Our model suggests some approaches to patient management which are of immediate practical importance. Both humoral (autoantibodies and CICs) and cellular (inversion of T4:T8 ratios and depressed NK activity) factors impair antiviral cytotoxic responses (Figure 1). Methods to remove humoral factors by plasmapharesis may deserve serious consideration. Cyclophosphamide may control increased immunoglobulin production, and in low dose may

preferentially inhibit T8 suppressor cells. Alternatively, these
cells may be selectively removed by appropriate monoclonal
antibodies. This subset also includes cytotoxic T lymphocytes, so
some obvious caution is required in such an approach. Improvement
might set in motion a process leading to recovery. Reduction in
CMV antigenic load could improve immune function (Figure 1).

The suggestion that any particular group carries a specific
infectious agent capable of causing severe immunodeficiency and
cancer is an assertion of tremendous seriousness. This labeling
is of more concern if the group in question is the object of
discriminatory practices. Given the potential repercussions of
such a suggestion, it is important that substantial evidence
become available (41).

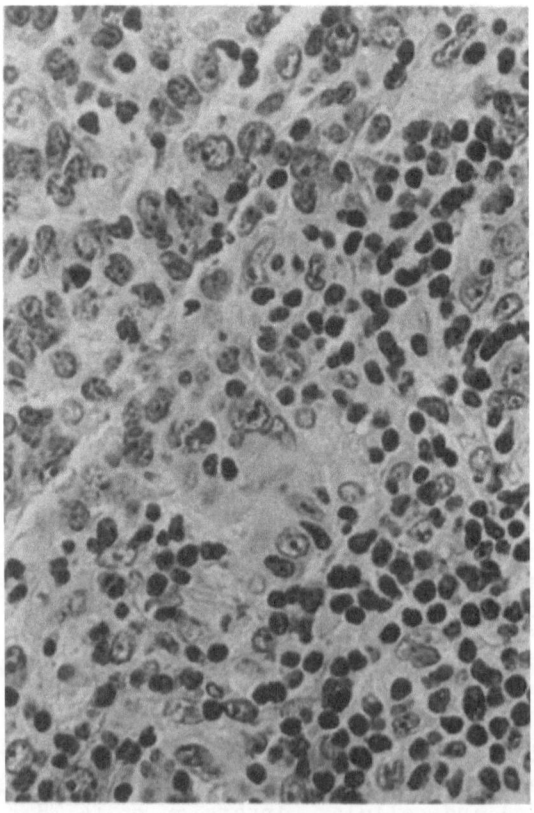

Fig. 3.   Photomicrograph of reactive lymph node from a patient
          with AIDS. A heterogeneous population of lymphoid cells.
          Approximately 17 genome copies/cell of EBV were present.
          Hematoxylin and eosin X450. (Courtesy of Dr. R. Tubbs.)

The notion that a new specific infectious agent is causing
AIDS derives from the following three assumptions: 1) that the
same disease is occuring in at least four disparate groups:
Haitians, IV drug users, hemophiliacs, and homosexual men; 2) That
it is spread by contagion between these groups; and 3) That the
disease is new in all these groups. We thus have one hypothesis
(that of a specific infectious agent) based on two hypotheses: An
identical disease in at least four disparate groups, and its new
occurrence in all.

A further source of support for the specific infectious
etiology comes from the report that a cluster of patients with KS
or PCP could be interconnected through sexual contact (42). The

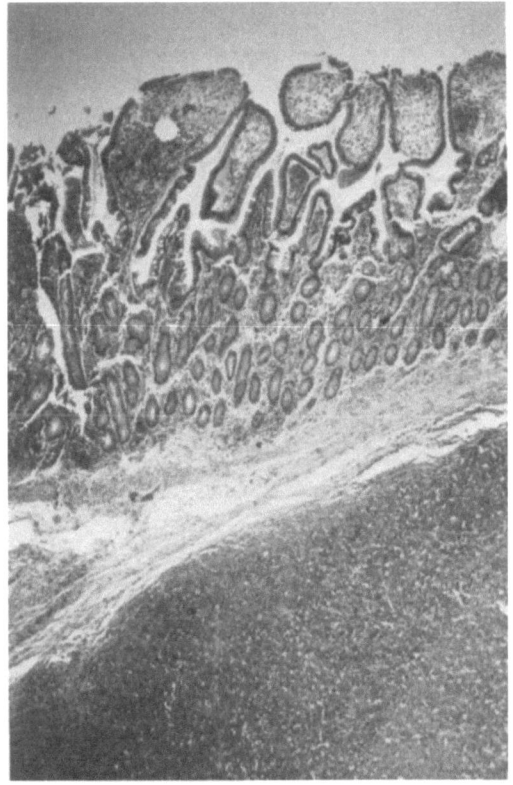

Fig. 4.   Photomicrograph of Burkitt lymphoma involving terminal
          ileum from a patient with AIDS. Hematoxylin and eosin
          X50. Two EBV genome equivalents/cell were identified.
          A mu kappa monoclonal, EBNA positive tumor cell line
          carrying 14q+ was established from the lymphoma.
          (Courtesy Dr. R. Tubbs.)

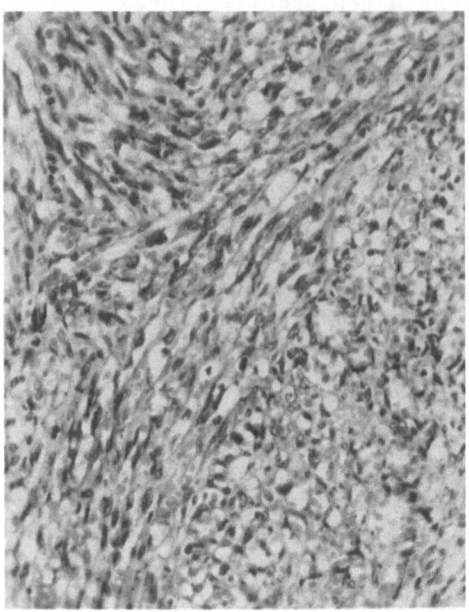

Fig. 5. Kaposi's sarcoma of patient with AIDS. Hematoxylin and
         eosin X750.

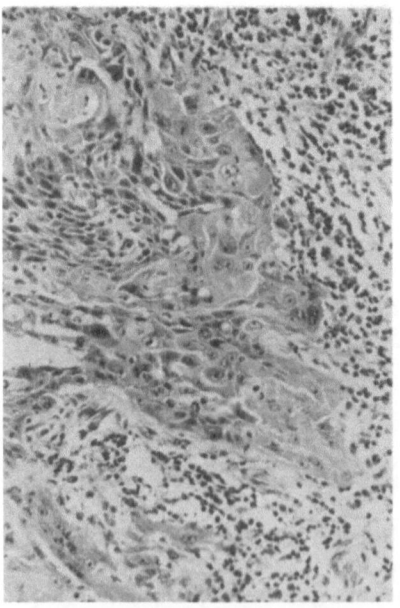

Fig. 6. Photomicrograph of squamous cell carcinoma involving
         anus. Hematoxylin and eosin X250.

interpretation that the spread of AIDS could be brought about by a single exposure to an infectious agent rests on the simplistic assumption that homosexual men constitute a homogeneous population whose members have sexual contact with the same number of different partners each year. (The number cited was a median of 13.5 to 50 different sexual partners for homosexual men between 18 and 64.) Available evidence indicates that many of the cases of AIDS have occurred in a probably rather small subgroup of homosexual men who have had sexual contact with an unusually large number of different partners (2).

Malignancies in AIDS

The spectrum of infections and malignancies (Figures 3,4,5,6) seen in promiscuous homosexual men have long been familiar as consequences of an impairment predominantly of cell-mediated immunity, whatever its causes. Already mentioned, the group most resembling these men are renal transplant recipients. The cancers in RTR occurring in high frequency and the virus likely responsible are identical to AIDS patients: B cell lymphomas (EBV), KS (CMV), and squamous cell carcinoma (papilloma virus) (43). Two patients with AIDS who developed lymphoma exhibited 8;14 and 8;22 translocations commonly found in EBV-associated Burkitt's lymphoma (44,45). Some other well-known situations in which similar infections include some primary disorders of T cell function, protein-calorie malnutrition, Hodgkin's disease, and in patients subjected to the aggressive use of corticosteroids. We thus have examples of congenital, neoplastic, and iatrogenic immunodeficiency disorders wherein a spectrum of infectious and neoplastic diseases occur similar to that seen in AIDS. Despite clinical similarities, a common infectious cause has never been suggested in these situations.

While there can be little doubt that AIDS is a new phenomenon among homosexual men, this cannot be said with confidence for the Haitians and IV drug users. Nutritional factors, as well as some indigenous tropical infections might underlie the immunosuppression among Haitians (46). There are known immunologic consequences to the use of opiates (47). Multiple infections associated with IV drug abuse could be the pathway to immunosuppression in drug users. In any group, unless suspected, pneumocystis pneumonia will not be detected. Diagnosis requires biopsy and use of special stains. A re-examination of histology sections from old autopsies for the presence of pneumocystis and CMV could clarify this point. This approach has been employed successfully in finding a specific bacterium in lungs stored for years. It is well known that recipients of blood transfusions are at risk of exposure to CMV. If transfusions are repeated, occasional exposure to this virus in addition to multiple allogeneic antigens (as in homosexual men) may lead to immuno-

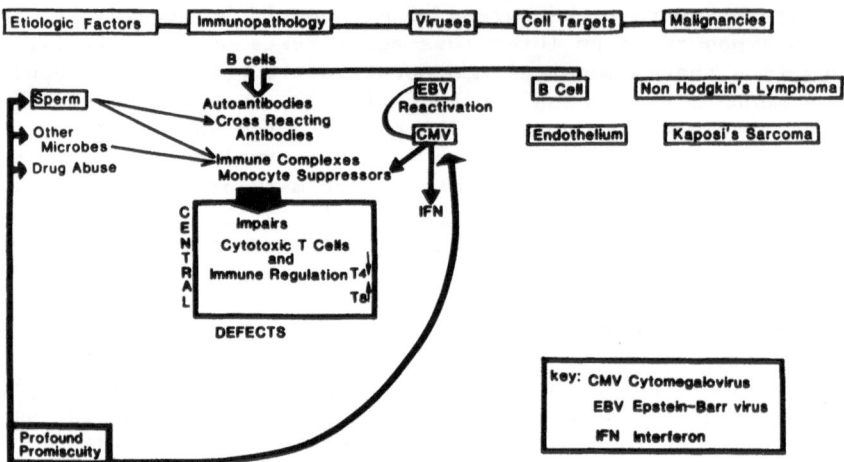

Fig. 7.   Summary of hypothesis of acquired immune deficiency
           syndrome (AIDS in male homosexuals. Repeated sexual
           encounters expose these men to repeated cytomegalovirus
           (CMV) infections and exposures to allogeneic semen.
           Immune responses to these agents are deleterious and
           lead to the phase of acquisition of immunodeficiency.
           Formation of cross-reacting antibodies and immune
           complexes impaires immune regulation and surveillance.
           If exposure is sustained, disease progresses. Opportu-
           nistic infections and viral-induced malignant neoplasms
           can then develop. EBV indicates Epstein-Barr virus,
           INF, interferon. (From: Sonnabend, J. et al. Acquired
           immunodeficiency syndrome, opportunistic infections, and
           malignancies in male homosexuals. J. Am. Med. Assoc.,
           249:2370, 1983. Copyright 1983, America Medical Assoc.)

suppression. The underlying disease requiring transfusion may
also produce immunodeficiency. The consequences of an impaired
immune response may be similar, although the pathways that lead to
it can be diverse.

SUMMARY AND CONCLUSIONS

     Figure 7 summarizes our hypothesis regarding the etiology of
AIDS in a subset of male homosexuals. This model is being
investigated in our laboratory. It offers potentials for
prevention by limiting exposure to sperm and ubiquitous viruses
by use of condoms and decreasing sexual activity. Basic understanding of the mechanisms of viral oncogenesis are also being
elaborated by these studies

REFERENCES

1. Centers for Disease Control, Acquired immune deficiency
    syndrome (AIDS): precautions for clinical and labora-
    tory staffs. Morbidity and Mortality Weekly Report,
    31:577, 1982.
2. Marmor, M., Laubenstein, L., William, D.C., Friedman-Kien,
    R.D., Byrum, R.D., D'Onofrio, S., and Dubin, N. Risk
    factors for Kaposi's sarcoma in homosexual men. Lancet,
    i:1083, 1982.
3. Carney, W.P., Rubin, R.H., Hoffman, R.A., Hansen, W.P.,
    Healey, K., Hirsch, M.S. Analysis of T cell subsets in
    cytomegalovirus mononucleosis. J. Immunol., 126:2114,
    1981.
4. Reinherz, E.L., O'Brien, C., Rosenthal, P., and Schlossman,
    S.F. The cellular basis for viral induced immuno-
    deficiency: analysis by monoclonal antibodies. J.
    Immunol., 125:1269, 1980.
5. Carney, W.P. and Hirsch, M.S. Mechanisms of immuno-
    suppression in cytomegalovirus mononucleosis. II.
    Virus-monocyte interactions. J. Infect. Dis.,
    144:47, 1981.
6. Kantor, G.L., Goldbey, L.S., and Johnson, B.L. Immuno-
    logical abnormalities induced by postperfusion cyto-
    megalovirus infection. Ann. Int. Med., 73:553, 1970.
7. Olding, L.B., Kingsbury, D.T., and Oldstone, M.B.A.
    Pathogenesis of cytomegalovirus infection. Distribution
    of viral products, immune complexes and autoimmunity
    during latent murine infection. J. Gen. Virol.,
    33:267, 1976.
8. Keller, R., Peitchel, R., and Goldman, J.N. An IgG-Fc
    receptor induced in cytomegalovirus infected human
    fibroblasts. J. Immunol., 116:772, 1976.
9. Rahman, A.A., Teschner, M., Sethi, K.K., and Brandis, H.E.
    Appearance of IgG (Fc) receptor(s) on cultured human
    fibroblasts infected with human cytomegalovirus. J.
    Immunol., 117:253, 1976.
10. Lang, D.J. and Kummer, J.F. Demonstration of cytomegalovirus
    in semen. N. Engl. J. Med., 287:756, 1972.
11. Lang, D.J., Kummer, J.F., and Hartley, D.P. Cytomegalovirus
    in semen: persistence and demonstration in extracellular
    fluids. N. Engl. J. Med., 291:121, 1974.
12. Drew, W.L., Mintz, L., Miner, R.C., Sands, M., Ketterer, B.
    Prevalence of cytomegalovirus infection in homosexual
    men. J. Infect. Dis., 143:188, 1981.
13. Drew, W.L., Conant, M.A., Miner, R.C., Huang, E.-S.,
    Ziegler, J.L., Groundwater, J.R., Gullett, J.H.,
    Volberding, P., Abrams, D.I., and Mintz, L.
    Cytomegalovirus and Kaposi's sarcoma in young homosexual
    men. Lancet, ii:125, 1982.

14.   Stagno, S., Pass, R.F., Dworsky, M.E., Henderson, R.E.,
      Moore, E.G., Walton, P.D., and Alford, Ch.A. Congenital
      cytomegalovirus infection: the relative importance of
      primary and recurrent maternal infection. N. Engl. J.
      Med., 306:945, 1982.

15.   Oill, P., Fiala, M., Schofferman, J., Byfield, P.E., and Guze,
      L.B. Cytomegalovirus mononucleosis in a healthy adult.
      Association with hepatitis, secondary Epstein-Barr virus
      antibody response and immunosuppression. Am. J. Med.,
      62:413, 1977.

16.   Jondal, M. and Klein, G. Surface markers on human T and B
      cells. VI. Presence of Epstein-Barr virus receptors on
      human B lymphocytes. J. Exp. Med., 138:1378, 1973.

17.   Rosen, A., Gergely, P., Jondal, M., and Klein, G.
      Polyclonal Ig production after Epstein-Barr virus infec-
      tion of human leukocytes in vitro. Nature, 267:52, 1977.

18.   Fong, S., Vaughan, J.H., Tsoukas, C.D., Carson, D.A.
      Selective induction of autoantibody secretion in human
      bone marrow by Epstein-Barr virus. J. Immunol.,
      129:1941, 1982.

19.   Gottlieb, M.S., Schrott, R., Schanker, H.M., Weisman, J.D.,
      Fan, D.T., Wolf, R.A., and Saxon, A. Pneumocystis
      carinii pneumonia and mucosal candidiasis in previously
      healthy homosexual men: evidence of a new acquired
      cellular immunodeficiency. N. Engl. J. Med., 305:1425,
      1981.

20.   Bird, A.G., Britton, S., Ernberg, I., and Nilsson, K.
      Characteristics of Epstein-Barr virus activation of
      human B lymphocytes. J. Exp. Med., 154:832, 1981.

21.   Purtilo, D.T. and Sakamoto, K. Epstein-Barr virus and human
      disease: immune responses determine the clinical and
      pathologic expression. Human Pathol., 12:677, 1981.

22.   Tosato, G., Magrath, I.T., and Blaese, R.M. T cell mediated
      immunoregulation of Epstein-Barr virus (EBV) induced B
      lymphocyte activation in EBV seropositive and EBV sero-
      negative individuals. J. Immunol., 128:575, 1982.

23.   Meuer, S.C., Schlossman, S.F., and Reinherz, E.L. Clonal
      analysis of human cytotoxic T lymphocytes: T4+ and T8+
      effector T cells recognize products of different major
      histocompatibility complex regions. Proc. Natl. Acad.
      Sci. USA, 79:4590, 1982.

24.   Quinnan, G.F. Jr., Kirmani, N., Rook, A., Manischewitz, J.F.,
      Jackson, L., Moreschi, G., Santos, G.W., Saral, R.,
      and Burns, W.H. Cytotoxic T cells in cytomegalovirus
      infection HLA-restricted T-lymphocytes and non-T lympho-
      cyte cytotoxic responses correlate with recovery from
      cytomegalovirus infection in bone marrow-transplanted
      recipients. N. Engl. J. Med., 307:7, 1982.

25.   Bird, A.G., McLachlan, S.M., and Britton, S. Cyclosporin A
      promotes spontaneous outgrowth in vitro of Epstein-Barr
      virus induced B cell lines. Nature, 289:300, 1981.

26. Crawford, D.H., Sweny, P., Edwards, J., Janossy, G., and Hoffbrand, A.V. Long-term T cell-mediated immunity to Epstein-Barr virus in renal allograft recipients receiving cyclosporin A. Lancet, $\underline{1}$:10, 1981.

27. Magrath, I.T., Pizzo, P.A., Novikovs, L., Levine, A.S. Ehancement of Epstein-Barr virus replication in producer cell lines by a combination of low temperature and corticosteroids. Virology, $\underline{97}$:477, 1979.

28. Abrams, D. Lymphoproliferative diseases in homosexual males. In: D.T. Purtilo (ed.), Immune Deficiency and Cancer: Epstein-Barr Virus and Lymphoproliferative Malignancies. New York: Plenum Press, 1983.

29. Gaston, J.S.H., Richardson, A.B., and Epstein, M.A. Epstein-Barr virus specific T-cell memory in renal allograft recipients under long term immunosuppression. Lancet, $\underline{1}$:923, 1982.

30. Hanto, D.W., Sakamoto, K., and Purtilo, D.T. The Epstein-Barr virus in the pathogenesis of post-transplant lymphoproliferative disorders. Surgery, $\underline{90}$(2):204, 1981.

31. Ziegler, J.L., Drew, W.L., Miner, R.C., Mintz, L., Rosenbaum, E., Gershow, J., Lennette, E.T., Greenspan, J., Shillitoe, E., Beckstead, J., Casavant, C., and Yamamoto, K. Outbreak of Burkitt-like lymphoma in homosexual men. Lancet, $\underline{ii}$:631, 1982.

32. Stahl, R.E., Freidman-Kien, A., Dubin, R., Marmor, M., and Zolla-Pazner, S. Immunologic abnormalities in homosexual men. Am. J. Med., $\underline{73}$:171, 1982.

33. Morris, L., Distenfeld, A., Amorosi, E., and Kaspatkin, S. Autoimmune thrombocytopenic purpura (ATP) in homosexual men. Am. Intern. Med., $\underline{96}$:714, 1982.

34. Charlesworth, J.A., Quin, J.W., MacDonald, G.J., Lennane, R.J., and Boughton, C.-R. Complement, lymphotoxins and immune complexes in infectious mononucleosis: serial studies in uncomplicated cases. Clin. Exp. Immunol., $\underline{34}$:241, 1978.

35. DeStefano, E., Friedman, R.M., Friedman-Kien, A.E. et al. Acid labile human leukocyte interferon in homosexual men with Kaposi's sarcoma and lymphadenopathy. J. Inf. Dis,

36. Witkin, S. and Sonnabend, J.A. Immune responses to spermatozoa in homsexual men. Fertil. & Steril. 1983, in press.

37. Mather, S., Gaust, J.M., Williamson, H.O., and Fudenberg, H.H. Cross reactivity of sperm and T lymphocyte antigens. Am. J. Reproductive Immunol., $\underline{1}$:113, 1981.

38. Beck, B.N., Gillis, S., and Henney, C.S. Display of the neutral glycolipid ganglio-N-tetraosylceramide (Asialo GM_1) on cells of the natural killer and T lineages. Transplantation, $\underline{33}$:118, 1982.

39. Witkin, S.S., Sonnabend, J., Richard, J.M., and Purtilo,
     D.T. Induction of antibody to asialo GM$_1$ by spermatozoa
     and its occurrence in the sera of homosexual men with the
     acquired immune deficiency syndrome. Lancet, in press.

40. Sonnabend, J., Witkin, S.S., and Purtilo, D.T. Acquired
     immunodeficiency syndrome, opportunistic infections, and
     malignancies in male homosexuals. A hypothesis of
     etiologic factors in pathogenesis. J. Am. Med. Assoc.,
     249:2370, 1983.

41. Purtilo, R., Sonnabend, J., and Purtilo, D.T.
     Confidentiality, informed consent and untoward social
     consequences in research on a "new killer disease"
     (AIDS).

42. Centers for Disease Control. A cluster of Kaposi's sarcoma
     and Pneumocystis carinii pneumonia among homosexual male
     residents of Los Angeles and Orange Counties, California.
     Morbidity and Mortality Weekly Report, 31:305, 1982.

43. Purtilo, D.T. Viruses, tumors, and immune deficiency.
     Lancet, 1:684, 1982.

44. Chaganti, R.S.K. Significance of chromosome change to
     hematopoietic neoplasms. Blood, 61:1269, 1983.

45. Rowley, J.D. Identification of the constant chromosome
     regions involved in human hematologic malignant disease.
     Science, 216:479, 1982.

46. Purtilo, D.T. Nutritional considerations in the epidemiology
     of lymphoma. In: M. Hutchinson and C.E. Butterworth, Jr.
     (eds.), Nutritional Factors in the Induction and
     Maintenance of Malignancy. Academic Press, Inc., in
     press.

47. McDonough, R.J., Madden, J.J., Falek, A., Shafer, D.A.,
     Pline, M., Gordon, D., Bokos, P., Kuehnle, J.C., and
     Mendelson, J. Alteration of T and null lymphocyte fre-
     quencies in the peripheral blood of human opiate
     addicts: in vivo evidence for opiate receptor sites
     on T lymphocytes. J. Immunol., 125:2539, 1980.

LYMPHOPROLIFERATIVE DISEASES AND KAPOSI'S SARCOMA

IN HOMOSEXUAL MALES

Donald Abrams

Cancer Research Institute
University of California San Francisco
San Francisco, CA 94143

INTRODUCTION

On July 3, 1981, the Centers for Disease Control (CDC) in Atlanta, Georgia reported ten cases of Pneumocystis carinii pneumonia (PCP) and 22 cases of Kaposi's sarcoma (KS) in previously healthy young homosexual men (1). A syndrome of acquired immunodeficiency (AIDS) underlies the appearance of these often fatal illnesses in this subpopulation of male homosexuals (2-9). The problem has reached epidemic proportions with 1.2 new cases being reported to the CDC daily. More men have died as a consequence of this syndrome than the combined total of all deaths from toxic shock syndrome and the initial outbreak of Legionnaire's disease. With the recognition of AIDS in heterosexual patients predominantly intravenous drug abusers, Haitian nationals and refugees, and a few hemophiliacs (10,11) - investigations to define the etiology of the underlying immune dysfunction have been intensified. Clustering of cases in the homosexual community has implied a transmissible agent is responsible for AIDS (12). A viral etiology seems most plausible. The possibility of an underlying genetic predisposition to aberrant handling of a common viral infection is reminiscent of the model of Purtilo's X-linked lymphoproliferative syndrome (13-16).

In addition to KS, an unusual cluster of diffuse undifferentiated non-Hodgkin's lymphoma (DUNHL)(Burkitt's-like) occurs in the homosexual men (17). Other severe opportunistic infections besides Pneumocystis carinii pneumonia (PCP) have included cryptococcal meningitis and central nervous system toxoplasmosis in young, previously healthy homosexual men. A less virulent condition recognized by physicians caring for large numbers of

385

urban homosexuals is the syndrome of diffuse persistent lymphadenopathy of unknown etiology (18). In a retrospective analysis,
44% of 73 KS patients, 23% of 61 PCP patients and all four of the
DUNHL patients had a history of antecedent lymphadenopathy prior
to the diagnosis of their ultimate illness. Prospective studies
of these patients are ongoing at the University of California San
Francisco, and at medical centers in New York and Los Angeles.
Uncovering the connection between these various conditions could
greatly increase our understanding of the interaction between
immunodeficiency, viral infection, and oncogenesis.

    Evaluation of homosexual men with KS in the Kaposi's Sarcoma
Clinic at the University of California San Francisco and the
syndrome of diffuse persistent lymphadenopathy in the Lymphoma
Clinic of the Cancer Research Institute have generated much
information. Directions for further studies to unlock the
mysteries of this unprecedented epidemic have been generated.
Historical information and results of our immunologic and virologic studies will be reviewed.

Kaposi's sarcoma

    Kaposi's sarcoma, a neoplasm of vascular endothelial origin
(Figure 1), was first described as "multiple idiopathic pigmented
hemangiosarcoma" by Moricz Kaposi in 1872 (19,20). The tradi-

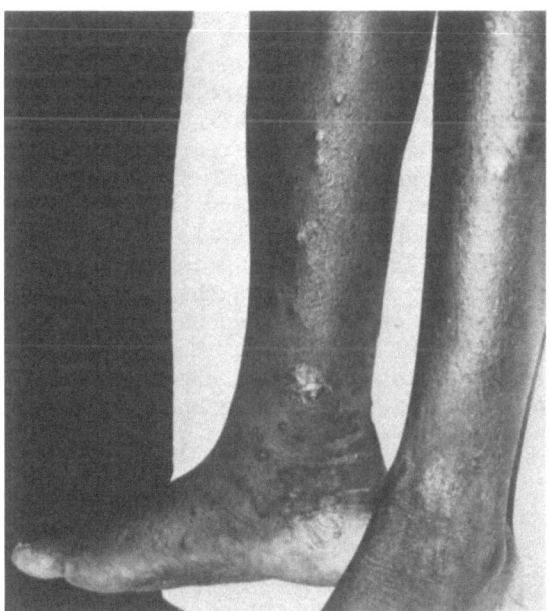

Fig. 1.   Kaposi's sarcoma involving legs. Raised purple-red
          lestions measure up to 1.5 cm in diameter.

tional form of the malignancy has been seen in elderly Italian and
Jewish men. Although tumor has been found in internal organs at
autopsy, primarily indolent cutaneous violaceous nodular lesions
occur on the lower extremities. Patients survive many years with
or without therapeutic intervention and usually die of a disease
unrelated to their malignancy. The annual incidence in the United
States had been 0.02-0.06/100,000. In the twenty-year period
ending in 1979, only three cases of KS in men less than fifty
years of age had been registered in the New York City Tumor
Registry. The sudden appearance of the cancer in young homosexual
men was easily recognized as an aberrant phenomenon.

    KS accounts for 10% of all cancers in Uganda. Noteworthy is
the partial overlap in locale with Burkitt's lymphoma. A virulent
form of KS is found in adolescent black males in Uganda where the
male to female ratio is 25:1 (20). These young men have an
aggressive tumor involving visceral organs and lymph nodes.
Despite initial responses to aggressive chemotherapy, early
relapse tends to occur and survival is only approximately three
years.

    Iatrogenically immunosuppressed patients also have an in-
creased incidence of KS (21,22). For example, renal transplant
recipients on immunosuppressive therapy or patients with collagen
vascular disease undergoing immunosuppressive treatment develop
KS. Only in patients with autoimmune defects does the KS affect
females and males with equal frequency. The KS tends to resemble
the African form rather than the traditional form, i.e., tendency
toward marked visceral involvement and early death. Case reports
of remission of KS on discontinuing the immunosuppressive therapy
appear in the literature (23).

    In the fourteen months since the initial report of 22
patients, two hundred men in twenty-seven states and seven foreign
countries have developed KS. Over half of the reported patients
lived or live in New York City, with an additional 25% divided
between San Francisco and Los Angeles (24). The average age of
the affected population is 35 years and 92% of the patients in the
20-50 age group. The current outbreak of KS among homosexual men
most closely resembles cases seen in Africans and immunosuppressed
patients. No apparent increased predilection for Italian, Jewish
or black homosexuals is found. Eighty percent of the patients
present with skin or mucous membrane lesions. Lesions may appear
at any site, unlike the tendency to restriction to the lower
extremity in traditional KS. Isolated oral mucosal lesions
without skin involvement may be an initial presentation. Patients
often experience a prodrome of fatigue, weight loss, fever and
night sweats. This is especially true of the subset solely with
lymphadenopathy who lack cutaneous involvement. Suspicion of
lymphoma prompts lymph node biopsy and diagnosis of lymph-

adenopathic KS (25,26). Splenomegaly and retroperitoneal involvement are also common in this subgroup. Most of these patients develop classical cutaneous lesions later despite chemotherapy.

The mortality rate from KS among homosexual men has been 25% during the first year AIDS has been recognized. Most patients have died secondary to opportunistic infections. This is likely due to their underlying immunodeficiency, perhaps exacerbated by the effects of cytotoxic chemotherapy. Postmortem examination reveals widespread visceral involvement with tumor in lungs, liver, spleen, throughout the gastrointestinal tract and in thyroid, pancreas, adrenal glands, testes, kidneys and vertebral bone marrow.

Traditional KS has been associated with second malignancies in up to 37% of patients (27,28) including lymphoreticular cancers in 58% of cases, i.e., Hodgkin's or non-Hodgkin's lymphoma or acute lymphocytic leukemia. Of 35 patients evaluated to date in the Kaposi's Sarcoma Clinic at the University of California San Francisco, a large cell lymphoma was discovered as an incidental finding at autopsy in one patient who died with widely disseminated KS. The increased tendency for immunosuppressed renal transplant patients to develop this primary central nervous system lymphoma is well recognized suggesting similarities in the underlying immunodeficiency in the two groups of patients.

Non-Hodgkin's Lymphoma

Four young homosexual men in San Francisco have developed diffuse, undifferentiated non-Hodgkin's lymphoma (17). This rare B-cell neoplasm is often difficult to distinguish histologically from Burkitt's lymphoma. Two of these patients initially presented with jaw involvement reminiscent of Burkitt's lymphoma. All patients had widespread malignancy at diagnosis and expired despite early response to aggressive chemotherapy. All of the patients had antecedent lymphadenopathy and 3 of the 4 had splenomegaly prior to the diagnosis. Epstein-Barr nuclear antigen (EBNA) was detected by immunofluorescence in tumor specimens from two of the four patients (Ziegler et al., Lancet in press). Cases of DUNHL have subsequently been reported from Chicago and New York in men with previously diagnosed by biopsies to have had benign reactive lymphadenopathy.

Diffuse Lymphadenopathy

In 1979, the year in which the first cases of KS and PCP presented, physicians caring for large numbers of homosexual men became aware of a new syndrome in this population. Young sexually active homosexuals with a past history of multiple sexually transmitted diseases were being referred, to physicians engaged in hematology-oncology practices, with diffuse lymphadenopathy and splenomegaly. The purpose of referral was to rule out lymphoma. Prior evaluation by primary care physicians failed to uncover an etiology for the enlarged nodes. Biopsies generally revealed benign reactive follicular hyperplasia. Polyclonal increases in gammaglobulin correlated with the B cell hyperactivity seen in biopsy specimens. Due to the lack of yield, cost-benefit analysis often dictated against biopsies in men with this presentation. Half of these patients were asymptomatic and sought medical attention only after discovering an enlarged node. The other half suffered from vague fatigue, intermittent unexplained febrile episodes, night sweats, and weight loss. With the recognition of the epidemic of KS and opportunistic infection in young homosexual men and the awareness of a purely lymphadenopathic presentation of KS, interest in further definition of this syndrome heightened. Speculation as to whether the lymphadenopathy syndrome was premalignant or an evolutionary stage in the development of more severe immunodeficiency was sparked by the retrospective reporting of prior lymph node enlargement in KS, DUNHL, and PCP patients (18). A longitudinal prospective analysis of a cohort of these patients is ongoing in centers across the country. Currently, 70 patients are enrolled in a study at the University of California San Francisco. Four to six new patients are seen each week.

Demographic similarities prevail between patients with benign lymphadenopathy and KS. The mean age of 45 patients under study is 33 years. The year of onset of the lymphadenopathy was prior to 1979 in eight patients. Additional cases are accruing in parallel to the increasing incidence of KS and PCP. Lymph node biopsy in all men in this group have revealed benign reactive hyperplasia. In the general population, this nonspecific diagnosis is made in one-third to one-half of all node biopsies done in adults, excluding patients with known primary malignancies (29,30). The etiologic agent responsible for the lymphadenopathy is found in less than 10% of patients with this pathologic diagnosis. Various series report that 25-50% of these patients develop a disorder related to lymph node enlargement within one year of the nonspecific biopsy. Nearly 20% develop a lymphoma, especially following atypical lymphoid hyperplasia. To date, none of our patients with the lymphadenopathy syndrome have progressed to more malignant disorders. The longest period of follow-up is less than one year. Investigators in New York report five of 46 patients developing KS (R. Enlow - personal communication) and one of 45 developing KS and two each developing PCP and DUNHL in another series (C. Metroka, personal communication).

Immunologic Profiles

Investigations performed under the direction of Arthur Ammann in the Pediatric Immunology Laboratory at the University of

California San Fancisco have identified a spectrum of immune
dysfunctions in the subpopulations of homosexual men (31).
Employing monoclonal antibody identification of T cell subsets and
routine in vitro techniques for evaluating T cell function
(including phytohemagglutinin - PHA stimulation and mixed leukocyte culture - MLC), defects in cell-mediated immunity were
demonstrated in all subgroups. By comparison, a small group of
elderly heterosexual patients with traditional KS displayed normal
T cell subsets and functional studies. Immunoglobulin concentrations in the elderly KS group were also within normal limits,
suggesting aberrant immune response is not obvious in patients
with classical KS.

A reversal of the helper to suppressor T cell ratio was
demonstrated by use of the OKT-4 and OKT-8 monoclonal antibodies
in all the homosexual men. The normal ratio of 15 healthy
heterosexual controls for OKT-4:OKT-8 was 2.2 ± 0.3. Eight
patients with PCP or other opportunistic infections displayed
severe reversal of the ratio to 0.4 ± 0.3. The reversal among the
homosexual patients reflects both a marked decrease in OKT-4 to
14% (controls 50-62%) and an equally significant increase in the
suppressor cell population to 49% (controls 23-31%). Both the PHA
and MLC responses in this group were depressed to 10% of the
control values.

Nine KS patients pre-treatment had a helper to suppressor
ratio of 0.9 with a depressed PHA response, but no significant MLC
impairment. In a group of 11 patients post-treatment (not
necessarily the same as the pre-treatment group in all cases), the
ratio fell to 0.7. Also a significant impairment in MLC was noted
concurrently with the decreased PHA response. Eight lymphadenopathy patients studied showed a depressed ratio to 1.1 with a
slight but significant impairment in PHA response. Most surprisingly, the group of ten healthy homosexual controls also demonstrated a similar ratio, i.e., 1.2. However, functional studies
are normal (32). The decreased percentage of helper T cells
despite the normal number of T cell rosettes in all of these
groups accounts for the reversal of the ratio.

Coincident with evidence of ratio reversal and functional
T cell impairment, homosexual patients with KS and the lymphadenopathy syndrome demonstrated elevated serum immunoglobulin
concentrations when compared to normal heterosexual and healthy
homosexual controls. Significant elevations in both IgG and IgA
isotypes were found in KS patients. Of note, the elevation in IgA
in the KS patients reflects tumor involvement of gastrointestinal
tract. The lymphadenopathy group demonstrated even high IgG
concentrations. IgA, IgM, and IgE were also increased. Both KS
and lymphadenopathy patients had elevated total hemolytic complement levels and normal C3 and C4. No detectable circulating
immune complexes via Clq assay were found.

The implications of these immunologic aberrations is unclear.
Certainly, a spectrum of impaired immunity from healthy homosexuals through those with severe opportunistic infections occurs.
The earliest detectable abnormality is a reversal of the helper to
suppressor ratio in the healthy homosexual control group. It is
accepted that viral infections, including cytomegalovirus,
Epstein-Barr virus (EBV), and hepatitis B virus produce a transient reversal of the ratio secondary due to activated suppressor
cell fractions (33,34). Similarly, viral infection may activate
B cells and produce viral-specific antibodies accounting for the
immunoglobulin elevations in these populations.

The Role of Cytomegalovirus

Cytomegalovirus (CMV) has been implicated as a causative
factor in KS (35). Electron micrographs of tissue culture cell
lines derived from Ugandan tumor specimens have demonstrated
herpes-like viral particles that cross-reacted with high titer
anti-CMV sera (36). Seroepidemiologic studies of European
patients with KS reveal an increased CMV titer and in some
patients very high titers are found (37,38). No significant
increase in titers against other herpesviruses were found,
suggesting a generalized immunosuppression. CMV-antigens and CMV
RNA and DNA has been detected in tumor specimens confirming the
suspected association between CMV and KS (39,40). Immunosuppressed renal transplant patients are known to be vulnerable to
CMV and KS further supporting this association.

Studies done by W. Lawrence Drew et al. show CMV IgG antibody
in 94% of sexually active homosexual men in San Francisco (39-41)
versus 54% of heterosexual men in the same venereal disease
clinic. Similarly, 57% of the homosexual men demonstrated a CMV
IgM antibody, indicating recent infection or re-activation of
latent infection. This isotype was found in only 4% of the
heterosexuals. CMV viruria was found in 14% of homosexual men,
less than 30 years old, or 7.4% among 190 homosexuals studied.
None of the heterosexual men excreted the virus. On the basis of
the past links between CMV and KS and the high incidence of past
and present CMV infection in homosexual men, extensive studies
have been performed to evaluate the role of this virus in the
current epidemic. Drew was able to culture CMV from at least on
excretion in 7 of 10 KS patients (42) and viral cultures of KS
tumor specimens were negative in 8 of 8 patients. Using an anti-
complementary immunofluorescence technique, CMV-related antigen
was detected in tumor tissue from 6 of 9 patients. Adjacent
normal skin from three patients was similarly processed as an
internal control. None of the normal specimens demonstrated the
antigen. In situ hybridization techniques documented CMV RNA in
two tumor specimens and was questionable in a third. Viral DNA is
currently being probed in tumors with fragments of CMV DNA genome
to document integration of viral DNA into host genetic material.

One hundred percent of men with persistent lymphadenopathy
studied to date have elevated CMV IgG titers. CMV IgM is detected
in one-half of the lymphadenopathy patients as comparable to other
sexually active homosexual men. Semen is a rich source of CMV.
In men with lymphadenopathy who were cultured, the virus was
present in a single semen specimen of 10 of 25 patients. This is
five fold more than the overall incidence of viruria in the VD
clinic population. However, the data may reflect increased yield
semen rather than urine samples. In any event, 40% positivity of
CMV in the semen of homosexual men with lymphadenopathy and
immunosuppressive impact of CMV itself, suggests a possible
mechanism for the acquired immunodeficiency syndrome. Homosexual
men who are the passive recipients of semen inoculations from
multiple potentially CMV-infected partners are at risk for
sequential CMV infections, each upsetting their helper and
suppressor T cell compartments. The absence of the virus in the
heterosexual population explains why heterosexual women
(especially prostitutes) have apparently not been at risk for
developing the immunodeficiency syndrome through venereal routes.
This data has prompted many of our patients to re-evalute their
lifestyles and sexual practices.

The Role of Epstein-Barr Virus

Few oncologists can deny the association between EBV and
Burkitt's lymphoma and nasopharyngeal carcinoma (43-47). The work
of Purtilo points strongly to the role of this virus in the
development of lymphoproliferative disorders in individuals wth
the X-linked lymphoproliferative syndrome and immunosuppressed
renal transplantation patients (48-51). Despite previous seroepidemiologic studies which suggested no correlation between KS
and EBV titers (37,38), the marked male predominance in the
current epidemic of KS and the similarities between the immune
dysfunction in the male homosexuals and iatrongenically immunosuppressed renal transplant patients led our group to obtain EBV

Table 1. EBV Serologies in Two KS Patients

	Patient #1	Patient #2	Controls
VCA IgG	1280	2560	80
VCA IgM	<5	<5	<5
VCA IgA	80	160	<5
EA-D	20	40	<5
EA-R	<5	160	<5
EBNA	80	80	20

serologies on all men being evaluated with these disorders. EBV serology performed by Evelyne Lennette on two of our initial KS patients were provocative. The presence of an anti-EBNA ruled out a variant of XLP. High titer VCA IgG and the presence of anti-EA-R were reminiscent of Burkitt's lymphoma. The presence of IgA anti-VCA and EA-D were suggestive of the profile seen in nasopharyngeal carcinoma. Whether these data confirm aberrant handling of an ongoing EBV infection, a reactivation of a latent infection, or reflect impaired cell-mediated immune responses in these patients remains unclear (52,53). Analysis of EBV titers of 20 KS patients reveals an average VCA IgG titer two dilutions above the controls. Five of twenty patients demonstrate an IgA anti-VCA. Thirteen patients had antibody to an early antigen, with one patient demonstrating both R and D components. Anti-EBNA was within normal limits in 18/20 patients, with two patients demonstrating low values.

Results of attempts to detect EBNA by fluorescent techniques in KS tumor specimens are not available at this time. Two specimens have been analyzed for the presence of EBV DNA by Georg Bornkamm, Freiburg. The results were negative.

The syndrome of diffuse persistent lymphadenopathy has been thought to be a form of chronic infectious mononucleosis. Heterophiles have been positive in only 3 of 50 patients. The follicular hyperplasia pattern seen in lymph node biopsy specimens in these patients is not entirely consistent with the mixed pattern seen in nodes of patients with acute infectious mono- nucleosis. In the latter cases effacement of the normal architec- ture and marked paracortical involvement is found.

EBV titers in the lymphadenopathy patients are almost indistinguishable from those of the Kaposi's sarcoma patients except for the absence of IgA anti-VCA antibodies. Elevated VCA IgG titers and antibodies to EA-D are also seen in the lymphade- nopathy patients. Again, EBNA is generally normal with a few patients showing slightly elevated titers and a similar number slightly depressed.

SUMMARY AND HYPOTHESES

Data to date suggests that the lymphoproliferative diseases observed in homosexual men are most probably due to an interac- tion between defective immune system and a persistent viral infec- tion (or infections). Many aspects of the puzzle remain to be

clarified. Which virus is responsible for the immunodeficiency?
Is it herpesvirus or an unidentified new agent? Is it a mutant
of a common virus? Is it a RNA virus? Is activation of an
oncogene occurring due to integration of viral genomes at
critical sites in host DNA (54)? Is a virus actually responsible
for the immune deficiency or present as a manifestation of a
primary immune defect? Is the immune deficiency acquired, as it
is widely presumed to be, or do all of these men have an underlying genetic predisposition manifest due to lifestyle?
Researchers in New York have demonstrated an increased incidence
of HLA-DR5 in their patients with KS (55). San Francisco patients
do not show this association.

Other possible explanations of the immune deficiency have
been postulated. One group has suggested that nitrite inhalants,
popular in the homosexual community, could alter the helper to
suppressor ratio (56). However in the small study all but one
patient had high CMV titers and a majority of the patients using
nitrite also demonstrated lymphadenopathy. Either of these
factors alone could account for the ratio reversal, independent
of the nitrite use.

Seminal plasma has been implicated as an immunosuppressive
agent (59). Women have been exposed to this substance for eons,
through vaginal, rectal and oral mucosa, and they do not show
profound AIDS. Anal trauma combined with the use of vasocilatory
nitrites in substantial numbers of homosexual men may allow semen
to gain access to the systemic circulation. New York researchers
have demonstrated the presence of anti-sperm antibodies in the
sera of homosexual men with AIDS. They suggest that anti-sperm
antibodies may cross-react with antigens on the OKT4 lymphocytes
accounting for the decimation of helper cells in the homosexuals.

Another intriguing hypothesis suggests that a form of graft-
versus-host disease (GVHD) may be the underlying pathophysiologic
mechanism in these disorders (3). Skin, gut, liver and the immune
system are targets affected in these homosexual men as is seen in
bone marrow transplant patients with GVHD (58). Immune profiles
of transplant patients with GVHD are very similar in both patients
(59-61). The graft in this instance could be immunocompetent
lymphocytes donated in semen. The viable lymphocyte could wreak
havoc on a host previously compromised by prior viral infections
and their associated immunosuppression.

The plethora of hypotheses confirms that the solution to this
problem remains elusive. The ultimate breakthrough will not only
add to our understanding of the interactions of immune deficiency,
viral infection and oncogenesis, but will also shed light on
modalities optimal for treatment and measures for prevention of
lymphoproliferative disorders in man.

REFERENCES

1. Friedman-Kien, A., Laubenstein, L., Marmor, M. et al. Kaposi's sarcoma and Pneumocystis pneumonia among homosexual men - New York City and California. Morbid. Mortal. Week. Rev., 30:305, 1981.

2. Gottlieb, M.S., Schroff, R., Schanker, H., Weisman, J.D., Peng, T.F., Wolf, R.A., and Saxon, A. Pneumocystis carinii pneumonia and mucosal candidiasis in previously healthy homosexual men. Evidence of a new acquired cellular immunodeficiency. N. Engl. J. Med., 305:1425, 1981.

3. Levine, A.S. The epidemic of acquired immune dysfunction in homosexual men and its sequelae - opportunistic infections, Kaposi's sarcoma, and other malignancies: an update and interpretation. Cancer Treat. Rep., 66:391, 1982.

4. Masur, H., Michelis, M.A., Greene, J.B., Onorato, I., Vande Stouwe, R.A., Holzman, R.S., Wormser, G., Brettman, L., Lange, M., Murray, H.W., and Cunningham-Rundles, S. An outbreak of community-acquired Pneumocystis carinii pneumonia. Initial manifestation of cellular immune dysfunction. N. Engl. J. Med., 305:1431, 1981.

5. Siegal, F.P., Lopez, C., Hammer, G.S., Brown, A.E., Kornfeld, S.J., Gold, J., Hassett, J., Hirshman, S.Z., Cunningham-Rundles, C., Adelsberg, B.R., Parham, D.M., Siegal, M., Cunningham-Rundles, S., and Armstrong, D. Severe acquired immunodeficiency in male homosexuals, manifested by chronic perianal ulcerative herpes simplex lesions. N. Engl. J. Med. 305:1439, 1981.

6. Gottlieb, G.J., Ragaz, A., Vogel, J.V., Friedman-Kien, A., Rywlin, A.M., Weiner, E.A., and Ackerman, A.B. A preliminary communication on extensively disseminated Kaposi's sarcoma in young homosexual men. Am. J. Dermatopathol., 3:111, 1981.

7. Hymes, K.B., Greene, J.B., Marcus, A., William, D.C., Cheung, T., Prose, N.S., Ballard, H., and Laubenstein, L.J. Kaposi's sarcoma in homosexual men - A report of eight cases. Lancet, ii:598, 1981.

8. Mildvan, D., Mathur, U., Enlow, R.W., Romain, P.L., Winchester, R.J., Colp, C., Singman, H., Adelsberg, B.R., and Spigland, I. Opportunistic infections and immune deficiency in homosexual men. Ann. Intern. Med., 96:700, 1982.

9. Follansbee, S.E., Busch, D.F., Wofsy, C.B., Coleman, D.L., Gullet, J., Aurigemma, G.P., Ross, T., Hadley, W.K., and Drew, W.L. An outbreak of Pneumocystis carinii pneumonia in homosexual men. Ann. Intern. Med., 96:705, 1982.

10. Hensley, G.T., Moskowitz, L.B., Pitchenik, A.E. et al. Opportunistic infections among Haitians in the United States. Morbid. Mortal. Week. Rev., 31:353, 1982.

11.   Ehrenkranz, N.J., Rubini, J., Gunn, R. et al. Pneumocystis
      carinii pneumonia among persons with hemophilia A.
      Morbid. Mortal. Week. Rep., 31:365, 1982.

12.   Fannin, S., Gottlieb, M.S., Weisman, J.D. et al. A cluster
      of Kaposi's sarcoma and Pneumocystis carinii pneumonia
      among homosexual male residents of Los Angeles and
      Orange Counties, California. Morbid. Mortal. Week.
      Rep., 31:305, 1982.

13.   Purtilo, D.T., Paquin, L., DeFlorio, D., Virzi, F., and
      Sakhuja, R. Immunodiagnosis and immunopathogenesis of
      the X-linked recessive lymphoproliferative syndrome.
      Sem. Hematol., 16:309, 1979.

14.   Purtilo, D.T. Epstein-Barr virus-induced oncogenesis in
      immune-deficient individuals. Lancet, 1:300, 1980.

15.   Purtilo, D.T. Immune deficiency predisposing to Epstein-
      Barr virus-induced lymphoproliferative diseases: the
      X-linked lymphoproliferative syndrome as a model. Advan.
      Cancer Res., 34:279, 1981.

16.   Purtilo, D.T. and Klein, G. Introduction to Epstein-Barr
      virus and lymphoproliferative diseases in immunodefi-
      cient individuals. Cancer Res., 41:4209, 1981.

17.   Ziegler, J.L., Wagner, G., Greenspan, J.S. et al. Diffuse
      undifferentiated non-Hodgkin's lymphoma among homosexual
      males - United States. Morbid. Mortal. Week. Rev.,
      31:277, 1982.

18.   Mildvan, D., Mathur, U., Enlow, R. et al. Persistent,
      generalized lymphadenopathy among homosexual males.
      Morbid. Mortal. Week. Rep., 31:249, 1982.

19.   Kaposi, M. Idiopathigches multiples pigment sarcom der
      Haut. Arch. Dermatol. Syph., 4:265, 1872.

20.   Safai, B. and Good, R.A. Kaposi's sarcoma: a review and
      recent developments. Cancer, 31:2, 1981.

21.   Harwood, A.R., Osoba, D., Hofstader, S.L., Goldstein, M.B.,
      Cardella, C.J., Holecek, M.J., Kunynetz, R., and
      Giammarco, R.A. Kaposi's sarcoma in recipients of renal
      transplants. Am. J. Med., 67:759, 1979.

22.   Klepp, O., Dahl, O., and Stenwig, J.T. Association of
      Kaposi's sarcoma and prior immunosuppressive therapy. A
      5-year material of Kaposi's sarcoma in Norway. Cancer,
      42:2626, 1978.

23.   Myers, B.D., Kesler, E., and Levi, J. Kaposi's sarcoma in
      kidney transplant recipients. Arch. Int. Med., 133:307,
      1974.

24.   Auerbach, D.M., Bennett, J.V., Brachman, P.S. et al.
      Epidemiologic aspects of the current outbreak of
      Kaposi's sarcoma and opportunistic infections. N. Engl.
      J. Med., 306:248, 1982.

25.   Bhana, D., Templeton, A.C., Master, S.P., and Kyalwazi, S.K.
      Kaposi sarcoma of lymph nodes. Br. J. Cancer, 24:464,
      1970.

26. Finkbeiner, W.E., Egbert, B.M., Groundwater, J.R., and Sagebiel, R.W. Kaposi's sarcoma in young homosexual men. Arch. Pathol. Lab. Med., 106:261, 1982.

27. Safai, B., Mike, V., Giraldo, G., Beth, E., and Good, R.A. Association of Kaposi's sarcoma with secondary primary malignancies. Possible etiopathogenic implications. Cancer, 45:1472, 1980.

28. Ulbright, T.M. and Santa Cruz, D.J. Kaposi's sarcoma: relationship with hematologic, lymphoid, and thymic neoplasia. Cancer, 47:963, 1981.

29. Sinclair, S., Beckman, E., and Ellman, L. Biopsy of enlarged, superficial lymph nodes. J. Am. Med. Asoc., 228:602, 1974.

30. Schroer, K.R. and Franssila, K.O. Atypical hyperplasia of lymph nodes. A follow-up study. Cancer, 44:1155, 1979.

31. Ammann, A., Abrams, D., Conant, M., Chudwin, D., Cowan, M., Volberding, P., Lewis, B., and Casavant, C. Acquired immune dysfunction in homosexual men: immunologic profiles. Clin. Immunol., 1982.

32. Stahl, R.E., Friedman-Kien, A., Dubin, R., Marmor, M., and Zolla-Pazner, S. Immunologic abnormalities in homosexual men. Relationship to Kaposi's sarcoma. Am. J. Med., 73:171, 1982.

33. Reinherz, E.L., O'Brien, C., Rosenthal, P., and Schlossman, S.F. The cellular basis for viral-induced immunodeficiency: analysis by monoclonal antibodies. J. Immunol., 125:1269, 1980.

34. Tosato, G., Magrath, I., Koski, I., Dooley, N., and Blaese, M. Activation of suppressor T cells during Epstein-Barr-virus-induced infectious mononucleosis. N. Engl. J. Med., 301:1133, 1979.

35. Giraldo, G., Beth, E., Coeur, P. et al. Kaposi's sarcoma: a new model in the search for viruses associated with human malignancies. J. Natl. Cancer Inst., 49:1495, 1972.

36. Giraldo, G., Beth, E., and Haguenau, F. Herpes-type virus particles in tissue culture of Kaposi's sarcoma from different geographic regions. J. Natl. Cancer Inst., 49:1509, 1972.

37. Giraldo, G., Beth, E., Kourilsky, F.M., Henle, W., Henle, G., Mike, V., Huraux, J.M., Andersen, H.K., Gharbi, M.R., Kyalwazi, S.K., and Puissant, A. Antibody patterns to herpesviruses in Kaposi's sarcoma: serological association of European Kaposi's sarcoma with cytomegalovirus. Int. J. Cancer, 15:839, 1975.

38. Giraldo, G., Beth, E., Henle, W., Mike, V., Safai, B., Huraux, J.M., McHardy, J., and De The, G. Antibody patterns to herpesviruses in Kaposi's sarcoma. II. Serological association of American Kaposi's sarcoma with cytomegalovirus. Int. J. Cancer, 22:126, 1978.

39.   Giraldo, G., Beth, E., Hammerling, U., Tarro, G., and
      Kowrilsky, F.M. Detection of early antigens in nuclei
      of cells infected with cytomegalovirus or herpes simplex
      virus type 1 and 2 by anti-complement immunofluorescence,
      and use of a blocking assay to demonstrate their
      specificity. Int. J. Cancer, 19:107, 1977.

40.   Giraldo, G., Beth, E., and Huang, E.-S. Kaposi's sarcoma
      and its relationship to cytomegalovirus (CMV). III.
      CMV DNA and CMV early antigens in Kaposi's sarcoma.
      Int. J. Cancer, 26:23, 1980.

41.   Drew, W.L., Mintz, L., Miner, R.C., Sands, M., and Ketterer,
      B. Prevalence of cytomegalovirus infection in homo-
      sexual men. J. Infect. Dis., 143:188, 1981.

42.   Drew, W.L., Miner, R.C., Ziegler, J.L., Gullet, J.H.,
      Abrams, D.I., Conant, M.A., Huang, E.-S., Groundwater,
      J.R., Volberding, P., and Mintz. L. Cytomegalovirus and
      Kaposi's sarcoma in young homosexual men. Lancet,
      ii:125, 1982.

43.   Ziegler, J.L., Magrath, I.T., Gerber, P., and Levine, P.H.
      Epstein-Barr virus and human malignancy. Ann. Intern.
      Med., 86:323, 1977.

44.   de The, G., Geser, A., Day, N.E., Tukei, P.M., Williams,
      E.H., Beri, D.P., Smith, P.G., Dean, A.G., Bornkamm,
      G.W., Feorino, P., and Henle, W. Epidemiological evi-
      dence for causal relationship between Epstein-Barr virus
      and Burkitt's lymphoma from Ugandan prospective study.
      Nature, 274:756, 1978.

45.   Ziegler, J.L. Burkitt's lymphoma. N. Engl. J. Med.,
      305:735, 1981.

46.   Henle, G., Henle, W., Clifford, P., Diehl, V., Kafuko, G.W.,
      Kirya, B.G., Klein, G., Morrow, R.H., Munube, G.M.R.,
      Pike, P., Tukei, P.M., and Ziegler, J.L. Antibodies to
      Epstein-Barr virus in Burkitt's lymphoma and control
      groups. J. Natl. Cancer Inst., 43:1147, 1969.

47.   Klein, G., Giovanella, B.C., Lindahl, T., Fialkow, P.J.,
      Singh, S., and Stehlin, J.S. Direct evidence for the
      presence of Epstein-Barr virus DNA and nuclear antigen
      in malignant epithelial cells from patients with poorly
      differentiated carcinoma of the nasopharynx. Proc.
      Natl. Acad. Sci. USA, 71:4737, 1974.

48.   Purtilo, D.T., Bhawan, J., Hutt, L.M., DeNicola, L.,
      Szymanski, I., Yange, J.P.S., Boto, W., Maier, R., and
      Thorley-Lawson, D. Epstein-Barr virus infections in the
      X-linked recessive lymphoproliferative syndrome. Lancet,
      i:798, 1978.

49.   Hanto, D.W., Frizzera, G., Gajl-Peczalska, K.J., Sakamoto,
      K., Purtilo, D.T., Balfour, H.H., Jr., Simmons, R.L.,
      and Najarian, J.S. Epstein-Barr virus-induced B-cell
      lymphoma after renal transplantation. N. Engl. J. Med.,
      306:913, 1982.

50. Purtilo, D.T., Sakamoto, K., Saemundsen, A.K., Sullivan, J.L., Synnerholm, A.-C., Anvret, M., Pritchard, J., Sloper, C., Sieff, C., Pincott, J., Pachman, L., Rich, K., Cruzi, F., Cornet, J.A., Collins, R., Barnes, N., Knight, J., Sandstedt, B., and Klein, G. Documentation of Epstein-Barr virus infection in immunodeficient patients with life-threatening lymphoproliferative diseases by clinical, virological, and immunopathological studies. Cancer Res., 41:4226, 1981.

51. Saemundsen, A.K., Purtilo, D.T., Sakamoto, K., Sullivan, J.L., Synnerholm, A.-C., Hanto, D.W., Simmons, R., Anvret, M., Collins, R., and Klein, G. Documentation of Epstein-Barr virus infection in immunodeficient patients with life-threatening lymphoproliferative diseases by Epstein-Barr virus complementary RNA/DNA and viral DNA/DNA hybridization. Cancer Res., 41:4237, 1981.

52. DeSchryver, A., Klein, G., Henle, G., Henle, W., Cameron, H.M., Santesson, L., and Clifford, P. Virus associated serology in malignant disease: antibody levels to viral capsid antigens (VCA), membrane antigens (MA) and early antigens (EA) in patients with various neoplastic conditions. Cancer, 9:353, 1972.

53. Levine, P.H., Connelly, R.R., Herberman, R.B., McCoy, J.L., and Fabrizio, P.L. Humoral and cellular immunity to EBV and lymphoid cell line antigens in human lymphoma. In: G. de The, H.A. Epstein, and H. zur Hausen (eds.), Oncogenesis and Herpesvirus II, Part 2: Epidemiology, Host, Response Control. pp. 225-235. Lyon: International Agency for Research on Cancer, 1975.

54. Payne, G.S., Bishop, J.M., and Varmus, H.E. Multiple arrangements of viral DNA and an activated host oncogene in bursal lymphomas. Nature, 295:209, 1982.

55. Friedman-Kien, A.E., Laubenstein, L.J., Rubinstein, P., Buimovici-Klein, E., Marmor, M., Stahl. R., Spigland, I., Kwang, S.K., and Zolla-Pazner, S. Disseminated Kaposi's sarcoma in homosexual men. Ann. Intern. Med., 96:693, 1982.

56. Goedert, J.J., Wallen, W.C., Mann, D.L., Strong, D.M., Neuland, C.Y., Greene, M.H., Murray, C., Fraumeni, J.F., Jr., and Blattner, W.A. Amyl nitrite may alter T lymphocytes in homosexual men. Lancet, 1:412, 1982.

57. Shearer, G.M. and Hurtenbach, U. Is sperm immunosuppressive in male homosexuals and vasectomized men? Immunol. Today, 3:153, 1982.

58. Shulman, H.M., Sullivan, K.M., Weiden, P.L., McDonald, G.B., Striker, G.E., Sale, G.E., Hackman, R., Tsoi, M.-S., Storb, R., and Thomas, E.D. Chronic graft-versus-host syndrome in man. Am. J. Med., 69:204, 1980.

59.   Reinherz, E.L., Parkman, R., Rappeport, J., Rosen, F.S., and
      Schlossman, S.F. Aberrations of suppressor T cells in
      human graft-versus-host disease. N. Engl. J. Med.,
      300:1061, 1979.
60.   Saxon, A., McIntyre, R.E., Stevens, R.H., and Gale, R.P.
      Lymphocyte dysfunction in chronic graft-versus host
      disease. Blood, 58:746, 1981.
61.   Friedrich, W., O'Reilly, R.J., Koziner, B., Gebhard, D.F.,
      Jr., Good, R.A., and Evans, R.L. T-lymphocyte reconsti-
      tution in recipients of bone marrow transplants with and
      without GVHD: imbalances of T-cell subpopulations having
      unique regulatory and cognitive functions. Blood,
      59:696, 1982.

MENDELIAN PREDISPOSITION TO LYMPHOMAGENESIS

Henry T. Lynch and Guy S. Schuelke

School of Medicine, Department of Preventive Medicine
Creighton University
Omaha, Nebraska

INTRODUCTION

More than 100 inherited cancer and precancer syndromes show simple Mendelian inheritance (81). Of the commonly occurring hereditary breast (82) or colon cancers (90), several differing genotypes give rise to the respective hereditary cancer syndromes. A voluminous literature on etiology of lymphomas is emerging linking genetics, immunology, and variable environmental factors.

Immunological factors probably play an etiological role in some cancers. However, the extent to which immunological factors under genetic control modulate carcinogenesis remains enigmatic. Inherited immunodeficiency disorders are associated with more than a 100-fold higher cancer occurrence (69,146). The natural history of an immunodeficiency syndrome, including cancer evolution, unfolds during a short time period (69).

The recent informational explosion in genetics, immunology, virology and cancer in general has shed light on lymphomagenesis as summarized in Table 1.

A primary question to be addressed is, "To what degree do qualitative and/or quantitative immunological aberrations occur in inherited lymphomageneses?" Alternatively, we might ask the equally thorny question, "In classical Mendelian inherited forms of lymphomageneses, to what degree are immunological parameters of any type primary ('drivers') vs. secondary-epigenetic ('passengers') in the etiologic chain of events leading to carcinogenesis?"

Table 1. Genetically Inherited Lymphomagenesis Susceptibility

Disorder	Malignancies

Inheritance
Sex-linked Recessive

Agammaglobulinemia	Lymphomas
Wiskott-Aldrich syndrome	Lymphomas, myelogenous leukemia, astrocytoma
Immunodeficiency with hyper-IgM	Lymphoproliferative malignancies
X-linked lymphoproliferative syndrome	malignant lymphoma

Autosomal Recessive

Ataxia telangiectasia (Louis-Bar syndrome)	Lymphocytic leukemia, Hodgkin's disease, reticulum cell sarcoma, glioma, medulloblastoma gastric carcinoma and other cancers increased in heterozygotes
Bloom's syndrome	Leukemia, lymphoma, esophageal cancer, adenocarcinoma of colon
Chediak-Higashi syndrome	Lymphoproliferative malignancy
Common variable immunodeficiency (may also be X-linked)	Lymphoreticular malignancies, thymomas, and gastrointestinal malignancies
Sjögren's syndrome	Lymphoma and adenocarcinoma of parotid gland

Autosomal Dominant

Systemic lupus erythematosus	Lymphoma and thymoma
Kaposi's sarcoma (very infrequent)	Malignant lymphoma and multiple other primary cancers
Hodgkin's disease	Multiple other malignancies
Lymphoma	Lymphoma and other cancers
FAMMM syndrome	Malignant melanoma, lymphoreticular and epithelial malignancies

Cardinal features of hereditary cancer and pertinent to those associated with lymphomagenesis include: a) early age of onset; b) tendency to an excess of multiple primary cancers; c) distinctive histologic cancer patterns; d) physical signs and/or biological markers of cancer-prone genotypes; and e) in certain forms of cancer improved survival vs. sporadic cases (81,82,90). Collectively, such cancer-prone kindreds provide powerful models for studying genetic, immunological and other possible etiological factors in oncogenesis.

Survey and Perspective

Hereditary lymphomageneses with variable immunological associations will be reviewed in the following genetically associated contexts: 1) genetically unclassified kindreds prone to lymphomageneses; 2) lymphomageneses that may be associated with other cancers which constitute a syndrome; 3) lymphomageneses and the cancer-associated genodermatoses; 4) specific immunologic deficiency wherein IgA deficiency will serve as a prototype model; 5) lymphomas; 6) autoimmune disorders; and 7) the X-linked lymphoproliferative syndrome which links genetics, immunology, and viruses with human lymphoid malignancy.

These categories enable investigation of identifiable landmarks; i.e., chromosomal breakage syndromes which have cutaneous signs, and predispose to lymphomageneses and immune abnormalities. Examples of hereditary lymphomas will be mentioned. Clinical/laboratory features will be discussed to elicit clues for testing hypotheses unifying genetics, immunology, and lymphomageneses.

Unclassified Families Prone to Lymphomas

Table 2 summarizes the data available on seven kindreds with multiple cases of both lymphoreticular and other types of cancer. These family studies suggest that identification of as yet unclassified familial cancer aggregations, inclusive of lymphoid malignancies may provide opportunities to investigate relationships between genetically determined cancer susceptibility, immune parameters, and environmental interactions.

An Integrative Viral and Genetic Hypothesis

An individual's genetic makeup would, by analogy with animal systems, be expected to profoundly influence susceptibility to putative human oncogenic viruses. The immune system is one mechanism which might be important in resisting such viruses. Differing genotypes produce individuals with various degrees of susceptibility to viruses (or other carcinogenic agents). Different phenotypes (clinical disease) are conceptually possible with various degrees of genetically determined immune resistance and exposures to a given virus. Viral exposure of a genetically resistant individual during times of physiological (50), environmental (104), iatrogeneic (100), or emotionally (133) induced immune suppression could conceivably result in a phenotype

Table 2.   Summary Data on Kindreds with
Unclassified Cancer Susceptibility

Cancer Type	Relation to Proband	Reference
(a)meningiosarcoma	proband	98
lymphoma	sibling	
cecal adenocarcinoma	sibling	
osteogenic sarcoma	sibling	
leukemia	maternal uncle	
(b)chronic lymphocytic leukemia	proband	9
chronic lymphocytic leukemia	sibling	
chronic lymphocytic leukemia	sibling	
lymphoma	child	
(c)Waldenstrom's macroglobulinemia	proband	10
Waldenstrom's macroglobulinemia	child	
Waldenstrom's macroglobulinemia	child	
Waldenstrom's macroglobulinemia	child	41
(d)Waldenstrom's macroglobulinemia	proband	42
lymphoma	sibling 1	
lymphoma	sibling 2	
lymphoma	sibling 3	
lymphoma	sibling 4	
Hodgkin's disease	child of sibling 2	
lung adenocarcinoma	child of sibling 2	
acute lymphocytic leukemia	5 year old grandson of lung cancer subject	
(e)Lymphoreticular malignancies	6 of 10 siblings	110
(f)Multiple primary cancers	proband	55
lymphocytic lymphoma	brother	
(g)Lymphoreticular	healthy members of multiple families were studied	31

Additional findings:

(a)Early age of cancer onset in the 4 affected siblings (9 total), fragile chromosome #16 in father and 2 normal siblings, high EBV antibodies in 2 sisters.
(b)Depression of immunoglobulin production, PHA responses and mixed leukocyte
responses in several family members.
(c)Both kappa and lambda light chains associated with the different IgM parapro-
teins, autoimmune findings prevalent, all with cancer and/or autoantibodies
possessed HLA-A2, B8, DRW-3 antigens.
(d)Nine total siblings in proband generation, impaired PHA responses in family
members associated with polyclonal IgM elevations and/or elevated EBV titers.
(e)Multiple other malignancies in kindred; of 4 subjects tested all were low in
IgG, 2 were low in IgA, and 2 had depressed skin tests and in vitro PHA
responses.
(f)Both were IgA deficient.
(g)Elevated average IgM levels, depressed skin tests and Con A response in
patients' relatives.

(clinical disease) routinely associated with a high susceptible
genotype (Figure 1).

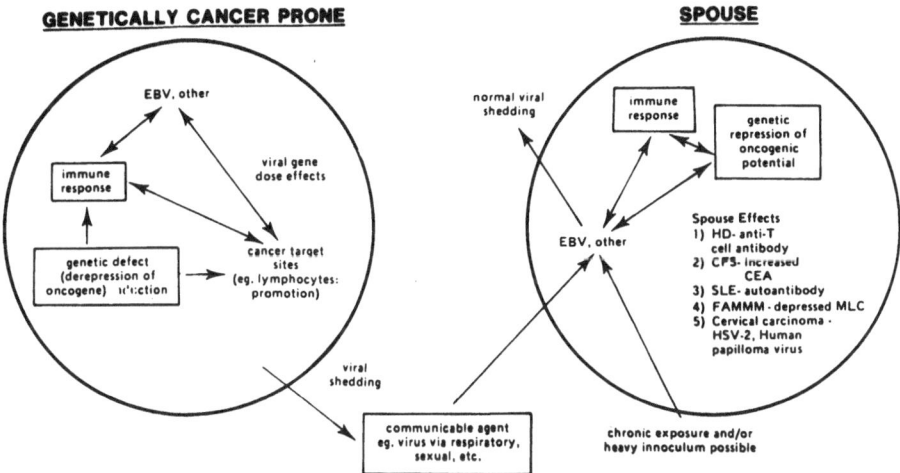

Fig. 1.   Schematic diagram integrating a genetic-viral-immuno-
          logical hypothesis to partially explain susceptibility
          to lymphomagenesis and/or other malignancies. Complex
          interactions between inherited predisposition to cancer,
          viruses, and the immune system culminating in lymphomage-
          nesis are postulated. Contributions from the spouse are
          included. (From: Lynch, H.T. and Guirgis, H.A. Child-
          hood cancer and the SBLA syndrome. Med. Hypoth. $\underline{5}$:15,
          1979. Churchill Livingstone, Inc., publishers.

Lymphomagenesis and the Cancer-Associated Genodermatoses

Immunological abnormalities may associate with cutaneous
stigmata in several hereditary cancer-associated genodermatosis
(84) (Table 1). For example, Wiskott-Aldrich syndrome (WAS) is a
sex-linked disorder characterized by a triad of thrombocytopenia
with bleeding, increased susceptibility to infections, and an
eczematous skin eruption. Approximately 12% of WAS patients
develop lymphoreticular malignancies (84,132). Myelogenous
leukemia and astrocytoma also has been reported.

WAS lacks a specific immunologic abnormality, although
defective immune function is uniformly present (146).
Investigators have speculated that there is a group of related
disorders consonant with WAS which, show similar clinical features
and different immunological abnormalities consistent with genetic
heterogeneity. Meuwissen elsewhere in this monograph considers
WAS with respect to EBV and bone marrow transplantation.

Ataxia telangiectasia (AT) (Louis-Bar syndrome) is an autosomal recessively inherited disease characterized by progressive
cerebellar ataxia and oculocutaneous telangiectasia (80,107,120,

136,140). The autosomal recessive mode of inheritance was
indicated among 64 families with AT by: 1) no affected children
having affected parents; 2) approximately 25% of siblings of index
cases were affected; and 3) frequent consanguinity (76). Patients
may manifest recurrent severe sinopulmonary infection. IgA is
lacking (146) perhaps accounting for the susceptibility to
repeated sinopulmonary infection. Autopsy has revealed thymic
aplasia and dysplasia, with absence of Hassall's corpuscles (3).
Lymph nodes showed poorly developed lymphoid cuffs about the
germinal centers. Reticulum cell hyperplasia or lymphopenia may
also occur.

Subjects with AT show frequent lymphoid and gastric cancers
(65). Haere et al. (54) studied gastric carcinoma in a mother
(obligate heterozygote) and in two of her five AT affected
offspring. Onset of gastric carcinoma in the AT patients was
unusually early (19-21 years). Also, carcinoma of the ovary, basal
cell carcinoma, and central nervous system neoplasms have been
noted in a review by Lynch and Fusaro (84). The possibility of
cancer excess in heterozygous carriers of the deleterious AT gene
has been discussed by Swift (136). Finally, AT is also characterized by chromosomal instability, as is Fanconi's anemia and
Bloom's syndrome leading to their characterization as chromosome-
breakage syndromes (126).

Bloom's syndrome is an autosomal recessively inherited disease
characterized by facial telangiectatic erythema, photosensitivity,
and dwarfism with doliocephaly (13,14,30,45,46,63,126). Within
three years of life, facial erythema develops, involving the
butterfly region of the face, forehead, lips, ears, and eyelid
margins. The erythema may be exacerbated by sunlight exposure in
sunburned regions. Several patients have had abnormally low
concentrations of IgA and IgM along with depressed in vitro
mitogen responsiveness (63). These patients show chromosomal
abnormalities including breaks, rearrangments, sister chromatid
exchanges, quadraradial configurations and decreased DNA replication.

Bloom's syndrome patients have a high incidence of leukemia
and lymphoma, squamous cell cancer of the esophagus, and adenocarcinoma of the colon (46). Investigation of potential viral
involvement in the lymphomas and squamous carcinomas seen in these
patients would help to further elucidate the etiology of these
cancers.

Chediak-Higashi (CH) syndrome is inherited as an autosomal
recessive (84) and is discussed in detail by Merino in this book.
The phenotype comprises decreased pigmentation of the hair and
eyes, photophobia, nystagmus and abnormal susceptibility to
infection. These patients have low natural killer (NK) activity
(1) and frequently succumb with lymphoproliferative disorders.

Primary Immune Deficiencies

Selective immunoglobulin A (IgA) (135) deficiency is the most frequent of the primary immunodeficiencies (132). Various modes of inheritance have been described (3,146). Evaluation of autoimmune diseases and asthma of early onset may uncover IgA deficiency.

Recently, Schuelke et al, (121,122) described autosomal dominant transmission of ovarian carcinoma with depressed serum IgA levels among relatives at risk. In addition, one of three kindreds with the Cancer Family Syndrome showed abnormally low IgA levels suggesting that this aberration might be etiologic in some families with inherited susceptibility to non-lymphoid malignancies.

Common variable immunodeficiency (CVI) is second in frequency to selective IgA deficiency among the aggregate of primary immunodeficiency diseases (146). However precise delineation of CVI is difficult and hence many disorders are grouped in this category. CVI shows defective maturation of B cells into functional immunoglobulin-secreting cells and T-cell defects (often progressive) (146).

Thymomas, epithelial malignancies, and lymphoreticular cancer have been described in CVI. The cancer spectrum is similar to that found in IgA deficiency. The genetics of CVI remains enigmatic. However, an increased incidence of cancer in relatives of CVI patients has been described (132).

The X-linked immunodeficiency of Bruton is characterized by onset of recurrent infections of multiple organs with bacteria, parasites, and viruses (146). The immunological defect in this disorder arises from an arrest in lymphocyte development at a pre B stage. Typically, all of the serum immunoglobulin classes are either reduced or absent. Lymphomas occur infrequently in this disease.

Selective IgM deficiency is relatively rare and the mode of inheritance has not been delineated. Recurrent meningeal, upper respiratory and upper gastrointestinal tract infections due to multiple types of bacteria occur. A significant reduction or absence of IgM with normal levels of IgG, IgA, IgD and IgE are found (146). B cells show a reduced or absent IgM response. Predominant cancers in this disease are lymphoreticular, although others have been described.

Reduced concentration of IgG and IgA but normal to markedly elevated IgM and IgD are detected in X-linked immunodeficiency with hyper-IgM (146). "Acquired" forms have been described.

Recurrent pyogenic respiratory tract infections occur in infancy. Hepatosplenomegaly and lymphadenopathy are common. The B cells in these patients secrete IgM but fail to switch to synthesize IgG and IgA. Lymphomas are the predominant malignancy in this disorder (146).

Familial Hodgkin's Disease

A "two-disease hypothesis" is based on the bimodal age distribution of Hodgkin's disease (HD) (24). Occupational, racial, and ethnic factors contribute to international variations in incidence. Familial and/or genetic as well as environmental factors, have been implicated in its etiology (7,16,18,24,25,39, 51,53,62,88,89,93,94,95,98,103,108,117,118,128,144,145).

Strongly supporting a primary genetic influence on HD susceptibility are the suggested associations in families with HLA antigens B5, BW35, and B37 (7,39,53,84,93,145). An autosomal recessive inheritance has even been suggested in the most extensive HD prone kindred reported (117). Observed instances of HD in concordance monozygote twins (51) also compatible with a primary genetic susceptibility. Malignancies reported in addition to HD in kindreds include other lymphoid and epithelial cancers (18,25,62). This raises the possibility that some instances of multiple HD cases in kindreds are an expression of broader genetically determined cancer susceptibility syndrome (81) and accents the need to search for cancer of all anatomic sites for the duration of the subjects' lives in hereditary cancer. Obviously, such familial observations do not prove genetic HD susceptibility since a shared environment complicates the observations.

Immunological studies on relatives of HD patients have also provided clues as to possible etiology of HD and associated immune findings. Suggestive lines of evidence include: 1) abnormal cell mediated activities in surviving monozygotic and dizygotic twins of HD patients (8); 2) abnormal anti-EBV antibody responses (128); and 3) recurrent herpes or infectious mononucleosis in 2 cancer free sibs of 3 HD patients (95). These findings might indicate a primary genetically determined immune defect predisposing to HD. Anti-T cell auto-antibodies in non-bloodline family members (98) are moreover compatible with an environmental agent. Cautious interpretation of such results is needed since cause-effect type relationships between cancer and immune parameters are difficult to establish.

Discussed in detail by Linder, Purtilo and Krueger in this book, is the etiological relation of EBV to African Burkitt's lymphoma and nasopharyngeal carcinoma (29,36,113,148). Also discussed in detail by Johnson in this book are cotton-topped

marmosets and owl monkeys which, when inoculated with EBV, develop
fatal lymphoproliferative diseases (37,127). In addition,
virtually all African patients afflicted with Burkitt's lymphoma
and Chinese patients manifesting nasopharyngeal carcinoma, have
high EBV antibody titers (57,58). Monkeys and humans with XLP
(112,125,127,138) who are susceptible to EBV-induced lymphomagenesis do not develop high titer antibodies to EBV antigens
(99,111). Moreover, risk of developing BL in endemic areas is
increased if the individual develops high titer antibodies (35).

Epstein-Barr Virus (EBV) and Familial Cancer

Levine et al. (75) studied antibody titers to Epstein-Barr
virus (EBV) associated antigens in relative from 21 families with
lymphomas and other cancers. They prospectively studied normal
individuals at high cancer risk. Antibody titers to the EB viral
capsid antigen (VCA) and early antigen (EA) were significantly
higher in 83 affected members from the 21 subject families. The
highest antibody titers were found in families where the predominant tumors were carcinoma, soft tissue sarcoma, and lymphoma.
They suggested that the high EBV titers in certain patients
represented an abnormal immune response which might be related to
familial cancer susceptibility.

Genetic Predisposition to Burkitt's Lymphoma (BL)

Other authors in this publication have discussed the evidence
for etiologic involvement of EBV with human malignancy. We will
discuss evidence for inherited predisposition to BL. BL has been
described in siblings in Africa (26,102,147) leading to speculation about a genetic susceptibility to an oncogenic agent
(61,134). Two seronegative sisters from Indiana have had American
BL (D. Purtilo - personal communication). The surviving sister
developed infectious mononucleosis (IM) while she was in remission
from the BL. An 8 year old boy with XLP and BL succumbed to IM
many years after onset of BL (D. Purtilo - personal communication). There is a 2:1 male to female occurrence of BL. This
suggest relative immune deficiency of males compared to females.

Five Tanzanian families with multiple cases of BL in familial
association with other forms of cancer have been reported (17).
One of these families included a woman with nasopharyngeal
carcinoma (NPC) whose daughter had BL. Other associations
include: 1) a boy with BL whose sister developed chronic myelogenous leukemia (CML); 2) a man with CML whose son developed
BL; and 3) two brothers and a half-brother with BL. Attention was
given to these familial occurrences, particularly the association
of BL with NPC and CML among close relatives. These observations
are noteworthy since NPC and CML are relatively rare in Tanzania.
Genetic factors may be etiologic to these forms of cancer in the

subject's family. However, the possibility that the cancer
clustering might have been the result of shared environmental
factors or chance occurrences cannot be excluded.

Jones et al. (66) studied HLA in 78 patients with BL and 70
controls from Ghana. An increased relative risk in BL patients
with DR7, HLA-A1 and B12 (Bw44) was observed.

Primary Immunodeficiencies

Kersey and colleagues describe malignancies with primary
immunodeficiency in another portion of this book. The Minnesota
group reviewed 35 lymphoreticular disorders in patients from the
Immunodeficiency Cancer Registry (ICR) focusing on ataxia telangiectasia (AT) and Wiskott-Aldrich syndrome (WAS) (42). Of 267
cases of malignancies and PID reported from their registry, 70% of
neoplasias diagnosed in the entire series were lymphoreticular.
Approximately one-third of these lesions had been "unclassifiable"
by conventional categories. Thirty-one of 35 patients manifested
lymphoreticular malignancies; 3 were undefined lymphoreticular
disorders, and 1 was "reactive lymphoid hyperplasia." Twenty-one
were non-Hodgkin's lymphomas (NHL), 8 were Hodgkin's disease, and
only 2 were acute lymphoblastic leukemias. Thus a striking
prevalence of NHL over leukemia (65% vs. 8%, excluding adult
patients) was found. In contrast, in the general pediatric
population NHL accounts for 13.5% and the leukemias for 76% of
hematopoietic malignancies. Moreover, the NHL were diffuse in
pattern and a significant portion (38%) were B-cell immunoblastic
sarcomas. According to a review by Frizzera (42), only 4.2% of
lymphoreticular cancers are of this entity.

Other aspects were the 50% prevalence of the lymphocytic
depletion type of HD and the occurrence in very young patients.
In the general population the depletion type is the rarest (5-15%)
and it occurs in middle-aged or elderly individuals.

Autoimmune Disorders

Sjögren's syndrome is the complex of dry eyes and mouth, i.e.,
keratoconjunctivitis, arthritis (130) and sometimes progressive
systemic sclerosis, Raynaud's phenomenon, polyarteritis, poly-
myositis, chronic active hepatitis, primary biliary cirrhosis, and
occasionally SLE (67,81). Hypergammaglobulinemia and other immune
phenomena may also occur (28). Lymphomas have been noted in
excess in patients with Sjögren's syndrome (79,115,141).
Adenocarcinoma of the parotid gland has also been described in
these patients.

Possibly autosomal recessive transmission occurs (27,79) and
an increased association with HLA-B8 has been observed (23,43,47,

129,139).   HLA-B8 is increased approximately 4.4 fold (from combined data) with Sjogren's syndrome (43) and the relative risk of
other associated diseases with HLA-B8 were: juvenile diabetes
2.1; Graves' disease 3.6; chronic active hepatitis 3.6; dermatitis
herpetiformis 4.3; myasthenia gravis 4.5; celiac disease 11.1; and
idiopathic Addison's disease 12 fold.   These authors reasoned that
an autoimmunity locus in linkage dysequilibrium with HLA-B8 might
predispose to these disorders.

SLE is a multisystem disease with protean manifestations.
Immunological deficiency, lymphoma, connective tissue disorders,
and dysgammaglobulinemia have been reported in a patient with SLE
(131).   More than 10 patients with SLE and lymphoma are recorded.
Larsen (71,72,73) demonstrated increased concentrations of IgG in
relatives of probands with SLE.   Moreover, 41 (12%) of 340
patients with SLE had affected relatives.   Individual pedigrees
show several possible modes of inheritance.   Abnormal serologic
patterns in patients with SLE (5,32,33,72) and dermatoglyphic
similarities in patients (40) are found.   Familial prevalence of
SLE is recognized (4,12,19).

Green et al. (52) described impaired delayed hypersensitivity
and T and B cell defects in SLE.   In NZB/BL mice, spontaneously
SLE-like-disease and a high incidence of lymphomas emerges with
time.   Furthermore, current concepts favor suppressor T cell
dysfunction as predisposing to abnormal B cell proliferation in
response to an extrinsic antigens or autoantigens.   Most
non-Hodgkin's lymphomas are thought to be of B cell origin (53).

SBLA Syndrome

Lymphomageneses occurs in the SBLA syndrome as an apparent
autosomal dominant trait involving all three germinal layers
including Sarcoma, Breast and brain tumors, Leukemia, lymphoma,
laryngeal and lung cancers, and Adrenal cortical carcinoma
(85,86).   This diverse spectrum of cancer occurs at an early age
of onset.   Li and Fraumeni (77,78) proposed a hypothesis involving
genetic predisposition to exongenous factors (oncogenic virus?) as
being etiologic.

Cancer occurs during childhood and a second peak during early
adulthood and middle age (86).   Congenital cancer may occur in
progeny of affected mothers (85).   We hypothesize interaction of
the SBLA genotype (Figure 2) (first hit) and other etiologic
events (putative oncogenic virus, derepressed oncogene, tumor
specific antigens, and immunologic changes associated with
pregnancy) which cross the placenta contributing to cancer in the
fetus (second hit).   This theory is based on the supposition that
the mothers have already sustained both 'hits' (germinal and
somatic) and the fetuses received the germinal 'hit' at concep-

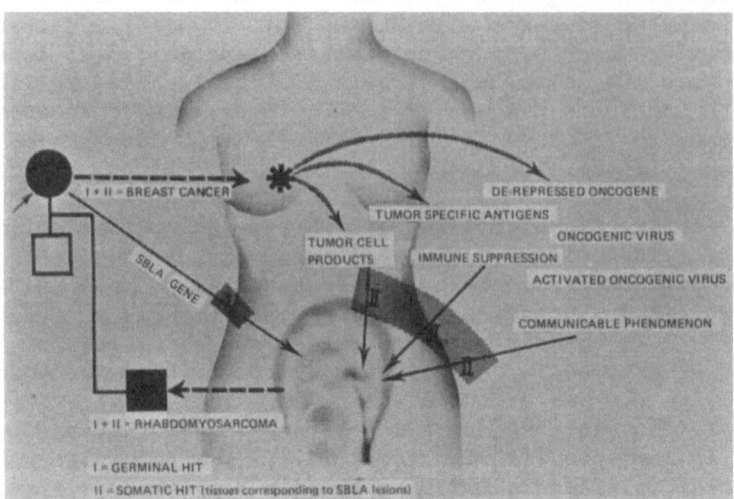

Fig. 2. Diagram of "two hit" hypothesis to partially explain
         cancer development. (From: Lynch, H.T. and Guirgis, H.A.
         Childhood cancer and the SBLA syndrome. Med. Hypothesis,
         5:15-22, 1979. Churchill Livingstone, Inc., publisher.)

tion, but they sustain the second 'hit' transplacentally (Figure
2). This hypothesis will require extensive testing in families
manifesting the SBLA syndrome.

Familial Adult T Cell Leukemia

Imamura (64) described two brothers who almost simultaneously
developed adult T cell leukemia (ATL). The leukemia cells
possessed no B cell markers. Studies in Japan (143) from the T
and B cell malignancy study group revealed that 11 of 102 patients
with ATL showed a familial involvement suggesting more frequent
occurrence of familial T cell than B cell malignancies.
Seroepidemiological studies in Japan support a postulated association between human T cell lymphomas and a retrovirus (22,59,60,
101,114).

Kaposi's Sarcoma

Kaposi's sarcoma (KS) is a multifocal neoplastic disorder
characterized by cutaneous, subcutaneous, and visceral tumors
(20,92,119). The tumor is associated with Hodgkin's disease, NHL,
mycosis fungoides, leukemia, and multiple myeloma. There is also
a tendency to multiple primary cancers and increased incidence
among young Africans, northern Italians, and eastern European Jews

(15,92,96,119). Rare reports of KS affecting several members of a family with vertical transmission have suggested the possibility of autosomal dominant inheritance (34,38,83,96,142,149). An HLA association (6,21) has also been found. Recent work has suggested that this tumor might result from a generalized defect in regulation of proliferation of lymphocytes and other cell types (6).

Abrams discusses KS in male homosexuals and Penn describes the prevalence of the tumor in renal transplant recipients in other chapters in this book. Some investigators have postulated an infectious etiology (2,48,116). These patients also develop opportunistic B cell lymphomas (EBV?) and squamous cell carcinomas (papilloma or herpes viruses?).

Hepatitis B Virus (HBV) and Hepatocellular Carcinoma (HC)

While not immediately linked to lymphomagenesis, HC is another example of a virus associated with a complex etiology that probably involves multiple factors (genetics, immune susceptibility) and other environmental exposures (liver flukes?). HC appears to be linked to HBV (56). Family studies show early infection which is transmitted by a HBV-carrier mother. Persistent infection with HBV is associated with chronic active hepatitis, postnecrotic cirrhosis, and HC, especially in males in southeast Asian areas endemic for HBV. Lynch et al. (87) have shown a high degree of concordance between HBV and HC in an informative family. Future research will possibly disclose other human malignancies might be attributable to a viral involvement in the etiology of the diseases. Immunological intervention with vaccines (56) raises hope that certain human malignancies, including lymphomas, may be prevented or cured (112).

SUMMARY AND CONCLUSIONS

We have discussed throughout this review diverse immunological abnormalities associated with lymphomas. The immune abnormalities might be a consequence of the lymphoma or alternatively, they may be etiologically linked to lymphomagenesis. Etiologic links could be derived from several mechanisms:

1) Basic cellular metabolism (68) and/or structural changes (70) that might by themselves predispose to malignancy in lymphocytes and/or other cells. Such defects might alter events after viral infection of susceptible cells (44).

2) Defective immune regulation. Ineffective immune responses are mounted to viruses and/or viral antigens on malignantly transformed cells. The genes may be linked to the major histocompatibility locus (74,105,106) or other chromosomes.

3) Environmental influences which are immunosuppressive might occur in Burkitt's lymphoma (35), adult T cell leukemia (60), and certain homosexuals (48,116).

Any or all of these mechanisms may etiologically link immune defects with lymphomagenesis in context with genetic factors. Formal proof of any etiologic link could be difficult. Potentially confounding factors include: 1) chance avoidance of contact with viruses and/or carcinogens; 2) absence (genetically determined?) of viral receptors (49,123); and 3) transfer of maternal T lymphocytes to some immunodeficient individuals in utero (109).

In reviewing the immune surveillance theory, Schwartz (124) notes contradictions of the hypothesis. Predilection of immunodeficient patients to lymphoreticular malignancy does, however, raise questions regarding the theory. Chronic antigen stimulation in the absence of efficient control of lymphocyte proliferation might lead to lymphomagenesis (Figure 1). Viral stimulation of lymphocytes might also partly explain the predilection to lymphoreticular malignancy. Finally, it is conceivable that a genetically inherited defect in some basic cellular function might predispose to both cancer and immune impairments.

A logical extension of the immune surveillance theory is the proliferation of virally infected cells in a host with defective immune responses as in polyoma virus in animals (124). In the XLP syndrome immune abnormalities to EBV predispose to lymphomagenesis. Continued investigations in populations with immunodeficiencies may reveal additional viral agents.

Ability to predict susceptibility to both lymphoid and other malignancies needs to be accomplished. This book offers much information to begin to define this objective with regards to EBV-induced lymphomas. Retrospective and prospective evaluation of groups of patients might reveal subgroups genetically prone to malignancy as a result of environmental and/or iatrogenic exposures (e.g. transplant recipients). Such predictability would be useful in patient management. Evaluation of the cancer history in kindreds of both the patients who do and do not develop malignancy after an environmental/iatrogenic exposure could reveal a means of cancer predictability.

In conclusion, we think that understanding of lymphomagenesis would be enhanced significantly by studying families prone to these disorders. This inquiry should include laboratory studies to test specific hypotheses relevant to genetic-environmental interaction.

REFERENCES

1. Abo, T., Roder, J.C., Abo, W., Cooper, M.D., and Balch, C.M. Natural killer (HNK-1+) cells in Chediak-Higashi patients are present in normal numbers but are abnormal in function and morphology. J. Clin. Invest., 70:193, 1982.

2. A cluster of Kaposi's sarcoma and Pneumocystis carinii pneumonia among homosexual male residents of Los Angeles and Orange Counties, California. MMWR, 31(#23):305, 1982.

3. Ammann, A.J. and Hong, R. Disorders of the T cell system. In: E.R. Steihm and V.A. Fulginiti (eds.), Immunologic Disorders in Infants and Children. pp. 314. Philadelphia, Pa: W.B. Saunders Co., 1980.

4. Ansell, B.M. and Lawrence, J.S. A family study in lupus erythematosus, abstracted. Arth. Rheum., 6:260, 1963.

5. Arnett, F.C. and Shlman, L.E. Studies in familial systemic lupus erythematosus. Medicine, 55:313, 1976.

6. Ben-Chetrit, E., Ben-Amitai, D., and Levo, Y. The association between Kaposi's sarcoma and dysgammaglobulinemia. Cancer, 49:649, 1982.

7. Berberich, F.R., Berberich, M.S., Engleman, E.G., Grumet, F.C., and King, M.-C. Hodgkin's disease susceptibility linked to the HLA locus: classical linkage analysis and a new concordance method. Abstract #174, Am. Soc. Hum. Genet., 33d Ann Mtg, Detroit, Sept. 29 - Oct. 2, 1982.

8. Bjorkholm, M., Holm, G., DeFaire, U., and Mellstedt, H. Immunological defects in healthy twin siblings to patients with Hodgkin's disease. Scand. J. Haematology, 19:396, 1977.

9. Blattner, W.A., Dean, J.H., and Fraumeni, J.F. Familial lymphoproliferative malignancy: clinical and laboratory follow up. Ann. Int. Med., 90:943, 1979.

10. Blattner, W.A., Garber, D.L., Mann, L., Fisher, W., Bauman, A.W., and Fraumeni, J.F. Macroglobulinemia and autoimmune disease in a family. Abstract for Ann Mtg ASCO, C-505:413, 1979.

11. Blattner, W.A., Lubiniecki, A.S., Mulvihill, J.J., Lally, P., and Fraumeni, J.F. Genetics of SV40 T-antigen expression: studies of twins, heritable syndromes and cancer families. Int. J. Cancer, 22:231, 1978.

12. Block, S.R., Winfield, J.B., Lockshin, M.O., D'Angelo, W.A., and Christian, C.L. Studies of twins with systemic lupus erythematosus. A Review of the literature and presentation of 12 additional sets. Am. J. Med., 59:533, 1975.

13. Bloom, D. and German, J. The syndrome of congenital telangiectatic erythema and stunted growth. J. Ped., 68:103, 1966.

14.   Bloom, D. and German, J.   The syndrome of congenital
      telangiectatic erythema and stunted growth.   Arch.
      Derm., 103:545, 1971.
15.   Bluefarb, S.M. Kaposi's Sarcoma.   Springfield IL., Charles
      C. Thomas, 1957.
16.   Bowers, T.K., Moldow, C.F., Bloomfield, C.D., and Yunis,
      E.J.   Familial Hodgkin's disease and the major histocom-
      patibility complex.   Vox. Sang., 33:273, 1977.
17.   Brubaker, G., Levin, A.G., Steel, C.M., Creasley, G.,
      Cameron, H.M., Linsell, C.A., and Smith, P.G.   Multiple
      cases of Burkitt's lymphoma and other neoplasms in
      families in the north Mara district of Tanzania.   Int.
      J. Cancer, 261:165, 1980.
18.   Buehler, S.K., Firme, F., Fodor, G., Fraser, G.R., Marshall,
      W.H., and Vaze, P.   Common variable immunodeficiency,
      Hodgkin's disease, and other malignancies in a
      Newfoundland family.   Lancet, 1:195, 1975.
19.   Bywaters, E.G.   Family studies of rheumatoid arthritis and
      lupus erythematosus in Great Britain.   In: J.H. Kellgren
      (ed.), The Epidemiology of Chronic Rheumatism.   A sym-
      posium organized by the Council for International
      Organization of Medical Sciences.   Vol. 1, pp. 294-258.
      Philadelphia: Davis Co., 1963.
20.   Byrk, D., Farman, J., Dallemand, S., Meyers, M.A., and
      Wecksell, A.   Kaposi's sarcoma of the intestinal tract:
      roentgen manifestations.   Gastrointes. Radiol., 3:425,
      1975.
21.   Walker, M., Rubinstein, P., Carrier, C., Carpenter, C.,
      Krassner, J., and Friedman-Kien, A.   The HLA system in
      patients with Kaposi's sarcomas.   Abstract of Annual
      AACHT meeting, 1982.   Human Imm., 5(#2):178, 1982.
22.   Catovsky, D., Rose, M., Goolden, A.W.G., Shite, J.M.,
      Bourikas, G., Brownell, A.I., Blattner, W.A., Greaves,
      M.F., Galton, D.A.G., McCluskey, D.R., Lampert, I.,
      Ireland, R., Bridges, J.M., and Gallo, R.C.   Adult T
      cell lymphoma-leukemia in blacks from the West Indies.
      Lancet, 1:827, 1982.
23.   Chused, T.M., Kassan, S.S., Opelz, G., and Moutsopoulos,
      H.M. Sjogren's syndrome associated with HLA-Dw3.   N.
      Engl. J. Med., 296:895, 1977.
24.   Cole, P., MacMahon, B., and Aisenberg, A.   Mortality from
      Hodgkin's disease in the United States: evidence for the
      multiple aetiology hypotheses.   Lancet, ii:1371, 1968.
25.   Creagan, E.T. and Fraumeni, J.F., Jr.   Familial Hodgkin's
      disease.   Lancet, ii:547, 1972.
26.   Dalldorf, G., Linsell, C.A., and Barnhart, F.E.   An epide-
      miological approach to the lymphomas of African children
      and Burkitt's sarcoma of the jaws.   Perspect. Biol.
      Med., 7:435, 1964.

27. Delaney, W.E. and Balogh, K. Carcinoma of the parotid gland associated with benign lymphoepithelial lesion (Mikulicz's disease) in Sjogren's syndrome. Cancer, 19:853, 1966.

28. Denko, C.W. and Gergenstal, D.M. The Sicca syndrome (Sjögren's syndrome): a study of sixteen cases. Arch. Int. Med., 105:849, 1960.

29. DeThé, G., Ambrosioni, J.C., Ho, H., and Kwan, H.C. Lymphoblastoid transformation and presence of herpes-type viral particles in a Chinese nasopharyngeal tumor cultured in vitro. Nature, 221:770, 1969.

30. Dicken, C.H., Dewald, G., and Gordon, H. Sister chromatid exchanges in Bloom's syndrome. Arch. Derm., 114:755, 1978.

31. Dworsky, R., Baptista, J., Parker, J., Chandor, S., Noble, G., Herrmann, K., Henle, W., and Henderson, B. Immune function in healthy relatives of patients with malignant disease. J. Natl. Cancer Inst., 60:27, 1978.

32. Dubois, E.R. Lupus Erythematosus. In: A Review of the Current Status of Discoid and Systemic Lupus Erythematosus and Their Variants. Un. of S. California Press, Los Angeles, 1974, 2nd edition.

33. Dubois, R.W., Weiner, J.M., and Dubois, E.L. Dermatoglyphic study of systemic lupus erythematosus. Arth. Rheum., 19:83, 1976.

34. Epstein, E. Kaposi's sarcoma and parapsoriasis en plaque in brothers. J. Am. Med. Assoc., 219:1377, 1972.

35. Epstein, M.A. and Achong, B.G. The relationship of the virus to Burkitt's lymphoma. In: M.A. Epstein and B.G. Achong (eds.), The Epstein-Barr Virus. New York: Springer-Verlag, 1979.

36. Epstein, M.A., Achong, B.G., and Barr, Y.M. Virus particles in cultured lymphoblasts from Burkitt's lymphoma. Lancet, 1:702, 1964.

37. Epstein, M.A., Hunt, R.D., and Rabin, H. Pilot experiments with EB virus in owl monkeys (Aotus trivirgatus). I. Int. J. Cancer, 12:309, 1973.

38. Finlay, A.Y. and Marks, R. Familial Kaposi's sarcoma. Br. J. Dermatol., 100:323, 1979.

39. Forbes, J.F. and Morris, P.J. Analysis of HLA antigens in patients with Hodgkin's disease and their families. J. Clin. Invest., 51:1156, 1972.

40. Fraga, A., Armendares, S., Mintz, G., Mora, J., and Cortes, R. Dermatoglyphic patterns in systemic lupus erythematosus (SLE) and their changes in patients with increased fetal wastage. J. Rheum., (Suppl 1):35, 1974.

41. Fraumeni, J.F., Wertelecki, W., Blattner, W.A., Jensen, R.D., and Leventhal, B.G. Varied manifestations of a familial lymphoproliferative disorder. Am. J. Med., 59:145, 1975.

42.   Frizzera, G., Rosai, J., Dehner, L.P., Spector, B.D., and
      Kersey, J.H. Lymphoreticular disorders in primary
      immunodeficiencies: new findings based on an up-to-date
      histologic classification of 35 cases. Cancer, 46:692,
      1980.

43.   Fye, K.H., Terasaki, P.I., Moutsopoulos, H., Danials, T.E.,
      Michalski, J.P., and Talal, N. Association of Sjogren's
      syndrome with HLA-B8. Arth. Rheum., 19:883, 1976.

44.   Gallo, R.C. and Wong-Staal, F. Retroviruses as etiologic
      agents of some animal and human leukemias and lymphomas
      and as tools for elucidating the molecular mechanism of
      leukemagenesis. Blood, 60(3):545, 1982.

45.   German, J. Genetic disorders associated with chromosomal
      instability and cancer. J. Inves. Derm., 60:427, 1973.

46.   German, J., Bloom, D., and Passarge, E. Bloom's syndrome.
      V. Surveillance for cancer in affected families. Clin.
      Genet., 2:162, 1977.

47.   Gershwin, M.E., Terasaki, P.I., Graw, R. et al. Increased
      frequency of HL-A8 in Sjogren's syndrome. Tis. Ant.,
      6:432, 1975.

48.   Gerstoft, J., Malchow-Moller, A., Bygbjerg, I., Dickmeiss,
      E., Enk, C., Halberg, P., Haahr, S., Jackobsen, M.,
      Jensen, K., Mejer, J., Nielsen, J.O., Thomsen, H.K.,
      Sondergaard, J., and Lorenzen, I. Severe acquired immu-
      nodeficiency in European homosexual men. Br. Med. J.,
      285:17, 1982.

49.   Gervias, F., Wills, A., Leyritz, M., Lebrun, A., and Joncas,
      J.H. Relative lack of Epstein-Barr virus (EBV) recep-
      tors on B cells from persistently EBV seronegative
      adults. J. Immun., 126:897, 1981.

50.   Gill, T.J. and Repetti, C.F. Immunologic and genetic fac-
      tors influencing reproduction. Am. J. Pathol., 95:465,
      1979.

51.   Gracz, K., Kofman, S., and Economou, S.G. Hodgkin's disease
      in monozygotic twins: a case report. J. Surg. Oncol.,
      12:221, 1979.

52.   Green, J.A., Dawson, A.A., and Walker, W. Systemic lupus
      erythematosus and lymphoma. Lancet, ii:753, 1978.

53.   Greene, M.H., McKeen, E.A., Li, F.P., Blattner, W.A., and
      Fraumeni, J.F. HLA antigens in familial Hodgkin's
      disease. Int. J. Cancer, 23:777, 1979.

54.   Haerer, A.F., Jackson, J.F., and Evers, C.G. Ataxia
      telangiectasia with gastric adenocarcinoma. J. Am. Med.
      Assoc., 210:1884, 1969.

55.   Hamoudi, A.B., Ertel, I., Newton, W.A., Reiner, C.B., and
      Clatworthy, H.W. Multiple neoplasms in an adolescent
      child associated with IgA deficiency. Cancer,
      33:1134, 1974.

56.   Hann, H.L., Kim, C.Y., London, W.T., Whitford, P., and
      Blumberg, B.S. Hepatitis B virus and primary hepato-

cellular carcinoma: family studies in Korea. Int. J.
Cancer, 30:47, 1982.

57. Henle, G., Henle, W., Clifford, P., Diehl, V., Kafuko, G.W.,
      Kirya, B.G., Klein, G., Morrow, R.H., Munube, G.M.A.,
      Pike, P., Tukei, P.M., and Ziegler, J.L. Antibodies to
      Epstein-Barr virus in Burkitt's lymphoma and control
      groups. J. Natl. Cancer Inst., 43:1147, 1969.

58. Henle, W., Henle, G., Ho, H., Burtin, P., Cachin, Y.,
      Clifford, P., Schryver, A.P., DeThe, G., Diehl, V., and
      Klein, G. Antibodies to Epstein-Barr virus in
      nasopharyngeal carcinoma, other head and neck neoplasms
      and control groups. J. Natl. Cancer Inst., 44:225,
      1970.

59. Hinuma, Y., Komoda, H., Chosa, T., Kondo, T., Kohakura, M.,
      Takenaka, T., Kikuchi, M., Ichimaru, M., Yunoki, K.,
      Sato, I., Matsuo, R., Takiuchi, Y., Uchimo, H., and
      Hanaoka, M. Antibodies to adult T cell leukemia-virus-
      associated antigen (ATLA) in sera from patients with ATL
      and controls in Japan: a nation-wide seroepidemiologic
      study. Int. J. Cancer, 29:631, 1982.

60. Hinuma, Y., Nagata, K., Hanaoka, M.A., Nakai, M., Matsumoto,
      T., Kinoshita, K., Shirakaw, S., and Miyoshi, I. Adult
      T cell leukemia: antigen in an ATL cell line and detec-
      tion of antibodies to the antigen in human sera. Proc.
      Natl. Acad. Sci. USA, 78:6476, 1981.

61. Hirshaut, Y., Cohen, M., and Stevens, D. Serological dif-
      ferences between American and African Burkitt's
      lymphoma. Fed. Proc., 30:301, 1971.

62. Horbar, J.D., Dickerman, J.D., Allen, E.F., and Albertini,
      R.J. Hodgkin's disease following acute lymphocytic
      leukemia in a patient from a cancer-prone family: a case
      report. Med. Ped. Oncol., 9:219, 1981.

63. Hutteroth, T.H., Litwin, S.D., German, J. Abnormal immune
      responses of Bloom's syndrome lymphocytes in vitro. J.
      Clin. Invest., 56:1, 1975.

64. Imamura, N., Kozanemaru, S., and Kuramoto, A. T cell
      leukemia a few months apart in two brothers. Lancet,
      1:1361, 1982.

65. Jackson, J.F. Ataxia telantiectasia. In: H.T. Lynch
      (ed.), Skin, Heredity, and Malignant Neoplasms. pp.
      94-103. New York: Medical Examination Publishing, 1972.

66. Jones, E.H., Biggar, R.J., Nkrumah, F.K., and Lawler, S.D.
      Study of the HLA system in Burkitt's lymphoma. Hum.
      Immun., 3:207, 1980.

67. Kassan, S.S. and Gardy, M. Sjögren's syndrome: an update
      and overview. Am. J. Med., 64:1037, 1978.

68. King, M.C., Go, R.C.P., Elston, R.C., Lynch, H.T., and
      Petrakis, N.L. Allele increasing susceptibility to
      human breast cancer may be linked to the glutamate-
      pyruvate transaminase locus. Science, 208:406, 1980.

69.   Kirkpatrick, C.H.   Cancer and immunodeficiency diseases.
       Birth Defects, 12:61, 1976.
70.   Kopelovich, L., Lipkin, M., Blattner, W., Fraumeni, J.F.,
       Lynch, H.T., and Pollack, R.E.   Organization of actin-
       containing cables in cultured skin fibroblasts from
       individuals at high risk of colon cancer.   Int. J.
       Cancer, 26:301, 1980.
71.   Larsen, R.A.   Family studies in systemic lupus erythematosus
       (SLE).   VI. Presence of rheumatoid factors in relatives
       and spouses.   J. Chron. Dis., 25:191, 1972.
72.   Larsen, R.A.   Family studies in systemic lupus erythematosus
       (SLE).   VII. Serum immunoglobulins: IgG concentrations in
       relatives of selected SLE probands.   J. Chron. Dis.,
       25:215, 1972.
73.   Larsen, R.A.   Family studies in systemic lupus erythemato-
       sus (SLE).   IX. Thyroid diseases and antibodies.   J.
       Chron. Dis., 25:225, 1972.
74.   Legrand, L., Rivat-Perrah, L., Huttin, C., and Dausset, J.
       HLA and Gm linked genes affecting the degradation rate
       of antigens (sheep red blood cells) endocytized by
       macrophages.   Human Imm., 4:1, 1982.
75.   Levine, P.H., Fraumeni, J.F., Jr., Reisher, J.L., and
       Waggoner, D.E.   Antibodies to Epstein-Barr virus asso-
       ciated antigen in relatives of cancer patients.   J.
       Natl. Cancer Inst., 52:1037, 1974.
76.   Levin, S., Gottfried, E., and Cohen, M.   Ataxia
       telangiectasia: a review with observations on 47 Israeli
       cases.   Ped., 6:135, 1977.
77.   Li, F.P. and Fraumeni, J.F., Jr.   Soft tissue sarcomas,
       breast cancer, and other neoplasms.   A familial
       syndrome?   Ann. Int. Med., 71:747, 1969.
78.   Li, F.P. and Fraumeni, J.F., Jr.   Familial breast cancer,
       soft tissue sarcomas, and other neoplasms.   Ann. Int.
       Med., 83:834, 1975.
79.   Lichtenfeld, J.L., Kirschner, R.H., and Wiernick, P.H.
       Familial Sjögren's syndrome with associated primary
       salivary gland lymphoma.   Am. J. Med., 60:286, 1976.
80.   Louis-Bar (Mme.)   Sur un syndrome progressif comprenant des
       telangiectasies capillaires cutanees et conjonctivales
       symetriques a disposition naevoide et des trobules cere-
       belleux.   Confinia. Neurol., 4:32, 1971.
81.   Lynch, H.G.   Cancer Genetics.   Springfield: Charles C.
       Thomas Co., 1976.
82.   Lynch, H.T.   Breast Cancer Genetics.   New York: Van Nostrand
       Reinhold Co., 1981.
83.   Lynch, H.T. and Frichot, B.C.   Skin, heredity and cancer.
       Sem. Oncol., 5: 67, 1978.
84.   Lynch, H.T. and Fusaro, R.M.   Cancer Associated
       Genodermatoses.   New York: Nostrand Reinhold Co., 1982.

85. Lynch, H.T. and Guirgis, H.A. Childhood Cancer and the SBLA syndrome. Med. Hypoth., 5:15, 1979.

86. Lynch, H.T., Mulcahy, G.M., Harris, R.E., Guirgis, H.A., and Lynch, J.F. Genetic and pathologic findings in a kindred with hereditary sarcoma breast cancer, brain tumors, leukemia, lung, laryngeal, and adrenal cortical carcinoma. Cancer, 41:2055, 1974.

87. Lynch. H.T., Petcharin, S., Kannika, P., and Lynch, J.F. Familial hepatocellular carcinoma in an endemic area of Thailand. Cancer Gen. and Cytogen., in press.

88. Lynch, H.T., Purtilo, D., Schuelke, G., Lynch, J.F., and Danes, B.S. Familial Hodgkin's disease. In preparation, 1982.

89. Lynch, H.T., Saldivar, V.A., Guirgis, H.A., Terasaki, P.I., Bardawil, W.A., Harris, R.E., Lynch, J.F., and Thomas, R. Familial Hodgkin's disease and associated cancer: a clinical-pathological study. Cancer, 38:5:2033, 1976.

90. Lynch, P.M. and Lynch. H.T. Colon Cancer Genetics. New York: Van Nostrand Reinhold Co., in press, 1983.

91. MacMahon, B. Epidemiology of Hodgkin's disease. Cancer Res., 26:1189, 1966.

92. Mann, S.G. Kaposi's sarcoma. Experience with ten cases. AJR, 121:793, 1974.

93. Marshall, W.H., Barnard, J.M., Buehler, S.K., Grumley, J., and Larsen, B. HLA in familial Hodgkin's disease: results and a new hypothesis. Int. J. Cancer, 19:450, 1977.

94. Marshall, W.H., Buehler, S.K., Grumley, J., Salmon, D., Landre, M.F., and Frazser, G.R. A familial aggregate of common variable immunodeficiency, Hodgkin's disease and other malignancies in Newfoundland. I. Clinical features. Clin. Inves. Med., 2:153, 1980.

95. McBride, A. and Fennelly, J.J. Immunological depletion contributing to familial Hodgkin's disease. Eur. J. Cancer, 316:549, 1977.

96. McGinn, J.T., Ricca, J.J., and Currin, J.F. Kaposi's sarcoma following allergic angitis. Ann. Int. Med., 42:921, 1955.

97. Meisner, L.F., Gilbert, E., Ris, H.W., and Haverty, G. Genetic mechanisms in a cancer predisposition: a report of a cancer family. Cancer, 43:679, 1979.

98. Mendius, J.R., DeHoratius, R.J., Messner, R.P., and Williams, R.C. Family distribution of lymphocytotoxins in Hodgkin's disease. Ann. Int. Med., 84:151, 1976.

99. Miller, G. Biology of Epstein-Barr virus. In: G. Klein (ed.), Viral Oncology. pp. 713-738. New York: Raven Press, 1980.

100. Mitchison, N.A., Kinlen, L.J., Akagi, T., Ohtsuki, Y., Shiraishi, Y., Nagata, K., and Hinuma, Y. Present concepts in immune surveillance. In: M. Fougereau and J.

Gausset (eds.), Immunology 80. pp. 641-650. New York: Academic Press, 1980.

101. Miyoshi, I., Kulonishi, I., Yoshimoto, S. et al. Type C virus particles in a cord T cell line derived by co-cultivating normal human cord leukocytes and human leukemic T cells. Nature, 294:770, 1981.

102. Morrow, R.H., Pike, M.C., Smith, P.G., Ziegler, J.L., and Kisuule, A. Burkitt's lymphoma: a time-space cluster of cases in Bwamba county of Uganda. Br. Med. J., 2:491, 1971.

103. Nunez-Roldan, A., Martinez-Guibelalde, F., Gomez-Garcia, P., Gomez-Pereira, C., Nunez-Ollero, G., and Torres-Gomez, A. Possible HLA role in a family with Hodgkin's disease. Tis. Ant., 13:377, 1979.

104. Oppenheim, T.J., Sandberg, A.L., Altman, L.C., Hook, W.A., and Dougherty, S.F. Relationship of mitogen and tannins in walnuts to suppression of lymphocyte transformation after ingestion of walnuts. In: K. Lindahl-Kiessling and D. Osoba (eds.), Lymphocyte Recognition and Effector Mechanisms. pp. 79-84. New York: Academic Press, 1974.

105. Pandey, J.P., Johnson, A.H., Fudenberg, H.H., Amos, D.B., Gutterman, J.U., and Hersh, E.M. HLA antigens and immunoglobulin allotypes in patients with malignant melanoma. Human Imm., 2:185, 1981.

106. Pellegris, G., Illeni, M.T., Rovini, D., Vaglini, M., Cascinelli, N., and Chidoni, A. HLA complex and familial malignant melanoma. Int. J. Cancer, 29:621, 1982.

107. Peterson, R.D., Cooper, M.D., and Good, R.A. Lymphoid tissue abnormalities associated with ataxia telangiectasia. Am. J. Med., 41:342, 1966.

108. Plouffe, J.F., Silvan, J., Schwartz, R.S., Callen, J.P., Kane, P., Murphy, L.A., Goldstein, I.J., and Fekety, R. Abnormal lymphocyte responses in residents of a town with a cluster of Hodgkin's disease. Clin. Exp. Imm., 35:163, 1979.

109. Pollack, M.S., Kirkpatrick, D., Kapoor, N., Dupont, B., and O'Reilly, R.J. Identification by HLA typing of intrauterine-derived maternal T cells in four patients with severe combined immunodeficiency. N. Engl. J. Med., 307:662, 1982.

110. Potolsky, A.I., Heath, C.W., Buckley, C.E., and Rowlands, D.T. Lymphoreticular malignancies and immunologic abnormalities in a sibship. Am. J. Med., 50:42, 1971.

111. Purtilo, D.T. Malignant lymphoproliferative diseases induced by Epstein-Barr virus in immunodeficient patients, including X-linked, cytogenetic, and familial syndromes. Cancer Genet. & Cytogenet., 4:251, 1981.

112. Purtilo, D.T. and Klein, G. (eds.) Introduction to Epstein-Barr virus and lymphoproliferative diseases in immunodeficient individuals. Cancer Res., 41:4209, 1981.

113. Reedman, G.M. and Klein, G. Cellular localization of an Epstein-Barr virus (EBV)-associated complement-fixing antigen in producer and nonproducer lymphoblastoid cell lines. Int. J. Cancer, 11:499, 1973.

114. Robert-Guroff, M., Nakao, Y., Notake, K., Ito, Y., Sliski, A. and Gallo, R.C. Natural antibodies to human retrovirus HTLV in a cluster of Japanese patients with adult T cell leukemia. Science, 215:975, 1982.

115. Rothman, S., Block, M., and Hauser, F.V. Sjogren's syndrome associated with lymphoblastoma and hypersplenism. Arch Derm. Syph., 63:642, 1951.

116. Safai, B. and Good, R.A. Kaposi's sarcoma: a review and recent developments. Ca-A. Ca. J. Clinicians, 31(#1):2-12, 1982.

117. Salmon, D., Landre, M.F., Fraser, G.R., Buehler, S.K., Grunley, J., and Marshall, W.H. A familial aggregate of Hodgkin's disease, common variable immunodeficiency, and other malignancy cases in Newfoundland. II. Geneological analysis and conclusions regarding hereditary determinants. Clin. Inves. Med., 4:175, 1979.

118. Salimonu, L.S., Bryant, D.G., Buehler, S.K., Chandra, R.K., Grumley, J., and Marshall, W.H. Immunoglobulins in familial Hodgkin's disease and immunodeficiency in Newfoundland. Int. Arch. Allergy Appl. Imun., 63:52, 1980.

119. Samitz, M.H. Dermatologic gastrointestinal relationships. In: H.L. Bockus (ed.), Gastroenterology. pp. 426-473. Philadelphia, PA: W.B. Saunders, 1976.

120. Sawitsky, A., Bloom, D., and German, J. Chromosomal breakage and acute leukemia in congenital telangiectatic erythema and stunted growth. Ann. Int. Med., 65:487, 1966.

121. Schuelke, G.S., Lynch, H.T., Lynch, J.F., Chaperon, E.A., Recabaren, J.A., Grabner, B., and Albano, W.A. Cellular immune function study in an ovarian cancer-prone kindred. Br. J. Cancer, in press, 1982.

122. Schuelke, G.S., Lynch, H.T., Lynch, J.F., Fain, P.R., and Chaperon, E.A. Low serum IgA in a familial ovarian cancer aggregate. Cancer Gen. & Cytogen., 6:231, 1982.

123. Schwaber, J.F., Klein, G., Ernberg, I., Rosen, A., Lazanes, H., and Rosen, F.S. Deficiency of Epstein-Barr virus (EBV) receptors on B lymphocytes from certain patients with common variable agammaglobulinemia. J. Immunol., 124:2191, 1980.

124. Schwartz, R.S. Another look at immune surveillance. N. Engl. J. Med., 293:181, 1975.

125. Seeley, J.K., Sakamoto, K., Ip, S.H., Hansen, P.W. and Purtilo, D.T. Abnormal lymphocyte subsets in X-linked lymphoproliferative syndrome. J. Immunol., 127:2618, 1981.

126. Setlow, R.B. Repair deficient human disorders and cancer.
      Nature 271:713, 1978.
127. Shope T., Dechairo, D., and Miller, G. Malignant lymphoma
      in cotton-topped marmosets following inoculation of
      Epstein-Barr virus. Proc. Natl. Acad. Sci. USA,
      70:2487, 1973.
128. Shope, T.C., Khalifa, S., Smith, S.T., and Cushing, B.
      Epstein-Barr virus antibody in childhood Hodgkin's
      disease. Am. J. Dis. Child., 136:701, 1982.
129. Sinkovics, J.G., Trujillo, J.M., Pienta, R.J., and Ahern,
      M.J. Leukemagenesis stemming from autoimmune disease.
      In: Genetic Concepts and Neoplasia. A Collection of
      Papers Presented at the Twenty-Third Annual Symposium on
      Fundamental Cancer Research. pp. 138-190. Baltimore:
      Williams & Wilkins, 1970.
130. Sjogren, H. Zur kenntnis der keratoconjunctivities sicca
      (keratitis filiformis bei hypofunktion der tranendrusen).
      Acta. Oph., (Suppl) 2:1, 1933.
131. Smith, C.K., Cassidy, J.T., and Bole, G.G. Type I dysgam-
      maglobulinemia, systemic lupus erythematosus, and
      lymphoma. Am. J. Med., 48:113, 1970.
132. Spector, B.D., Perry, G.S. and Kersey, J.H. Genetically
      determined immunodeficiency diseases (GDID) and
      malignancy: report from the Immunodeficiency Cancer
      Registry. Clin. Immunol. Immunopath., 11:12, 1978.
133. Stein, M., Keller, S., and Schleifer, S. Role of the
      hypothalamus in mediating stress effects on the immune
      systems. In: B.A. Stoll (ed.), Mind and Cancer
      Prognosis. pp. 85-101. John Wiley & Sons, Ltd, 1979.
134. Stevens, D.A., O'Connor, G.T., Levine, P.H., and Rosen, R.B.
      Acute leukemia with "Burkitt's lymphoma cells" and
      Burkitt's lymphoma. Ann. Int. Med., 76:967, 1972.
135. Stiehm, E.R. The B lymphocyte system. In: E.R. Stiehm and
      V.A. Fulginiti (eds.), Immunologic Disorders in Infants
      and Children. 2nd edition, pp. 52-81. Philadelphia:
      W.B. Saunders, 1980.
136. Swift, M. Malignant disease in heterozygous carriers.
      Birth Defects, 12:133, 1976.
137. Swift, M. and Chase, C. Cancer in families with xeroderma
      pigmentosum. J. Natl. Cancer Inst., 62:1415, 1979.
138. Sullivan, J.L., Byron, K.S., Brewster, F.E., and Purtilo,
      D.T. Deficient natural killer cell activity in X-linked
      lymphoproliferative syndrome. Science, 210:543, 1980.
139. Svejgaard, A. HLA and disease. In: N.R. Rose and H.
      Friedman (eds.), Manual of Clinical Immunology. 2nd
      Edition, pp. 1049-1058. Washington, D.C.: American
      Society for Microbiology, 1980.
140. Tadjoedin, M.K. and Fraser, F.C. Heredity of ataxia
      telangiectasia (Louis-Bar syndrome). Am. J. Dis. Child.,
      110:64, 1965.

141. Talal, N. and Bunim, J.J. The development of malignant lymphoma in the course of Sjögren's syndrome. Am. J. Med., 36:529, 1964.

142. Templeton, A.C. and Dhru, D. Kaposi's sarcoma in half-brothers. Trop. Geogr. Med., 17:324, 1975.

143. The T and B cell malignancy study group. Statistical analysis of immunologic, clinical and histopathologic data on lymphoid malignancies in Japan. Japan J. Clin. Oncol., 11:15, 1981.

144. Thompson, E.A. Pedigree analysis of Hodgkin's disease in a Newfoundland genealogy. Ann. Hum. Genet., 45:279, 1981.

145. Torres, A., Martinez, F., Gomez, P., Gomez, C., Garcia. J.M., and Nunez-Roldan, A. Simultaneous Hodgkin's disease in three siblings with identical HLA genotype. Cancer, 46:838, 1980.

146. Vance, J.C. Immune system evaluation in genetic immunodeficiency diseases associated with malignancies. In: H.T. Lynch and R.M. Fusaro (eds.), Cancer-Associated Genodermatoses. pp. 300-365. New York: Van Nostrand Reinhold, 1982.

147. Wright, D.H. The epidemiology of Burkitt's tumors. Cancer Res., 27:2424, 1967.

148. Wolf, H., zur Hausen, H., and Becker, V. EB viral genomes in epithelial nasopharyngeal carcinoma cells. Nature New Biol., 244:245, 1973.

149. Zeligman, I. Kaposi's sarcoma in a father and son. Bull. Johns-Hopkins Hosp., 107:208, 1960.

CHROMOSOMAL DEFECTS AND THEIR ROLE IN LYMPHOMAGENESIS

Avery A. Sandberg

Roswell Park Memorial Institute

Buffalo, New York 14263

INTRODUCTION

The major thrust of this book, i.e., lymphoproliferative disorders in subjects rendered immunodeficient either through therapy or inheritance and, thus, more susceptible to infections with viruses (particularly Epstein-Barr virus, EBV), raises a number of crucial questions regarding the role of chromosomal changes at various stages of these complex events. An attempt will be made to relate known cytogenetic events and changes in lymphoma to their possible role in lymphomagenesis in immune deficiency disorders. The terms cytogenetic, chromosomal and karyotypic will be used interchangeably.

Cell Type and Lymphomagenesis

Lymphomagenesis is characterized by involvement of a number of different types of tissues and cells. Examination of the phenotypic characteristics of lymphoid cells usually reveals the cells to be of B, T or "common" cell origin, with each category having a number of possible subpopulations. Thus, the origin of lymphoproliferative disorders is usually expressed in terms of the cell type constituting the original precursor cell and a number of phenotypic manifestations, including such aspects as sheep erythrocyte rosette formation, surface immunologic markers, and enzymatic characteristics. The varied cellular background to lymphoproliferative neoplasias makes them both complex and interesting, for there is always the likelihood, as has been shown for a number of other diseases (6,12,17,18), that each neoplastic lesion, depending on its cellular origin, may be characterized by specific chromosomal changes, thus allowing not only application to

427

diagnosis, but also supplying basic information regarding lymphoma-genetic mechanisms. Moreover, B cells can be involved in neoplasia outside the realm of lymphoma, e.g., multiple myeloma. However, some myelomas may have cytoge-netic characteristics of frank lymphoma (12).

Mitogens and Karyotyping of Lymphoid Neoplasia

Determining differences in the types of lymphoid cells involved in neoplasia may raise practical problems. In those cases in which sufficient metaphases are not available for analysis, particularly in chronic lymphocytic leukemia (CLL), a mitogen specific for the cell type is required for karyotyping. Until a few years ago, only T cell mitogens were available for the study of human neoplasia, the most common being phytohemagglutinin (PHA). In recent years, mitogenic agents stimulating B cells (and some of them also T cells) have been introduced. Some of them may show specificity for subgroups of B cells, though this has not been established with certainty. A list of these mitogens is shown in Table 1. Still unknown is whether all types or only certain subtypes of B or T cells, particularly the former, are stimulated by the mitogens shown in Table 1. Also, there is no assurance that a mitogen stimulating normal B cells will be mitogenic for neoplastic B cells, particularly lymphoma cells. This aspect must be investigated rigorously to ascertain the type of cells (neoplastic or normal) being stimulated by the mitogens. For example, for many years CLL cells were stimulated with PHA and the karyotype in this disease was thus regarded as normal diploid. Obviously, the cells stimulated under these conditions were normal T cells (12). Once B cell mitogens were introduced, cytogenetic changes were found in most cases of CLL, including nonrandom, specific changes. The effect of these mitogens in various lymphomas, particularly those where metaphases are sparse or nil, requires further study. Even in those lymphomas in which meta-phases are plentiful, ascertainment as to whether the mitogens stimulate the neoplastic and/or normal lymphoid elements is

Table 1. Mitogens of Human Lymphocytes

Phytohemagglutinin (PHA) (T cells)
Leukoagglutinin (LA) (T cells)
Sodium metaperiodate (NaIO) (T cells)
Pokeweed mitogen (PWM) (T & B cells)
Protein A from Staph. aureus (STA) (B cells)
Calcium Ionophore (A 23187) (B & T cells)
Liposaccharide B from E. coli (LPS) (B cells)
Epstein-Barr virus (EBV) (B cells)

---

needed. Thus, a comparison can be made of the cytogenetic changes
with specific pathologic and clinical features.

EBV and Chromosome Changes

     To date, in vitro studies with the EB virus (EBV) have not
pointed to a specific or characteristic karyotypic change
resulting from infection of B cells with EBV. Thus, in cell
cultures obtained from lymphoid tissue, chromosome exchanges
leading to the formation of marker chromosomes, pseudodiploidy,
and an occasional dicentric chromosome were the most common.
Later, when the cells became polyploid, markers were more common.
Banding has revealed that these markers were of different origin.
In a study of hybrid clones derived from fused human lymphoblastoid cells and unique mouse fibroblastic cells grown under special
conditions, the findings suggested that the resident EBV genome
was closely associated with chromosome #14 and the presence of
this chromosome was sufficient for the maintenance and expression
of EBV infection in human lymphoblastoid cells (21). A few reports
indicate that effects may be produced by EBV on chromosomes #7 or
#14; generally, this has not been a universal experience and
except for usual changes (gaps, breaks and other disruptive
manifestations of chromosomal structure), the karyotypic changes
observed have been rather disappointing. The findings have not
deciphered the relation of the karyotypic changes observed in
Burkitt lymphoma (BL) having a strong association with EBV, and
the type of changes observed in vitro. This lack of specific
chromosome changes induced by EBV has been also true of established cell lines of B cell origin produced through infection with
EBV. However, the possibility remains that were appropriate cells
to be infected with EBV, such as those involved in BL and other
lymphomas, the karyotypic changes observed might be more specific
than those observed to date with other cell types.

     Chromosomal changes in infectious mononucleosis (IM), a
disease due to EBV, have been neither consistent nor specific,
though a study in depth utilizing a number of different time
schedules and mitogens, thus yielding observations on the chromosome changes in a number of different cell types, has not been
accomplished to date. In one study cells were examined after 2
and 24 hours (11) and others after incubation without PHA and
after 48 hrs with PHA. A total of 21 consecutive IM cases (7-32
yrs. in age) were studied 4-27 days after the onset of symptoms.
No karyotypic abnormalities were seen using a trypsin-Giemsa
banding procedure. On the other hand, in another study (20) on
blood cells obtained immediately after laboratory confirmation of
the diagnosis in 10 cases, definite chromosomal changes were found
in samples incubated (without a mitogen) for 24 and 72 hrs. The
authors stated that in addition to the changes typical of viral
infection (chromosome breakage and aberrations), a few cells were

consistently found to harbor a deleted #22 similar to a Ph1. This
finding has not been confirmed and its significance remains
unknown. Needed are studies at various times during the disease,
utilizing mitogens which stimulate B or T cells (shown in Table
1), unstimulated cells, and using appropriate banding techniques.

Bearing on this subject is the report by Abo et al. (1) of a
30-month-old Japanese boy who since the age of 1 year had chronic,
recurrent IM manifested by repeated episodes of severe cough. He
had high fever accompanied by marked lymphadenopathy and hepatosplenomegaly and high EBV antibody titers. Ultimately, the boy
developed a Burkitt-type lymphoma which was shown to have a
reciprocal translocation between chromosomes #10 and #17.
Apparently, this type of tumor differed from the usual type of
Burkitt's lymphoma in which the preponderant number of cases have
involvement of chromosome #8 and either chromosome #2, #14, or
#22. Thus, in my opinion, the chromosomal changes observed in
this particular case, though they are not of the same type as
those observed in BL, may be related to the EBV. The case is of
considerable interest, since it indicates that if EBV is related
to the causation of BL and if it was also responsible for the

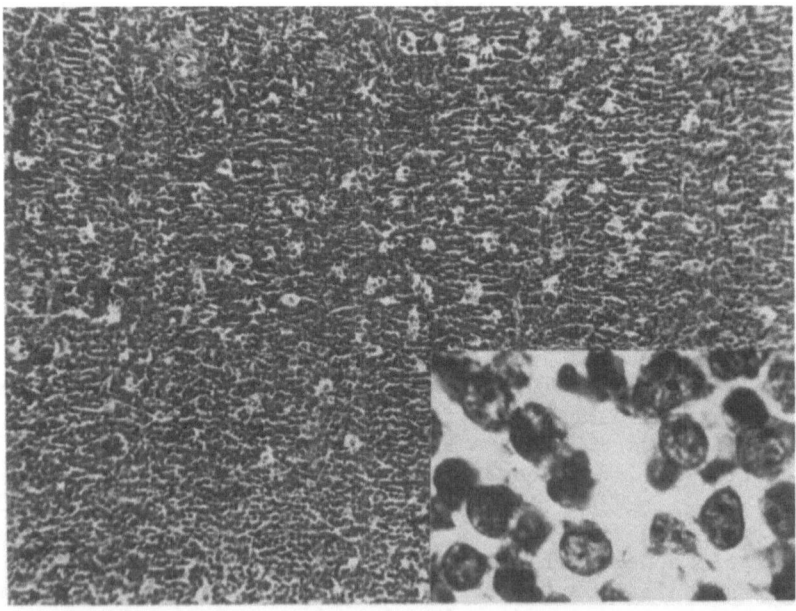

Fig. 1. Histologic and cytologic (inset) appearance of nonendemic
         Burkitt lymphoma (BL). The "starry night" pattern of
         the histology is typical of the endemic and nonendemic
         disease.

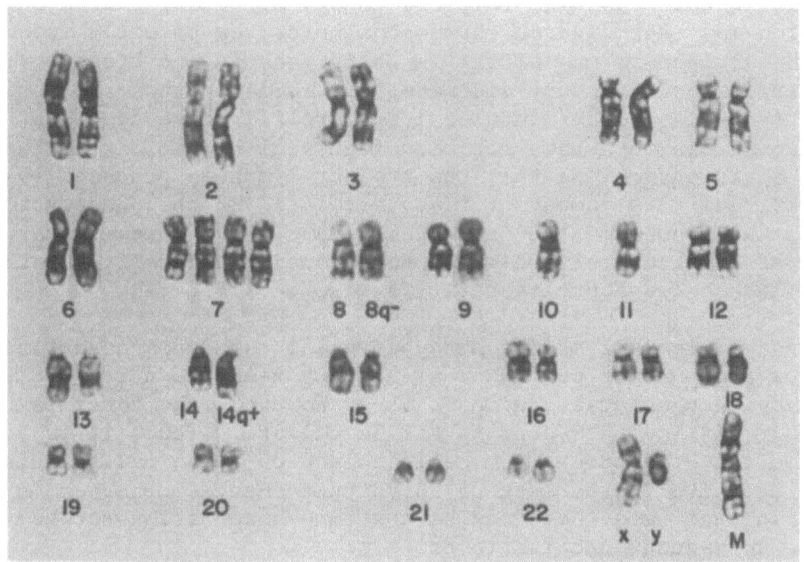

Fig. 2. Karyotype (G-banded) of a cell with 47 chromosomes of the BL tumor shown in Fig. 1. A t(8;14) is present; this karyotypic anomaly is present in the majority of BL, though variant translocations, i.e., 2;8 and 8;22 (see Fig. 4), are being described. Other changes, probably secondary, consist of +7,+7,-10,-11, and a marker (m). The possible origin of the marker is shown in Fig. 3.

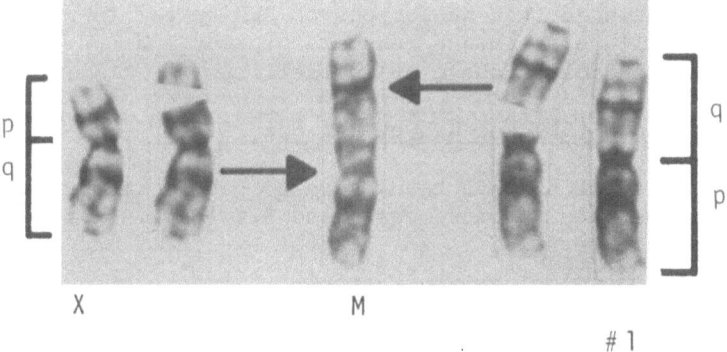

Fig. 3. Possible origin of the marker chromosome present in the BL shown in Figs. 1 and 2. The marker appears to have originated from the #1 and X chromosomes.

lymphoma in this Japanese boy, the tumors originating from such an infection may show diverse chromosomal pictures possibly indicative that lymphomas may differ in their genesis and biology. Also, in immunodeficiency diseases, particularly those X-linked, which predispose to EBV-induced lymphoproliferative diseases, the chromosomal findings have not been identical or similar to those of BL, again indicating that the type of lymphoma produced by EBV may vary, due to a number of factors related to the phenotypic and genetic background of the individuals involved. However, karyotyping of lymphoma cells has not been done on tumors from patients with X-linked lymphoproliferative syndrome (XLP).

Another example is the nasopharyngeal carcinoma associated with the presence of EBV DNA. It has not been shown to have the karyotype changes observed in BL (19), however, the tumor is extremely difficult to grow in tissue culture. Thus, it is possible that the progenitor cell in each of these malignancies may be decisive in the type of karyotypic changes observed, even though in each case there may be a strong association between EBV and the subsequent neoplastic process.

XLP (discussed elsewhere in this volume by Purtilo) is a disease wherein affected males fail to mount effective immune responses to EBV, with fatal IM, aplastic anemia, agammaglobulinemia or malignant lymphoma ensuing (2). An examination of the chromosome changes in lymphoblastoid cell lines and in PHA and PWM stimulated lymphocytes from males with XLP syndrome, their obligate carrier mothers and normal subjects, revealed increased non-specific changes (particularly in D-group chromosomes), including polyploidy, in the cell lines from cells of affected males and carrier females of the XLP syndrome as compared to those of controls. The sister chromatid exchange (SCE) levels in the cell lines were lower than in stimulated lymphocytes of XLP, the latter showing SCE levels similar to those of controls. Yet, the authors (2) concluded that phenotypes of XLP appear to arise chiefly from failure of immune responses to EBV and not from intrinsic chromosomal breakage or instability.

Burkitt's Lymphoma (BL) and Karyotypic Specificity

The majority of BL have been shown to have a reciprocal translocation between chromosomes #8 and #14 (Figs. 1-3). Other aspects of BL are reviewed in the chapter by Linder and Purtilo. However, more and more cases with variant translocations involving chromosomes #8 and #2 or #22 are being described (3,13,15). The crucial event in the genesis of Burkitt lymphoma is deletion of the long arm of chromosome #8 at band q24 (q24;13). The chromosome to which the material is translocated is either chromosome #14 (band q32), chromosome #2 (band p12) or chromosome #22 (band q12) (Fig. 4). The biological features do not differ significantly,

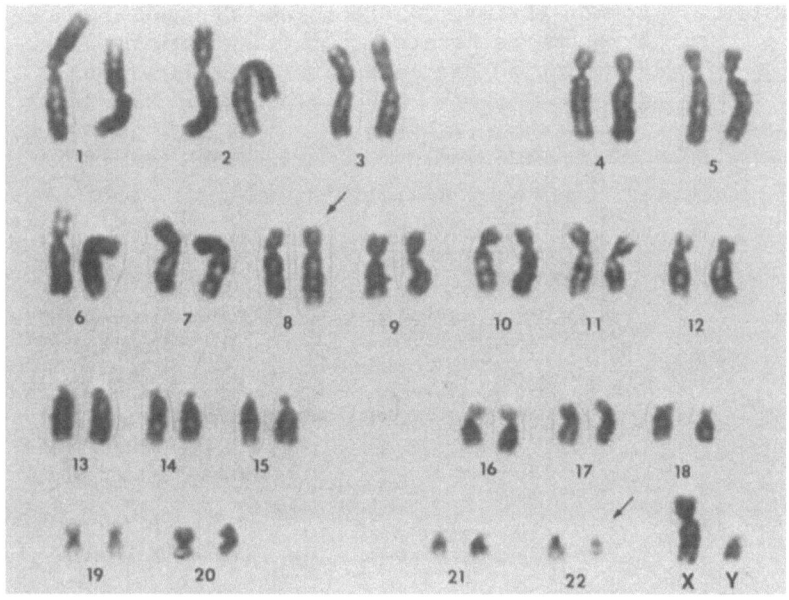

Fig. 4. Variant translocation in a Burkitt leukemia cell, i.e.,
t(8;22) (q24;q12). The break in #8 is the same as in
other translocations of BL involving this chromosome.

but phenotypic expression of the surface light chains (i.e.,
translocations involving chromosome #2 expressing kappa light
chains and those involving chromosome #22 lambda light chains,
exclusively) are governed by the specific rearrangements. These
observations pinpoint the location of genes for immunoglobulins
and serve to define the type of changes, both from a genetic and
biologic viewpoint, affecting such tumors. Changes other than the
typical translocations in BL are also present in a majority if not
in almost all cases of this cancer. Possibly these secondary
changes play a role in the biologic behavior of the tumors,
providing differences in the clinical pictures of endemic and
nonendemic BL, tumor spread, response to therapy, and survival of
the patients (14).

A number of BL, even though associated with karyotypic
changes, show no evidence of EBV infection, possibly indicating
that the virus _per se_ may not be responsible for the karyotypic
changes. Mechanisms other than infection with EBV may be responsible for the development of BL. This lack of association with
EBV is characteristic of non-endemic BL cases and might indicate
that EBV plays a secondary role in the causation of BL, at least
in non-endemic areas. Once lymphomagenesis occurs, the chromosomal changes appear to be the same in endemic as in nonendemic

Table 2. Common (Primary?) Chromosome Changes in Human
Lymphoma as Related to the New International
Formulation and Rappaport Classifications

Chromosome Change	International Formulation of Malignant Lymphomas	Rappaport Classification of Malignant Lymphomas
	Low Grade	
+12,14q+	A. <u>Small lymphocytic</u>	Well differentiated lympho-cytic, diffuse
	Consistent with CLL plasmacytoid	
t(14;18)	B. <u>Follicular, predominantly small cleaved cell</u>	Poorly differentited, lympho-cytic, nodular, diffuse
	Sclerosis	
t(14;18)	C. <u>Follicular, mixed, small cleaved and large cells</u>	Mixed, nodular
	Diffuse areas sclerosis	Mixed, nodular, diffuse
	Intermediate Grade	
t(14;18)	D. <u>Follicular, predominantly large Cell</u>	Histiocytic, nodular
	Diffuse areas Sclerosis	Histiocytic, nodular, diffuse
?	E. <u>Diffuse, small cleaved cell</u>	Poorly differentiated lympho-cytic, diffuse
	Sclerosis	
?t(12;14)	F. <u>Diffuse, mixed, small and large cell</u>	Mixed, diffuse
	Sclerosis Epithelioid cell component	Non-Hodgkin's lymphoma with epithelioid reaction
t(8;14) and ?t(11;14)	G. <u>Diffuse, large cell</u>	Histiocytic, diffuse
	Cleaved cell Non-cleaved cell Sclerosis	
	High Grade	
t(8;14),6q-	H. <u>Large cell, immunoblastic</u>	
	Plasmacytoid Clear cell	Histiocytic, diffuse
	Polymorphous Epithelioid cell component	Mixed, diffuse Non-Hodgkin's lymphoma with epithelioid reaction
?1q+,6q-,9q+	I. <u>Lymphoblastic</u>	Malignant lymphoma, lympho-blastic
	Convoluted cell Non-convoluted cell	Convoluted nuclei Non-convoluted nuclei
t(8;14),t(1;8),t(8;22)	J. <u>Small non-cleaved cell</u>	Undifferentiated
	Burkitt's	Undifferentiated, Burkitt's type
	Follicular areas	

BL. These chromosomal changes may be closely associated with the development of tumors. The key cytogenetic event in the karyotypic changes in BL appears to be the deletion of the long arm of chromosome #8, which may be the locus for BL development. One view is that activation of an oncogene at this site might cause the cell to proliferate.

Cytogenetic Changes in Non-Burkitt Lymphoma

Cytogenetic information regarding lymphomas developing in patients with immunodeficiency and EBV infection or cases developing secondarily to chemo- and/or radiotherapy is scarce. Hanto et al. describe evidence elsewhere in this volume that conversion from polyclonal to monoclonal B cell proliferation in renal transplant recipients is associated with cytogenetic errors in the cells containing EBV. Will the chromosomal picture relate to the EBV infection or to the type of lymphoma? I would predict that the latter is more likely, though secondary leukemia under similar circumstances has shown karyotypic changes which in many cases are different from those seen in de novo acute leukemias.

The karyotypic findings in other forms of lymphoma (i.e., non-Burkitt lymphomas) have not been established with the precision and characteristics of BL. Pathologists have not agreed on a uniform system for classifying the lymphomas, thus often making correlations with karyotypic findings difficult. However, recent attempts at bringing the classification of non-Burkitt lymphomas into a homogeneous system (9) have led to definite correlations. Possibly the chromosome findings may be more specific for characterizing a lymphoma. Karyotypes may provide more information than most of the other phenotypic parameters. Furthermore, as shown in Table 2, correlations between the karyotypic changes, the type of lymphoma and phenotypic characteristics are already appearing; there is little doubt that ultimately detailed correlations will reveal specificity for the cytogenetic findings in lymphoma, akin acute and chronic leukemias (12).

Table 3. Translocations Involving Chromosome
#14 In Non-Burkitt Lymphoma

t(1;14)(q23;q32)
t(8;14)(q22;q32)
t(10;14)(q24;q32)
t(11;14)(q13;q32)
t(12;14)(q13;q32)
t(14;14)(q24;q32)
t(14;18)(q32;q21)
t(Y;14)(q12;q24?)

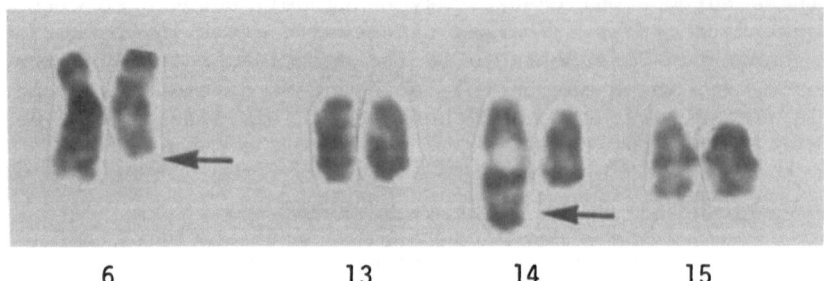

Fig. 5. Partial karyotype of a cell from a hairy cell leukemia
indicating the possible relationship of this disease to
lymphoma, particularly of the B cell variety, based on
the presence of 2 of the most common chromosome changes
in lymphoma, i.e., 6q- and 14q+.

The 14q+ and 6q- Anomalies in Lymphoma

Outstanding among the changes in lymphoma is the presence of
the 14q+ anomaly. The band involved is very similar in most cases
(12). However, the donor chromosome involved, when it can be
identified or when present, has shown considerable variability
(Table 3). This variability has to be sorted out as uniform
morphologic classifications of lymphomas are developed. Certain
lymphomas are more often than not involved by a translocation between chromosomes #14 and #8 or between #11 and #14. Several other
lymphomas may have different types of translocations not involving
#14 or the other chromosomes. Why is chromosome #14 a common
recipient chromosome among these lymphomas? Band q32 on #14 is
vulnerable to breakage and reunion with material involved in
reciprocal and non-reciprocal translocations. This site contains
the locus which codes for heavy chains of immunoglobulin. It seems
that the behavior of the genetic material translocated to or
becoming contiguous with #14 assumes a major role in the genesis
of lymphoma. The secondary karyotypic changes, as pointed out for
BL, may possibly play a major role in the biologic behavior of the
tumors (14). Thus, chromosome analysis in every case of lymphoma
may ultimately reveal that a specific cytogenetic change affects
each specific type of lymphoma (Fig. 5).

A rather common change in lymphoma is deletion of the long arm
of chromosome #6 (6q-), originally described by us in acute
lymphoblastic leukemia (ALL) (12). It is one of the most common
changes in lymphoma, though its biologic and clinical significance
is yet to be determined. ALL with 6q- carries a relatively good
prognosis. Do lymphomas in which the 6q- anomaly is found show
good prognoses? Other common changes in lymphoma are shown in

Table 4, though their exact significance remains to be determined. In my opinion these changes play an important role in the biologic behavior of the tumors (12) including spread, response to therapy and/or radiation, and ultimately in the prognosis.

Chromosome Changes in Chronic Lymphocytic Leukemia (CLL)

Chronic lymphocytic leukemia (CLL) shows informational gaps as compared to other leukemias and lymphomas regarding cytogenetic characteristics. In the Western world, CLL is preponderantly a B cell disease. The introduction of mitogens for B cells has allowed karyotyping of CLL cells. It appears that trisomy #12 (+12) is the most common anomaly in CLL, followed by 14q+ (15). Involvement of chromosome #12 has been ascribed by Gahrton et al. (7) to be a key event in development of lymphoproliferative disorders. Incidentally, +12 is a common anomaly in some forms of lymphoma, possibly indicating that CLL is akin to some lymphomas. Recently, prognostic aspects have been ascribed to trisomy 12 in CLL (15), though undoubtedly many more cases will have to be examined before this is established with certainty. The phenotypic manifestations, particularly at the cellular level, of the trisomy 12 are also being investigated (15). In addition, the possibility has been raised that segment q13 to q22 on chromosome #12 carries important genes that are duplicated in those lymphoproliferative disorders characterized by trisomy of the chromosome (7).

Karyotypic Changes in T Cell Lymphoma

A cytogenetic definition of T cell lymphomas has not reached the same level of information as that of B cell malignancies. The cytogenetic findings in T cell cancers have been obtained primarily on cells from cutaneous T cell lymphomas and T cell CLL (4,8,10). In the latter, 14q+ has been found in a few cases, and an occasional T cell lymphoma. However, generally the karyotypic changes in T cell disorders are complex. No specific or non-

Table 4.   Common Karyotypic Changes
in Malignant Lymphomas

14q+
Del(1)
Del(3)
Del(6)
+18
Del(18)
Del(8)
+7

random changes characterizing an entity within this group of
diseases has emerged.

Lymphomas of T cell origin may have the 14q+ anomaly, though
in most cases the origin of the extra material is unknown. In any
case, the 14q+ anomaly characterizes a wide range of cells in the
lymphoid system, even though phenotypically the cells may differ
in their characteristics. The 6q- anomaly was also found in
several cutaneous T cell lymphomas (10), again pointing to a
sharing of karyotypic similarities by lymphoid disorders of
different cellular origin. Noteworthy, T cell lymphomas have not
yet been reported in immunodeficient subjects, however, T cell ALL
has been described in patients with ataxia telangiectasia (AT).

Karyotypic Hypothesis of Lymphomagenesis (and Oncogenesis)

DNA rearrangement, rather than point mutation, is an emerging
explanation for carcinogenesis, at least in some forms of cancer
(5,16), even though there is no direct evidence supporting this
hypothesis. However, Bloom's syndrome, a disorder of spontaneous
chromosomal rearrangements is associated with a very high rate of
cancer, thus indicating that genetic rearrangements at the
chromosomal level rather than chemical mutagens may be a cause of
some human cancers. Even though the cancer incidence is significantly increased in Bloom's syndrome and similar disorders, it is
so only at specific organ sites, which are often not the most
common sites for cancer in the general population in the age range
of these patients. However, in Bloom's syndrome and ataxia
telangiectasia (AT), DNA rearrangement could be implicated as a
possible cause of the malignancy, particularly of the lymphoid
variety. In AT translocation involving chromosome 14 at a band
different from that seen in lymphoma may predispose the individuals to certain lymphoproliferative malignancies. The role played
by the compromised immunologic system in AT patients in the
development and behavior of lymphoid malignancies remains to be
established. Also, the significance of specific karyotypic changes
in the non-neoplastic and neoplastic cells needs clarification in
this condition (12). Translocations observed in lymphoma may by
themselves lead to rearrangements of DNA which per se may be
responsible for the development of the malignancy or at least the
biologic manifestations of the disorder (Fig. 6). Changes in DNA
function, possibly leading to lymphoma development, through mechanisms such as oncogene activation or mutagenic susceptibility, may
result from events including trisomy 12 in CLL; the presence of
extra material on chromosome #14 at band 32 in BL; and deletion of
the long arm of chromosome #6 (6q-) in lymphoma. Inherent in each
one of these mechanisms is an expression of DNA function in the
direction of neoplasia of the lymphoid system. Possibly, some
specificity is manifested by the karyotypic changes in various
types of lymphoid cells.

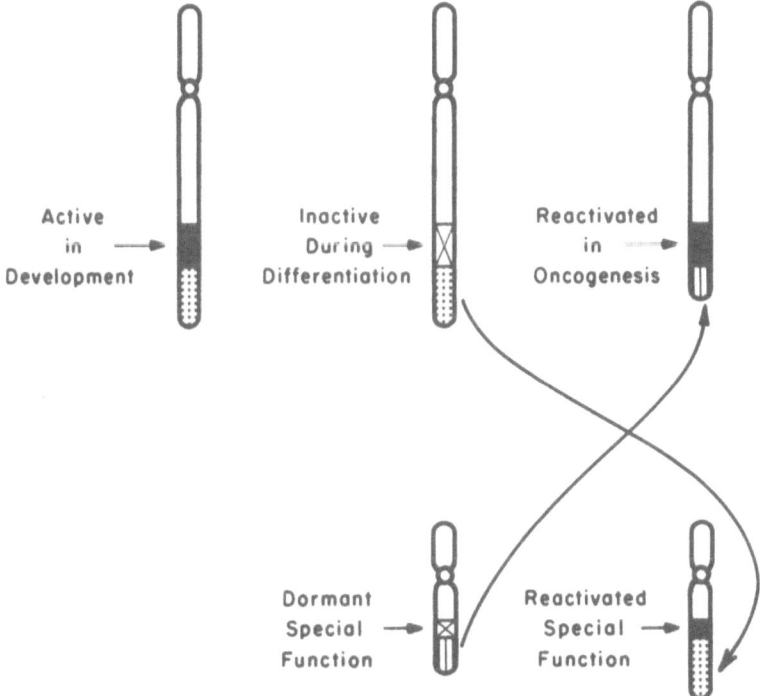

Fig. 6. Schematic presentation of possible chromosome alterations leading to oncogenesis. A region active genetically during embryogenesis is shown in black and the future translocation is stippled. The genes active in development becomes inactive during the differentiated life. However, when a translocation takes place, the genes contiguous with the inactivated segment of the larger chromosome assumes functions it had during embryogenesis. Conversely, a segment of the smaller chromosome contiguous with the chromosome translocated to the larger one, allows the specialized function to be expressed, i.e., ACTH synthesis by lung or other cancers. A similar result may occur when a chromosome is deleted in toto or in part or acquires extra material without obvious translocation.

SUMMARY AND CONCLUSION

I have discussed some chromosome changes implicated in lymphomagenesis. Certain lymphomas and CLL are characterized by karyotypic changes which can be considered specific, if not characteristic, for each particular lymphoid cancers (20). Undoubtedly, as information is obtained, the specificity and significance of these chromosomal changes will be established.

Shown in Table 2 are specific chromosomal abnormalities
correlated with specific histopathologic types of non-Hodgkin's
lymphomas.

Many lymphomas to date have not been characterized by specific
translocations or non-random chromosomal changes. Thus, it is
possible that the nature and genesis of these lymphomas may reside
in factors not identical or similar to those of lymphomas which are
characterized thus far by karyotypic changes. Cytogenetic studies
in lymphoma remain a challenge and offer a fruitful field in which
correlations between chromosomal changes and histological, immunologic, enzymatic, and other phenotypic characteristics, and
prognosis will reveal the significance of these changes. Thus,
etiologic factors involved in the genesis of these malignancies
will be further understood.

ACKNOWLEDGEMENTS

    This work was supported in part by grants CA-14555 and CA-
28853 from the National Cancer Institute.

REFERENCES

1. Abo, W., Kamada, M., Motoya, T., Imamura, M., Motoya, T.,
        Iwanga, M., Aya, T., Yano, S., Nakao, T., Osato, T.
        Evolution of infectious mononucleosis into Epstein-Barr
        virus-carrying monoclonal malignant lymphoma. Lancet,
        1:1272, 1982.
2. Barnabei, V.M., Sakamoto, K., Seeley, J.K., and Purtilo,
        D.T. Chromosomal breakage and sister chromatid exchange
        in peripheral blood lymphocytes and lymphoblastoid cell
        lines in the X-linked lymphoproliferative syndrome.
        Cancer Genet. & Cytogenet., 6:313, 1982.
3. Berger, R. and Bernheim, A. Cytogenetic studies on
        Burkitt's lymphoma-leukemia. Cancer Genet. &
        Cytogenet., 1:231, 1982.
4. Edelson, E.L., Berger, C.L., Raafat, J., and Warburton, D.
        Karyotype studies of cutaneous T cell lymphoma: evidence
        for clonal origin. J. Invest. Dermatol., 73:548, 1979.
5. Feinberg, A.P. and Coffey, D.S. Organ site specificity for
        cancer in chromosomal instability disorders. Cancer
        Res., 42:3252, 1982.
6. First International Workshop on Chromosomes in Leukaemia,
        1977. Chromosomes in acute non-lymphocytic leukaemia.
        Br. J. Haematol., 39:311, 1978.
7. Gahrton, C., Robert, K.-H., Friberg, K., Juliusson, G.,
        Biberfeld, P., and Zech, L. Cytogenetic mapping of the
        duplicated segment of chromosome 12 in lymphoprolifera-
        tive disorders. Nature, 297:513, 1982.

8. Liang, J.C., Gaulden, M.E., and Herndon, J.H. Chromosome
       markers and evidence for clone formation in lymphocytes
       of a patient with Sezary syndrome. Cancer Res.,
       40:3426, 1980.

9. National Cancer Institute sponsored study of classifications
       of non-Hodgkin's lymphomas. Summary and description of
       a working formulation for clinical usage. The
       non-Hodgkin's lymphoma pathologic classification project.
       Cancer, 49:2112, 1982.

10. Nowell, P.C., Finan, J.B., and Vonderheid, E.C. Clonal
       characteristics of T cell lymphomas: cytogenetic evidence
       from blood, lymph nodes, and skin. J. Invest.
       Dermatol., 78:69, 1982.

11. Philip, P., Ernst, P., and Wantzin, G.L. Karyotypes in
       infectious mononucleosis. Scand. J. Haematol., 15:201,
       1975.

12. Sandberg, A.A. The Chromosomes in Human Cancer and Leukemia,
       pp. 776. New York: Elsevier North-Holland, Inc., 1980.

13. Sandberg, A.A. Chromosome changes in the lymphomas. Human
       Pathol., 12:531, 1981.

14. Sandberg, A.A. Chromosomal changes in human cancer:
       specificity and heterogeneity. In: A.H. Owens, Jr.,
       P.S. Coffey and S.B. Baylin (eds.), Tumor Cell
       Heterogeneity: Origins and Implications. Vol. 4. New
       York: Academic Press, 1982.

15. Sandberg, A.A. Cytogenetic abnormalities in lymphoid
       neoplasia. In: I.T. Magrath and B. Ramot (eds.),
       Influence of the Environment on Leukemia and Lymphoma
       Subtypes. New York: Raven Press, 1982.

16. Sandberg, A.A. Perspectives in cytogenetics on human
       lymphomas and solid tumors. In: S. Tura (ed.), 2nd
       International Course on Theoretical and Practical
       Aspects of Oncologic Cytogenetics, 1982.

17. The Second International Workshop on Chromosomes in
       Leukemia, 1979. Cancer Genet. & Cytogenet., 2:89, 1980.

18. The Third International Workshop on Chromosomes in Leukemia,
       1980. Cancer Genet. & Cytogenet., 4:95, 1981.

19. Utsumi, K.R., Yoshida, T.A. A chromosome survey on tissue
       culture cells derived from nasopharyngeal cancer. Gann,
       10:291, 1971.

20. Watt, J.L., Page, B.M., and Davidson, R.J.L. Cytogenetic
       study of 10 cases of infectious mononucleosis. Clin.
       Genet., 12:267, 1977.

21. Yamamoto, K., Mizuno, F., Matsuo, T., Tanaka, A., Nonoyama,
       M., and Osato, T. Epstein-Barr virus and human
       chromosomes: close association of the resident viral
       genome and the expression of the virus-determined
       nuclear antigen (EBNA) with the presence of chromosome
       14 in human/mouse hybrid cells. Proc. Natl. Acad. Sci.
       USA, 75:5155, 1978.

22.   Yunis, J.J., Oken, M.M., Kaplan, M.E., Ensrud, K.M, Howe
      R.R., and Theologides, A. Distinctive chromosomal
      abnormalities in histologic subtypes of non-Hodgkin's
      lymphoma. N. Engl. J. Med., 307:1231, 1982.

INTERFERON THERAPY IN HERPES VIRUS INFECTIONS

Milan Fiala and
Satya N. Chatterjee

Department of Surgery
University of California
Davis, CA

INTRODUCTION

Interferon (IFN's) are a family of proteins secreted by
vertebrate cells antigenic or mitogenic stimulation, or stimulation by synthetic compounds, intracellular infection, microbial
polysaccharides, or endotoxins. They show broad, partially
species-specific antiviral activity by inducing certain cellular
enzymes. Additionally, IFN exerts many regulatory functions (1).

The three types of IFN are:

1) IFN-alpha species are produced in leukocytes on induction
by viruses, double-stranded RNA, synthetic polymers, microbial
polysaccharides or endotoxin, or by simple molecules such as
substituted pyrimidines. IFN-alpha species are relatively stable
to pH 2 and heat. IFN-alpha preparations include a dozen of
species each with 165 or 166 amino acids. At least 10 genes of
IFN-alpha with 85-95% sequence homology are known (2). The
primary structure of natural IFN-alpha species lacks ten
COOH-terminal amino acids as is suggested by their DNA gene
sequence. The molecular weight (MW) was determined by
SDS-acrylamide gel electrophoresis at 18,000-20,000 daltons,
however, multimeric forms are found. Natural human IFN species
are glycoproteins (glycosylation is more extensive with IFN beta
than IFN alpha) but recombinant molecules lack the sugar moiety
although the biological activities are preserved.

2) IFN-beta is produced in fibroblasts on stimulation by
viruses and other inducers as is IFN-alpha. IFN-beta is coded by

a single gene (IFN-betal) which shares about 30% DNA sequence
homology with the IFN alpha genes. Its MW is estimated between
20,000 and 26,000 (3).

3) IFN-gamma is produced either by T lymphocytes on antigenic
stimulation or by T or B lymphocytes on mitogenic stimulation. It
is pH 2 and heat-labile and its MW is estimated at 20,000 or
25,000 (4). IFN gamma cDNA has been cloned and expressed. The
nucleotide sequence indicates its composition of 146 amino acids
with MW of 17,000 (5).

Regulatory Functions of Interferons

In addition to antiviral properties, IFN exerts regulatory
functions (1) including growth inhibition (6), effects on cellular
differentiation, cell surface, and immune functions including
stimulation or inhibition of antibody formation (7), in vitro
stimulation (8) but in vivo depression (9) of NK cell activity and
in vitro and in vivo enhancement of monocyte function (8,9). The
effects on NK cell function in patients depends on the time of
sampling with increased activity at 24 hours following the
injection (10). Interferon suppresses antibody production, if
given before the antigenic challenge, but enhances antibody
production if administered after the challenge (11). Interferon
also enhances phagocytosis in vivo.

Antiviral Properties - Pre-Clinical Studies

Leukocyte-derived IFN alpha (and more recently, recombinant
IFN-alpha subtypes) have been tested in cell culture and animals
regarding their relative antiviral activity. In tissue cell
culture, herpes simplex Type 2 virus (HSV-2) was more sensitive
and herpes simplex Type 1 virus (HSV-1) less sensitive than
vesicular stomatitis virus to the three interferon types, alpha,
beta, and gamma (12). IFN-alpha subtype AD was more active in
mice against encephalomyocarditis virus than subtype D. The
activity occurred only when IFN-alpha was administered before the
infection, not after (13). Because the currently available
antiviral therapy in man frequently falls short of expectations
(14), interferon has been tested in combination with Acyclovir®.
This combination was synergistic on HSV (15) and cytomegalovirus
(CMV) (16). In man a combined regimen with adenine arabinoside
has been used successfully in hepatitis B virus infection (17).
In rabbit IFN-alpha-suppressed epithelial damage from HSV-1
keratitis when given topically one day before or two days after
the infection at a daily dose of 5×10^5 U per eye (18).

Whether prolonged antiviral therapy can eradicate HSV latency
has been studied in several model systems. A rabbit ocular model
has been a reliable indicator of drug efficacy in the treatment of

human keratitis. Polyinosinic polycytidylic acid administered topically to rabbits with recurrent ocular infection decreased virus isolation rate (19), but only during its administration. Acyclovir® and interferon prevent reactivation of HSV in animals (20) and in explanted mouse sensory ganglia (21). However, they have not eradicated the latent infection during the quiescent phase. Defects in cell-mediated immunity are considered a key to

Table 1. Clinical Studies on Systemic Interferon
in Herpes Virus Infections

IFN*Dose	Treatment duration	Patient population	Targeted viruses	Clinical results	
equivalent to 35 x 10^{6}U	8 days or longer	Herpes zoster in in cancer patients	VZV ref. 29	Progression (1°derm)^{xx} PL 3.9 days (50%) IFN 1.6 days (31%) ***Visceral compl. PL 6/45 IFN 1/45	Dissemination 3.6 days 0.0 days postherpetic pain PL 5/14
2.5 x 10^5/kg bid	2 days	Herpes zoster in cancer patients	VZV ref. 30	Progression (1°derm)^{xx} N.S.	Dissemination PL 5/15 IFN 1/17
Equivalent to a) 3 to 14x10^{6}U b) 21 x 10^{6}U I.M. daily (q 12 hr)	3-11 days	Children with cancer and varicella (therapy)	VZV ref. 27	New lesions (days) PL* 5.3 IFN 3.8	Mortality or life threatenting disseminating PL 6/21
5 x 10^5 U/kg day	5 days	Monkeys during epizootic (prophlaxis)	VZV ref. 28	Attack rate PL 8/13 IFN 2/14	
15-42 x 10^6 U/day	2-29 days	Bone marrow transplant recipients	CMV pneumonia ref. 35	All 8 patients died No toxicity to granulocyte progenitor cells	
1.5 x 10^6 U/day	21 days	6 y/o boy with fatal lympho-proliferation	EBV ref. 40	IFN-inducible chromosomal defect Reduced NK cells Reduced T gamma cells	
1 x 10^6 U/day	21 days	3 y/o girl with adenopathy, hepatospleno-megaly, pannicu-litis	EBV Hirsch 1982	Resolution of adenopathy, fever, panniculitis	
3 x 10^6 2x/wk	8 wks	Renal transplant recipients (RT)	CMV (EBV, HSV) ref. 33	Viremia: IFN 5/11 Placebo 9/10	
3 x 10^6 2x/wk	8 wks	RT	EBV ref. 41	EBV excretion decreased	
3 x 10^6 3x/wk plus 3 x 10^6 2x/wk	6 wks plus 8 wks	RT	CMV (EBV, HSV) ref. 34	CMV syndrome: IFN 1/20 Placebo 7/20	
about 5 x 10^6	5 days	Surgical patients for decompression of trigeminal sensory root	HSV ref. 24	Throat wash: PL 42% HSV IFN 9% HSV	

*PL = placebo; IFN = interferon
**1° derm. = primary dermatome (% area of)
***Visceral compl. = visceral complications such as pneumonia, hepatitis, D.I.C. etc.
N.S. = not signficant

reactivation of HSV. Defective IFN-gamma production by lymphocytes may predict more frequent recurrences of herpes labialis
(22). The combination therapy with IFN-alpha and gamma may
simulate physiological mechanisms (23).

Clinical Studies with Interferon

Leukocyte-derived IFN-alpha has been tested to some degree in
all herpesvirus infections of man (Table 1):

1. **Herpes labialis and genitalis**: Interferon was administered to patients operated on for trigeminal neuralgia by decom-
pression of the trigeminal sensory root. The frequency of
reactivation as measured by lesions or positive throat cultures
was reduced (24). Interferon administered at a low dose to
patients with initial herpes genitalis may have an effect on virus
shedding and time to healing.

Topical IFN-alpha accelerates healing and shortens HSV
shedding when given after debridement or in combination with
triflurothymidine in acute herpetic keratitis. Interferon
preparation with 30×10^6 U/ml was significantly better than one
with 1×10^6 U/ml in reducing healing time to 2.9 days compared to
5.3 days (25). Human IFN-beta has been used for this indication
with equal success as IFN-alpha (26).

2. **Varicella**: Higher dose (3.5×10^5 U per kg) was more
effective than a lower dose ($0.4 - 2.5 \times 10^5$ U per kg) in termi-
nating new lesions and preventing life-threatening dissemination
(27). Interferon will probably be effective in the prophylaxis of
varicella in immunodeficient patients, even late in the incubation
period, as prophylaxis has been accomplished during an epidemic in
a monkey colony (28).

3. **Herpes zoster**: Only the higher dose (5.1×10^5 U per kg),
not the lower dose (1.7×10^5 U per kg) was effective in reducing
the progression of zoster in primary dermatome and cutaneous
dissemination. Both doses reduced the frequency and intensity of
post-herpetic neuralgia (29). Corollary to this study was an
abbreviated trial (2 days compared to 5-7 days in the previous
study) in which viral dissemination was reduced but progression
in the primary dermatome was noted (30). Possibly the virus
contained in leukocytes during the viremic phase is unusually
susceptible to even a low dose of interferon. Antiviral therapy
of CMV infection with Acyclovir® was efficacious when administered
in the stage of viremia, but not on an established organ infection
such as CMV pneumonia (32). Perhaps it should not be surprising
that the large doses (36×10^6 U per day) of interferon are
required systemically, since in the human body this dose provided
only a minute fraction of interferon unit per cell. In the

vesicle fluid several thousand units of interferon are present when dissemination is arrested (31).

4) <u>Cytomegalovirus infections</u>: IFN-alpha has been used for the prophylaxis of CMV infections after renal and bone marrow transplantation and in isolated cases for the therapy of CMV pneumonia. In a prophylactic study of renal transplant recipients receiving azathioprine and prednisone, interferon was administered at a dose of 3×10^6 U twice weekly for 6 weeks. Serum levels reached 17-200 U per ml 4-12 hours after administration. The drug delayed CMV excretion and reduced the incidence of viremia. The positive effect was not seen in the group receiving additional immunosuppression with antithymocyte globulin (33). When the duration of therapy was extended to 14 weeks, and the dose raised to 3 million U three times a week, a significant reduction in the incidence of CMV syndrome was observed, in addition to the reduction of viremia (34).

Interferon, used prophylactically in bone marrow transplant recipients in doses up to 20×10^6 U does not appear to be as efficient as in the renal transplant population, but has been surprisingly well tolerated during bone marrow engraftment. Use of IFN in treating CMV pneumonia has been disappointing (35). Leukocyte interferon may transiently depress CMV excretion in urine of patient with congenitally acquired CMV or with CMV retinitis related to cancer or acquired immunodeficiency syndrome (AIDS) in homosexual patients. Long-term clinical benefits of such treatment are not clear (36).

Another potential indication for the use of interferon is the AIDS of homosexuals, possibly related to CMV or another virus with immunosuppressive effects. Recently, a defect in the <u>in vitro</u> production of interferon by mononuclear cells upon stimulation with HSV has been described as the earliest sign of immunodeficiency, differentiating between patients with the defect who develop opportunistic infections and those without the defect who may develop Kaposi's sarcoma (37).

5) <u>Epstein-Barr virus (EBV)</u>: Since interferon inhibits the outgrowth of EBV-infected lymphocytes <u>in vitro</u> (38), it may limit EBV-induced lymphoproliferation <u>in vivo</u>.

Therapeutic strategies are likely to differ according to whether the patient is immunodeficient or immunologically normal. In immunodeficient individuals, current therapy with immune gammaglobulin, immune plasma and Acyclovir® has not been effective (14) and in one patient, monoclonal B-cell lymphoma developed during the therapy (39). Hanto describes this case in a renal transplant recipient elsewhere in this book. Interferon could be useful as suggested by resolution of fever, subcutaneous nodules,

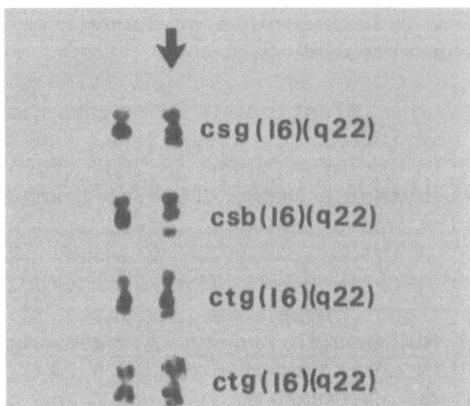

Fig. 1. Karyotype of peripheral blood leukocyte. Chromosome
         16 (arrow) developed a breakpoint when interferon was
         added to culture media. (From: Thestrup-Pederson,
         K. et al. Epstein-Barr virus-induced lymphoproliferative
         disorder converting to fatal Burkitt-like lymphoma in
         a boy with interferon-inducible chromosomal defect.
         Lancet, ii:997, 1980.)

lymphadenopathy, and hepatomegaly in a child with EBV infection
during interferon therapy (Hirsch, M., personal communication).
In another study, interferon was administered to a child with
EBV-induced lymphoproliferative disorder. This patient developed
a defect in the long arm of the chromosome in pair #16 (Figure 1)
during the therapy but the disease progressed to lymphoma. This
patient had low NK cell activity which was not increased by
interferon (40).

     In renal transplant recipients, EBV is an important pathogen,
especially in patients receiving anti-thymocyte globulin.
Elsewhere in this monograph Hanto summarizes EBV-induced lymphoproliferative diseases in renal transplant recipients. Interferon
reduced virus shedding in the throat but had no effect on EBV EA
(R) antibody responses (41). Circulating interferon levels have
been measured at as high as 640 U/ml in a study of bone-marrow
transplant patients (42) whereas, in renal transplant recipients
no interferon was detected (43).

Toxicity of Interferon

     IFN-alpha prepared in leukocytes by induction with Sendai
virus, as described by Cantell (44), has been the standard drug in
most clinical studies before 1982. In the near future, inter-

ferons produced by recombinant DNA techniques will be introduced
into experimental antiviral therapy. Preliminary results in
cancer studies with IFN-alpha clone A produced in E. coli have
been published (45).

1) Toxicities of IFN-alpha (Cantell's leukocyte-derived):

    a) Influenza-like symptoms, headache, malaise, fever,
        chills, fatigue, myalgia, backache and arthralgia, have
        an onset 4 hours after the injection, peak at 8 hours
        and wane after 10 hours (46). In the course of long-
        term administration, fever greater than 38.3°C occurred
        mainly during the first 3 days and after the 7th day
        patients were generally afebrile (47).

    b) The neutrophil count and the total WBC count were
        depressed 24 hours after the injection, whereas, at 8
        hours, the lymphocyte count fell (46). In a long-term
        study hematological toxicity occurred in most patients;
        leukopenia (to $1300/mm^3$) and granulocytopenia (to
        $585/mm^3$) were most pronounced in the first 4 weeks (47).

    c) Fatigue, loss of appetite, and weight loss were more
        frequent with higher doses.

    d) A child with EBV-induced lymphoproliferative disorder had
        abnormal chromosomal fragility (Figure 1) on exposure to
        interferon in vivo and in vitro (40) but IFN-alpha does
        not seem to have such an effect in general (Thestrup-
        Pedersen, K., personal communication) and neither has
        IFN-beta (48).

    e) At least one male with malignancy procreated a child
        while on long-term treatment. The child was normal
        (Strander, H., personal communication).

    f) Reversible increases in SGOT levels occurred frequently.
        Also, hepatic cytochrome p450 is depressed by interferons
        with antiviral activity.

2) Toxicities of IFN-alpha clone A:

The side effects were similar, but not identical, to IFN-
alpha (45). Fatigue was dose-dependent and dose-limiting. In a
few patients, paresthesias and numbness were dose-limiting.
Gastrointestinal side-effects were encountered at high dose
levels. The influenza-like symptoms were more severe at higher
doses and attenuated after the first week. Hematological toxicity
included leukopenia, relative lymphocytosis and absolute neutropenia but was not dose-limiting, and was rapidly reversible on

discontinuation of interferon. Increased SGOT was encountered
only rarely, as compared to daily administration of IFN-alpha.

Antibody IFN-alpha clone A was detected following therapy in
one quarter of the patients (45). Interferon antibodies have also
been detected in patients receiving fibroblast IFN-beta (49),
patients treated with Cantell's IFN-alpha, in a patient with
systemic lupus erythematosus (50), as well as in some sera
obtained before therapy. No untoward side-effects of IFN-alpha
antibodies have been noticed.

Pharmacokinetics of Interferons

1) Cantell's IFN-alpha is well absorbed after intramuscular
administration of a dose of 3×10^6U resulting in peak serum
levels of 65 to 133 U/ml. No accumulation of interferon occurred
over 5 weeks. The half-life of elimination was 7.3 hours (47).
After intravenous injection into rats and monkeys IFN-alpha was
found in the mitochondrial lysosomal fraction together with two
types of inactivating enzymes. No interferon was found in the
urine (51). 2) Recombinant IFN-alpha clone A - The time of
maximum observed serum concentrations was 4.6 hours after 3
million units intramuscularly and 6.1 hours after 72 million
units. The half-life of elimination was 4.6 hours after 3 mill U
and 6.1 hours at 72 mill U given intramuscularly. The half-life
of elimination was 8.2 hours (45).

Future Plans for Interferon Therapy

IFN is considered an important factor in recovery from acute
herpes virus infections (52) and in control of latent herpes virus
infections (23,53). The site and sequence of time involved in
interferon production and interactions between IFN-alpha and gamma
are not understood. During acute CMV infections in mice, mainly
IFN-alpha is produced, whereas later, both IFN-alpha and gamma are
produced (54). IFN-gamma, in combination with IFN-alpha or
IFN-beta are synergistic in their antiviral activities (55).
IFN-gamma is considered more important as an immunoregulatory than
as an antiviral agent (56). Thus, it is conceivable that in
future studies IFN-alpha may be given either with or before
IFN-gamma. IFN-alpha may be effective by its direct antiviral
effect. IFN-gamma may enhance cellular immunity and potentiate
the antiviral effect of IFN-alpha. Relatively large doses (25-36
million U daily) of IFN-alpha have been effective in varicella-
zoster virus infections. It remains to be seen whether smaller
doses (103 million U daily) might be efficacious in some infections, such as recurrent Herpes genitalis or labialis without the
unpleasant side effects seen in interferon given in high doses.

SUMMARY AND CONCLUSIONS

Three types of interferons (IFN's), alpha, beta, and gamma, are produced in vertebrate cells in response to intracellular infection or foreign molecules. After virus stimulation IFN's alpha (a mixture of a dozen species) are made in leukocytes, and IFN beta in fibroblasts. IFN's are glycoproteins with MW 18,000-26,000. IFN's are used experimentally in antiviral and cancer therapy for their antiviral and growth-inhibitory properties but their immunoregulatory and other functions may also be important. In most clinical studies leukocyte-derived IFN-alpha mixture has been used. Recently, single IFN-alpha 2 clone made by genetic engineering has been given to patients with cancer. IFN-alpha mixture is effective in high doses (20-40 million U daily) in the therapy of varicella and zoster. Anecdotal reports in herpes genitalis, CMV and EBV infection anecdotal reports suggest beneficial results with doses in the range of several million units daily. In CMV infections, IFN has been of benefit only prophylactically but not therapeutically. Side-effects of high doses are troublesome, ie., fever and flu-like symptoms, fatigue and leukopenia. The long-term consequences of IFN antibodies produced against the recombinant IFN in some patients on therapy are unknown (57).

REFERENCES

1.   Vilcek, J., Gresser, I., and Merigan, T.C. Regulatory
         functions of interferons. Annals NY Acad. Sci., 350:,
         1980.
2.   Lawn, R.M., Gross, M., Houck, C.M., Franke, A.E. et al. DNA
         sequence of a major human leukocyte interferon gene.
         Proc. Natl. Acad. Sci., 78:5435, 1981.
3.   Ohno, S. and Taniguchi, T. Structure of a chromosomal gene
         for human interferon beta. Proc. Natl. Acad. Sci. USA,
         78:5305, 1981.
4.   Yip, Y.K., Barroclough, B.S., Urban, C., and Vilcek, J.
         Molecular weight of human gamma interferon is similar to
         that of other human interferons. Science, 215:411,
         1982.
5.   Gray, P.W., Leung, D.N., Yelverton, E. et al. Expression of
         human immune interferon cDNA in E. coli and monkey
         cells. Nature, 295:503, 1982.
6.   Gresser, I. On the varied biological effects of interferon.
         Cell. Immunol., 40:406, 1977.
7.   Harfast, B., Muddlestone, J.R., Casali, P., Merigan, T.C.,
         and Oldstone, M.B.A. Interferon acts directly on human
         B lymphocytes to modulate immunoglobulin synthesis. J.
         Immunol., 127:2146, 1981.

8.   Herberman, R.B., Ortaldo, J.R., Mantovani, A. et al. Effect
      of human recombinant interferon on cytoxic activity of
      natural killer (NK) cells and monocytes. Cell.
      Immunol., 67:160, 1982.
9.   Maluish, A.E., Ortaldo, J.R., Sherwin, S. et al.
      Immunological monitoring of patients receiving recom-
      binant leukocyte A interferon. Abstracts of the 1982
      ASCO meeting, St. Louis, 1982.
10.   Troyl, M. Enhanced human NK cell activity following treat-
      ment with interferon in vitro and in vivo. In:
      Mediation of Cellular Immunity in Cancer by Immune
      Modifiers.
11.   Sonnenbeld, G. and Merigan, T.C. A regulatory role for
      interferon in immunity. Annals NY Acad. Sci., 332:345,
      1979.
12.   Overall, J.C., Yeh, T.J., and Kern, E.R. Sensitivity of
      Herpes simplex virus types I and II to three prepara-
      tions of human interferon. J. Infect. Dis., 142:943,
      1980.
13.   Weck, P.K., Rinderknecht, E., Estell, D.A., and Stebbing, N.
      Antiviral activity of bacteria-derived human alpha
      interferons against encephalomyocarditis virus infection
      of mice. Infect. Immunol., 35:660, 1982.
14.   Sullivan, J.L., Byron, K.S., Brewster, F.E., Sakamoto, K.,
      Shaw, J.E., and Pagano, J.S. Treatment of life-
      threatening Epstein-Barr virus infections with
      Acyclovir®. Am. J. Med., 73:262, 1982.
15.   Hammer, S.M., Kaplan, J.C., Lowe, B.R., and Hirsch, M.S.
      Alpha interferon and Acyclovir treatment of Herpes
      simplex virus in lymphoid cell cultures. Antimicrob.
      Ag. Chemother., 21:634, 1982.
16.   Spector, S.A., Tyndall, M., and Kelley, E. Effect of
      Acyclovir-combined with other antiviral agents on human
      cytomegalovirus. Am. J. Med., 73:36, 1982.
17.   Smith, C.I., Kitchen, L.W., Scullard, G.H., Robinson, W.S.,
      Gregory, P.B., and Merigan, T.C. Vidarabine mono-
      phosphate and human leukocyte interferon in chronic
      hepatitis B infection. J. Am. Med. Assoc., 247:2261,
      1982.
18.   Smolin, G., Stebbing, N., Friedlaender, M., Friedlaender,
      R., and Okumoto, M. Natural and cloned human leukocyte
      interferon in herpes virus infections of rabbit eyes.
      Arch. Ophtalmol, 100:481, 1982.
19.   Nesburn, A.B. and Ziniti, P.J. Long-term topical poly 1:C
      in experimental chronic ocular herpes simplex infection.
      Am. J. Ophthalmol., 72:821, 1971.
20.   Trousdale, M.D., Dunkel, E.C., and Nesburn, A.B. Effect of
      Acyclovir on acute and latent herpes simplex virus
      infections in the rabbit. Invest. Ophthalmol. Vis. Sci.
      19:1336, 1980.

21.   Wohlenberg, C., Openshaw, H., and Notkins, A.L. In vitro
         system for studying the efficacy of antiviral agents in
         preventing the reactivation of latent herpes simplex
         virus. Antimicrob. Ag. Chemother., 15:625, 1979.
22.   Merigan, T.C. and Cunningham, A.L. Interferons as markers
         for immune response in man to viral antigens. Presented
         at the WHO Scientific Group on the Relevance of Recent
         Progress in Vaccines and Antiviral Drugs to the
         Prevention and Control of Viral Disease, London 5-9,
         July 1982.
23.   Merigan, T.C. Present appraisal and future hopes for the
         clinical utilization of interferons. In: I. Gresser
         (ed.), Interferon III. New York: Academic Press, 1981.
24.   Pazin, G.J., Armstrong, J.A., Lam, M.T., Tarr, G.C.,
         Janetta, P.J., and Ho, M. Prevention of reactivated
         herpes simplex infection by human leukocyte interferon
         after operation on the trigeminal root. N. Engl. J.
         Med., 301:225, 1979.
25.   Sundmacher, R., Cantell, K., and Neumann-Haefflin, D.
         Combination therapy of dendritic keratitis in
         trifluorothymidine and interferon. Lancet, ii:687,
         1978.
26.   Sundmacher, R., Cantell, K., Skoda, R., Hallermann, C., and
         Neumann-Haefelin, D. Human leukocyte and fibroblast
         interferon in a combination therapy of dendritic kera-
         titis. Albrecht von Graefes Arch. Klin. Ophthalmol.
         208:229, 1978.
27.   Arvin, A.M., Kushner, J.H., Feldman, S., Baehner, R.L.,
         Hammond, D., and Merigan, T.C. Human leukocyte inter-
         feron for the treatment of varicella in children with
         cancer. N. Engl. J. Med. 306:761, 1982.
28.   Arvin, A.M., Martin, D.P., and Merigan, T.C. Interferon
         prophyulaxis for varicella infection in Erythrocebus
         patas monkeys. J. Infect. Dis., in press, 1982.
29.   Merigan, T.C., Rand, K.H., Pollard, R.B., Abdallah, P.S.,
         Jordan, G.W., and Fried, R.P. Human leukocyte inter-
         feron for the treatment of herpes zoster in patients
         with cancer. N. Engl. J. Med., 298:981, 1978.
30.   Merigan, T.C., Gallagher, J.G., Pollard, R.B., and Arvin, M.
         Short-course human leukocyte interferon in treatment of
         herpes zoster in patients with cancer. Antimicrob. Ag.
         Chemother., 19:193, 1981.
31.   Stevens, D.A. and Merigan, T.C. Interferon, antibody and
         other host factors in herpes zoster. J. Clin. Invest.
         51:1170, 1972.
32.   Balfour, H.H., Bean, B., Mitchell, C.D., Sachs, G.W., Boen,
         J.R., and Edelman, C.K. Acyclovir in immunocompromised
         patients with cytomegalovirus disease. A controlled
         trial at one institution. Am. J. Med., 73:241, 1982.

33. Cheeseman, S.H., Rubin, R.H., Stewart, J.A., Tolkoff-Rubin, N.E., Cosimi, A.B., Cantell, K., Gilbert, J., Winkle, S., Herrin, J.T., Black, P.H., Russell, P.S., and Hirsch, M.S. Controlled clinical trial of prophylactic human-leukocyte interferon in renal transplantation. N. Engl. J. Med., 300:1345, 1979.

34. Hirsch, M.S., Schooley, R.T., Rubin, R.H., Tolkoff-Rubin, N., and Cantell, K. Interferon in renal transplant recipients. Presented at the Interferon meeting, Squaw Valley, March 1982.

35. Meyers, J.D., McGuffin, R.W., Neumann, P.E., Singer, J.W., and Thomas, E.D. Toxicity and efficacy of human leukocyte interferon for treatment of cytomegalovirus pneumonia after marrow transplantation. J. Infect. Dis., 141:555, 1980.

36. Chou, S. and Merigan, T.C. Preliminary observations on the effect of human leukocyte interferon on viral excretion in CMV retinitis. Abstracts of the 6th Cold Spring Harbor meeting on herpes viruses, 1982.

37. Lopez, C., Fitzgerald, P.A., and Siegal, F.P. Severe acquired immunodeficiency syndrome in male homosexuals: diminished capacity to make interferon-alpha in vitro is associated with susceptibility to opportunistic infections. Submitted for publication 1982.

38. Thorley-Lawson, D. The transformation of adult but not newborn human lymphocytes by Epstein-Barr virus and phytohemagglutinin is inhibited by interferon: the early suppression by T cells of Epstein-Barr infection is mediated by interferon. J. Immunol., 126:829, 1981.

39. Hanto, D.W., Frizzera, G., Gajl-Peczalska, K.J., Sakamoto, K., Purtilo, D.T., Balfour, H.H., Simmons, R.L., and Najarian, J.S. Epstein-Barr virus-induced B-cell lymphoma after renal transplantation: Acyclovir therapy and transition from polyclonal to monoclonal B cell proliferation. N. Engl. J. Med., 306:913, 1982.

40. Thestrup-Pederson, K., Esmann, V., Bisballe, S., Jensen, J.R., Pallesen, G., Hastrup, J., Madsen, M., Thorling, K., Grazia-Masucci, M., Saemundsen, A.K., and Ernberg, I. Epstein-Barr virus-induced lymphoproliferative disorder converting to fatal Burkitt-like lymphoma in a boy with interferon-inducible chromosomal defect. Lancet, ii:997, 1980.

41. Cheeseman, S.H., Henle, W., Rubin, R., Tolkoff-Rubin, N.E., Cosimi, B., Cantell, K., Winkle, S., Herrin, J.T., Black, P.H., Russell, P.S., and Hirsch, M.S. Epstein-Barr virus infection in renal transplant patients: effect of antithymocyte globulin and interferon. Ann. Intern. Med., 93:39, 1980.

42. Rhodes-Feuillette, A., Canivet, M., Devergie, A., Gluckman, E., Mazeron, M.-C., Perol, Y., and Peries, J.

Circulating interferon after marrow transplant in cytomegalovirus infection. Lancet, 1:1217, 1981.

43. Chatterjee, S.N. and Jordan, G.W. Interferon in the circulation of renal transplant recipients. J. Inf. Dis.,
in press, 1982.

44. Cantell, K. and Hirvonen, S. Large-scale production of
human leukocyte interferon containing 10^8 units per ml.
J. Gen. Virol., 39:541, 1978.

45. Gutterman, J.U., Fine, S., Quesada, J., Horning, S.J.,
Levine, J.F., Alexonian, R., Bernhardt, L., Kramer,
M., Spiegel, H., Colburn, W., Trown, P., Merigan, T.C.,
and Dziewanowski, Z. Recombinant leukocyte A
interferon: pharmacokinetics, single-dose tolerance and
biological effects in cancer patients. Ann. Intern.
Med., 96:549, 1982.

46. Scott, G.M., Secher, D.S., Flowers, D., Bate, J., Cantell,
K. and Tyrrell, D.A.J. Toxicity of interferon. Br.
Med. J., 282:1345, 1981.

47. Gutterman, J.U., Blumenschein, G.R., Alexanian, R., Yap,
H-Y., Buzdar, A.U., Cabanellas, F., Hortobagyi, G.N.,
Hersh, E.M., Rasmussen, S.L., Harmon, M., Kramer, M.,
and Pestka, S. Leukocyte interferon-induced tumor
regression in human metastatic breast cancer, multiple
myeloma and malignant lymphoma. Ann. Int. Med., 93:399,
1980.

48. Bartram, C.R., Morier, W., and Schmidt, A. Human fibroblast
interferon does not induce chromosomal abnormalities.
Lancet, 1:1372, 1981.

49. Valibracht, A., Treuner, J., Flehmig, B., Joesters, K.E.,
and Niethammer, D. Interferon-neutralizing antibodies
in a patient treated with human fibroblast interferon.
Nature, 289:496, 1981.

50. Panem, S., Check, I.J., Henriksen, D., and Vilcek, J.
Antibodies to alpha-interferon in a patient with systemic lupus erythematosus. Submitted, 1982.

51. Bino, T., Edery, H., Gertler, A., and Rosenberg, H.
Involvement of the kidney in catabolism of human leukocytes interferon. J. Gen. Virol., 59:39, 1982.

52. Spruance, S.L., Green, J.A., Chiu, G., Yeh, T.J.,
Wenerstrom, G., and Overall, J.C. Jr. Pathogenesis of
herpes simplex labialis: correlation of vesicle fluid
interferon with lesion age and virus titer. Infect.
Immunol., 36:907, 1982.

53. O'Reilly, R.J., Chibbaro, A., Anser, E., and Lopez, C.
Cell-mediated immune responses in patients with
recurrent herpes simplex infections. II. Infection
associated deficiency of lymphokine production in
patients with recurrent herpes labialis or herpes pro-
gentialis. J. Immunol., 118:1095, 1977.

54.   Kelsey, D.R., Overall, J.C. Jr., and Glasgow, L.A.
         Production of alpha and gamma interferons by spleen
         cells from cytomegalovirus-infected mice. Infect.
         Immunol., 36:651, 1982.
55.   Fleischmann, W.R., Georgiades, J.A., Osborne, L.C., and
         Johnson, H.M. Potentiation of interferon activity by
         mixed preparations of fibroblastic and immune inter-
         feron. Infect. Immunol., 26:248, 1979.
56.   Sonnenfeld, G., Salvin, S.B., and Younger, J.S. Cellular
         source of interferons in circulation of mice with
         delayed hypersensitivity. Infect. Immunol., 18:283,
         1977.
57.   Trown, P.W., Dennine, R.A., Kramer, M.J., Connell, E.V.,
         Palleroni, A.V., Quesada, J., and Gutterman, J.U.
         Antibodies in human leucocyte interferons in cancer
         patients. Lancet, 1:81, 1983.

EPSTEIN-BARR VIRUS AND MARROW TRANSPLANTATION RECIPIENTS

Hilaire J. Meuwissen[1], and David T. Purtilo[2]

[1]Birth Defects Institute, Center for Laboratories
Research, Albany, NY
[2]Department of Pathology & Laboratory
42nd & Dewey Avenue
Omaha, NE 68105

INTRODUCTION

We focus on the role of Epstein-Barr virus (EBV) as an agent
potentially causing acute infectious complications in bone marrow
transplant patients (MTP). Secondly we consider EBV as a possible
contributor to the lymphoid malignancies developing in these
patients. We limit our discussion to marrow transplants performed
with sibling donors who are matched at the major histocompatibility (MHC) locus with the recipient. Patients receiving
marrow not matched at the major histocompatibility locus (MHC)
seldom survive for more than a few months.

Techniques for elimination of T cells from haplotype-identical
parental marrow have recently been used successfully. The number
of cases so far is small and their survival following the transplant procedure is therefore of limited duration (1,2).

Successful marrow transplant with allogeneic MHC-matched
sibling marrow was first described in 1968 in two patients: one
with severe combined immune deficiency (SCID) (3), and one with
the Wiskott-Aldrich syndrome (WAS) (4). In the accompanying
chapter, Neudorf and colleagues discuss the lack of lymphomas in
SCID and WAS patients successfully reconstituted by bone marrow
transplantation. Patients with SCID can be transplanted with
MHC-matched sibling marrow because they do not, as a rule, reject
the transplant. Fortunately, the graft-vs-host disease (GVHD) is
rarely fatal. However, patients with conditions other than SCID

require intensive immunosuppressive and myeloablative treatment to
obtain stable functioning marrow grafts. As clinical experience
has accumulated, the long-term survival of MTP patients has
improved (5). The procedure is successfully used to correct
congenital disorders, involving immunocytes, granulocytes,

Table 1. Epstein-Barr Virus Antibody Titers in
a Family with Wiskott-Aldrich Syndrome

Subject	Age/sex	Date	Anti-Epstein-Barr Virus Titers					
			Anti-VCA			Anti-EA		
			IgM	IgA	IgG	DR	D	EBNA
Father	39/M	1/12/82	<2	<2	80	<5	<5	20
		4/22/82	<2	<2	40	<5	<5	20
		7/17/79	<2	<2	80	<5	<5	40
		12/28/79	<2	<2	160	<5	<5	20
Mother	39/F	1/12/82	<2	<2	640	<5	<5	20
		4/22/82	<2	<2	160	<5	<5	40
Patient 1	1/M	1/17/71	<2	80	640	160	160	5
		2/7/72	<2	80	640	160	80	5
		10/24/79	<2	80	>1200	>160	>160	20
		5/6/80	<2	80	>1280	>160	>160	20
		2/3/81	<2	40	>1280	>160	>160	20
	15/M	1/12/82	<2	<2	1280	80	80	20
		4/22/82	<2	40	640	160	160	10
Patient 2	1/M	12/14/71	<2	<2	seronegative			
Patient 3	2 1/2M	1/25/79	Seronegative					
		2/12/80	<2	<2	80	$\leq$5	<5	<5
		8/5/80	<2	<2	640	>40	40	10
		5/5/81	<2	$\leq$5	<1280	>40	40	10
	5 1/2M	1/12/82	<2	$\leq$2	640	40	40	20
		4/22/82	<2	10	320	40	40	10
Controls			<2	<2	20–160	<5	<5	$\geq$10
Seronegative			<2	<2	<5	<5	<5	<5

Abbreviations: M, male; F, female; VCA, viral capsid
antigen; EA, early antigen; EBNA, EB
nuclear-associated antigen.
*Effector/target cell ratio

erythrocytes, and osteoblasts. In addition, aplastic anemia and
various forms of leukemia are treated by marrow transplantation.

Epstein-Barr Virus and Marrow Transplantation.

Many conditions for which MTP may now be curative are not
associated with marked degrees of immunodeficiency. Data is not
available that EBV causes more overt infections in patients with
aplastic anemia, leukemias, or hemoglobinopathies than in normal
subjects. EBV is not a pathogen known to cause disease in
patients with primary immunodeficiency disease (IDD) who have been
treated with MTP (primarily SCID and WAS). Notably, infectious
mononucleosis (IM) in these patients pre and post MTP is very low.
X-linked lymphoproliferative syndrome (XLP) is a notable exception
to this rule. XLP is characterized by unusual vulnerability to
EBV. Harada and Purtilo describe XLP in detail elsewhere in this
text. Marrow transplantation has not yet been recorded for XLP.

The paucity of reports of IM-like illnesses does not mean that
patients with IDD do not manifest other disorders due to EBV. Two
studies of patients with ataxia telangiectasia (AT) revealed
markedly increased antibodies to EBV early antigen (EA) and viral
capsid antigen (VCA) as compared to controls (6,7).

We have studied three patients with WAS experiencing many
serious infections but never having had an IM; two of the brothers
have produced EA antibodies over many years in conjunction with
IgA antibodies to VCA and abnormally high titers of IgG anti-VCA
(8) (Table 1). These two WAS patients had primary infections with
EBV which were either asymptomatic or atypical. However, they
were unable to prevent repeated reactivation of the virus.
Production of antibodies against EBV has continued until a
host-virus detente was achieved. Comparisons of XLP and WAS are
summarized in Table 2.

Similar studies have been done in patients with various IDD.
Harada summarizes some of these results elsewhere in this book and
Erickson describes EBV in patients with SCID who have received
thymic epithelial transplants.

Unrecognized EBV infection in IDD

Possibly patients with primary immunodeficiencies have
unrecognized infections with EB virus? In the first place, data
presented in this text by Tobi reveals that atypical EBV infections occur even in subjects who do not suffer from IDD.
Secondly, patients with IDD have immunologic abnormalities which
may diminish or alter the symptoms and signs which are typical for
diagnosing certain infections. Patients with SCID, for instance,
do not produce a typical rash after a measles infection, probably

Table 2. Comparison of Patients with X-linked Lymphoproliferative Syndrome (XLP) and Wiskott-Aldrich Syndrome (WAS)

Characteristic	WAS	XLP
Inheritance	X-linked	X-linked
Fatal Infectious mononucleosis	None?	66%
Malignant lymphoma	15%	35%
Hypo- and dysgammaglobulinemia	Catabolism	19% hypo X
Aplastic anemia	Rare	17%
Persistent Active EBV	?	Yes
Anti-VCA	Elevated to normal	Absent to normal
Anti-EA	Elevated to absent	Low or absent
Anti-EBNA	Normal	Absent or Low
Maternal EBV antibodies	Elevated?	Elevated 85% carriers
NK Activity Pre EBV	?	Normal
NK Activity Post EBV	Reduced	Reduced
Regression autologous LCL	Absent to weak	Absent to weak

Abbreviations: WAS, Wiskott-Aldrich syndrome; XLP, X-linked lymphoproliferative syndrome; EBV, Epstein-Barr virus; NK, natural killer cell; LCL, lymphoblastoid cell line.

because of their impaired T cell function. In the same way, it is
conceivable that EB virus infections in patients with IDD may not
be associated with atypical lymphocytosis, lymphadenomegaly, and
rash because of their immunologic impairment. Thirdly, techniques
that demonstrate EB virus in blood and tissues and special
techniques for demonstrating EBV antibodies are not generally
available. Therefore, often the necessary diagnostic determinations are not utilized in patients with IDD and fevers of
unknown etiology. We consider that EBV infections with manifestations other than those of the classical IM are probably more
frequently occurring in these patients than has been suspected.

If patients with primary immunodeficiencies have frequent
reactivation of EB virus, it is tempting to speculate that they
may be more likely to develop EBV-associated malignancies. Data
regarding this point is scant.

Patients with WAS, AT, SCID, and common variable hypogammaglobulinemia have a markedly increased incidence of malignancies
(9), especially B cell lymphomas. [See Kersey's contribution in
this monograph.] Recent studies indicate that many of the
lymphomas in WAS patients are B cell lymphomas (10).
Unfortunately, the tissues available from these patients in the
past have not been studied for EBV genome. Furthermore, the
number of patients who suffer from primary IDD is small. Several
years will be required to determine whether their B cell lymphomas
are EBV-associated as they are in patients post renal or heart
transplantation. A single patient with ataxia telangiectasia has
recently been described who had an EBV-carrying lymphoma (11).
Careful scrutiny of all new instances of B cell malignancies in
patients with primary IDD is indicated.

EBV in marrow transplant patients

The degree of immunologic deficit seen in MTP patients is
profound, particularly in the immediate post-transplant period:

(a)   The disease for which MTP is performed may be associated with
      significant immunologic deficiency, i.e., SCID or WAS.

(b)   In diseases such as leukemia and other malignancies the
      primary disease may have been treated with therapeutic agents
      which suppress not only the malignant cells but also the
      patient's immune system.

(c)   In most marrow transplants, immunosuppression and myeloabla-
      tive treatment is given, with combinations of cyclophospha-
      mide, 6-thioguanine, daunorubicin, X-irradiation, and other
      agents. Only in a few patients with SCID can this therapy be
      omitted. Immunosuppressive treatment inhibits the recipient's

capacity to reject donor cells and myeloablative treatment
is thought to create marrow "space" for donor stem cells (12).

Except in cases of transplantation with syngeneic identical twin donors, the marrow donors are allogeneic to the
recipient even though matched at the MHC locus; they remain
mismatched at non-MHC loci. Graft-versus-host disease,
therefore, is a common sequel in allogeneic marrow transplantation. The condition, if severe, is associated with the
destruction of the regenerating lymphoid system and continued
long-lasting immunologic depression (13).

(d)   If graft-versus-host disease (GVHD) occurs, current treatment
      regimens use immunosuppressive drugs such as Methotrexate,
      antithymocyte globulin, and prednisone for treatment, again
      aggravating the immunodeficient state (14).

(e)   Finally, many infections occur in MTP patients associated with
      immune depression, notably cytomegalovirus (CMV) (15).

The recipient's immune system gradually recovers in the post-
transplantation period depending on the occurrence of complications such as infection or GVHD (16). The capability to produce
immunoglobulins and antibodies returns 2-3 months following the
transplant and gradually expands to include a full range of antibody specificities. The levels of immunoglobulins may even become
supranormal, and the immunoglobulins may show restricted heterogeneity (17); both abnormalities are normalized with time. Delayed
hypersensitivity and mitogen responsiveness take longer to
recover, i.e., it may remain abnormal 6-12 months following the
transplant. Regulatory T cell abnormalities persist for months.
In patients with severe infections and chronic GVHD, the immunologic recovery process is more delayed. In patients who have not
received pre-transplant immunosuppressive and myeloablative
therapy (patients with SCID), immunologic reconstitution is relatively rapid.

Few reports of documented EBV-induced infections are available
in MTP patients. This is surprising given their extraordinary
susceptibility to infections. Early in the post-transplant period
pyogenic, fungal, and protozoal infections predominate. Later on,
pneumocystis, CMV, and herpesvirus infections are threats (15).
The same caution must be used in interpreting this dearth of
reports on EB virus infections in MTP patients as in individuals
with primary immunodeficiencies. Clinical manifestations of EBV
infection may depend on the immune status of the patient. For
example, if the donor is EBV seropositive, transfused and en-
grafted B cells begin to produce antibodies in memory B cells
residing in the donor before the transplant continue to function
in the recipient. The recipient is protected from EBV infection

by passively transfused EBV antibodies given to the recipient from
the EBV-positive marrow donor or from random blood, platelet,
granulocyte, or plasma transfusions: antibodies neutralize EBV
preventing spread of the virus. The recipient may be incapable of
producing EBV antibodies because of their compromised immunity
(donor B cells may be immunosuppressed by the prophylaxis for GVHD
or by infections).

      Lange et al. (18) studied 50 MTP patients, seven of whom were
seronegative recipients of seronegative donor marrow. Data was
presented on only one of the latter group: this patient produced
autologous EBV antibodies 4 months after transplantation and had
no clinical evidence of IM or GVHD. IgM anti-VCA or heterophile
antibody was not produced, the IgG anti-VCA was abnormally high,
and antibodies to EA and EBNA were produced slowly. Similar
findings were found in five of eight seropositive MTP recipients
who were studied for more than one year. These unusual antibodies
were not derived from passive immunization. None of the patients
developed an IM-like illness. No uniform association was observed
between the serologic response to EBV and GVHD. In the early
post-transplant period, all patients had passively transmitted EBV
antibodies which were apparently protective. They may have
obviated clinically overt EBV infection.

      In one instance, an EBV infection was diagnosed in an EBV
seronegative marrow transplant recipient whose MHC-matched
brother had developed infectious mononucleosis several weeks
before the transplant (19). Serologic evidence of EBV infection
coincided with severe GVHD. Whether the virus was an "innocent
by-stander", triggered or even caused GVHD, remains an unresolved
question.

      As discussed previously, EBV has been associated with malig-
nant B cell lymphoma in transplant patients (see Hanto's, Penn's
and Bieber's chapters in this volume) and the incidence of
EBV-associated malignancy in MTP is therefore of interest. The
total number of malignancies occurring following marrow transplantation is 9; four patients had leukemia recurring in donor cells,
while one patient each had glioblastoma multiforme and cancer of
the colon (2). Three patients had B cell lymphomas (21).

EBV-induced Lymphoma Complicating MT for Leukemia

      One major support for a viral etiology of lymphoma/leukemia is
the malignancy occurring in donor bone marrow in patients being
treated for leukemia. To our knowledge only three cases of
malignant lymphoma have been recorded, all in MTP being treated
for leukemia. Recently, a Seattle group (22) has reported an
EBV-carrying monoclonal B cell lymphoma in a boy who received
marrow from his sister. Karyotype of the lymphoma showed two X

chromosomes. DNA of fibroblasts derived from donor and recipient
were compared using molecular hybridization techniques. The
finding of a similar polymorphic gene in donor and lymphoma, which
was different than the recipient, further confirmed donor origin
of the lymphoma. EBV genome was detected in the lymphoma. The
lymphomas in MTP have all been of donor origin. This is not
surprising, since few recipient's B cells are expected to survive
the intense chemotherapy and X-irradiation given to prepare the
patients for transplantation.

The number of MTP patients from the Immunodeficiency-Cancer
Registry and the Marrow Transplantation Registry who have experienced long-term survival with donor marrow is estimated at between
250-300. Comparing the incidence of B cell lymphoma in patients
with MTP with those receiving renal transplant (i.e., 5-6%) and
cardiac transplant recipients (10-15%) [see the data of Israel
Penn and Charles Bieber in this volume], the incidence appears to
be lower. For strict comparison, the number of patients' years at
risk needs to be considered in these calculations.

Striking differences are found regarding immune competence and
frequency of opportunistic lymphoma in patients transplanted with
solid organs as compared to marrow:

(a) The immunosuppressive therapy which marrow transplant patients
     receive is intense. The patients immune system is almost
     completely obliterated with lethal doses of chemotherapeutic
     drugs and lethal total body irradiation, particularly in cases
     of patients with leukemia. Once the period of maximum danger
     of GVHD has passed (the first 100 days), all immunosuppressive
     therapy is discontinued, unless chronic GVHD appears. In
     contrast, other organ transplantation patients do not require
     the intense immunosuppression at the beginning of the trans-
     plant which marrow transplant patients receive. However,
     cardiac and renal transplant recipients remain on immuno-
     suppressive drugs virtually for the life of the graft, unless
     the donor is syngeneic. When rejection crises occur during
     the post-graft period, immunosuppressive therapy is often
     intensified.

(b) The second major difference is in the match between donor and
     recipient. The great majority of renal transplant patients and
     all hepatic and cardiac transplant patients receive
     MHC-mismatched non-sibling grafts, often from unrelated
     donors. Virtually all long-term survivors of marrow
     transplant grafts have grafts from siblings matched at MHC.

In marrow transplantation, therefore, immunodeficiency
following the graft is profound but usually transient (recovery to
a normal status occurs) while grafting of other organs is often

associated with marked histocompatibility differences between donor and recipient. This difference dictates continued suppression of the recipient's immune system. Drugs used for this purpose include Imuran, prednisone, antithymocyte globulin, and Cyclosporin A. The latter two agents are associated with development of lymphoma even in patients not receiving grafts (23). That immunosuppression and drug treatment are intimately linked to development of lymphoma, may be deduced by reports of the disappearance of a malignancy following discontinuation of drugs (24). Our view is that the patient regains cytoxic responses against EBV-specific antigens on the surface of B cells.

Noteworthy, patients who had developed B cell lymphoma following marrow transplantation were mismatched at the MHC. In one patient, at the HLA-A locus and the other at HLA-D. Both patients developed severe GVHD (25). Data on the frequency of B cell lymphomas in recipients of MHC matched sibling kidneys as compared to mismatched cadaver kidneys is not available for comparison. These data should be obtained because experimental data suggest that chronic antigenic exposure is associated with development of lymphoma.

Antigenic disparity, treatment with immunosuppressive drugs, and possibly infections probably play a role in development of B cell lymphoma. EB virus is associated with B cell lymphoma originating in marrow transplant patients just as it does in recipients of solid organ grafts.

CONCLUSIONS AND SUMMARY

Infections caused by EBV have only rarely been described in patients who have received MHC-identical marrow transplants or in patients with primary immunodeficiencies for which marrow transplants often are used. Nevertheless, growing evidence suggests that patients with primary immunodeficiencies - in particular, ataxia telangiectasia and Wiskott-Aldrich syndrome - have immunologic defects which lead to chronic reactivation of EBV.

B cell lymphomas are particularly common in recipients of solid organ grafts and in patients with primary immunodeficiencies. In the former group, these malignancies are associated with EBV. Evidence is now accumulating that this may also be the case in patients with AT and WAS. Although B cell lymphomas occur in MTP, they appear infrequently compared to renal and cardiac transplant recipients. If patients with primary immunodeficiencies are transplanted with unmatched thymic epithelium, the incidence of B cell lymphomas (some of which are associated with EBV) is comparable (26) to that in renal transplant recipients (27). Marrow graft recipients transplanted with MHC-identical sibling donor marrow may escape B cell lymphomas because of their close matching of HLA and shorter duration of immunosuppressive drugs. Further careful study of lymphomas in patients with immunodeficiencies, marrow transplants, and solid tissue transplants with histologic immunochemical and hybridization techniques is warranted.

ACKNOWLEDGEMENTS

We thank Mrs. Leah Taub for secretarial assistance.

REFERENCES

1.   Reisner, Y., Kapoor, N., Kirkpatrick, D. et al. Transplantation for acute leukemia with HLA-A and B nonidentical parental marrow cells fractionated with soybean agglutinin and sheep red blood cells. Lancet, 1:327, 1981.

2.   Reinherz, E.L., Geha, R., Rappeport, J.M et al. Reconstitution after transplantation with T-lymphocyte-depleted HLA haplotype-mismatched bone marrow for severe combined immunodeficiency. Proc. Natl. Acad. Sci., 79:6047, 1982.

3.   Gale, R.P. Progress in bone marrow transplantation in man. Surv. Immunol. Res., 1:40, 1982.

4.   Bach, F.H., Albertini, R.H., Anderson, J.L., Joo, P., and Bortin, M.M. Bone-marrow transplantation in a patient with the Wiskott-Aldrich syndrome. Lancet, ii:1364, 1968.

5.   Gatti, R.A., Meuwissen, H.J., Allen, H.D., Hong, R., and Good, R.A. Immunologic reconstitution of sex-linked lymphopenic immunologic deficiency. Lancet, ii:1366, 1968.

6.   Kapoor, N., Kirkpatrick, D., Blaese, R.M. et al. Reconstitution of normal megakaryocytopoiesis and immunologic functions in Wiskott-Aldrich syndrome by marrow transplantation following myeloablation and immunosuppression with busulfan and cyclophosphamide. Blood, 57:692, 1981.

7.   Thomas, E.D., Fefer, A., Buckner, C.D., and Storb, R. Current status of bone marrow transplantation for aplastic anemia and acute leukemia. A critical review. Blood, 49:671, 1977.

8.   Buckley, R.H. Transplantation. In: E.R. Stiehm and V.A. Fulginiti (eds.), Immunologic disorders in infants and children. pp. 795. Philadelphia: WB Saunders, 1980.

9.   Joncas, J., Lapointe, N., Gervais, F., and Leyritz, M. Unusual prevalence of Epstein-Barr virus early antigen

(EBV-EA) antibodies in ataxia telangiectasia. J. Immunol., 119:1857, 1977.

10. Berkel, A.I. et al. Epstein-Barr virus (EBV) carrying lymphoma in a patient with ataxia telangiectasia (AT) and review of immune responses to EBV in AT patients. Submitted for publication.

11. Purtilo, D.T., Bechtold, T., Harada, S., Yetz, J., Rogers, G., and Meuwissin, H.J. Epstein-Barr virus in a family with Wiskott-Aldrich syndrome. J Ped., in press.

12. Hoyer, J.R., Cooper, M.D., Gabrielson, A.E., and Good, R.A. Lymphopenic forms of congenital immunologic deficiency diseases. Medicine, 47:201, 1968.

13. Filipovich, A.H, Spector, B.D, and Kersey, J. Immunodeficiency in humans as a risk factor in the development of malignancy. Prevent Med., 9:252, 1980.

14. Frizzera, G., Rosai, J., Dehner, L.P., Spector, B.D., and Kersey, J.H. Lymphoreticular disorders in primary immunodeficiencies: new findings based on an up-to-date histologic classification of 35 cases. Cancer, 46:692, 1980.

15. Saemundsen, A.K. Epstein-Barr virus-carrying lymphoma in a patient with ataxia-telangiectasia. Brit. Med. J., 282:425, 1981.

16. Graze, P.R. and Gale, R.P. Chronic graft-versus-host disease: a syndrome of disordered immunity. Am. J. Med., 66:611, 1979.

17. Howard, R.J., Miller, J., and Najarian, J.S. Cytomegalovirus-induced immune suppression. II. Cell-mediated immunity. Clin. Exp. Immunol., 18:119, 1974.

18. Witherspoon, R.P., Storb, R., Ochs, H.D. et al. Recovery of antibody production in human allogeneic marrow graft recipients: influence of time post-transplantation, the presence or absence of chronic graft-versus-host disease, and antithymocyte globulin treatment. Blood, 58:360, 1981.

19. Lum, L.G., Seigneuret, M.C., Storb, R.F., Witherspoon, R.P., and Thomas, E.D. In vitro regulation of immunoglobulin synthesis after marrow transplantation. I. T-cell and B-cell deficiencies in patients with and without chronic graft-versus-host disease. Blood, 58:431, 1981.

20. Atkinson, K., Farewell, V., Storb, R. et al. Analysis of late infections after human bone marrow transplantation: role of genotypic nonidentity between marrow donor and recipient and of nonspecific suppressor cells in patients with chronic graft-versus-host disease. Blood, 60:714, 1982.

21. Radl, J., Dooren, L.J., Eijsvoogel, V.P., Van Went, J.J., Hijmans, W. An immunological study during post-transplantation follow-up of a case of severe combined immunodeficiency. Clin. Exp. Immunol., 10:367, 1972.

22.   Clift, R.A., Buckner, C.D., Fefer, A. et al.   Infectious
      complications of marrow transplantation.   Transplant.
      Proc., 6:389, 1974.

23.   Lange, B., Henle, W., Meyers, J.D., Yang, L.C., August, C.,
      Koch, P., Arbeter, A., and Henle, G.   Epstein-Barr virus
      related serology in marrow transplant recipients.   Int.
      J. Cancer, 26:151, 1980.

24.   Sullivan, J.L., Wallen, W.C., and Johnson, F.L.   Epstein-Barr
      virus infection following bone marrow transplantation.
      Int. J. Cancer, 22:132, 1978.

25.   Data obtained from the Statistical Center of the Inter-
      national Bone Marrow Transplant Registry.   The analysis
      has not been reviewed or approved by the Advisory
      Committee of the Registry.

26.   Gossett, T.C., Gale, R.P., and Fleischman, H.   Immunoblastic
      sarcoma in donor cells after bone-marrow transplantation.
      N. Engl. J. Med., 300:904, 1979.

27.   Schubach, W.H., Hackman, R., Neiman, P.E., Miller, G., and
      Thomas, E.D.   A monoclonal immunoblastic sarcoma in donor
      cells bearing Epstein-Barr virus genomes following allo-
      geneic marrow grafting for acute lymphoblastic leukemia.
      Blood, 60:180, 1982.

28.   Dr. Israel Penn (personal communication).

29.   Fialkow, P.J., Thomas, E.D., Bryant, J.E., and Neiman, P.E.,
      Leukaemic transformation of engrafted human marrow cells
      in vivo.   Lancet, 1:251, 1971.

30.   Thomas, E.D., Bryant, J.I., Buckner, C.D. et al. Leukaemic
      transformation of engrafted human marrow cells in vivo.
      Lancet, 1:1310, 1972.

31.   Goh, K. and Kemperer, M.R.   In vivo leukemic transformation
      cytogenetic evidence of in vivo leukemic transformation
      of engrafter marrow cells.   Am. J. Hematol, 2:283, 1977.

32.   Elfenbeing, G.J., Brogaonkar, D.S., Bias, W.B. et al.   Cyto-
      genetic evidence for recurrence of acute myelogenous
      leukemia after allogeneic bone marrow transplantation in
      donor hematopoietic cells.   Blood, 52:627, 1978.

33.   Newburger, P.E., Latt, S.A., Pesando, J.M. et al.   Leukemia
      relapse in donor cells after allogeneic bone marrow
      transplantation.   N. Engl. J. Med., 304:712, 1981.

34.   Buckley, R.H.   Transplantation.   In: E.R. Stiehm and
      V.A. Fulginiti (eds.), Immunologic Disorders in Infants
      and Children.   pp. 776-804.   Philadelphia: WB Saunders,
      1980.

35.   Dr. C. Dean Buckner (personal communication)

36.   Hanto, D.W., Frizzera, G., Purtilo, D.T., Sakamoto, K.,
      Sullivan, J.L., Saemundsen, A.K., Klein, G., Simmons,
      R.L., and Najarian, J.S.   Clinical spectrum of
      lymphoproliferative disorders in renal transplant
      recipients and evidence for the role of Epstein-Barr
      virus.   Cancer Res., 41:4253, 1982.

37. Reece, E.R., Gartner, J.G., Seemayer, T.A., Joncas, J.H., and Pagano, J.S. Epstein-Barr virus in a malignant lymphoproliferative disorder of B-cells occurring after thymic epithelial transplantation for combined immunodeficiency. Cancer Res., 41:4243, 1982.

38. Walford, R.L. Increased incidence of lymphoma after injections of mice with cells differing at weak histocompatibility loci. Science, 152:78, 1966.

39. Louie, S. and Schwatz, R.S. Immunodeficiency and the pathogenesis of lymphoma and leukemia. Sem. Hematol., 15:117, 1978.

40. Floersheim, G.L., Nassenstein, D., and Torhorst, J. Growth of human tumors in mice after short-term immunosuppression with procarbazine, cyclophosphamide, and antilymphocyte serum. Transplantation, 30:275, 1980.

41. Herra, G.A. and Head, D.R. Histiocytic lymphoma arising at the site of injection of antilymphocytic globulin: necropsy follow-up of previously reported case. Milit. Med., 146:652, 1981.

42. Matas, A.J., Simmons, R.L., and Najarian, J.S. Chronic antigenic stimulation, herpesvirus infection, and cancer in transplant recipients. Lancet, 1:1277, 1975.

IMMUNORECONSTITUTION BY BONE MARROW TRANSPLANTATION DECREASES LYMPHOPROLIFERATIVE MALIGNANCIES IN WISKOTT-ALDRICH AND SEVERE COMBINED IMMUNE DEFICIENCY SYNDROMES

Steven M.L. Neudorf,
Alexandra H. Filipovich and
John H. Kersey

Department of Pediatrics and Laboratory Medicine
University of Minnesota
Minneapolis, MN 55455

INTRODUCTION

Data linking immunodeficient individuals to a high incidence of malignancy has been collected through the analysis of outcomes in renal allograft recipients (1) and patients with naturally occurring immunodeficiency states such as severe combined immune deficiency (SCID), Wiskott-Aldrich syndrome (WAS) and ataxia telangiectasia (2-4). The mechanisms involved in the pathogenesis of malignancy in patients with naturally occurring or acquired immunodeficiencies are poorly understood. In large part this is due to the heterogeneity in the scope and severity of immune deficiency in these patients. In addition, some patients are exposed to potentially oncogenic agents, such as Epstein-Barr virus (EBV), that may influence the development of malignancy. Despite the complexity of these patients, certain aspects of the relationship between naturally occurring immune deficiency and malignancy can be studied. Many patients with SCID and WAS have been successfully immunoreconstituted by bone marrow transplantation (BMT). Therefore, it has become possible to ask whether immunoreconstitution prevents the development of malignancy in these patients. This chapter addresses this question by analyzing cases of malignancy in immunodeficient individuals that have undergone either BMT or thymus transplantation. These data will be compared to previously reported cases of malignancies in untransplanted immunodeficient patients.

Patients

Data concerning cases of malignancies and the results of BMT in SCID and WAS patients were obtained from three sources: the Immunodeficiency Cancer Registry (ICR), the International BMT Registry (IBMTR), and published and unpublished data from individual investigators.

The ICR, established at the University of Minnesota in 1973, collects data concerning malignancies in naturally occurring immunodeficiency states. These data have been obtained using ICR generated surveys and through abstraction from published case reports. Using these data, incidence figures for malignancies, in particular, immunodeficiency states have been estimated. Data concerning over four hundred patients have been registered. Limitations of the data stem from our inability to account for undiagnosed immunodeficient patients in the community or due to failure of physicians to complete ICR surveys. In addition, we cannot account for the period of observation nor quantify the period of risk individual patients have who do not develop malignancy. Thus, the actual incidence of immunodeficiency states, as well as the actual incidence figures for malignancies occurring in immunodeficient patients worldwide, have not been established.

The IBMTR has collected data from seventeen BMT centers in North America and Europe. Forty-eight patients have received BMT between 1968-1976 as therapy for SCID. These patients were heterogeneous with respect to specific diagnoses, conditioning regimen used, histocompatibility differences between donor and recipient and dose and route of administration of bone marrow cells.

The remainder of cases were obtained from previously published case reports, including personal communications to investigators to obtain follow-up data concerning transplant recipients.

Severe Combined Immune Deficiency

Table 1 compares the frequency of malignancy in SCID patients that did not undergo BMT to the frequency of malignancy in SCID patients that received bone marrow or thymus transplants. Twenty-four cases of malignancy occurring in untransplanted SCID patients have been reported to the ICR (3). The most commonly reported histologic type of malignancy was non-Hodgkin's lymphoma (NHL) accounting for 50% of cases. In addition, 25% of cases were leukemias, 4% were Hodgkin's disease, 4% were carcinomas and 17% specific diagnoses were not available. The median age of the SCID patients at diagnosis of malignancy was 1.83 years with a range of 0.08 - 5.0 years of age (ICR unpublished data).

Table 1.   The Effect of Immunoreconstitution on the Development of Malignancies in Patients with Severe Combined Immunodeficiency

Method of Immunoreconstitution	Reported Cases of Malignancy	Age (years) at diagnosis of Malignancy (1)	Age (years) of Surviving Patients (1)	Years Post BMT (1)	References
None attempted	24	1.83 (0.08-5.0)	NA(3)	---	3, ICR unpublished data
Bone Marrow Transplant (n=48)	0	---	6.1 (1-8)	4.8 (0.75-7.75)	5
Thymus Transplant(2) (n=24)	4	3.7 (1.75-4.6)	NA(3)	2.5 (1 - 4)	6,7

[1] Median (range)
[2] Includes fetal thymus and cultured thymic epithelium transplants
[3] NA - not available

Forty-eight patients with SCID treated with BMT were reported
to the IBMTR as of June, 1976 (5). Fifteen patients survived a
minimum of 0.75 years post transplant with the median interval
post BMT being 4.8 years (range 0.75 - 7.75 years). The median
age of surviving patients was 6.1 years (range 1 - 8 years). None
of the fifteen surviving patients developed lymphoreticular
malignancies and all patients had immunoreconstitution. Although
the number of patients is relatively small, the median follow-up
time post BMT exceeded the median age at which untransplanted SCID
patients developed malignancy.

Twenty-four patients with SCID received thymus transplants in
the form of either fetal thymus or cultured thymic epithelium
implants (6). Eight of these patients have survived a minimum of
one year post transplant with a median of about 2.5 years (range 1
- 4 years) post transplant (R. Hong, personal communication).
Four of twenty-four recipients died as a result of polyclonal B
cell lymphomas. Three of the cases have been published previously
(7). The fourth case occurred subsequent to the initial report
(R. Hong - personal communication). These patients were 3 - 7
years old when malignancies developed. The published cases developed lymphoma at 2, 9 and 24 months post thymus transplant. All
three patients were severely immunodeficient throughout their post
transplant course.

Wiskott-Aldrich Syndrome

Table 2 compares the frequency of malignancy occurring in non-
transplanted and transplanted WAS patients. Sixty-two WAS
patients with malignancy were reported to the ICR (3). Non-
Hodgkin's lymphoma accounted for 71% of malignancies in WAS.
More than 60% of cases of non-Hodgkin's lymphoma were classified
as B-immunoblastic sarcomas. Many cases presented as localized
extranodal infiltrates, especially in the central nervous system
and liver (8). For example, an 18 year old patient with WAS developed a B immunoblastic sarcoma in brain (Figure). The median
age at which WAS patients developed malignancy was 5.95 years
(range 0.24 - 32.85 years) (ICR - unpublished data). Other
malignancies seen in WAS patients included leukemias (10% of
cases), Hodgkin's disease (5%), carcinomas (3%) and unspecified or
unclassified lesions (11%).

Follow-up information has been obtained for fifteen patients
with WAS treated with BMT. Nine cases have been reported previously (9 - 13). Data concerning six additional WAS patients
treated with BMT were obtained through personal communications.
Twelve patients are currently alive, a median age of 3.7 years
(range 0.7 - 14 years) post BMT. The median age of surviving
patients is 5.3 years (range 1.5 - 16 years) which is similar to
the age when untransplanted patients developed malignancies.

Table 2. The Effect of Immunoreconstitution on the Development of
Malignancy in Wiskott-Aldrich Syndrome Patients

Method of Immunoreconstitution	Reported Cases of Malignancy	Age (years) at diagnosis of Malignancy (1)	Age (years) of Surviving Patients (1)	Years Post BMT (1)	References
None attempted	62	5.95 (0.24 - 32.85)	---	---	3, ICR unpublished data
Bone Marrow Transplant (n=15)[2]	0	---	5.3 (1.5 - 16)	3.7 (0.7 - 14)	9-13

[1]Median (range)
[2]Include twelve surviving patients

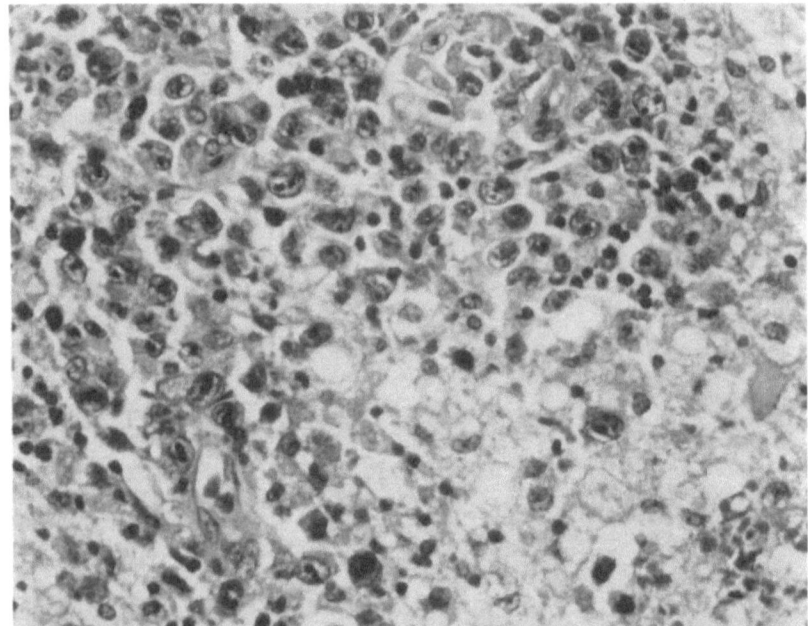

Fig. 1.   Photomicrograph of immunoblastic sarcoma from the brain
           of an 18 year old patient with Wiskott-Aldrich syndrome.
           Hematoxylin and eosin X450.

Malignancy has not been reported in any surviving patient nor has
malignancy contributed to the cause of death in the three non-
surviving WAS patients.

DISCUSSION

    This retrospective analysis was performed to investigate
whether immunoreconstitution with BMT has decreased the occurrence
of malignancy and specifically lymphoproliferative tumors in
patients with SCID and WAS. We have reported a high incidence of
malignancy in untransplanted patients with SCID and WAS (2-4).
These observations were compared to the frequency of malignancy in
immune deficient patients after BMT (or thymus transplant in some
cases of SCID). None of the patients with SCID or WAS that underwent successful BMT have developed malignancies. In contrast,
some patients with SCID that received thymus transplants and
remained severely immunodeficient developed lymphoproliferative
tumors. These results are consistent with the hypothesis that

immunoreconstitution may prevent the development of malignancy.

Our hypothesis that immunoreconstitution may prevent development of malignancy is further supported by data concerning renal allograft recipients undergoing immunosuppressive therapy to prevent graft rejection. When compared to the general population, renal allograft recipients had about a 100 fold increase in malignancy (1). About 20% of the malignancies are lymphomas. Like patients with SCID and WAS, renal allograft recipients tend to develop lymphomas in extranodal sites (14). Elsewhere in this book, Penn describes these cancers in detail. At least two patients who developed lymphoma following renal transplantation demonstrated spontaneous resolution of their malignancies associated with discontinuation of immunosuppressive drugs (14) suggesting that immunoreconstitution may prevent or reverse aberrant lymphoproliferation in susceptible hosts.

Although results of our analysis suggest that immunoreconstitution may prevent the development of malignancies in SCID and WAS patients, these results are preliminary and should be interpreted cautiously because of the short interval of time post BMT for these patients. In addition, the lack of a known population base in the SCID and WAS patients prevents us from calculating accurate expected malignancy data in these diseases.

Several issues remain to be examined. Short follow-up time does not permit us to speculate whether BMT may delay rather than prevent the expression of malignancies in SCID or WAS patients. The role of the underlying lymphocyte abnormalities (not yet defined in most patients with naturally occurring immunodeficiencies) or other mechanisms of oncogenesis in the pathogenesis of malignancy are unknown. In some patients abnormal host response to viruses, e.g., EBV has been postulated to be important in the pathogenesis of malignancy (15). This view is expressed in the chapter by Meuwissen and Purtilo in this book. Patients with ataxia telangiectasia are postulated to have defective DNA repair mechanisms making these patients susceptible to x-irradiation and perhaps irradiation induced malignancies (16). These patients develop many types of tumors and the degree of immunodeficiency does not appear to correlate with any one tumor type (17).

Finally, the cellular mechanisms involved in the prevention of malignancies in BMT recipients are unknown. Patients who undergo BMT for malignancies or aplastic anemia are severely immunodeficient during the first year post BMT (reviewed in 18), yet few, de novo malignancies have been reported. One possible explanation for this is that immune function of patients following BMT is generally improving throughout the first year post-BMT so that the period of greatest risk for the development of malignancy, on the basis of severe immunodeficiency, may be relatively short.

New methods to study mechanisms of oncogenesis and characterize the nature of immunodeficiency states are currently under development. These new understandings coupled with continued encouraging results of BMT in SCID and WAS patients should enhance our ability to study and eventually prevent malignancies in these patients.

SUMMARY AND CONCLUSIONS

A retrospective analysis was performed comparing the occurrence of malignancies in patients with severe combined immunodeficiency and Wiskott-Aldrich syndrome who were immunoreconstituted with similar patients who were not transplanted. Our hypothesis is that immunoreconstitution may prevent the occurrence of malignancy in these susceptible hosts. Data from the Immunodeficiency-Cancer Registry showed that 62 cases of malignancy occurring in WAS patients and 24 cases of malignancies occurring in SCID patients were reported. In contrast, none of the 48 SCID patients that received bone marrow transplants (including 15 long-term survivors) developed malignancy. All surviving patients had evidence of immunoreconstitution. Four SCID patients that received a thymus transplant and remained immunodeficient developed lymphoproliferative tumors.

Although these results are preliminary with respect to low numbers of surviving patients and short interval post transplant, they suggest that immunoreconstitution may prevent the occurrence of malignancy in susceptible hosts.

ACKNOWLEDGEMENTS

The authors wish to acknowledge Dr. R. Hong, University of Wisconsin; Dr. R. O'Reilly, Memorial Sloan-Kettering Institute; Dr. R. Parkman, Sidney Farber Cancer Institute; and Dr. H. Meuwissen, University of Albany Medical Center for providing current data concerning the post transplant course of their patients. The authors also wish to acknowledge Dr. G. Frizzera who provided the photomicrograph and Ms. K. Pyne for assistance in the preparation of this manuscript.

REFERENCES

1. Penn, I. Malignancies associated with immunosuppressive or cytotoxic therapy. Surgery, 83:294, 1978.
2. Kersey, J., Spector, B., and Good, R. Primary immunodeficiency diseases and cancer: the Immunodeficiency-Cancer Registry. Int. J. Cancer, 12:333, 1973.

3.   Filipovich, A.H., Zerbe, D., Spector, B., and Kersey, J.
     Lymphomas in persons with naturally occurring immunode-
     ficiency disorders. In: I.T. Magrath (ed.), The
     Influence of the Environment on Leukemia and Lymphoma
     Subtypes. New York: Raven Press, 1983.
4.   Spector, B.D., Perry, G., and Kersey, J.H. Genetically
     determined immunodeficiency diseases (GDID) and
     malignancy: report from the Immunodeficiency-Cancer
     Registry. Clin. Immunol. Immunopathol., 11:12, 1978.
5.   Bortin, M. and Rimm, A. Severe combined immunodeficiency
     disease. Characterization of the disease and results of
     transplantation. J. Am. Med. Assoc., 238:591, 1977.
6.   Hong, R. Present and future status of thymus transplan-
     tation. Ann. Clin. Res., 13:350, 1981.
7.   Borzy, M.S., Hong, R., Horowitz, S.D., Gilbert, E., Kaurman,
     D., De Mendonca, W., Oxelius, V.A., Dictor, M., and
     Pachman, L. Fatal lymphoma after transplantation of
     cultured thymus in children with combined immunodefi-
     ciency disease. N. Engl. J. Med., 301:565, 1979.
8.   Frizzera, G., Rosai, J., Dehner, L., Spector, B.D., and
     Kersey, J.H. Lymphoreticular disorders in primary
     immunodeficiencies: new findings based on an up-to-date
     histologic classification of 35 cases. Cancer, 46:692,
     1980.
9.   Kapoor, N., Kirkpatrick, D., Blaese, R., Oleske, J.,
     Hilgartner, M., Changanti, R., Good, R., and O'Reilly, R.
     Reconstitution of normal megakaryocytopoiesis and
     immunologic functions in Wiskott-Aldrich syndrome by
     marrow transplantation following myeloablation and immu-
     nosuppression with busulfan and cyclophosphamide.
     Blood, 57:692, 1981.
10. Bach, H.F., Albertini, R.J., Joo, P., Anderson, J.L.,
     and Bortin, M.M. Bone marrow transplantation in a
     patient with the Wiskott-Aldrich syndrome. Lancet,
     ii:1364, 1968.
11. August, C.S., Hathaway, W.W., Githens, J.H., Pearlman, D.,
     McIntosh, K., and Favara, B. Improved platelet function
     following bone marrow transplantation in an infant with
     Wiskott-Aldrich syndrome. J. Pediat., 82:58, 1973.
12. Meuwissen, H.J., Kieserman, E.G., Taft, B., Pollara, B., and
     Pickering, R.J. Marrow transplantation in Wiskott-
     Aldrich syndrome: T cell engraftment with cyclophospha-
     mide. Complete engraftment with total body irradiation.
     Pediat. Res., 12:483, 1978.
13. Parkman, R., Rappaport, D., Geha, R., Cassady, R., Levey,
     R., Nathan, D.G., Belli, J., and Rosen, F. Complete
     correction of the Wiskott-Aldrich syndrome by allogeneic
     bone marrow transplantation. N. Engl. J. Med., 298:921,
     1978.

14.   Hanto, D., Sakamoto, K., Purtilo, D.T., Simmons, R., and
Najarian, J. The Epstein-Barr virus in the pathogenesis
of post transplant lymphoproliferative disorders.
Surgery, 90:204, 1981.

15.   Thestrup-Pedersen, K., Esmann, V., Jensen, J.R., Hastrup,
J., Thorling, K., Saemundsen, A.K., Bisballe, S.,
Oallesen, G., Madsen, M., Grazia-Masucci, M., and
Emberg, I. Epstein-Barr virus-induced lymphoprolifera-
tive disorder converting to fatal Burkitt-like lymphoma
in a boy with interferon inducible chromosomal defect.
Lancet, ii:997, 1980.

16.   Taylor, A., Harnden, D., Arlett, C., Harcourt, S., Lehmann,
A., Stevens, S., and Bridges, B. Ataxia telangiectasia:
a human mutation with abnormal radiation sensitivity.
Nature, 258:427, 1975.

17.   Filipovich, A.H. and Spector, B.D. Immunodeficiency (ID) as
a susceptibility factor for malignancy in ataxia
telangiectasia (AT): report from the Immunodeficiency-
Cancer Registry (ICR). Pediat. Res., 15(4):A806, 1981.

18.   Tsoi, M. Immunological mechanisms of graft-versus-host
disease in man. Transplantation, 33:459, 1982.

CONTRIBUTORS

Donald Abrams, M.D.
Cancer Research Institute
University of California
San Francisco, CA 94143

Emma Anisimova, Ph.D.
Institute of Sera and Vaccines
Department of Experimental
  Virology
108 W. Pieck Street
101 03, Prague 10
Czechoslovakia

Charles Bieber, M.D.
Senior Research Associate
Department of Cardiac Surgery
Stanford University Medical
  Center
Stanford, CA 94305

Satya N. Chatterjee, M.D.
Department of Surgery
University of California,
  Davis
Davis, CA

Michael Cleary, M.D.
Stanford University School of
  Medicine
Department of Pathology
Laboratory of Experimental
  Oncology
300 Pasteur Drive
Stanford, Ca 94305

Milan Fiala, M.D.
Department of Surgery
University of California
  Davis
Davis, CA

Alexandra H. Filipovich, M.D.
Department of Pediatrics
  and Laboratory Medicine
University of Minnesota
Minneapolis, MN 55455

Glauco Frizzera, M.D.
Departments of Surgery and
  and Laboratory Medicine,
  Pathology
University of Minnesota
  Health Sciences Center
Minneapolis, MN 54555

Kazimiera J. Gajl-Peczalska,
  M.D., Ph.D.
Departments of Surgery and
  Laboratory Medicine,
  Pathology
University of Minnesota Health
  Sciences Center
Minneapolis, MN 54555

Douglas Hanto, M.D.
Departments of Surgery and
  Laboratory Medicine, Pathology
University of Minnesota Health
  Sciences Center
Minneapolis, MN 54555

Shinji Harada, M.D.
Departments of Pathology and
  Laboratory Medicine, and
  the Eppley Institute for
  Research in Cancer and
  Allied Diseases
University of Nebraska Medical
  Center, Omaha, Ne 68105

Werner Henle, M.D.
Children's Hospital of
  Philadelphia
34th St. and Civic Center Blvd.
Philadelphia, PA 19104

Richard L. Heberling, M.D.
Department of Cardiovascular
  Surgery
Stanford Medical Center
Stanford, California 94305

S.W. Jamieson
Department of Cardiac Surgery
Stanford University Medical Ctr.
Stanford, CA 94305

Donald R. Johnson, Ph.D.
Departments of Pathology and
  Laboratory Medicine and
  the Eppley Institute for
  Research in Cancer and
  Allied Diseases
University of Nebraska Medical Ctr.
Omaha, NE 68105

John H. Kersey, M.D.
Department of Pediatrics and
Laboratory Medicine
University of Minnesota
Minneapolis, MN 55455

George Klein, M.D.
Department of Tumor Biology
Karolinska Institute
Stockholm, Sweden

Gerhard R.F. Krueger, M.D.
Immunopathology Section
Pathology Institute
University of Cologne
5000 Cologne 41
Federal Republic of Germany

James Linder, M.D.
Department of Pathology and
  Laboratory Medicine
University of Nebraska Medical
  Center
Omaha, Ne 68105

Helen L. Lipscomb, Ph.D.
Departments of Pathology and
  Laboratory Medicine and the
  Eppley Institute for Research
  in Cancer and Allied Diseases
University of Nebraska Medical
  Center
Omaha, NE 68105

Henry T. Lynch, M.D.
School of Medicine
Department of Preventive
  Medicine
Creighton University
Omaha, Nebraska

Fernando Merino, M.D., Ph.D.
Institute for Scientific
  Investigation
Caracas, Venezuela

Hilaire J. Meuwissen, M.D.
Birth Defects Institute
Center for Laboratories Research
Albany, NY

Abraham Morag, M.D.
Division of Clinical Virology
Section of Virology
Hadassah-Hebrew University
  Medical School
Jerusalem, Israel

Steven M.L. Neudorf, M.D.
Department of Pediatrics and
  Laboratory Medicine
University of Minnesota
Minneapolis, MN 55455

Phillip E. Oyer, M.D.
Department of Cardiovascular
  Surgery
Stanford Medical Center
Stanford, CA 94305

Paul K. Pattengale, M.D.
Departments of Pathology and
  Microbiology
USC School of Medicine
2025 Zonal Avenue
Los Angeles, CA 90033

Israel Penn, M.D.
Department of Surgery
University of Cincinnati
  Medical Center
Veterans Administration Medical
  Center
3200 Vine Street
Cincinnati, Ohio 45220

Katerina Prachova, Ph.D.
Institute of Sera and Vaccines
Department of Experimental
  Virology
108 W. Pieck Street
101 03, Prague 10
Czechoslovakia

Ruth Purtilo, Ph.D.
Department of Humanities and
  Jurisprudence
University of Nebraska Medical
  Center
Omaha, Nebraska 68105

David T. Purtilo, M.D.
Departments of Pathology and
  Laboratory Medicine,
  Pediatrics, and the Eppley
  Institute for Research in
  Cancer and Allied Diseases
University of Nebraska Medical
  Center
Omaha, Nebraska 68105

Jaroslav Roubal, Ph.D.
Institute of Sera and Vaccines
Department of Experimental
  Virology
108 W. Pieck Street
101 03, Prague 10
Czechoslovakia

Ari Saemundsen, Ph.D.
Department of Microbiology
University of Iceland
P.O. Box 855
101 Raykjavik, Iceland

Avery A. Sandberg, M.D.
Roswell Park Memorial Institute
Buffalo, New York 14263

Guy S. Schuelke, Ph.D.
School of Medicine
Department of Preventive
  Medicine
Creighton University
Omaha, Nebraska

Richard L. Simmons, M.D.
Departments of Surgery and
  Laboratory Medicine,
  Pathology
University of Minnesota Health
  Sciences Center
Minneapolis, MN 54555

Joseph Sonnabend, M.D.
49 West 12th Street
New York, New York 10011

E. B. Stinson, M.D.
Department of Cardiovascular
  Surgery
Stanford Medical Center
Stanford, CA 94305

Bill Sugden, Ph.D.
McArdle Laboratory
University of Wisconsin
Madison, WI 53706

Eiji Tatsumi, M.D.
Departments of Pathology and
  Laboratory Medicine and the
  Eppley Institute for Research
  in Cancer and Allied Diseases
University of Nebraska Medical
  Center
Omaha, Nebraska 68105

Martin Tobi, M.B., Ch.B.
Department of Internal Medicine
University of Chicago
Chicago, IL 60637
Present Address:
Laboratory Immunology
NCI, NIH
Bethesda, MD 20205

David J. Volsky, Ph.D.
Departments of Pathology and
  Laboratory Medicine and the
  Eppley Institute for Research
  in Cancer and Allied Diseases
University of Nebraska Medical
  Center
Omaha, Nebraska 68105

Roger Warnke, M.D.
Assistant Professor
Department of Pathology
Stanford University Medical
  Center
Stanford, CA 94305

Steven S. Witkin, M.D.
Department of Obstetrics and
  Gynecology
The New York Hospital
Cornell Medical Center
525 East 68th Street
New York, NY 10021

Hans Wolf, Ph.D.
Max von Pattenkofer Institute of
  Hygiene and Microbiology
University of Munich
Munich, West Germany